Collaboration:

A Health Care Imperative

Notice

Medicine is an ever-changing science. As new research and clinical experience broaden our knowledge, changes in treatment and drug therapy are required. The editor and the publisher of this work have checked with sources believed to be reliable in their efforts to provide information that is complete and generally in accord with the standards accepted at the time of publication. However, in view of the possibility of human error or changes in medical sciences, neither the editor nor the publisher nor any other party who has been involved in the preparation or publication of this work warrants that the information contained herein is in every respect accurate or complete, and they are not responsible for any errors or omissions or for the results obtained from use of such information. Readers are encouraged to confirm the information contained herein with other sources. For example and in particular, readers are advised to check the product information sheet included in the package of each drug they plan to administer to be certain that the information contained in this book is accurate and that changes have not been made in the recommended dose or in the contraindications for administration. This recommendation is of particular importance in connection with new or infrequently used drugs.

Collaboration:
A
Health
Care
Imperative

Toni J. Sullivan, EdD, RN, FAAN

PROFESSOR AND DEAN

Sinclair School of Nursing
University of Missouri—Columbia
Columbia, Missouri

New York St. Louis San Francisco Auckland Bogotá Caracas **McGraw-Hill**
Lisbon London Madrid Mexico City Milan Montreal Health
New Delhi San Juan Singapore Sydney Tokyo Toronto Professions
Division

McGraw-Hill

A Division of The McGraw·Hill Companies

1 2 3 4 5 6 7 8 9 0   DOCDOC   9 9 8 7

ISBN 0-07-063350-9

This book was set in Perpetua by V&M Graphics, Inc.
The editors were John Dolan and Peter McCurdy;
the production supervisors were Heather Munro and Catherine Saggese;
the cover designer was Ed Schultheis and the index was prepared by Southwest Indexing.
RR Donnelley & Sons was printer and binder.

This book is printed on acid-free paper.

CATALOGING-IN-PUBLICATION DATA IS ON FILE FOR THIS TITLE AT THE LIBRARY OF CONGRESS.

Contents

Contributors

Primary Author and Editor

Toni J. Sullivan, EdD, RN, FAAN
Professor and Dean
Sinclair School of Nursing
University of Missouri–Columbia
Columbia, Missouri

Contributing Authors

Jane M. Armer, PhD, RN,
Associate Professor of Nursing
Co-Director Office of Research
Sinclair School of Nursing
University of Missouri–Columbia

Julie Bailey, MS(N)c, RN
Teaching Associate
Sinclair School of Nursing
University of Missouri–Columbia

Patricia J. Blair, MD
President
A Call To Serve, International (ACTS, INT)
Columbia, Missouri and San Jose, California

James D. Campbell, PhD
Associate Professor of Family and Community Medicine
Department of Family and Community Medicine
School of Medicine
University of Missouri–Columbia

Julie Clawson, PhDc, RN
Associate Professor of Nursing
Department of Nursing
Central Missouri State University, Warrensburg, Missouri
Doctoral Candidate, Sinclair School of Nursing
University of Missouri–Columbia

Marcia Flesner, MS(N), PhD student, RN
Nursing Administrator
Sinclair School of Nursing Nursing Center at Moberly Area Community College
Clinical Instructor of Nursing
Sinclair School of Nursing
University of Missouri–Columbia

Victoria T. Grando, PhD, RN
Assistant Professor of Nursing
Sinclair School of Nursing
University of Missouri–Columbia

Genevieve Gray
Deputy Vice Chancellor (Planning)
Professor of Nursing
University of Western Sydney
Australia

Belinda Heimerichs, MS(N), RN
Executive Director
Missouri Nurses Association
Jefferson City, Missouri

Daryl J. Hobbs, PhD
Professor of Rural Sociology
Director
Office of Social and Economic Data Analysis
University of Missouri–Columbia

Alice F. Kuehn, PhD, RN, CS, FNP\GNP
Associate Professor of Nursing
Sinclair School of Nursing
University of Missouri–Columbia

Afaf Ibrahim Meleis, PhD, RN, FAAN
Professor
Department of Community Health Systems
School of Nursing
University of California, San Francisco
San Francisco, California

Susan Morgan, PhD, RN
Professor of Nursing
Department of Nursing
Central Missouri State University
Warrensburg, Missouri

Rosemary Porter, PhD, RN
Associate Professor ard Associate Dean
Sinclair School of Nursing
University of Missouri–Columbia

Jill Scott, PhDc, RN
Instructor of Clinical Nursing
Sinclair School of Nursing
University of Missouri–Columbia

Research Assistants
Marcia Flesner, PhD student
Jill Scott, PhDc

Preface

Collaboration, simply defined as working together for a common goal, is easy to extol and difficult to achieve. To be other than an apple pie and motherhood concept, collaboration must be made operational by at least two or more people acting in tandem in pursuit of shared goals.

It is in the design and practice of collaboration that the challenges begin. Collaboration requires of its practitioners the acquisition and application of a complex constellation of values and abilities. When the two or more collaborators *share* values and *agree upon* plans and actions a mutually satisfying and productive collaborative relationship may result. Such relationships, while not rare, are neither readily achieved nor maintained. Their occurrence is recognized as cause for commendation and celebration.

The literature clearly documents that nurses and other health professionals, individually and collectively, are establishing collaborative relationships among themselves or with colleagues from other disciplines. While the need for multidisciplinary, multiinstitutional, and international collaboration within transforming American health care delivery and educational systems and within dynamic international arenas has arguably never been greater, the effectiveness and success of these collaborative ventures cannot be readily assured.

The nursing and health services management literature, and to a lesser extent, the medical literature on collaboration is extensive, particularly concerning RN–MD collaboration. It is surprisingly more data-based than one might expect. This abundant attention positions the topic as one of central interest to nursing and perhaps medicine in my judgment. It also squares with my experience. Collaboration is central to my functioning as a dean within the academic health center and to my activities as a member of several boards, committees, and task forces in the university, state, and nation.

The aims for this book are ambitious and are rooted in a passionate commitment to widespread successful collaborative relationships within health care delivery and health professions education between health care providers and within integrated health care coalitions and delivery systems. The book aims to be an authoritative treatment of the subject by organizing a comprehensive and lively scholarly presentation of the extensive work reported to date. The topic is also enlivened by the inclusion of several small studies, designed and conducted for the book by selected guest researchers and authors. In addition, a select few leading scholars on collaboration are contributing state-of-the-art chapters in their areas of renown. I am honored by their participation.

Collaboration: A Health Care Imperative will be useful to nurse, physician, and other health professions educators, practitioners, and scholars studying any one of a number of areas of collaboration or related practices and processes. It will be useful to nursing and other health professions education administrators, health services executives, or nurse managers who are fostering collaborative practices or program models in their settings or interorganizationally. Faculty teaching in graduate nursing and other health professions education programs should find the book rich in conceptual, theoretical, and research-based insights. Graduate students committed to advancing nursing or another health science in collaborative models in the new health care delivery and health professions paradigms of the future will find this book indispensable. Nurses and other providers on the front lines in community or hospital-based settings with responsibilities for designing or participating in collaborative models of practice will, hopefully, find this book to be an indispensable ally and teacher. It is expected that physicians and other colleagues will find many useful chapters in this book. In short, anyone committed to working together with others toward common health care goals will profit from *Collaboration: A Health Care Imperative*.

Acknowledgements

This book is a collaborative work. A work of this size and magnitude could not be accomplished by one person acting alone. No one person has the breadth and depth required in so many facets of this complex subject to 'go it alone'. Moreover, as a busy dean who was attempting to meet major position obligations during most of the 15 months spent writing or editing this volume, it would be unthinkable that I complete this task without the collaboration, assistance, and support of many wonderful colleagues. I am indebted to them. I appreciate their sharing in this labor of love with me more than they can ever know.

I want to express my heartfelt thanks to all of the contributing authors. They enrich this volume immeasurably. I am honored by their presence. The two research assistants, Marcia Flesner and Jill Scott were sensational. Marcia spent the best part of a year entering 318 books\articles into *Papyrus*. Jill spent endless hours in the library conducting literature searches and tracking down wayward resources that I just had to have. She also served as second reader on several reliability and validity exercises. I am delighted they both have chapters in the book, thus getting some of the credit they have so richly earned.

Special thanks are due to Rose Porter, Associate Dean, who covered for me so many times while I was off writing. I didn't doubt for one minute that she would do an outstanding job of taking charge of the school in my absences. No one ever had a better associate. Sooner or later most of the faculty and staff of the school had a chance to show their support of the Dean and her book.

No one ever fell short. I want to especially thank Elaine Litwiller who in the beginning was my secretary and then received a promotion to Administrative Assistant in the school. Nevertheless, in the beginning and throughout the project, Elaine was my computer guru and the one who put the finishing touches on the chapters. She saved my life more than once such as when the computer files got lost or the computer locked up or any one of a hundred different crises. Susan Hatfield, my Executive Staff Assistant, made the whole thing possible. She ruled my calendar and my time. She managed my mail better than anyone else ever has. She offered endless words of encouragement. Susan is simply the best there is!

I want to voice special thanks to Ed Sheridan, Provost of the University. He kindly approved my 3 month research leave, Summer '96, which got me off to a great start. He also turned a blind eye to my writing schedule this year. In fact, he offered many words of encouragement, and even read draft material. I am very grateful to him.

The editors and executive staff at McGraw-Hill have been terrific. They offer much encouragement within a very professional and goal-directed framework. This is exactly the approach I need. I've learned to have great confidence in them and I'm glad they are the publishers of this book. A special word of thanks to Gail Gavert, who was the first to have faith in me and offered me a contract. Thanks are due to John Dolan who has nurtured me and this project every step of the way. Peter McCurdy has brought me and this manuscript down the stretch. He is a tough man, but I wouldn't trade him for another. Thank you.

My family deserves a special note of thanks and love. My adult children, Jim and Jill, and Eric, my son-in-law, are proud of their mom and always let me know it. My husband Jim, has lived the book with me. He is always, always there. He knows all the ups and the downs of the entire challenging and wonderful process. He lived them. He owns a piece of this book. He is my main partner. He is special and so is the time we had together doing this work. Those who know me will expect me to acknowledge the supportive presence of a special little creature. Sheena was always there, chasing my mouse and blinking at the wonder of it all, from the keyboard, of course. Somehow, I think she knows how much I loved having her there.

Dedication

This book is dedicated to all those health care providers who are practicing collaboration or transformational leadership, and to the patients and consumers and students who are fortunate to have you working with them. You know who you are. Thank you.

Introduction

Although collaboration has long been a working companion of mine, the first stage of my current work with collaboration began four years ago when I accepted an appointment as Co-Chair of the Collaborative Practice Task Force in the state of Missouri. Over the ensuing three years my nurse and physician colleagues and I struggled to reach agreement on guidelines for RN–MD (and DO) collaborative practice in Missouri. Deeply dissatisfied with our woefully slow (or absent) progress and feeling hurt or angry most of the time, I was mobilized into action. I began to systematically study the subject of collaboration in the professional literature. Surprised by the extensiveness of the literature and confused by the jumble of meanings and descriptions put forward by collaborators and scholars of collaboration, I decided it was imperative that I extend my focus to scholarly work. Metaphorically speaking, the roadways were gridlocked. I wanted to bring order to the traffic congestion.

The book *Collaboration: A Health Care Imperative* begins the second leg of my journey through busy and heavily traveled roadways. The heavy traffic is analogous to the literature on collaboration, which is abundant and even rich, but leaves one feeling intellectually dissatisfied. There must be avenues one can travel to understanding. At the very least new avenues for exploration can be plotted.

The literature on collaboration, as already noted, is large. The extensive data base of literature compiled for the foundational and theoretical chapters of this volume, described here, reflects the vastness of the literature. It forms the basis, for the most part, of data used to develop Part I of the book, as well as Chapters 10 and 11 in Part III. Four primary sources of data were searched and organized. CINAHL (Cumulative Index Of Nursing And Allied Health Literature) was searched using the key word *collaboration* from 1982 to March,1996.The scope of the term was defined in CINAHL as: pooling of resources and ideas within or across disciplines for innovation and problem-solving. For articles published prior to 1989 researchers are instructed to "see under Interpersonal Relations, Interprofessional Relations, and Intraprofessional Relations."

CINAHL provides comprehensive coverage of English language journals related to nursing and 15 allied health disciplines. Material from over 650 journals is included in CINAHL A total of 1361 articles were listed using the key words identified. Careful scanning revealed that 239 of these addressed collaboration in some substantive way and were within the nursing and/or nursing and medical disciplines. Articles focusing primarily on clinical practice or clinical programs and those merely indicating that people were working together in care delivery were eliminated. Also eliminated were articles on collaboration within and among the 15 allied health disciplines. The 239 articles were entered into the computer program *Papyrus*; hard copies were also made.

The second computer database accessed was MEDLINE. This database covers the international literature on biomedicine, including the allied health fields and the biological and physical sciences, humanities and information science as they relate to medicine and health care. Information is indexed from approximately 3600 journals published worldwide. The timeframe for articles searched was 1992 to May, 1996. The heading *collaboration* was not indexed prior to 1992. The heading available for use after 1991 was *collaboration as cooperative behavior*, defined in MEDLINE as the interaction of two or more persons or organizations directed toward a common goal which is mutually beneficial; an act or instance of working or acting together for a common purpose or benefit.

The listing contained 300 articles; the great majority were clinical in nature and simply were identified in the list because two or more persons were sharing in the care delivery or research being reported upon. I reviewed each title and abstract carefully, selecting all articles that might focus upon collaboration as the primary topic. This process yielded 23 articles, all of which were entered into *Papyrus*. Hard copies were also made and filed.

The third source of literature accessed was the *New England Journal of Medicine*. Searched from 1992 to July, 1995 using the code terms *collabo-*

ration and *collaboration with nurses*. The term *collaboration* yielded 81 articles. The term *collaboration with nurses* yielded 1 article. An analysis of the titles and abstracts, looking for articles focusing upon MD–RN or MD–MD collaboration as the substantive topic, led to a selection of 9 articles. The 9 were entered into *Papyrus* and hard copies were placed on file.

These three sources, totaling 271 articles, were then supplemented by scholarly books, documents, reports known to me or recommended by colleagues or research assistants. Several of the articles from CINAHL, MEDLINE, or *NEJM* were separated out as they became known as landmark or classic publications. In addition, as articles were reviewed, citations were noted. Articles that were cited over and over again were added to the data base. At present *Papyrus* contains 318 listings.

All other chapters in this volume are equally rigorous in their searches of the literature, as appropriate to each chapter's topic. These data bases are rich and variable and are described at the beginning of each chapter. In several cases, such as Chapters 14, 16, and 17, the literature searches build on the foundational searches presented in the foundational chapters.

Collaboration: A Health Care Imperative is organized in 6 parts and totals 21 chapters. The book is organized so that from beginning to end the reader may systematically study the topic with its many permutations and applications. For those who are serious students of the subject, this approach is recommended. The reader with a more targeted purpose for turning to the book will profit from studying the chapters specific to their interests and needs, along with the study of one or several foundations chapters. This approach should enable the reader to gain a current and orderly understanding of this rich topic that is responsive to their specific needs. Part I focuses upon conceptual, historical, and theoretical foundations of collaboration. Part II focuses upon interdisciplinary person-to-person collaboration, especially RN–MD collaboration encompassing advanced practice nurse and physician practice teams. Part III studies interorganizational collaboration. Part IV studies international collaboration, although international collaboration permeates all of the topical areas in the book. Part V is composed of six chapters that focus upon ways to facilitate collaboration, including collaborative learning and transformational leadership. The latter three chapters in the section address consumers as partners in health care. Part VI is focused upon collaboration as value-laden and as an imperative for societal and health-care functioning in the new millennium.

Part I

Part I, comprised of 5 chapters, takes the reader on a journey of the conceptual, historical, and theoretical foundations for collaboration between and among individuals, disciplines, and organizations: in health professions education and research, health care delivery, and intra- and inter-organizational arrangements. As a reflection of the literature, however, the random sampling of literature does focus the majority of its attention on collaboration between and among people, rather than collaboration between and among organizations.

The concept analysis of collaboration is divided between two chapters to ease the burden on the reader and incorporates all of the attributes of collaborators and collaboration derived from an evolutionary approach to concept analysis, such as antecedents, consequences, and references. This dynamic approach is extra sensitive to capturing a current understanding of a concept and to assessing its developmental status with an eye to future possibilities and desired strategies for achieving the preferred future. Those who are students of collaboration or would be users of collaboration will benefit from in-depth study of these chapters.

Chapter 3, a theoretical and contextual analysis, incorporates a historical framework for both the theoretical and contextual perspectives. The complexity of collaboration, viewed over time, has increased greatly while at the same time pat formulas or simple lists of "must dos" to achieve collaboration have fallen from favor. The influence of both role and systems theories on collaborative models of practice is especially focused.

What are the societal contexts within which collaboration has or has not flourished? Has the societal context for collaboration, in fact, varied over time? Does it matter? The contextual analysis offers 'food for thought' concerning these important questions. Concerning these questions and others throughout the book, reasoned positions are offered. In all cases, the reader is invited to engage in intelligent discourse with the text on these topics. This chapter, sandwiched between more conceptually and theoretically substantive chapters, is essential reading for reflective students of the subject including those who wish to put collaboration within a framework of societal well-being.

Chapter 4, a logical outcome of Chapters 1 and 2, offers a beginning systems model of collaboration. Using systems modeling and systems thinking, a symbolic presentation of a systems model of collaboration is made, along with beginning sets of relational statements. The model is preceded by an overview of systems concepts amd systems thinking, especially as described by Senge (1990). Those designing and testing collaborative programs or interventions or designing evaluation research studies on collaboration will hopefully find the model and propositions invaluable.

Chapter 5, an integrated research review of published studies on collaboration, is a comprehensive presentation and analysis of research on collaboration in the health sciences—education, practice, research, and intra- and interorganizational arrangements—to date. Program planners, researchers, academicians, and graduate students will find this chapter very useful for finding evidence or lack of evidence for pursuing their work in this field.

Overall, Part I offers a set of maps or blueprints for furthering the journey toward understanding the landscape of collaboration.

Part II

Part II, comprised of 3 chapters, focuses on collaboration between people—one or more persons in intra-inter-multidisciplinary collaborative arrangements. These chapters are skewed toward advanced practice nurses (APNs)–medical doctors (MD or DO) collaborative practices, because this coupling in collaborative practice arrangements is so important to health care in the 1990s and because the literature is so filled with it.

Campbell's Chapter 6 is a fine research-based journey through the 1980s with relationships to the present developed. Both the methods employed and the substantive findings in the body of work he reviews offer indispensable knowledge and knowledge-applications insights for practitioners, educators, and researchers of APN–MD collaboration. Chapter 6 visits the recent past, but points toward the future.

Chapters 7 and 8 are qualitative research studies completed for this book. One of them, Chapter 7 (Flesner and Clawson), reports on the different clinical care management approaches of APNs and MDs. The other, Chapter 8 (Bailey and Armer), tells the stories of successful APN–MD collaborative practices as told by these practitioner teams.

These three chapters document anew the breadth and depth of APN and MD practice and the richness of practice that occurs in collaborative practices. Campbell muses that something happens in collaborative practice between the providers that brings out the best practice qualities in each practitioner while also bringing their practice patterns and styles into harmony. The authors of Chapters 7 and 8 report similar findings. Those studying, contemplating, or engaging in collaborative practice will benefit from Part II.

Part III

Part III offers three provocative chapters on interorganizational collaboration. Each chapter intends to advance our thinking and our behaviors concerning interorganizational collaboration. Chapter 9 is a modified concept analysis and model design on coalition—formation and conduct. Building on Chapters 1, 2, and 4, it brings order and meaning to a vast and vastly confusing body of literature. Calling on both the literature and my own experience, a model useful for forming and conducting coalitions is put forward. It becomes very apparent in this important foundational chapter that the would-be collaborators cannot focus too much time, attention, and energy on the formation component of coalition work. The model is also useful for designing research on coalition formation and conduct and for planning evaluation research of coalition activities and outcomes. Chapter 9 provides examples of 15 coalitions from the United States and other nations.

Porter, Scott, and Sullivan (Chapter 10) report on their qualitative research study of nurse executives and other health care executives developing coalitions to meet their many and varied needs. This study presents a new 'hub and spoke' model of collaboration that has not been present in the nursing and health care literature. Does this model represent a new reality or commonplace model? The answer to this question and its implications are speculated upon. This section of the book is must reading for those practicing in or contemplating involvement in coalitions—and that means most of us.

Chapter 11 is a qualitative study on conflict-induced collaboration incorporating a story-telling methodology along with more traditional phenomenological research methodology. In this chapter, *When Collaboration Is Legislatively Mandated* (Sullivan, Morgan, Heimerichs, Scott), the participants on a Task Force to develop state-wide collaborative practice guidelines for APN–MD practice tell of their experiences using an approach designed to elicit their subjective responses. Their very rich human stories provide many insights for improving, or preferably averting conflict-induced collaboration approaches. This chapter makes a strong case for using voluntary approaches to the formation of collaborative models between organizations and disciplines.

Part IV

Part IV is comprised of 2 chapters on international collaboration. Two leading practitioners of the art and science of international collaboration offer contributed chapters from their very different perspectives. Meleis (Chapter 12, writing with her international colleague, Gray), a leading nurse educator with a long history of leadership in international graduate nursing education provides a state-of-the-art presentation and analysis of international collaboration; opportunities, challenges, and principles, with recommendations for future collaboration.

Chapter 13, authored by Blair, a physician who has devoted the last 5 years of her life and career to improving health care in nations in transition, focuses on the building of international coalitions among nations and disciplines in order to begin to develop the human and material resources of countries left with devastated infrastructures due to the break up of the former Soviet Union. Her international, multidisciplinary work in the republic of Georgia and other nations offers a model for emulation by others. Blair uses the coalition model presented in Chapter 9 coupled with a community values model to organize her presentation of 3 sharply contrasted case studies. This orderly approach provides an excellent model for organizing, analyzing, and evaluating international coalitions.

Part V

In a way Part V, encompassing 6 chapters, comes closest to being a how-to section of the book. It offers several chapters on topics that are recognized as facilitators of collaboration. While not exhaustive several of the most important facilitators are included. One chapter (14) presents the state-of-the-art of collaborative learning within the health sciences. The author (Kuehn) has been creatively engaged in such education for years. Several case examples from the literature and from her experience are provided and critiqued.

Chapter 15 is an exploration and overview of leadership, especially transformational leadership, to assist the designers and users of collaborative practice models to successfully design, implement and sustain them. Other chapters sound the chord over and over again about how critical supportive leadership is to collaboration.

The ability to articulate one's discipline and assert its unique perspective within a collaborating partnership is focused by nurse historian Grando. In Chapter 17 she reports on her phenomenological findings gleaned from listening to the how and what of articulating nursing by several past and present eminent nurse leaders and collaborating practitioners.

Three chapters in Part V address consumers as important collaborators or beneficiaries of collaboration in their health care. Armer (Chapter 17) reports on her investigations of consumers as recipients of health care by Advanced Practice Nurses. Their knowledge, perceptions, and attitudes about advanced practice nursing, which are extensive, are explored in detail. The knowledge gained can be very helpful to those in practice, or contemplating practice to learn how to best communicate their practices to the consumers of their care.

Chapter 18 analyzes data derived from a focus group of mainly senior citizen activists to gain their insights into the critical elements of forming and conducting grass roots coalitions and coalitions that combine both grass roots and professional members, as well as their perspectives on personal health care and on the current United States health care delivery system, especially managed care. Their reactions are very knowledgeable and strongly opinionated. Chapter 19 explores the literature on consumers, consumer advocacy, and citizen activism, especially as it relates to personal health care and to health care delivery. The perspectives used in analysis of the literature are historical, political, economic, and social. The findings are very provocative in terms of future directions of health care in the United States and internationally, as influenced by consumers.

These 3 chapters add considerably to a scanty body of literature on consumer behaviors and membership in collaborative health care partnerships. Everyone interested in forming and conducting a coalition that can benefit from consumer involvement, or those taking care of people in their collaborative practices, or those engaged in designing and conducting integrated health care delivery and financing systems ought to study these chapters.

Part VI

Part VI, comprised of 2 future-directed and values-focused chapters, means to be both intellectually challenging and personally satisfying. The distinguished rural sociologist, Hobbs, in Chapter 21, brings his vast demographic and sociological expertise to bear as he considers the future context, the global information era, within which collaboration will, and must, occur. He makes a case for the imperativeness of collaboration in health care to the well-being of society in the future. This chapter, along with other chapters in this book intends to provoke its readers into a serious consideration of why collaboration is important—even imperative— to a society where the citizens have access to quality health care and to a society of healthy people. The discussions in Chapter 20 have social, political, economic, health, and moral implications. They mean to!

Chapter 21 is unabashedly value laden. It follows an overview of all findings and discussion sections of the preceding chapters. Without wanting to repeat prior presentations, the author searched for overarching theme(s). Values of and for collaboration, in several permutations, are noted as the theme that ties the various chapters together. The highly ethical nature of collaboration; the deeply valued commitment to collaboration and to collaborating partners and partnerships; the universally valued importance of open, honest, continual communications between collaborators, and the deeply held value by many of collaboration as more than a practice, rather as a state of being requiring integration into all facets of human and social functioning, are focused. All are interrelated in a systems presentation of collaboration as a health care imperative in the global information era of the next millennium.

Conceptual and Theoretical Foundations

Concept Analysis of Collaboration: Part I[1]

Toni J. Sullivan

In all spheres of nursing and health care—practice, education, administration, and research,—the concept of collaboration is receiving much attention in the literature and has for many years. The beginning of the modern focus can be dated to 1970 and the publication of The Lysaught Report, *An Abstract For Action,* which advocated among its recommendations the establishment of a National Joint Practice Commission of nurses and physicians along with state counterpart commissions. The American Nurses Association (ANA) and the American Medical Association (AMA) jointly developed such a Commission in 1971. Its purpose was to promote joint practice of physicians and registered nurses (RNs) (Ritter 1983, McKay 1983, Styles 1984). National demonstration projects to promote joint practice in hospital settings with partial funding by the W. K. Kellogg Foundation began in 1978, and the subject of collaboration was widely discussed and debated in the literature.

Although these demonstration projects wound down by the early to mid-1980s, and the ANA and the AMA engaged in conflict over issues only indirectly related to collaborative practice, joint or collaborative practice received continuing impetus from another source. Federal policymakers had widespread concerns about the shortage of primary care providers, especially generalist physicians. After studying the problem, the Surgeon General, however, issued a report recommending that nurses should be educated to provide primary care and that practicing in

---

[1]Chapter 2 constitutes Part II of the concept analysis of collaboration.

collaboration with their physician colleagues could be used for that purpose (Report of the Surgeon General 1963). This demonstration of confidence in the potential of nursing led to enthusiastic development of the Nurse Practitioner model of nursing education and practice by some nurse and medical educators. It also gave impetus to the education and utilization of nurse-midwives and nurse anesthetists. Direct focus was on preparing these providers to practice jointly with their physician counterparts.

Growing concern throughout the years about the high and constantly escalating costs of health care has led to societal mandates to constrain costs and has, as of this writing, led to a focus on managed care approaches to financing and organizing health care delivery. These approaches, demanding that patient care include the prevention of illness and maintenance of good health, have sparked explosive demand for Advanced Practice Nurses (as Nurse Practitioners, Clinical Nurse Specialists, Nurse Midwives, and Nurse Anesthetists are now formally known) to engage in collaborative practice with physician colleagues in providing cost-effective, high-quality primary health care.

Collaboration within and across organizational settings having both similar and disparate missions has expanded dramatically over the years. Joint ventures are flourishing as service and educational institutions cope with massive change and complexity.

Increasingly, our literature, as well as our behaviors in health care delivery and health professions education settings, shows that collaboration among all actors is a favored approach to providing patient care, leading organizations, educating future health professionals, and conducting health care research. Thompson (1967) is cited in Baggs et al. (1992) as proposing that when situations become more complex, collaboration becomes more important in coordinating work. Thompson then defines complex situations as "dynamic and unpredictable" (p. 23).

Extensive attention to collaboration and an intensive belief that collaboration is the approach of choice is borne out in the following quotes.

Addressing patient care:

Clearly everyone gains in a collaborative practice setting—nurses and physicians because their relationship allows them to become better professionals, and patients who are the true beneficiaries of this collaboration. Improved patient care is the reward for medicine and nursing (Ritter 1983, p. 35).

Addressing education:

It is clear that major change in nursing and medical education is essential as a strategy to develop collaborative behavior, and that the notion of cooperation should be seen as a first step in this learning strategy (Fagin 1992, p. 301).

With respect to research:

One of the most effective strategies for assuring that research findings will influence practice and administrative decision-making of our professional policy-makers is to collaborate on research with such individuals (Henry 1992, p. 218).

With regard to organization:

Shared governance [a surrogate term for collaboration] leads to better decisions regarding patient care because staff nurse experts have ownership of all practice decisions. (McMahon 1992, p. 56).

Concerning interorganizational collaboration, in one consortium, Coluccio (1994, p.68) reports that "each hospital is linked with every other hospital and all are linked with the educational institution. The result is a strong, broad-based network of professionals and resources, involvement, and support." Becker, President of the Maine Hospital Association is quoted by Cerne (1993) as stating that collaboration "is the right way to go to provide the best patient care to their [Maine hospital] communities and to insure continuing access to patient care." (27).

But what is collaboration? What are the characteristics of collaboration that present the would-be-users with parameters or markers for going about the business of collaborating. Currently, the literature is replete with myriad and varied descriptors that are snippets of definitions. Collaboration is described, for example, as "working together in a joint intellectual effort" (Arcangelo 1994, Baggs and Ryan 1990), and "as partners sharing a common philosophy of patient care" (King 1990). The theme of power sharing is often addressed: Mundinger (1994) speaks of "sharing authority for practice equally." Similarly, Henneman (1995) speaks of "power-sharing," but as "based in knowledge and expertise, rather than role or title." Collaboration is often described as a "process of mutual respect for differences in opinion and perspective" (Hills 1994, p. 220) and a "process of negotiation and compromise integral to making decisions" (Henry et al. 1992, p. 220), as well as an "interpersonal process in which participating members contribute to a common product or goal" (Henneman 1995).

The extensive use of collaboration in the current health care environment and the significance attached to it beg for a systematic analysis of the abundant expressions of the concept in order to define and clarify it. A comprehensive definition of collaboration, one that categorizes the innumerable expressions used to convey meaning about the concept, should greatly facilitate further understanding of the concept and enhance our ability to use the concept successfully in practice, education, research, or management. Moreover, Henneman (1995) asserts that the meaning of the concept is not stable. "Our task," she asserts, "is to describe the nature of the present, and ourselves in the present" (p. 362).

As a result of this concept analysis, *Collaboration is defined as a dynamic, transforming process of creating a power sharing partnership for pervasive application in health care practice, education, research, and organizational settings for the purposeful attention to needs and problems in order to achieve likely successful outcomes.*

METHOD

The story is told that after St. Paul's Cathedral in England was destroyed by fire in 1666, Sir Christopher Wren, the great architect, was commissioned by the royal family to rebuild the cathedral. He undertook the monumental task in 1675 along with an army of craftsmen. They completed the huge building in 1710. Queen Anne then visited the edifice amid great fanfare to make the initial inspection. Entourage in tow, she slowly circled the great space saying not a word. Finally, turning to Sir Christopher, who was beside himself with anxiety, the queen said, "You have outdone yourself, Sir Christopher. The cathedral is awful, amusing, and artificial!" Whereupon, Sir Christopher breathed a sigh of relief, for in the meaning of the time *awful* meant *awesome, amusing* meant *amazing*, and *artificial* meant *artful*.

Concepts—and the words to express them—change and evolve, as this graphic story so aptly demonstrates. A research method that recognizes this reality is the method of choice for this concept analysis of collaboration. In this philosophically based evolutionary approach, as described by Rodgers (1993), selected concepts are seen as dynamic and evolving, rather than as static and absolute. They are context dependent, rather than universally true.

Concepts, in this view, are recognized as private and individualized. Private views are symbolically expressed with words or artistic expression. It is the examination of these expressions that provides the means to explore underlying meanings by gathering, sorting, relating, and clustering the expressions or attributes. The ability to form clusters of meaning from this conceptually based data gives concepts descriptive and explanatory power and, therefore, contributes to knowledge development. "Ultimately, concepts can be used to characterize phenomena of interest, to describe situations, and to communicate effectively" (Rodgers 1993, p. 75).

Significance, use, and application of the concept are recognized as three distinct influences on concept development over time. Concepts that explain important human phenomena and help resolve important human problems will be widely used, emphasized, studied, and applied (Toulmin 1972, cited in Rodgers 1993). Concept analysis, in this method, seeks to identify what is common in use, rather than impose a strict set of criteria or boundaries for excluding data. Consensus about current meaning is sought, rather than a fixed and unchanging essence.

Emphasis is placed on an inductive discovery approach to data gathering and analysis. Consequently, actual analysis does not focus on the creation of model cases. One or more model cases may be discovered in the literature. A sample case that captures many of the attributes of the concept as it is used in many settings would represent an ideal exemplar. If cases are not present in the literature, that absence in and of itself may present important insight about the current state of the concept. Specifically, raw data are gathered on attributes, antecedents, consequences, surrogate terms, related concepts, and references. Table 1-1 is a listing of the working definitions of these terms.

Literature Search

The literature used for the concept analysis included a sample of 30 articles from the 239 Cumulative Index of Nursing and Allied Health Literature (CINAHL) articles dating from 1982 to 1995, which were entered in a computer program known as *Papyrus*. Using a table of random num-

Table 1-1. Definitions of Data Categories

Attributes: Expressions of the concept; they can form clusters. Rodgers suggests asking:"What is this thing the writer is discussing?" (1993, p. 83)

Antecedents: Situations, events, or phenomena that precede an example of the concept. Ask: "What happens before the concept happens?" (Rodgers, 1993, p. 83) "What seems to need to be present in order for the concept [collaboration] to be occurring?

Consequences: Situations, events, or phenomena that follow an example of the concept. Ask: "What happens after the concept happens?" In other words, "What seems to be the result of the concept happening?" (Rodgers, 1993, p. 83).

References: Actual situations in which the concept is being used or to which it is being applied. These situations are both tangible, as a hospital for example, or abstract, as a desire to improve a relationship for example (Rodgers, 1993).

Related concepts: "Concepts that bear some relationship to the concept of interest, but do not share the same set of attributes" (Rodgers, 1993, p. 83). Related concepts are part of the network of concepts that add context to the concept of interest and impart significance. Overall they provide a rich background.

Surrogate terms: means of expressing the concept other than the means selected by the researcher; they may be used interchangeably with the main term. It is often difficult to distinguish between concepts and surrogate terms. Rodgers (1993, p.83) points out the idea that there may be many ways to express a term.

---

bers, 30 articles were selected as 10% of the sample, which is purported to be adequate to ensure credibility of the findings (Rodgers 1989). As the vast majority of the articles date later than 1989, it is not surprising that 28 of the 30 are from 1992 to 1995, whereas only two are from 1990 to 1991; none predate 1990.

The entire MEDLINE sample consisted of 25 articles, all of which were included in the database for the concept analysis in an effort to achieve the most credible sample possible. Also, six articles from the *New England Journal of Medicine*, all published from 1992 to 1995, were entered into the *Papyrus* database and were included in the sampling.

Twenty landmark or classic articles and books were also included in the database as a purposive sample that would enhance the search for meaning. Of these, 15 were published between 1981 and 1990 and 5, between 1993 and 1995. The presence in this study of the landmark or classic literature published before 1993 enabled an analysis of change and evolution of the concept over time.

Of the CINAHL articles, 3 are authored by MDs and 27 are written by RNs. The MEDLINE articles include 12 of 25 authored or coauthored by MDs. The *New England Journal of Medicine* entries do not include any that are MD authored.

Two of the landmark or classic publications are MD authored. Thus, of the total sample of 81 articles and books, 17 are authored or coauthored by MDs. Although a larger sample would be preferred in order to draw disciplinary comparisons, the 17 constitute the total available body of literature in this extensive literature search and comparisons will be attempted.

Data Collection and Analysis

The articles were obtained from the University of Missouri–Columbia Health Sciences Library or, if they were unavailable at the library, by interlibrary loan. All the identified articles were obtained, entered into *Papyrus*, and given a code number. Data were retrieved by the researcher aided by two research assistants. Initially, each article was read for the purpose of identifying its type (i.e., whether research, theory development, or case study), the themes presented, and the scope of the work. This step provided the additional benefit of helping to immerse the researchers in the literature and substantially increase their knowledge of collaboration in general.

Next, phrases, themes, and direct quotes were recorded on individual "sheets of paper" using either actual paper or computer entries. Data were extrapolated according to whether they were *attributes, antecedents, consequences, references, related concepts, or surrogate terms*. In addition, past, present, and future data on theoretical or conceptual foundations, context, barriers, and facilitators of collaboration were also recorded. (For a discussion of the theory analysis or conceptual frameworks underpinning collaboration, see Chapter 3.)

As data were recorded, the coded article number from the *Papyrus* database was also recorded, along with the date of the article and the page number of the datum. This procedure readily enabled the researcher to return to the original source as necessary for reference or further clarification and also facilitated the researcher's verification of the consistency of approach among all three data recorders, thus diminishing the potential for bias.

Analysis of the data was accomplished exclusively by the researcher by completing a minimum of three rounds of data analysis for each characteristic. Ample time was given to this process in order not to manipulate the data prematurely and to allow the data categories to emerge from the data itself. The data were reviewed, then rereviewed, related, ordered, reordered, counted (in some instances), and categorized. Themes and patterns were identified, revised, and refined.

The raw data compiled in this review of the literature were displayed in a chart of voluminous pages and then categorized and collapsed slightly where overlap was very obvious. For the most part, however, data are reported as presented by the authors, but within the categories selected to best display the magnitude of these findings.

Initially, the medical literature and nursing literature were combined, as were the older and newer references, in order to gain the broadest possible scope of the data. After the initial analyses were completed, however, a cross-disciplinary comparison of the literature was undertaken to determine differences in meanings and perspectives of medicine and nursing. Also undertaken was a time-based analysis. Data predating 1990 were compared with data from 1990 and later. Findings in both instances should increase understanding of collaboration and may enhance its successful utilization.

FINDINGS

Several clear and strong overall findings beg to be articulated. Perhaps the strongest of these is that in 81 articles and books from the mainstream medical and nursing literature on collaboration, there is not one negative consequence of collaboration reported between or to anyone. This includes zero evidence of any case in which physician–nurse collaboration resulted in a malpractice suit. It appears that everyone involved in, and everything addressed by, collaboration can benefit from it. A second and closely related finding is that collaboration is a complex and time-consuming process, but one with a highly predictable success rate, as long as all components of the process are accomplished.

A third finding is that all of the authors were proponents of collaboration. Many felt very strongly and used hyperbolic expressions to emphasize their points. Thus they spoke of *real* partners, *true* partnership, *full* partners, *collegial* communications, *excellent* communication, and joint problem-solving as *a way of life*. The next finding is that collaboration in all spheres of health care services and education is indeed significant, as evidenced by the scope—breadth and depth—of the literature and the reported implementation of collaboration in practice. Authors continually discuss and stress the fifth finding, which is that one cannot overemphasize the importance of a supportive and developmental environment. It is their belief that to achieve true collaboration, both human and system supports must be consistently and dependably present.

The next finding captures a negative position. Competition in a market-driven economy as the dominant approach to the evolution of health care delivery and financing, with its concomitant view of power based in control of resources, knowledge, and systems, is a negative energy that stifles the creation of collaborative arrangements. This finding is more implicit than explicit. It is inferred in part because of the insistence by several authors of another view of power—one whereby power is based in competence. There also appears to be a fundamental contradiction between collaboration and competition.

The seventh finding is rather surprising: The majority of the literature on collaboration between RNs and MDs describes hospital-based practices rather than primary care or community-based settings. Perhaps the literature published over the next 2 to 5 years will change this imbalance.

Characteristics

Analyses of attributes, antecedents, consequences, and references were completed in order to provide a foundation for the attributes, or characteristics, that constitute collaboration as defined earlier here. Despite the strong opinions and beliefs expressed by the various authors, there was consensus on many characteristics of collaboration, which enabled this definition.

Nurses and physicians expressed substantial, substantive agreement on the numerous characteristics undergirding the definition of collaboration. Throughout the period from 1981 to the time of this writing, there also has been substantive agreement. Consequently, the RN-authored literature and the MD-authored literature were combined for this analysis, as were the older references combined with the newer. Those differences that do exist are explored later in this chapter.

A few authors used the word *dynamic* to speak of dynamic process. *Transforming*, as a term was used by one author (Evans 1994) to describe a supportive environment, especially the leadership in the environment, and by others (Collucio and Kelley 1994) to describe a transformative educational model. The term *process* was used several times with respect to many different facets of collaboration, such as team building or planning. *Power* was a commonly used term with respect to authority, autonomy, decision making, or equality. The term *pervasive* was not used, nor was the word *purposeful*. The words *partners* or *partnership* were widely used by these scholars to best express the quality of the collaborative relationship.

Dynamic

Webster's New World College Dictionary, 3rd ed. (1996) defines dynamic as "moving energy," and as "marked by continuous usually productive activity or change" (p. 424). The recognition of energy and purposeful activity as elements of the term *dynamic* are why this word is part of the definition of collaboration. Authors speak of participants in collaborative arrangements as having high energy and as being enthusiastic and passionate. Evans (1994) states, "Collaboration does not exist without a measure of passion." Collaborators are flexible, changing to meet the varied needs of complex environments or interchanging their leadership roles depending on the expertise required at any given time. Collaborators are flexible in their distribution of status and authority.

The process of collaboration requires attention to shared planning, goal setting, decision making, interventions, and problem-solving. As collaborators arrange this continuously changing mosaic of activities, they are described as being open to negotiating differences of opinion, to putting aside their own agendas and status concerns and making decisions that are in the best interests of the patient, organization, or student, depending on the given situation. Collaboration, Weiss (1985) states, "requires a dynamic, flexible distribution of status and authority whereby responsibilities and influence vary from point to point depending on which individual or group has the superior competence required for a particular task" (p. 50).

Transforming

The term *transform* connotes substantial change in nature or composition, as when a caterpillar transforms itself into a butterfly. The butterfly is new and different from the caterpillar. It is not simply a caterpillar with a new outward appearance. The same is so for a collaborative relationship. It is new and different than a traditional relationship. As one nurse–physician collaborating partnership has written:

> Let's analyze the differences between traditional practices and collaborative practices. In the traditional model, health professionals function autonomously in a very static professional hierarchy dominated by physicians and administrators. Authority flows downward from administrators to physicians to Registered Nurses to ancillary staff to patients. The outcome is that care is provided incrementally by various individuals and often is disjointed and inconsistent. In collaborative relationship there is a team concept, with all parties sharing in the partnership of care. Because authority is shared, this effort results in more integrated and comprehensive care. (Miccolo and Spanier 1993, pp. 446–447).

Collaborative practice is defined by Weiss and Davis (1985 as "interaction between nurses and physicians that enable the knowledge and skills of both professionals to synergistically influence the patient care being provided" (p. 299).

In a transforming collaborative practice, collaborators share a value for collaboration. They have reached mutual agreement on philosophies and models of practice. They share concerns about patient or student or organizational welfare and ability of collaborators to better respond to presenting needs. As Iseminger (1996) states about their rural community-based practice, "We enjoy being where needed. We're not just doctors competing for patients. We have a philosophy of service to the underserved" (p. 28).

Those who collaborate have a commitment to change and a conviction that collaboration is needed. They have a passion and enthusiasm for the task of creating a collaborative approach or model of practice, education, research, or organizational management that is transforming. Evans (1994) speaks of collaboration as realigning "all traditional roles, stimulating interaction, and synergistically advancing thought in a communal pattern not achievable by other means. There is perhaps no more essential ingredient for its development than passion" (p. 30).

Collaborators describe feeling empowered by their working relationship. They report feelings of high self-esteem and of being highly motivated. They speak of honesty and integrity in their working relationship and of feeling comfortable in the partnership. They care about their partners. They engage in teaching and coaching behaviors at times and are generally very supportive of the best efforts of their partners. Collaborators recognize and appreciate their colleagues' contributions to the shared work. They attribute credit as it is due.

Disciplinary interests or personal agendas are secondary to the shared goals of the collaborators in a transforming partnership. One partner or teammate understands the perspectives and lived experience of the other(s). To develop a transforming collaborative relationship requires hard work and risk taking. As Pender (1992) states, "Collaboration is a human endeavor. There must be a willingness to express views openly, reveal areas of experience as well as inexperience, risk performing in the presence of others, and take criticism" (p. 249). Perhaps best of all in a transforming collaborative practice, people like each other and they like their work.

Process

Webster's New World College Dictionary, 3rd ed. (1996) describes *process* as a method of doing operations conducing to an end; as progression or advancement (p. 1072). It is on the basis of this meaning of the term process that collaboration is so defined. The scholars of collaboration refer to *process* frequently. As described earlier, however, this description is usually only in relation to component parts of collaboration, such as negotiation or team building. The overall conceptualization, design and building of a collaborative arrangement is, in the researcher's judgment and after analysis of the data, a highly complex process involving whole organizations and often myriad people. The different components of collaboration intersect and overlap in a dense tapestry. Antecedents of collaboration, such as supportive environments or problems to solve, become attributes, such as shared problem-solving and a transforming relationship. In turn, attributes of collaboration become consequences, such as problems solved or a deeply satisfying working relationship.

From a macro perspective, undertaking the development of collaborative arrangements is a multipart exercise involving several overlapping and semiorderly activities. Although no one describes a rigid set of steps to take, it is apparent that the process is one of building a foundation of a supportive environment and prepared providers or educators or staff—to ensure the subsequent successful undertaking of the tasks associated with whatever is the focus of the collaboration. Moreover, the participants are expected to do this through working together. These steps are preparation of the organization to achieve a supportive and conducive environment, preparation of the providers through education and socialization, taking first steps of working together by the would-be-collaborators, building collaborative model(s), and evaluating and nurturing the model(s) over time. None of this is easy. Warner et al. (1994) state that "[t]he process of collaboration is not easy and certainly not automatic" (p. 12).

Many authors devote much attention to the importance of a supportive environment being in place prior to starting collaborative practice. Jones (1994) asserts that "a change in style from managing others to leading others is a prerequisite to developing a collaborative model" (p. 33). Frequently mentioned are committed administrative leadership, supportive MD leadership, a stable workforce, sufficient resources and their efficient and flexible utilization, and a desire and commitment to collaboration by the staff who will be collaborating. Also focused are the abilities of the staff, RN or MD or other, in terms of their ability to work with others and their knowledge, skill, and expertise to engage in the work to be done. Ritter (1983) and others ask several key questions that they believe should be asked of organizations as part of an assessment of organizational readiness. Are necessary systems in place to support collaboration? Is the environment receptive? Is the timing right? Is there a stable workforce? Does the workforce have the necessary abilities to work collaboratively?

Particular attention is paid to the subject of assessing RN readiness to engage in collaborative practice with their MD counterparts. Registered nurse competence, assertiveness, legal status, self-esteem, self-confidence, self-sufficiency, ability to articulate issues, ability to hold one's own in the case of disagreements, and readiness to assume increased responsibility and be held accountable for one's actions are some of the many concerns identified regarding RN readiness to engage in collaborative practice. Clearly, physicians believe that nurse competence cannot be taken for granted.

Education for collaborative practice is considered a necessary part of the process of collaboration. The behaviors required to collaborate are considered to be learned—not automatic. Cinelli (1994) recommends teaching would-be-collaborators basic group process skills, leadership concepts, decision-making skills, and conflict management techniques. Others speak of a socializing education in which each learns about the other's discipline, perspectives, values, and expectations of the relationship. Devereux (1981) stresses the importance of conducting education for collaborative practice as a joint activity. As pointed out by Cowley (1994), education teaches collaborators to carry out similar tasks and functions, to develop underlying principles, and to develop transferable skills.

The ideal seems to be that once it is ascertained that the organization is ready for collaboration, and the potential collaborators have had their educational needs tended to, then the potential collaborators are ready to take their first steps in the process of becoming collaborators. Gaining insight into each other's views, understanding the concerns, practice perspectives, and approaches of the other(s), and building trust and communications are all first steps identified.

The notion of taking first steps in becoming partners or teammates does not mean that the process of creating a collaborative model of practice occurs in stages. It does intend to convey, however, the care and deliberateness with which the process ought to proceed. Building a collaborative practice model requires working together; spending time together; maintaining a high degree of contact over time; developing a partnership type of relationship even if the partners are several team members; and engaging together in shared planning, goal setting, decision making, and problem-solving.

Relationship building and shared decision making are, arguably, the two most monumental features of the entire process of collaboration. The relationship—one of partnership—is addressed in a later section. Decision making, as reflected by mention of the phrases *decision-making power for RNs, respecting the competence of providers, shared decision making, shared problem-solving, and influencing each other*, was identified and discussed approximately 50 times by these scholars. Moreover, an almost equal amount of attention was paid to the nature of the decision-making process. Decisions are arrived at through a negotiating process, a process of give and take, through consensus, and through a process of resolving disagreements with a high level of both assertiveness and cooperativeness. Weiss and Davis (1985) write that collaboration is a "negotiating process that builds and forms a new way of conceptualizing problems" (p. 299).

Two quotations that capture the significance of relationship and decision making to collaboration are as follows: 1) Referring to an education-service collaborative project: "This project was characterized by mutual respect for differences of opinion and perspectives, a longing for greater understanding of ideas and theoretical viewpoints, and a commitment to one another" (Hills 1994, p.222) and 2) Alt-White et al. (1983) state that "nurse–physician collaboration can be defined as the process whereby nurses and MDs work together in the delivery of quality care, jointly contributing in a balanced relationship characterized by mutual trust" (p. 8).

Power-Sharing

"Each partner in a collaborative model must develop a high level of clinical knowledge and expertise in order to enter the relationship as a partner" (Evans 1994, p. 28). Partners then engage in a joint intellectual effort to use their individual and collective expertise to solve or resolve important human problems or concerns. Is this attribute best described as *competency-based*? Frequent mention is made of knowledge, expertise, skills, and overall competence as foundations to the ability to engage in a collaborative practice. Trust is a significant attribute as well; it is identified by about 15 authors. Trust occurs as a result of the partner feeling confident about his or her partner's competence. The researcher clearly could have accepted competency-based as the identified attribute.

Is *authority-based* the best label for this attribute of ability to act as a partner on behalf of others in a collaborative practice? The second set of definitions of authority in *Webster's New World College Dictionary*, 3rd ed. (1996) specify authority as "the power to influence thought, opinion, and behavior" (p. 92). A few scholars do infer the term authority as the framework for acting as a functioning member of the collaborating partnership. Mundinger states: "Authority of the team rests on competence" (1994, p. 211). Another writer notes that nurses are not historically comfortable with the idea of the exercise of power. *Authority*, as the term to capture the equality of the nurse member(s) of the collaborative practice(s), is therefore, a more acceptable term than *power* would be (Henneman 1995). Only a few authors use the term *authority*; however, the researcher is not satisfied with the term because it doesn't capture the import of the topic to nurse collaborators.

Should the definition of collaboration be bold and embrace the term *power sharing* to best capture the idea of a partnership relationship in which two or more persons of differing but equally needed and respected abilities join together to address important human needs or problems? The researcher decided that the attribute had to incorporate the word *power*. The concept analysis evolutionary method gives weight to the "now time and this place." Given the level of change and turmoil in health care and health professions education, including the rapid and pervasive movement to managed care, which almost mandates collaborative approaches to care delivery in a highly competitive marketplace, the notion of power-sharing took on a level of insistence. Kappeli (1995, p. 254) states: "Power and its definition are central to the issue of cooperation." As well, the definition of power is also central to the whole process of collaboration. "Power is shared [in a collaborative practice]; it is based on knowledge and expertise rather than role or title" (Henneman 1994, p. 360).

The term *power* or power-related terms such as *empowered*, *autonomy*, *parity*, or *accountability* are used with great frequency in this body of literature and present a second strong rationale for selecting a term that included the word *power*. The meaning of the term and the related terms is compatible with the second set of meanings accorded power in *Webster's New World College Dictionary*, 3rd ed. (1996), wherein power is defined as "acting to produce an effect" (p. 1058). Weiss and Davis indicate three features of collaboration that operationally define power-sharing:

- the active and assertive contribution of each party,
- receptivity to and respect for the other party's contribution, and a
- negotiating process that builds upon the contributions of both parties to form a new way of conceptualizing the problem. (1985, p. 300).

Power sharing, based in competence, exists in order to accomplish the work to be done. The literature is replete with references to *sharing* work components. Collaborators engage in *shared* planning, development of philosophy, purpose, values, vision, and mission; goal setting, decision making, and problem-solving; rewards and satisfactions; and responsibility and accountability. The partners have complementary strengths and engage in a joint intellectual effort. Power is exercised responsibly by each in the process of making decisions. As previously discussed as a component of the attribute *process*, collaborators are able to work through their disagreements, engage safely in give-and-take concerning the work, negotiate differences of opinion to mutually agreeable conclusions, and often reach decisions by consensus.

Both physician and nurse authors accord importance to the use of the term *power* in describing collaboration. Miccolo and Spanier, RN and MD coauthors state: "Power on both sides (RN and MD partners) is valued by both, with recognition and acceptance of separate and combined spheres of activity and responsibility, mutual safeguarding of interests of each party and a commonality of goals" (p. 446). Katzman (1989), in reporting the findings of a descriptive, comparative study of nurse–physician attitudes and values toward collaboration, states that MDs agreed with nurses, but at a lower level of agreement; that nurses in a collaborative practice should have more authority than they perceive nurses usually have and as much say as MDs in patient care decisions (p. 211).

The literature does raise the issue, however, of MDs' concerns about RN competence. One crucial reason for nurses and physicians working together over time, besides getting to know each other, is to build a trusting relationship, which is in large measure based in confidence that the collaborating partner has the necessary knowledge, skills, and expertise. The competence of nurses is not taken for granted as it tends to be with MDs. Physicians may come to trust a particular nurse, but not all nurses. The physician considers this particular nurse to be special and not necessarily representative of all nurses. Prescott and Bowen (1985) report this finding in their descriptive study of RN and MD beliefs and values. "The issue of nurse competence presents problems for both" (p.132). Henneman (1994) makes the point in her analysis of the power sharing that occurs in a collaborative relationship "that the team members respect and trust the other's disciplines; have mutual recognition of knowledge and skills of each other's discipline" (p. 360).

Partnership

Collaboration is a dynamic, transforming process of creating a power-sharing partnership. "Partnership is the hallmark of true collaborative practice" (Miccolo and Spanier 1993, p.452). The attributes of dynamic, transforming, process, and power sharing all serve to modify the subject of partnership, which is the working relationship of two or more actors engaged in a collaborative arrangement. Because of the centrality of the partnership to the collaborators, it has not been possible to ignore discussion of the term to this point, nor would it be appropriate to do so. The top five most frequently identified attributes all address partnership. They are displayed in Table 1-2.

Webster's New World College Dictionary, 3rd ed. (1996) defines partner as "associate or colleague; one of two or more who work or play together" (p. 859) (The term *partnership* is simply defined as "the state of being a partner" [p. 859].) A second definition of partner is most interesting: "one of the heavy timbers that strengthen a ship's deck to support a mast." This latter meaning provides a graphic analogy for the strong support that collaborating partners provide each other in meeting the demands of their work. *Webster's* (p. 1994, 1983) defines relationship as "the state of being related or interrelated." Because *relationship* requires modifiers to imbue it with meaning, all references to *relationship* were combined with partnership by the researcher. Thus, the relationship that collaborators have with each other is one of partnership. All terms that modify the type of partnership also modify the nature of the relationship.

Collaborating partners have a strong relationship; they form a bond, a union. There is a noticeable cohesiveness in their relationship. They are comfortable working together and have an appreciation one for the other(s). All partners do their best in a collaborative relationship; they generously support each other and protect the interests of the other(s); they help each other. Communications among collaborators are excellent. Relationships are said to be open and honest. Partners respect and trust each other. Differences of opinion are negotiated within a context of respect, comfort, and honesty. Mutually satisfying resolution of differences is reached.

The collaborating partnerships can evolve into interdependence. Colucchio and Maguire (1983) express this by commenting that changes in communication patterns between primary care nurses and physicians

Table 1-2. Top 5 Partnership Attributes

Attribute	Frequency
Respecting each other	19
Communication	17
Working together	15
Partnership relationship	15
Trusting each other	13

Table 1-3. Shared Elements of Partnership

Element	Frequency
Shared Work	17
Shared decision making	13
Shared problem-solving	13
Shared responsibility	12
Shared goal setting	11
Shared vision, philosophy, values, ideas	8
Shared planning	4

occur in which mutual trust and respect have evolved into interdependence among the collaborators (cited in King et al. 1994, p. 174). Partners join together in what some call joint intellectual effort and joint practice. Information sharing among partners occurs as the information is used only to assist the partners in doing the work of their team.

The notion of sharing is of great importance to the partners in a collaborative relationship. As already briefly discussed under the attribute *process*, all elements of activity are shared; work and goal setting are two examples. Table 1-3 lists in descending order of frequency the shared elements identified by these experts. Clearly, the pattern of functioning within a collaborative practice is by sharing.

Partners have a balanced relationship in terms of their power and authority. They are colleagues; they share responsibility and authority; they respect each other and each other's competence. They are strong providers and a strong team. Miccolo and Spanier (1993) state that "[t]rue collaboration is a true partnership between parties, where mutual goal-setting occurs, where authority and responsibility for actions belong to individual partners, and where a deep commitment exists that patient care will be enhanced through working collaboratively" (p. 446).

Pervasive and Purposeful

"To become diffused, throughout every part of" is the definition of pervasive contained in *Webster's New World College Dictionary*, 3rd ed. (1996, p. 1009). In the case of collaboration, the diffusion is occurring throughout the health care arena—service, education, research, and management. This body of literature abundantly documents that collaborative arrangements are perceived as desirable and useful in myriad settings by professionally diverse, intradisciplinary and interdisciplinary sets of collaborating partners—in teams and in dyads. The focus for this attribute is on the *use* of collaboration. The question asked of this characteristic, or attribute, is What are the actual situations to which the concept is being applied? Most of the data responding to the question raised come from the analysis of data on the characteristic, or attribute, *references.*

Why collaboration is used so pervasively is addressed by discussion of the definitional attribute *purposeful*, which means "having a purpose or aim" (*Webster's* 1983, p. 957). No instances are reported in the literature in which collaborative activity was undertaken without a reason or purpose for doing so. Analysis of the data organized under the attribute *antecedents* reveals that either the collaborators have identified a problem or need to solve or meet, or they have a philosophical commitment to the approach of collaboration for their health and health-related endeavors. Usually, both are present—need and commitment. Because *use* and *purpose for use* are so closely linked, these two attributes are considered together. A quote from Gibbons et al. (1995) sets the stage for discussion: "In any setting, collaboration is a must for establishing a professional practice model to affect patient care positively" (p. 28).

Sample settings for collaborative service ventures include a variety of hospital departments and programs. Community hospitals and teaching hospitals, rural and urban hospitals, specialty hospitals and general hospitals, and American hospitals and Canadian, British, and Swiss hospitals are all representative of hospitals reporting the use of collaboration. An obstetric unit, a family birth center, an oncology unit, a hospital-based consumer health information center are some of the departments identified as using collaboration to accomplish their work. Others that are hospital-based include pediatric emergency transport services and a rehabilitation professional practice model with collaboration as its core feature.

Sample settings that are primarily community based include primary care office practices, community clinics, public health departments in the United States and Great Britain, and home health care organizations. All these identified settings report the successful use of collaborative practices. As was noted in the Findings section, this body of literature is heavily weighted toward collaborative practices occurring in hospitals or hospital-based and -owned services, although the entire range of possible settings and organizational sponsorship is encompassed.

Several collaborative ventures reported are a product of organization to organization collaboration to provide scarce, but needed services. Coalitions or joint ventures to pursue meeting a mutually agreed upon need are designed and developed to collaboratively provide services. Examples are a cardiac catheterization unit, an ambulatory care center, in- and out-patient psychiatric services, and an out-patient cancer treatment center.

Myriad collaborative programs reported in the literature are primarily education focused. Organizational sponsorship of these ventures is extremely diverse. Many are jointly sponsored by education and service institutions; others are supported by two or more colleges working together, or a school and a hospital within the same academic health center joining forces, or two or more departments within a hospital collaborating to plan and offer a clinically based academic program. The collaborators may be within one discipline and bring together various subdisciplinary expertise or the collaborators may represent two or more disciplines with their varying strengths and perspectives. The possibilities for organizational arrangements for collaboration appear to be almost endless.

Collaborative activity is most often undertaken to solve a perceived problem or defined need. The implementation of a collaborating interdisciplinary team to improve access to care in a remote rural region of Wisconsin is one example (Iseminger 1996). The many instances reported in the literature of nurturing of collaborative practices of RNs and MDs to improve quality of care in intensive care units, the joining together of several rural hospitals and a small university school of nursing to provide baccalaureate of science in nursing education for the working nurse, and the design of an interdisciplinary transport team to collaborate on pediatric emergency transport are all examples of needs or problems that precede a decision to focus on developing a collaborative model.

Usually, it is the person(s) who will be collaborating who are motivated to do so, rather than an external mandate. (This does not mean, however, that a supportive environment is not a necessary antecedent of collaboration as was discussed as part of the attribute *transforming*.) A MD might recognize, for example, that clinical needs are present in his or her practice that are outside of his or her practice expertise and might, therefore seek an advanced practice nurse as a practice partner. Knutsen (1994) reports that her obstetrician and nurse-midwifery colleagues came together in collaborative practice in order to provide their patients with the broadest range of maternity care possible. Another example might be of an interorganizational need. For example, one member of a 10-hospital consortium in Western Maine states, "The costs of health care in our communities is a problem for our communities and our businesses and we want to take a constructive approach together" (Cerne 1993, p. 27). Cerne then describes a variety of collaborative ventures among the hospitals.

Some further examples of the use and purposes of collaboration are the following. An urban university school of nursing in an academic health center and a small rural school of nursing are working in collaboration to meet the educational needs of the nurses residing in the rural area. A consortium of several health sciences schools in one academic health center was formed to increase interdisciplinary education and research in health policy. One tertiary care hospital in an academic health center and the university's school of nursing collaborate on a multitude of clinical teaching programs for graduate students. Interdisciplinary student preceptorships under the expert guidance of clinical adjunct faculty occur in clinical services for pregnant teens and their infants, radiation therapy patients, emergency patients, community residing incontinent elderly, depressed children and adolescents, early prenatal patients, multiorgan transport patients, and assessment and management of well children (examples noted are cited by Fagin 1992, p. 300).

Collaborative arrangements among researchers within and across disciplines are commonplace. Pender (1992) discusses the benefits of a partnership between research centers focused on health problems of children living in poverty. She suggests that such research programs targeted at communities in need may result in "research programs relevant to community interests and innovative community health programs for teenagers" (p. 249). The advancement of health policy and the bringing together of interdisciplinary social and health scientists to study and recommend integrated solutions to pressing social and health problems are purposes for collaborative research endeavors (Rosenfield 1992).

Numerous other, varied organizations also report using collaboration to pursue their ends. The American Board of Internal Medicine and The American Board of Pediatrics have joined forces, for example, to design a combined medical and pediatric residency. The national critical care nurses and the national critical care medicine groups, in another example, have developed and promulgated joint position statements on collaborative practice and on other topics since 1982. The Franciscan health care system, in yet another example, had a diverse and multidisciplinary team develop a curriculum on collaboration for use throughout their entire system to transform their management and clinical people from traditional to collaborative modes of behavior and functioning.

Clearly, the use of collaboration is pervasive, and without doubt, it is purposeful.

Likely Successful Outcomes

There is abundant evidence in this body of literature to overwhelmingly support asserting the term *successful outcomes* as the culminating attribute of the definition of collaboration. The modifier *likely* is used because there are, of course, no guarantees of success in achieving their goals when collaborators first start out. Yet these scholars clearly document that when a collaborative model has been collaboratively developed, is in place, and is fully operational, it is likely that successful outcomes will be achieved. In fact, these authors do not report any failures in collaborative situations in which they have engaged or observed. Achieving the goals collaborators set out to achieve, as well as many other related positive outcomes, is predictable as long as the collaborative process is not short-changed.

Tables 1-4 through 1-7 present the data supporting the definitional attribute of likely successful outcomes concerning patient, provider, and organizational outcomes that are of central concern within health care delivery. Citations of the authors naming the outcomes are also provided in the matrix tables to ease the reader in consulting the data.

Successful outcomes of education–service collaboration are reported in the literature by several scholars. Universities, in collaboration with service settings, are assisted in meeting their mission of service to society. They gain valuable practice expertise; they also gain practice settings for their faculty and students. Service settings gain the excitement of a learning environment; they also have available, knowledgeable providers from the faculty. Both the university and the service organization gain the ability to engage in activities that can only be accomplished as joint ventures, such as joint research projects or demonstration and development of model practices.

(Text resumes on page 31)

Table 1-4. Patient Outcomes/Author Matrix

	Baggs & Ryan, 90	Baggs, Phelps, Johnson, 92	Cinelli et al, 94	Devereux, 91	Evans, 94	Fagin, 92	Iseminger, 96	Jones (P.K.), 94	Kerfoot, 94	King, 90	Lyons, et al, 92	McEwen, 94	Miccolo & Spanier, 93	Mundinger, 94	Ritter, 83	Shore & Saba, 93
Improved quality of care					✓	✓			✓	✓	✓	✓		✓		
Increased patient satisfaction	✓			✓				✓	✓	✓	✓	✓		✓		
Fewer patient care errors	✓	✓						✓					✓		✓	
Lower mortality rates (Authors report on classic studies—see Chapter 4)					✓	✓										
Improved patient outcomes						✓										
Patients feel more important, secure, cared for, closer to nurses	✓		✓													✓

Table 1-5. All Providers Outcomes/Author Matrix

	Areangelo, et al, 94	Cinelli & Kelley, 94	Collucio et al, 94	Cowley, 94	Evans, 94	Fagin, 92	Gibbons, et al, 95	Henry et al, 92	Kerfoot, 94	King, 90	McKay, 83	Miccolo & Spanier, 93	Mundinger, 94	Organek & Hegedus, 93	Pender, 92	Ritter, 83	Sherwood, 94
Increased sharing of responsibility	✓		✓							✓	✓	✓			✓	✓	
Increased sharing of expertise							✓	✓					✓		✓		
Increase in more mutually satisfying problem solving							✓	✓		✓				✓			
Improved communications									✓	✓		✓					
Increased personal satisfaction		✓				✓											
Increased quality of professional life					✓												
Enhances trust and respect												✓					
Bridges care—cure dichotomy																✓	
Expands horizons of providers																	✓
Avoids redundant care; provides coverage				✓													
Empowers providers to influence health policy																✓	

27

Table 1-6. Registered Nurse and Physician Outcomes/Author Matrix

	Alt-White et al., 83	Baggs, et al, 92	Baggs, & Ryan, 90	Cinelli et al, 94	Collucio & Kelley, 94	Cowley, 94	Devereux, 91	Evans, 94	Fagin, 92	Gibbons, et al, 95	Henry, et al, 92
Registered Nurses											
Increased job satisfaction	✓	✓	✓			✓	✓				
Increased professional growth		✓	✓	✓	✓		✓		✓	✓	
Improved RN retention			✓		✓						
Increased RN involvement in decision making		✓			✓		✓	✓		✓	
RNs impact patient care policies							✓	✓		✓	
Reduces stress level			✓				✓				
Able to provide more individualized care											
Decreases burnout											
Supports ego									✓		
Improve credibility											✓
Improved career potential					✓						
Physicians											
Attractive practice model for primary care physicians											
Increases physician comfort working with RNs			✓								
Supports ego											
Increases job satisfaction									✓		
Increases professional growth				✓							

Table 1-6. Registered Nurse and Physician Outcomes/Author Matrix *(continued)*

	Hughes & Morgan, 94	Iseminger, 96	Jones, 94	King, 90	McEwen, 94	Miccolo & Spanier, 93	Mundinger, 94	Organek & Hegedus, 93	Ritter, 92	Sebas, 94	Styles, 84
Registered Nurses											
Increased job satisfaction	✓										
Increased professional growth				✓	✓			✓		✓	✓
Improved RN retention					✓	✓					
Increased RN involvement in decision making			✓						✓		
RNs impact patient care policies			✓								
Reduces stress level											
Able to provide more individualized care											
Decreases burnout						✓					
Supports ego											
Improve credibility											
Improved career potential											
Physicians											
Attractive practice model for primary care physicians		✓					✓				
Increases physician comfort working with RNs						✓					
Supports ego											
Increases job satisfaction										✓	
Increases professional growth		✓									

29

Table 1-7. Organizational Outcomes/Author Matrix

	Collucio								Miccolo						Shore		
	Collucio et al., 83	Alte-White, & Kelley, 94	Curran, 95	Devereux, 81	Evans, 94	Fagin, 92	Henry, et al., 92	Jones, 94	King, 90	McEwan, 94	& Spanier, 93	Mundinger, 94	Pender, 92	Ritter, 83	Rosenfield, 92	& Saba, 93	Styles, 84
Improved cost-effectiveness of care		✓	✓			✓	✓	✓	✓		✓*	✓	✓	✓			
Improves job performance and productivity of collaborators	✓						✓			✓		✓				✓	
Improved utilization of professional staff	✓								✓			✓					
Improved coordination of care	✓					✓											
Creativity dealing with rapid change	✓					✓											
Improved employer–employee relations	✓																
Balance and stability in organization; improved distribution of resources	✓																
More knowledgeable practitioners	✓												✓				
Increases funding for practice and research	✓																

*Recommends further study

Students in a collaborative environment gain an enriched education when they are taught by faculty in clinical practice or by clinical experts. Staff gain in an education–service collaborative setting; they often hold adjunct faculty appointments, providing opportunities for intellectual growth and development, career enhancement, and job enrichment. Faculty gain access to patients and to clinical problems that serve to meet their needs for both faculty practice and research. In addition, faculty have ready access to patients and systems for meeting the learning needs of their students.

The following excerpts or paraphrases add to an understanding of the attribute likely successful outcomes, as well as that of the definition of collaboration.

> Potential benefits of collaboration include: increased networking, information sharing and access to resources, involvement in an important cause, attaining the desired outcomes from the coalitions efforts, enjoyment of the coalition's work, receiving personal recognition, and enhancing one's skill (Butterfoss et al. 1993).

> Payoffs from partnering are synergy, cumulative energy, collaborative vision, expanded production capacity, and enhanced creative innovation (Pender 1992, p. 248).

> Success of hospitals is linked to the ability to facilitate the RN-MD relationship; care is made easier when physicians and nurses share concerns and rely on each other's professional competence (Dumont and Niziolek 1991, p. 331).

> The litmus test for this entire process (of a 10 hospital consortium) is whether we can view the interests of the communities ahead of the interests of individual hospitals (Donald MC Dowell, President, Maine Medical Center, Portland, cited by Cerne 1993, p. 26).

> [Collaboration among hospitals] is the right way to go to provide the best patient care to . . . communities and to ensure continuing access to care (Craig Becker, President, Maine Hospital Association, cited by Cerne 1993, p. 27).

> Clearly everyone gains in a collaborative practice setting. . . . (Ritter 1983, p. 68).

References

General

Arcangelo, V. P. (1994). The myth of independent practice. *Nursing Forum, 29*, 3–4.

Baggs, J. G. and Ryan, S. A. (1990). ICU nurse-physician collaboration & nursing satisfaction. *Nursing Economics, 8*, 386–392.

Baggs, J. G. Ryan, S. A., Phelps, C. E., Richeson, F., and Johnson, J. E. (1992). The association between interdisciplinary collaboration and patient outcomes in a medical intensive care unit. *Heart and Lung, 21*, 18–24.

Coluccio, M. and Kelley, L. K. (1994). Transformational partnership for delivery of RN baccalaureate education: A service/education leadership model. *Nursing Administration Quarterly, 18*, 65–71.

Fagin, C. M. (1992). Collaboration between nurse and physicians: No longer a choice. *Academic Medicine, 67*, 295–303.

Henneman, E. A. (1995). Nurse-physician collaboration: A poststructural view. *Journal of Nursing Administration, 22*, 359–363.

Henry, V., Schmitz, K., Reif, L., and Rudie, P. (1992). Collaboration: Integrating practice and research in public health nursing. *Public Health Nursing, 9*, 218–222.

Hills, M. D., Lindsey, E., Chisamore, M., Bassett-Smith, J., Abbott, K., and Fournier-Chalmers, J. (1994). University-college collaboration: Rethinking curriculum development in nursing education. *Journal of Nursing Education, 33*, 220–225.

King, M. B. (1990). Clinical nurse specialist collaboration with physicians. *Clinical Nurse Specialist, 4*, 172–177.

McKay, P. S. (1983). Interdependent decision making: Redefining professional autonomy. *Nursing Administration Quarterly, 7*, 21–30.

McMahon, J. M. (1992). Shared governance: The leadership challenge. *Nursing Administration Quarterly, 17*, 55–59.

Mundinger, M. O. (1994). Advanced practice nurse-good medicine for physicians? *Nursing Forum, 330*, 211–213.

Ritter, H. A. (1983). Collaborative practice: What's in it for medicine? *Nursing Administration Quarterly, 7*, 31–36.

Shore, W. B. and Saba, G. W. (1993). Toward a social policy for health. *New England Journal of Medicine, 329*, 1969.

Styles, M. M. (1984). Reflections on collaboration and unification. *Image: Journal of Nursing Scholarship, 16*, 21–23.

Surgeon General's Report. (1963) *Toward Quality in Nursing.*

REFERENCES BY CONCEPT ATTRIBUTE

Dynamic

Alt-White, A. C., Charns, M., and Strayer, R. (1983). Personal, organizational and managerial factors related to nurse-physician collaboration. *Nursing Administration Quarterly, 8*, 8–18.

Baggs, J. G. (1989). Intensive care unit use and collaboration between nurses and physicians. *Heart and Lung, 18*, 332–338.

Cinelli, B., Symons, C. W., Bechtel, L. and Rose-Colley, M. (1994). Applying cooperative learning in health education practice. *Journal of School Health, 64*, 99–102.

Coluccio, M. and Kelley, L. K. (1994). Transformational partnership for delivery of RN baccalaureate education: A service/education leadership model. *Nursing Administration Quarterly, 18*, 65–71.

Cowley, S. (1994). Collaboration in health care: The education link. *Health Visitor, 67*, 13–15.

Evans, J. A. (1994). The role of the nurse manager in creating an environment for collaborative practice. *Holistic Nursing Practice, 8*, 22–31.

Henry, V., Schmitz, K., Reif, LuA., and Rudie, P. (1992). Collaboration: Integrating practice and research in public health nursing. *Public Health Nursing, 9*, 218–222.

Iseminger, J. (1996). Going the distance. *On Wisconsin*, March/April, 26–30.

Jones, P. k. (1994). Developing a collaborative professional role for the staff nurse in a shared governance model. *Holistic Nursing Practice, 8*, 32–37.

Lyons, N., Reinke, C., Suthreland, K., Zelenkov, K. (1992). The ultimate birth center: A collaborative model for innovation. *Nursing Clinic of North America, 27*(1), 99–106.

Miccolo, M. A. and Spanier, A. H. (1993). Critical care management in the 1990s: Making collaborative practice work. *Critical Care Clinics, 9*, 443–453.

Pender, N. J. (1992). Partnerships: An alternative to rugged individualism. *Nursing Outlook, 40*, 248–249.

Webster's New World College Dictionary, 1996, Third Edition. MacMillan.

Weiss, S. J. and Davis, H. P. (1985). Validity and reliability of the collaborative practice scales. *Nursing Research, 34*, 299–305.

Transforming

Baker, C., and Diekelmann, N. (1994). Connecting conversations of caring: Recalling the narrative to clinical practice. *Nursing Outlook, 42*, 65–70.

Devereux, D. M. (1981). Essential elements of nurse-physician collaboration. *Journal of Nursing Administration, 1*(5), 19–23.

Donnelly, G. F., Warfel, W., and Wolf, Z. R. (1994). A faculty-practice program: Three perspectives. *Holistic Nursing Practice, 8*, 71–80.

Dumont, J., and Niziolek, C. (1991). The Cornerstones of Collaboration. *Journal of Professional Nursing, 7*, 331.

Evans, J. A. (1994). The role of the nurse manager in creating an environment for collaborative practice. *Holistic Nursing Practice, 8*, 22–31.

Fagin, C. M. (1992). Collaboration between nurse and physicians: No longer a choice. *Academic Medicine, 67*, 295–303.

Giardino, A. P., Giardino, E. R., and Burns, K. M. (1994). Same place, different experience: Nurses and residents on pediatric emergency transport. *Holistic Nursing Practice, 8*, 54–63.

Hills, M. D., Lindsey, E., Chisamore, M., Bassett-Smith, J., Abbott, K., and Fournier-Chalmers, J. (1994). University-college collaboration: Rethinking curriculum development in nursing education. *Journal of Nursing Education, 33*, 220–225.

Jones, P. k. (1994). Developing a collaborative professional role for the staff nurse in a shared governance model. *Holistic Nursing Practice, 8*, 32–37.

Kappeli, S. (1995). Interprofessional cooperation: Why is partnership so difficult. *Patient Education and Counseling, 26*, 251–256.

Miccolo, M. A., and Spanier, A. H. (1993). Critical care management in the 1990s: Making collaborative practice work. *Critical Care Clinics, 9*, 443–453.

Pender, N. J. (1992). Partnerships: An alternative to rugged individualism. *Nursing Outlook, 40*, 248–249.

Rosenfield, P. L. (1992). The potential of transdisciplinary research for sustaining and extending linkages between the health and social sciences. *Social Science Medicine, 35*, 1343–1357.

Warner, M., Ford-Gilboe, M., Laforet-Fliesser, Y., Olson, J., and Ward-Griffin, C. (1994). The teamwork project: A collaborative approach to learning to nurse families. *Journal of Nurisng Education, 33*, 5–13.

Weiss, S. J., and Davis, H. P. (1985). Validity and reliability of the collaborative practice scales. *Nursing Research, 34*, 299–305.

Process

Alt-White, A. C., Charns, M., and Strayer, R. (1983). Personal, organizational and managerial factors related to nurse-physician collaboration. *Nursing Administration Quarterly, 8*, 8–18.

Bruininks, R. H., Frenzel, M., and Kelly, A. (1994). Integrating services: The case for better links to schools. *Journal of School Health, 64*, 242–248.

Cerne, F. (1993). Joining forces: Maine hospitals find that cooperation brings results. *Hospitals, 67*, 26–27.

Cinelli, B., Symons, C. W., Bechtel, L., and Rose-Colley, M. (1994). Applying cooperative learning in health education practice. *Journal of School Health, 64*, 99–102.

Cowley, S. (1994). Collaboration in health care: The education link. *Health Visitor, 67*, 13–15.

Devereux, D. M. (1981). Essential elements of nurse-physician collaboration. *Journal of Nursing Administration, 1*(5), 19–23.

Eubanks, P. (1991). Quality improvement key to changing nurse-MD relations. *Hospitals, 65*(8), 26–30.

Evans, J. A. (1994). The role of the nurse manager in creating an environment for collaborative practice. *Holistic Nursing Practice, 8*, 22–31.

Fagin, C. M. (1992). Collaboration between nurse and physicians: No longer a choice. *Academic Medicine, 67*, 295–303.

Giardino, A. P., Giardino, E. R., and Burns, K. M. (1994). Same place, different experience: Nurses and residents on pediatric emergency transport. *Holistic Nursing Practice, 8*, 54–63.

Gibbons, K. B., Salter, J. P., Pierce, L. L., and Govoni, A. L. (1995). A model of professional rehabilitation nursing practice. *Rehabilitation Nursing, 20*, 23–28.

Henry, V., Schmitz, K., Reif, LuA., and Rudie, P. (1992). Collaboration: Integrating practice and research in public health nursing. *Public Health Nursing, 9*, 218–222.

Hills, M. D., Lindsey, E., Chisamore, M., Bassett-Smith, J., Abbott, K., and Fournier-Chalmers, J. (1994). University-college collaboration: Rethinking curriculum development in nursing education. *Journal of Nursing Education, 33*, 220–225.

Jones, P. k. (1994). Developing a collaborative professional role for the staff nurse in a shared governance model. *Holistic Nursing Practice, 8*, 32–37.

Kappeli, S. (1995). Interprofessional cooperation: Why is partnership so difficult. *Patient Education and Counseling, 26*, 251–256.

King, M. B. (1990). Clinical nurse specialist collaboration with physicians. *Clinical Nurse Specialist, 4*, 172–177.

McKay, P. S. (1983). Interdependent decision making: Redefining professional autonomy. *Nursing Administration Quarterly, 7*, 21–30.

Miccolo, M. A. and Spanier, A. H. (1993). Critical care management in the 1990s: Making collaborative practice work. *Critical Care Clinics, 9*, 443–453.

Prescott, P. A., and Bowen, S. A. (1985). Physician-nurse relationships. *Annuals of Internal Medicine, 103*, 127–133.

Ritter, H. A. (1983). Collaborative practice: What's in it for medicine? *Nursing Administration Quarterly, 7*, 31–36.

Styles, M. M. (1984). Reflections on collaboration and unification. *Image: Journal of Nursing Scholarship, 16*, 21–23.

Weiss, S. J., and Davis, H. P. (1985). Validity and reliability of the collaborative practice scales. *Nursing Research, 34*, 299–305.

Power-Sharing

Alt-White, A. C., Charns, M., and Strayer, R. (1983). Personal, organizational and managerial factors related to nurse-physician collaboration. *Nursing Administration Quarterly, 8*, 8–18.

Arcangelo, V. P. (1994). The myth of independent practice. *Nursing Forum, 29*, 3–4.

Baggs, J. G., and Ryan, S. A. (1990). ICU nurse-physician collaboration and nursing satisfaction. *Nursing Economics, 8*, 386–392.

Baker, C. M., Boyd, N. J., Stasiowski, S. A., and Simons, B. J. (1989). Interinstitutional collaboration for nursing excellence: Part 1, Creating the Partnership. *Journal of Nursing Administration, 19*, 8–12.

Cinelli, B., Symons, C. W., Bechtel, L., and Rose-Colley, M. (1994). Applying cooperative learning in health education practice. *Journal of School Health, 64*, 99–102.

Devereux, D. M. (1981). Essential elements of nurse-physician collaboration. *Journal of Nursing Administration, 1*(5), 19–23.

Evans, J. A. (1994). The role of the nurse manager in creating an environment for collaborative practice. *Holistic Nursing Practice, 8*, 22–31.

Fagin, C. M. (1992). Collaboration between nurse and physicians: No longer a choice. *Academic Medicine, 67*, 295–303.

Felton, G. (1994). Guest editorial: A response to the AMA. *Nursing Outlook, 42*, 84–87.

Henneman, E. A. (1995). Nurse-physician collaboration: A poststructuralist view. *Journal of Nursing Administration, 22*, 359–363.

Hills, M. D., Lindsey, E., Chisamore, M., Bassett-Smith, J., Abbott, K., and Fournier-Chalmers, J. (1994). University-college collaboration: Rethinking curriculum development in nursing education. *Journal of Nursing Education, 33*, 220–225.

Jones, P. k. (1994). Developing a collaborative professional role for the staff nurse in a shared governance model. *Holistic Nursing Practice, 8*, 32–37.

Jones, R. A. P. (1994). Nurse-physician collaboration: A descriptive study. *Holistic Nursing Practice, 8*(Suppl. 3), 38–53.

Kappeli, S. (1995). Interprofessional cooperation: Why is partnership so difficult. *Patient Education and Counseling, 26*, 251–256.

Katzman, E. M. (1989). Nurses and physicians perceptions of nursing authority. *Journal of Professional Nursing, 5*, 208–214.

King, M. B. (1990). Clinical nurse specialist collaboration with physicians. *Clinical Nurse Specialist, 4*, 172–177.

Miccolo, M. A., and Spanier, A. H. (1993). Critical care management in the 1990s: Making collaborative practice work. *Critical Care Clinics, 9*, 443–453.

Mundinger, M. O. (1994). Advanced practice nurse-good medicine for physicians? *Nursing Forum, 330*, 211–213.

Prescott, P. A., and Bowen, S. A. (1985). Physician-nurse relationships. *Annuals of Internal Medicine, 103*, 127–133.

Rosenfield, P. L. (1992). The potential of transdisciplinary research for sustaining and extending linkages between the health and social sciences. *Social Science Medicine, 35*, 1343–1357.

Weiss, S. J. (1985). The influence of discourse on collaboration among nurses, physicians, and consumers. *Research in Nursing and Health, 8*, 49–59.

Weiss, S. J., and Davis, H. P. (1985). Validity and reliability of the collaborative practice scales. *Nursing Research, 34*, 299–305.

Partnership

Alt-White, A. C., Charns, M., and Strayer, R. (1983). Personal, organizational and managerial factors related to nurse-physician collaboration. *Nursing Administration Quarterly, 8*, 8–18.

Arcangelo, V. P. (1994). The myth of independent practice. *Nursing Forum, 29*, 3–4.

Baggs, J. G., Ryan, S. A., Phelps, C. E., Richeson, F., and Johnson, J. E. (1992). The association between interdisciplinary collaboration and patient outcomes in a medical intensive care unit. *Heart and Lung, 21*, 18–24.

Baker, C., and Diekelmann, N. (1994). Connecting conversations of caring: Recalling the narrative to clinical practice. *Nursing Outlook, 42*, 65–70.

Bruininks, R. H., Frenzel, M., and Kelly, A. (1994). Integrating services: The case for better links to schools. *Journal of School Health, 64*, 242–248.

Cinelli, B., Symons, C. W., Bechtel, L., and Rose-Colley, M. (1994). Applying cooperative learning in health education practice. *Journal of School Health, 64*, 99–102.

Coluccio, M., and Kelley, L. K. (1994). Transformational partnership for delivery of RN baccalaureate education: A service/education leadership model. *Nursing Administration Quarterly, 18*, 65–71.

Cowley, S. (1994). Collaboration in health care: The education link. *Health Visitor, 67*, 13–15.

Donnelly, G. F., Warfel, W., and Wolf, Z. R. (1994). A faculty-practice program: Three perspectives. *Holistic Nursing Practice, 8*, 71–80.

Dumont, J., and Niziolek, C. (1991). The Cornerstones of Collaboration. *Journal of Professional Nursing, 7*, 331.

Eubanks, P. (1991). Quality improvement key to changing nurse-MD relations. *Hospitals, 65*(8), 26–30.

Evans, J. A. (1994). The role of the nurse manager in creating an environment for collaborative practice. *Holistic Nursing Practice, 8*, 22–31.

Fagin, C. M. (1992). Collaboration between nurse and physicians: No longer a choice. *Academic Medicine, 67*, 295–303.

Gibbons, K. B., Salter, J. P., Pierce, L. L., and Govoni, A. L. (1995). A model of professional rehabilitation nursing practice. *Rehabilitation Nursing, 20*, 23–28.

Gillick, M. R. (1992). From confrontation to cooperation in the doctor-patient relationship. *Journal of General Internal Medicine, 7*, 83–86.

Henneman, E. A. (1995). Nurse-physician collaboration: A poststructuralist view. *Journal of Nursing Administration, 22*, 359–363.

Hills, M. D., Lindsey, E., Chisamore, M., Bassett-Smith, J., Abbott, K., and Fournier-Chalmers, J. (1994). University-college collaboration: Rethinking curriculum development in nursing education. *Journal of Nursing Education, 33*, 220–225.

Jones, R. A. P. (1994). Nurse-physician collaboration: A descriptive study. *Holistic Nursing Practice, 8*(Suppl. 3), 38–53.

Kappeli, S. (1995). Interprofessional cooperation: Why is partnership so difficult. *Patient Education and Counseling, 26*, 251–256.

King, M. B. (1990). Clinical nurse specialist collaboration with physicians. *Clinical Nurse Specialist, 4*, 172–177.

Lyons, N., Reinke, C., Sutherland, K., Zelekov, K. (1992). The ultimate birth center: A collaborative model for innovation. *Nursing Clinic of North America, 27*(1), 99–106.

McEwen, M. (1994). Promoting interdisciplinary collaboration. *Nursing and Health Care, 15*, 304–307.

McMahon, J. M. (1992). Shared governance: The leadership challenge. *Nursing Administration Quarterly, 17*, 55–59.

Miccolo, M. A., and Spanier, A. H. (1993). Critical care management in the 1990s: Making collaborative practice work. *Critical Care Clinics, 9*, 443–453.

Prescott, P. A., and Bowen, S. A. (1985). Physician-nurse relationships. *Annuals of Internal Medicine, 103*, 127–133.

Reynolds, P. P., Giardino, A., Onady, G. M., and Siegler, E. L. (1994). Collaboration in the preparation of the generalist physician. *Journal of General Internal Medicine, 9*(Suppl. 1), S55–S63.

Rosenfield, P. L. (1992). The potential of transdisciplinary research for sustaining and extending linkages between the health and social sciences. *Social Science Medicine, 35*, 1343–1357.

Sabella, C. F., Neufeld, R., Ditzler, J., and Cooper, J. (1994). Improving professional collaboration in today's nursing home. *Nursing Homes, 43*, 32–38.

Sebas, M. B. (1994). Developing collaborative practice agreement for the primary care setting. *Nurse Practioner, 19*, 49–51.

Sherwood, G. (1994). Educational outreach in a rural underserved area. *Nursing Connections, 7*, 5–15.

Warner, M., Ford-Gilboe, M., Laforet-Fliesser, Y., Olson, J., and Ward-Griffin, C. (1994). The teamwork project: A collaborative approach to learning to nurse families. *Journal of Nursing Education, 33*, 5–13.

Weiss, S. J., and Davis, H. P. (1985). Validity and reliability of the collaborative practice scales. *Nursing Research, 34*, 299–305.

Pervasive

Baggs, J. G., Ryan, S. A., Phelps, C. E., Richeson, F., and Johnson, J. E. (1992). The association between interdisciplinary collaboration and patient outcomes in a medical intensive care unit. *Heart and Lung, 21*, 18–24.

Bruininks, R. H., Frenzel, M., and Kelly, A. (1994). Integrating services: The case for better links to schools. *Journal of School Health, 64*, 242–248.

Cerne, F. (1993). Joining forces: Maine hospitals find that cooperation brings results. *Hospitals, 67*, 26–27.

Coluccio, M., and Kelley, L. K. (1994). Transformational partnership for delivery of RN baccalaureate education: A service/education leadership model. *Nursing Administration Quarterly, 18*, 65–71.

Evans, J. A. (1994). The role of the nurse manager in creating an environment for collaborative practice. *Holistic Nursing Practice, 8*, 22–31.

Fagin, C. M. (1992). Collaboration between nurse and physicians: No longer a choice. *Academic Medicine, 67*, 295–303.

Giardino, A. P., Giardino, E. R., and Burns, K. M. (1994). Same place, different experience: Nurses and residents on pediatric emergency transport. *Holistic Nursing Practice, 8*, 54–63.

Gibbons, K. B., Salter, J. P., Pierce, L. L., and Govoni, A. L. (1995). A model of professional rehabilitation nursing practice. *Rehabilitation Nursing, 20*, 23–28.

Iseminger, J. (1996). Going the distance. *On Wisconsin*, March/April, 26–30.

Knudtsen, J. A. (1994). Nurse practitioners in primry care. *New England Journal of Medicine, 330*, 1537–1540.

Miccolo, M. A., and Spanier, A. H. (1993). Critical care management in the 1990s: Making collaborative practice work. *Critical Care Clinics, 9*, 443–453.

Sebas, M. B. (1994). Developing collaborative practice agreement for the primary care setting. *Nurse Practioner, 19*, 49–51.

Purposeful

Baggs, J. G. Ryan, S. A., Phelps, C. E., Richeson, F., and Johnson, J. E. (1992). The association between interdisciplinary collaboration and patient outcomes in a medical intensive care unit. *Heart and Lung, 21*, 18–24.

Bruininks, R. H., Frenzel, M., and Kelly, A. (1994). Integrating services: The case for better links to schools. *Journal of School Health, 64*, 242–248.

Cerne, F. (1993). Joining forces: Maine hospitals find that cooperation brings results. *Hospitals, 67*, 26–27.

Coluccio, M., and Kelley, L. K. (1994). Transformational partnership for delivery of RN baccalaureate education: A service/education leadership model. *Nursing Administration Quarterly, 18*, 65–71.

Donnelly, G. F., Warfel, W., and Wolf, Z. R. (1994). A faculty-practice program: Three perspectives. *Holistic Nursing Practice, 8*, 71–80.

Eubanks, P. (1991). Quality improvement key to changing nurse-MD relations. *Hospitals, 65*(8), 26–30.

Evans, J. A. (1994). The role of the nurse manager in creating an environment for collaborative practice. *Holistic Nursing Practice, 8*, 22–31.

Fagin, C. M. (1992). Collaboration between nurse and physicians: No longer a choice. *Academic Medicine, 67*, 295–303.

Giardino, A. P., Giardino, E. R., and Burns, K. M. (1994). Same place, different experience: Nurses and residents on pediatric emergency transport. *Holistic Nursing Practice, 8*, 54–63.

Gibbons, K. B., Salter, J. P., Pierce, L. L., and Govoni, A. L. (1995). A model of professional rehabilitation nursing practice. *Rehabilitation Nursing, 20*, 23–28.

Iseminger, J. (1996). Going the distance. *On Wisconsin*, March/April, 26–30.

Kappeli, S. (1995). Interprofessional cooperation: Why is partnership so difficult. *Patient Education and Counseling, 26*, 251–256.

Knudtsen, J. A. (1994). Nurse practitioners in primary care. *New England Journal of Medicine, 330*, 1537–1540.

Lyons, N., Reinke, C., Sutherland, K., Zelekov, K. (1992). The ultimate birth center: A collaborative model for innovation. *Nursing Clinic of North America, 27*(1), 99–106.

Miccolo, M. A., and Spanier, A. H. (1993). Critical care management in the 1990s: Making collaborative practice work. *Critical Care Clinics, 9*, 443–453.

Likely Successful Outcomes

Alt-White, A. C., Charns, M., and Strayer, R. (1983). Personal, organizational and managerial factors related to nurse-physician collaboration. *Nursing Administration Quarterly, 8*, 8–18.

Arcangelo, V. P. (1994). The myth of independent practice. *Nursing Forum, 29*, 3–4.

Baggs, J. G., and Ryan, S. A. (1990). ICU nurse-physician collaboration & nursing satisfaction. *Nursing Economics, 8*, 386–392.

Baggs, J. G., Ryan, S. A., Phelps, C. E., Richeson, F., and Johnson, J. E. (1992). The association between interdisciplinary collaboration and patient outcomes in a medical intensive care unit. *Heart and Lung, 21*, 18–24.

Cinelli, B., Symons, C. W., Bechtel, L., and Rose-Colley, M. (1994). Applying cooperative learning in health education practice. *Journal of School Health, 64*, 99–102.

Coluccio, M., and Kelley, L. K. (1994). Transformational partnership for delivery of RN baccalaureate education: A service/education leadership model. *Nursing Administration Quarterly, 18*, 65–71.

Cowley, S. (1994). Collaboration in health care: The education link. *Health Visitor, 67*, 13–15.

Curran, C. R. (1995). Collaboration needed for creative, flexible solutions. *Nursing Economics, 13*, 66–67.

Devereux, P. M. (1981). Essential elements of nurse-physician collaboration. *Journal of Nursing Administration, 1*(5), 19–23.

Donnelly, G. F., Warfel, W., and Wolf, Z. R. (1994). A faculty-practice program: Three perspectives. *Holistic Nursing Practice, 8*, 71–80.

Dumont, J., and Niziolek, C. (1991). The Cornerstones of Collaboration. *Journal of Professional Nursing, 7*, 331.

Evans, J. A. (1994). The role of the nurse manager in creating an environment for collaborative practice. *Holistic Nursing Practice, 8*, 22–31.

Fagin, C. M. (1992). Collaboration between nurse and physicians: No longer a choice. *Academic Medicine, 67*, 295–303.

Iseminger, J. (1996). Going the distance. *On Wisconsin*, March/April, 26–30.

Gibbons, K. B., Salter, J. P., Pierce, L. L., and Govoni, A. L. (1995). A model of professional rehabilitation nursing practice. *Rehabilitation Nursing, 20*, 23–28.

Henry, V., Schmitz, K., Reif, LuA, and Rudie, P. (1992). Collaboration: Integrating practice and research in public health nursing. *Public Health Nursing, 9*, 218–222.

Hughes, A. M., and Morgan, J. (1994). University-Hospital research collaboration provides meaningful experience for student learning. *Journal of Nursing Education, 33*, 365–367.

Jones, P. k. (1994). Developing a collaborative professional role for the staff nurse in a shared governance model. *Holistic Nursing Practice, 8*, 32–37.

Kerfoot, K. (1994). The theory of cooperation and the nurse manager's challenge. *Nursing Economics, 12*, 100–101.

King, M. B. (1990). Clinical nurse specialist collaboration with physicians. *Clinical Nurse Specialist, 4*, 172–177.

Knaus, W. A., Draper, E. A., Wagner, D. P., and Zimmerman, J. E. (1986). An evaluations of outcome from intensive care in major medical centers. *Annuals of Internal Medicine, 104*, 410–418.

Lyons, N., Reinke, C., Sutherland, K., Zelenkov, K. (1992). The ultimate birth center: A collaborative model for innovation. *Nursing Clinic of North America, 27*(1), 99–106.

McEwen, M. (1994). Promoting interdisciplinary collaboration. *Nursing and Health Care, 15*, 304–307.

Mechanic, D., and Aiken, L. H. (1982). A cooperative agenda for medicine and nursing. *New England Journal of Medicine, 307*, 747–750.

Miccolo, M. A., and Spanier, A. H. (1993). Critical care management in the 1990s: Making collaborative practice work. *Critical Care Clinics, 9*, 443–453.

Mundinger, M. O. (1994). Advanced practice nurse-good medicine for physicians? *Nursing Forum, 330*, 211–213.

Organek, N. (1993). Advanced practice: A model for neonatal/perinatal and women/childing nurse. *Advanced Practice Model, 4*(4), 631–636.

Pender, N. J. (1992). Partnerships: An alternative to rugged individualism. *Nursing Outlook, 40*, 248–249.

Ritter, H. A. (1983). Collaborative practice: What's in it for medicine? *Nursing Administration Quarterly, 7*, 31–36.

Rosenfield, P. L. (1992). The potential of transdisciplinary research for sustaining and extending linkages between the health and social sciences. *Social Science Medicine, 35*, 1343–1357.

Rubenstein, L. Z., Josephson, K. R., Wieland, G. D., English, P. A., Sayre, J. A., and Kane, R. L. (1984). Effectiveness of a Geriatric Evaluation Unit. *New England Journal of Medicine, 311*, 1664–1670.

Sebas, M. B. (1994). Developing collaborative practice agreement for the primary care setting. *Nurse Practioner, 19*, 49–51.

Sherwood, G. (1994). Educational outreach in a rural underserved area. *Nursing Connections, 7*, 5–15.

Shore, W. B., and Saba, G. W. (1993). Toward a social policy for health. *New England Journal of Medicine, 329*, 1969.

Styles, M. M. (1984). Reflections on collaboration and unification. *Image: Journal of Nursing Scholarship, 16*, 21–23.

Concept Analysis: Part II[1]

2

Toni J. Sullivan

SURROGATE TERMS

A surrogate term is an interchangeable way of expressing a concept. The surrogate term contains all of the same attributes as the main concept; it is simply another way to express it. A review of the literature did not reveal any surrogate terms that are interchangeable in all health care academic and service situations in which collaboration may occur. Three surrogate terms, however, are interchangeable with the term collaboration in specific settings or situations: *joint practice, shared governance,* and *coalition.*

Joint Practice

The term *joint practice* was the term of choice for collaborative practice between registered nurses (RNs) and physicians stemming from the National Joint Practice Commission (NJPC). The Commission stated that "Joint practice is physicians and nurses collaborating to provide patient care" (Ritter 1983, p. 33; see also Devereux 1981, King 1990, Styles 1984, Notkin 1983). Although the term's use was early in the current history of collaborative practice, at least implicit in it is the inclusion of all of the attributes of collaboration. According to Ritter (1983), the term

[1]Chapter 1 constitutes Part I of the concept analysis of collaboration.

joint practice proved problematic and became a buzzword to physicians. Consequently, the term was changed officially in all NJPC documents to *collaborative practice*, a term more acceptable to both physicians and nurses. The term, however, is not in wide usage at present—at least not in the body of literature used in this study.

A descriptive definition of joint practice is offered by King (1990): "Joint practice is physicians and nurses working together as partners, sharing a common philosophy of patient care delivery, each assuming full legal responsibility for his or her decisions and actions in the delivery of care" (p.174).

Shared Governance

The term *shared governance* is widely used to describe organizational structure and functioning that is highly participatory. Staff in such an organizational arrangement are empowered to function in highly collegial ways with both management and colleagues. Decision-making authority is assumed by those closest to the practice issues. This term is a surrogate term for *collaboration* when it is used to describe a model of organizational functioning that contains the attributes of collaboration.

Several model descriptions in the literature seem to fit the requirements for consideration as a surrogate term. Among them are the following two descriptive definitions: "Shared governance is a true partnership in which health care professionals discuss, debate, and work from the same data base . . . . The beginning elements for success are a shared vision and education of all participants who will be impacted by this collaborative model" (Jones 1994, p. 34); and "Shared governance is a process, a dimension beyond participatory management, it vests ownership of practice decisions with staff, it is a partnership model of teamwork, guided by leaders who empower. It can transform our institutions and positively influence the care that our patients receive" (McMahon 1992, p. 55).

Coalition

Currently, the term coalition seems to be widely used to describe two or more organizations joining forces to take joint action or resolve a mutually shared concern or reach a common goal. The term we find present in the daily news, however, is joint venture. Webster's Ninth New World College Dictionary, 3rd edition (1996) describes coalition as a temporary alliance for joint action (p. 267). The term is not widely used in the random body of literature for this concept analysis. The term is common, however, in the literature on community development (Butterfoss et al. 1993). (The term will gain in usage in later chapters of this book, particularly those chapters that are concerned with interorganizational relationships.)

Although the term *coalition* is encompassed here as a surrogate term for *collaboration*, it is used with some hesitation. The challenge in building and maintaining coalitions may be in the depth of the commitment by the participants from each organization. Will the commitment continue after the immediate concern is addressed? A similar term that also embodies organizations joining together to undertake an enterprise beyond the resources of any one member is *consortium* (*Webster's* 1996, p. 298). This term is used by Coluccio and Kelley (1994) to describe their rural education-service partnership for baccalaureate nursing education.

RELATED CONCEPTS

Related concepts are terms that bear some relation to the main concept but do not share all or the same set of attributes. There are many concepts related to the concept of collaboration, as would be expected because collaboration is such a complex and rich concept. *Cooperation, collegial, team or teamwork, working together, interdependence, and professionalism or professional and practice model* are all related concepts frequently used in the literature. Each is often used as a substitute for a component of collaboration. Here, the same has been done in describing the various attributes of collaboration. Each is briefly defined and discussed as to which attributes of collaboration the term substitutes for, if any. Also identified are the breadth of usage and the limitations of the term.

Cooperation

The term *cooperation*, widely used in the study literature, is defined in *Webster's* (1996) as "associated with another or other for mutual benefit;

acting or working with another for mutual benefit" (p. 306). Cooperation is defined by several of the scholars as "attempting to satisfy the other person's concerns" (Prescott and Bowen 1985, p.131; see also Baggs and Schmitt 1988). The term is often coupled with *assertiveness*, which is defined as attempting to satisfy one's own concerns. In a model credited to Kilman and Thomas (1977) and cited in Prescott and Bowen (1985), the two (*assertiveness* and *cooperation*) are combined to equal various possible levels of collaboration. A collaborative person encompasses a good measure of both attributes (Weiss and Davis 1985). "Collaboration involves a mutual give and take (cooperativeness) as well as active participation in resolution of disagreements (assertiveness)" (Prescott and Bowen 1985, p.131). Clifford (1994) asserts that cooperation and collegiality are first steps to the more complex collaboration, and that although very important, they are only the beginning.

Collegial

The term *collegial* is marked by power or authority vested equally in two or more persons who do not necessarily have equal stature in society; equal sharing of authority is the ideal represented by this term (Webster's, p. 274). Attitudes and behaviors that are collegial are considered by these scholars as important antecedents of collaboration. If collegiality is not achieved by all participants in a collaborative practice, those of lower status may defer to those of higher status. Shared decision-making thus does not occur and patient welfare and advocacy may suffer because the patient does not receive the benefit of the thinking of the two providers and their shared decisions. The relationship is not one of partnership; rather, it reverts to a superordinate–subordinate type (Baggs and Schmitt 1988, Weiss and Davis 1985).

Dumont and Niziolek (1991) state that "[m]utual respect among colleagues and open communication are the cornerstones of collaborative practice, a necessity for successful hospitals in this decade" (p. 331). With respect to faculty relationships, Copp (1994) states, "Collegiality is vital to becoming a company of scholars. Faculty relationships are based on collegiality. A collegial environment supports respect for persons and ideas" (p. 196). Finally, Baker and Diekelmann (1994) state that "[c]ollegiality and shared decision-making between all care-givers have been demonstrated to be integral to optimal patient care outcomes" (p. 65).

Working Together

The term *working together* is used over and over again to substitute for the term collaboration. Several authors quote various editions of Webster's dictionary definition of collaboration as "working jointly with others, especially in an intellectual endeavor." The term, although a useful short-hand version of collaboration, only conveys the momentary working together and does not necessarily convey the full meaning of the complex collaboration as defined in this study definition.

Team or Teamwork

Team is commonly used as a surrogate term for *collaborators*. It speaks to the partnership relationship attribute of a dyad or group of two or more persons working together in a collaborative arrangement. Although this analysis is confined to health care and health professions settings and providers, the concept of team, as well as the concept of partnership, has wider application. *Teamwork* simply refers to a team approach to care. Henry et al. (1992) defines collaboration "as a team endeavor" (p. 219). King (1990) views collaborators as a "well functioning team" (p. 172). Warner et al. (1994) also speaks of a team approach to collaborative care and of teamwork as facilitating positive patient outcomes.

Interdependence

The term *interdependence*, like *collegial*, has a basis in a concept of power or authority—shared power or shared authority. The term has been used by many scholars since the time of the NJPC to compare and contrast collaborative and traditional practice. It particularly refers to the shared processes from planning to assumption of responsibility in which collaborators engage. "Collaborative practice is the antithesis of traditional, independent practice. It exemplifies the growing interdependence among health care professionals" (King 1990, p. 174, citing Burchell et al. 1983). King (1990, p.174) also cites Coluccio and Maguire (1983) as speaking of "changes in patterns of communication between primary care nurses and physicians in which mutual respect and trust have evolved into interdependence and collaborative practice."

The meaning of the term relative to its impact on the authority basis of collaborative practice is not consistently agreed upon by these scholars. Evans (1994) states that "[i]t is critical to separate the concepts of interdependency and autonomy. Autonomy implies that each team member makes decisions in a singular, independent fashion. In collaboration, on the other hand, trust in one another and respect for the individual perspectives of each contributor facilitate a sharing of responsibility and accountability for patient care" (p. 23).

Arcangelo (1994, p. 3), however, states:

> I contend that no health professional is an independent practitioner. Everyone involved in the care of a patient has the responsibility to provide comprehensive services that require collaboration and utilization of expertise based on individual needs. The practice of nurses in advanced practice is autonomous and collaborative, but not independent.

It seems as though the confusion arises around the concept of autonomy and its meaning in relation to collaboration. Baggs and Schmitt (1988) point out that collaborating doesn't mean working together on every interaction or patient encounter. That misses the point. This topic warrants further study, but there can be little doubt that collaborators share an interdependent relationship.

Professionalism or Professional Practice Model

Three authors virtually equate the term professionalism or the phrase professional practice model with collaboration. They speak of professionalism as antecedent to collaboration or speak of collaboration as antecedent to professional practice.

Lyons et al. (1992, p. 99) describe a professional practice model in their birthing center. "The spirit of professionalism is permeating the center and the staff." Four characteristics present are the social significance of the work is recognized by all providers and administrators, staff daily give their ultimate performance by providing their best work with the greatest possible care, staff have a strong sense of collegiality and collectivity, and there is a celebration of accomplishments and values in healthy and explicit ways. The staff in this setting are a team of collaborating obstetricians and nurse midwives, and their collaboration undergirds their professionalism.

Miccolo and Spanier (1993) describe the relationship of professionalism and collaboration as follows:

> To date, hospital administrators, physicians, nurses, and other allied health professionals have sought to protect their own turf . . . each viewing the other as a potential threat or adversary, rather than an ally. A new enlightened era of professionalism must evolve, with all health care workers and administrators having input into decisions that impact their ability to deliver care to the critically ill. Collaboration is a fundamental part of this evolution and offers a solution to the seemingly insoluble problems in the current health care system (p. 443).

Last, Gibbons et al. (1995) describe a professional rehabilitation nursing model, a model developed through and within a shared governance model. The developers of the model assert that collaboration among all the providers is "a must for establishing a professional practice model to affect patient care positively" (p. 28).

SAMPLE CASES

Several cases of collaboration are present in this body of literature. Most often, however, they are presented in fragments and used as a starting point for the authors to accomplish an agenda other than case study. The literature conveys the strong impression, nevertheless, that there are many fully developed and successful practices in existence. Each of the three cases available as model cases, which are briefly presented here, seems to embody the attributes of collaboration, although the completeness of the presentations varies. The reader is directed to Lyons et al. (1992) for more in depth discussion of the first model, to Coluccio and Kelley (1994) for data concerning the second, and to Iseminger (1996) with respect to the third.

A Model Birthing Center

The Virginia Mason Birth Center is a hospital-based birth center that is one unit of a large medical center. Relatively small, the center delivers about 1,400 births annually, with a staff of approximately 24 providers—

obstetricians, nurse-midwives, and family practice physicians. The center handles both low- and high-risk pregnancies, and its patients are diverse, coming from all socioeconomic strata and from all childbearing age groups. Six birthing units, two surgical suites, and an 18-bed mother-and-baby unit make up the physical plant. The small size of the center is believed to contribute to the community spirit, trust, and respect all providers feel for the setting and each other.

The center came about because of a crisis in obstetric care in the medical center in the 1970s. Retiring physicians, a low volume of deliveries, and the costs of subsidizing a low-volume service gave impetus to planned change. A multimember, multidisciplinary planning committee was formed; data and input were widely gathered. A report was written that was persuasive enough to convince reluctant board members and physicians to revitalize the service rather than discontinue it. The plan called for developing a birthing service unlike any other in the region at that time. Although the article does not discuss the initial decision makers or leadership, one can surmise that excellent leadership was present and active.

Key nursing leaders were recruited and developed; a nurse-midwifery service was started. Concomitantly, one obstetrician took the lead in recruiting other obstetricians. Once the multidisciplinary staff was in place, further recruitment was then always conducted by a multidisciplinary team with all members having full say on the appointment of all colleagues. On an ongoing basis, all the clinical and administrative leadership worked closely to define and refine the services. "Communication and collaboration were key factors in the success of the evolution of the birth center. Because the vision was clearly laid out in the planning document and agreed on by all and the leadership had the necessary expertise, authority, autonomy, and administrative support, resistance to the planned changes was minimized" (Lyons et al. 1992, p. 101).

The guiding philosophy of the center has been, and continues to be, individualized care, with a preference for minimal medication and intervention. There is a fundamental respect for individuals and families as participants and decision makers in their care. The nurses, physicians, and nurse-midwives share the same philosophy and goals for the services and for the patients. The interdependence of the providers maximizes the commitment to the shared philosophy. To maintain this continuity of philosophy and approaches to care, ongoing communication is essential. Weekly multidisciplinary prenatal care conferences are held, monthly collaborative practice inservices are held on various topics pertinent to various disciplinary providers, and semiannual meetings are held including providers from the medical center. All these sessions reinforce the shared philosophy and also provide opportunities to learn together, exchange information, and strengthen relationships.

The center staff prides itself on its openness to new innovations in care delivery developed throughout the years. They attribute their continued enthusiasm for creativity and innovativeness to the organizational climate that is supportive of new and alternative approaches to care. In addition, the providers are committed to continual learning of new (and sometimes old) ways of doing things. Being responsive to a diverse population of patients also requires an atmosphere of innovation and flexibility.

Material and human resources are seen as integral to the mission. Over the years, a physical environment has been created that supports the birth center philosophy and mission, including private rooms for labor, delivery, and recovery where the mother can labor and be delivered of her infant while supported and assisted by the father and other support persons as she wishes. Any remodeling to the birth center is planned and designed with input by the entire team.

Although a strong and ongoing commitment to quality care is discussed at length, data are not provided on patient care outcomes. The providers have thrived in this practice environment. They have grown professionally and increased their self-esteem. "Collaboration occurs on many levels at Virginia Mason. There is collegial communication and mutual respect between and within the disciplines. There is cooperation between administrators and clinicians. Joint problem solving is a way of life" (Lyons et al. 1992, p. 104).

A Service/Education Leadership Model

The setting is a large, remote rural area in the Pacific Northwest encompassing 4045 square miles consisting of mainland and islands. In some instances, travel requires boat or ferry as well as automobile. A consortium of rural community hospitals and a small private university joined forces to design and offer a baccalaureate of science in nursing education to the 5000 associate-degree-in-nursing–prepared nurses living in the area.

A group of nurse executives working [in the region] shared a common vision to develop and sustain a community-wide system to promote accessible, high quality education for the employed RN who desires to achieve a bachelor of science in nursing. In the absence of such a program . . . they decided to affiliate with a major university in the adjacent city of Seattle to deliver this education on-site in the hospitals. The nurse executives actively committed to sharing the resources necessary to bring this vision to reality (Coluccio and Kelley 1994, p. 66).

A needs assessment validated the need for the program; a call for proposals to Seattle-based universities led to an agreement to collaborate with Seattle Pacific University (SPU).

The consortium members then began what became a 2-year planning process to design the academic program and work through the myriad details of program implementation. The consortium hospitals and university formed an executive board; its activities were shaped by the Seattle Pacific University North Consortium (SPUNC) vision. Emphasis was placed on developing the board. The educational model and the foundation upon which the academic program would be built included potential faculty, mentors for students, and the student applicant pool. The board met regularly, often monthly, at the various members' homes. Meetings were structured around a planned agenda. "Throughout these meetings board members continuously reaffirmed their common vision, solidified their shared purpose, crafted a statement of mission, committed to mutual goals and objectives, developed a marketing plan, and identified resources" (Coluccio and Kelley, p. 68). A SPUNC coordinator from one of the hospitals was appointed and began working together with the SPU appointed coordinator. They worked together to develop master's-prepared clinical staff as faculty, plan the clinical learning experiences, and recruit and admit students to the program.

The educational model itself is based in an agreement by all consortium members that a traditional model of program delivery whereby the educational institution stands apart from the service institutions would not work. Such a model would have a minimum amount of coplanning and interaction with service providers. All members agreed that a model involving coplanning and interaction with multiple service institutions would benefit all institutions and be most responsive to the educational needs of all RNs registered nurses in the region who chose to apply to the program. This model, named the transformational model,

represents a high degree of integration of education and service within an entire community. Each hospital is linked with every other hospital and all are linked with the educational institution. The result is the availability of a strong, broad-based network of professionals and resources, involvement and support (Colluccio and Kelley, p. 68).

At the time of this writing, benefits of this newly implemented model were anticipated to include more knowledgeable practitioners, increased professionalism of the nursing workforce, increased retention of the nursing staff, improved recruitment, and overall enhanced employer–employee relations. The university would enjoy fulfilling its mission through service to these communities, expanding the geographic boundaries of program delivery, reaching and educating a new and place-bound student population, increasing the clinical expertise of its faculty, and successfully bridging the all too typical gap between education and service.

Going the Distance

Distance in this case refers to a vast area of rural northern Wisconsin where the landscape is beautiful and raw but can be very forbidding. "In health care terms the low population density translates into what the federal government defines as an underserved area. There just aren't enough doctors to cover huge rural chunks of northern Wisconsin. That's where U[niversity of] W[isconsin]-Madison and the North Woods Community Health Centers of the Haywood-Minong area come in—and come together" (Iseminger 1996, p. 27). This area constitutes an Area Health Education Center region (AHEC), a state and federally funded program initiative both to accomplish community-health care provider collaboration in health care and to educate providers for primary health care practice in underserved areas. This AHEC is a collaboration of academic, community, and (primarily) medical partners designed to improve access to care in the state's rural areas.

Students in medicine, nursing, pharmacy, and social work spend 4 to 8 weeks practicing at North Woods clinics and other cooperating agencies in the region. The students live on site and gain a real sense of what it would be like to live and work in a remote rural area. They also gain varied and valuable clinical experience, and local doctors gain skilled assistance. The practicing physicians also benefit from the intellectual and social stimulation that comes from precepting students.

These collaborating physicians have a commitment to service. "We enjoy being where we're needed . . . . We're not just doctors competing for patients. We have a philosophy of service to the underserved" (Iseminger 1996, p. 28). "On the job, they see many patients who can't afford health insurance and are too proud to go on Medicaid" (p. 28). One expresses their commitment to educating students: "By giving our students a rural experience, we're trying to attract them to underserved areas once they have their own practice" (p. 28). They hope that by sending graduates forth who are committed to rural practice that the answer to the critical question, "Where's the nearest clinic?" can be a firm "Not far from here" (p. 30).

From the AHEC home away from home base, students drive each day to one of several practice sites. All told, more than 40 physicians share in this collaboration and work with the multidisciplinary students. One physician reports giving his physician assistant student a "lot of freedom to assess patients by herself, then react to her assessment" (Iseminger 1996, p. 29). A nurse practitioner student says of her physician preceptor, "Nina showed respect for my abilities and guided me gently" (p. 30). The nurse practitioner student continues: "I experienced massive professional growth in those six weeks," she says. "It was heaven" (p. 30).

TEMPORAL AND CROSS-DISCIPLINARY COMPARISONS

From 1981 to 1996, the period of time encompassed in this literature search, the literature has not undergone many substantial changes. The comprehensiveness of the iteration of the attributes of collaboration, however, has grown noticeably. Early discussions of attributes of collaboration were heavily influenced by the practice components required by the W. K. Kellogg National Joint Practice Commission funded project for implementing collaborative practice in four selected hospitals. One of the required five elements for a hospital to be included as one of the four was primary nursing. In this model of care delivery, a single nurse is the primary assigned and accountable nurse provider for a group of patients. Care responsibilities encompass everything from planning to evaluation of care and from admission to discharge. This model of care delivery, which was positively received by nurse executives and nurse clinicians, is not currently being used widely. It is considered to be too costly to have a well-salaried professional nurse providing all the care for a (small) group of patients. Clearly, therefore, this requirement of primary nursing is not a part of the literature of the 1990s. Several current articles (Arcangelo 1994; McEwen 1994; Mundinger 1994) identify advanced practice nurses as the nurse providers of choice, whereas others do not discuss either the qualifications or the specific assignments of the collaborating nurses. It is continually pointed out, however, that the nursing personnel are expected to be competent.

Several articles in the literature of the 1980s discuss various aspects of RN and physician roles—expansion, overlap, conflict, negotiation, and scope of practice. Several assert that it is essential to achieve consensus on the roles of all disciplinary providers and to identify and reduce disparate role expectations of each. (Devereux 1981, Katzman 1989, McKay 1983, Prescott and Bowen 1985, Weiss and Davis 1985) The literature of the 1990s rarely speaks of role as a determinant of practice. Despite the later articles greatly outnumbering the earlier articles, only two 1990s articles mention role as a factor in establishing a collaborative practice (Giardino 1994,; Miccolo and Spanier 1993). Instead, the authors discuss the need for flexibility, openness, and shared responsibility. Role concepts may be outmoded as attributes of collaborative practice.

The benefit of the reporting in the early literature of a handful of landmark studies is noticeable in the work of the later authors. The work of Knaus et al. (1986), Mechanikc and Aiken (1982), Prescott and Bowen (1985), Rubenstein et al. (1984), and Weiss (1983 and 1985), are widely cited in the years following their publication. Their findings of lowered mortality rates and higher quality care in collaborative models of care, along with their findings of increased provider satisfaction and competency, add depth robustness to the literature.

As already mentioned, the term *joint practice* fell out of favor with physicians. It was officially replaced by the term *collaborative practice* beginning in 1981 (Ritter 1983). Its use in the literature began to diminish in the mid-1980s.

The literature is surprisingly scant with respect to the negative influence of competition as a driving motivator for practice, although a review of the data gathered on barriers to collaborative research has not yet been completed. There appear to be but two current articles that raise the specter of competition. The physician comments in Iseminger (1996) about not being doctors who simply compete for patients is a reference to competition, and Arcangelo (1994) states, "In this era of health care reform, a conflict has arisen between medicine and nursing concerning the market share of primary care . . . ." (p. 3).

As has already been mentioned, this literature (both the older and newer) is surprisingly sparse in its discussion of primary health care collaborative practices. The reporting of community-based practices is a bit more substantial, but not much. Reports of hospital-based practice, including outreach services, continue to dominate the literature.

On a positive note was the discovery of virtually no conceptual or philosophical differences between those articles that were authored by nurses and those authored by physicians. Several of the articles were, in fact, coauthored by physician–nurse partnerships. It seems that those who are engaged in full-blown collaborative practices, regardless of disciplinary affiliation, share their partner's beliefs, values, and attitudes about the virtues of collaborative practice. One small difference was noted: Physicians spoke more about their concern with increasing access to care for people residing in rural areas or for those who could not afford care than their nurse colleagues did.

IMPLICATIONS

Collaboration, it was learned as a result of this concept analysis, is a complex and rich tapestry of purposeful action by two or more people working together to address important needs and problems in health care delivery, education, and research. We learned that its successful development, implementation, and maintenance requires the support and commitment of complex small or large organizations including the allocation of a good measure of human and material resources. The partnership relationship that is required for collaboration to occur is developed and nurtured over time, as is the supportive organizational environment. It was also learned that such efforts are predictably rewarded by successfully achieving the planned-for positive outcomes. Care delivery is improved noticeably, and organizations meet their planned goals for excellence in service or education or research. Clinicians are more satisfied with their practice; patients, with their care; and educators and students, with their education.

Collaboration is the vehicle for bringing disparate disciplines and organizations together to act in ways they could not act on their own to resolve needs and concerns they are not able to address on their own.

Specifically, in education and research, myriad activities and programs cannot occur unless a collaborative approach is used, such as faculty–staff cosponsored clinical research, or graduate students clinical preceptorships in advanced practice roles with expert practitioners. In service–service organizational collaboration or in mixed mission education–service collaboration, unless these organizations join forces to meet goals they could not meet on their own, they would be passed by in the current turbulent environment.

In practice, rehabilitation has arguably been the one practice area that by definition requires a collaborative caregiving model. In other areas of practice, the mandate for collaboration has not been as clear. This concept analysis, however, makes a powerful case that the kind and quality of practice appropriate for now and for the future cannot occur except in a collaborative practice arrangement. Also, as health care organizations join forces in coalitions and consortiums that will fashion a new health care delivery, education, and research infrastructure in the United States and internationally, they must be able to develop and sustain strong collaborative relationships. The stakes are high. Arguably, many health care organizations will not survive unless they partner with other organizations and providers. Some would argue that many should not survive, and those that should survive will. In response to this argument, it can be said that this concept analysis provides a useful basis for further developing the knowledge and skills of executives, educators, and providers as they deal with these very challenging issues. Their failure to survive should not be the result of their ignorance about collaboration.

The very positive picture of collaboration that emerges from this concept analysis could lead to the erroneous conclusion that all health care providers and educators embrace collaboration in their practices and organizations. Those in the field know that nothing could be further from the truth. Although the need for collaboration is pervasive, and collaborative approaches have been used successfully in myriad health care settings, collaborative models are not widely used. Barriers to collaboration are rampant. Perhaps the very complexity of collaboration, along with the intense commitment of human and material resources required to develop a collaborative model, is one major deterrent. Providers and organizations simply may not possess either the resources or the expertise to undertake the challenge of collaboration. Another major deterrent likely concerns perceptions of losses from both disciplinary and economic perspectives if one engages in a shared practice. Losses of income, of authority, and of independence or autonomy are samples of losses that one might fear. The list of possible deterrents to collaboration could be very long.

In 1966, Pellegrino, a noted health care policy analyst, stated:

> While some of our mutual concerns [nurses and physicians] are matters of resources and techniques, a more urgent concern is of human organization and relationships. The focal human problem that we have not yet solved is how best to employ the particular skills of each of the health professions synergistically to the benefit of the patient (cited in Prescott and Bowen 1985, p. 127).

Although the concept of collaboration has evolved significantly since 1966, there is still much wisdom in this quotation. To add to the challenges faced by current providers is the rapidity with which organizations and systems are evolving; indeed, the definition of collaboration itself is changing. Henneman (1995) describes the situation this way:

> [The m]eaning [of collaboration] is not stable. Our task is to describe the nature of the present, and ourselves in the present. Society is calling for a coordinated approach to health care requiring a reevaluation of independent and interdependent roles of health professions" (p. 362).

This concept analysis provides a solid foundation upon which to build additional research and scholarship. Some of the research issues or questions identified are addressed in later chapters of this book; others are not addressed here. The entire gamut of research and study—clinical, philosophical and theory-based— and policy and policy-related work is stimulated. Much of this work is overlapping or sequential, of course. Clinical research has theoretical and philosophical components; theory-based scholarship often has a clinical project as an outgrowth; and both have policy implications. Policy research, in turn, may have important repercussions for clinical practice, education, or research.

Clinical Research

The very strong data on consequences or outcomes of collaboration beg for further study to validate and amplify those findings. Patient mortality and morbidity data, gathered and analyzed with great care, must be added to the handful of studies already in the literature. Such data need to be gathered on a variety of patients from many diverse settings. Cost factors need to be incorporated into study designs. Given the current cost-conscious environment, cost–benefit ratios are an essential variable coupled with the quality indicators. Many more case studies coauthored by collaborating partners need to be presented in the literature. There is a particular need for case studies by primary health care providers in community settings. The practice challenges they are experiencing and the strategies that are working for them in a managed care environment need to be told. That body of information is virtually absent in the literature. Field data using a variety of research methods, both qualitative and quantitative, are also called for to explore and elucidate the attributes of the definition in varied practices and practice settings.

Philosophical or Theory-Based Research

Perhaps it is a reflection of the state of development of the health professions and their difficulties in coming together to engage in collaboration, or perhaps it is a product of an environment in turmoil, or perhaps it is a constellation of both. In any event, the list of needed philosophical and theory-based work is long. This concept analysis ought to be repeated or updated in 2 to 3 years. Both the complexity of collaboration and the pace of change require this almost immediate updating, and it is likely that many changes will have occurred during this period.

There is a central need for philosophical and theoretical analyses of the meaning of power and its influence on related concepts such as autonomy and independence. Relating this sensitive topic to the need for increased reporting of case studies in the literature, the presence of in-depth case studies documenting strong transforming partnerships can both further enlighten would-be-collaborators and scholars about the meaning and import of power in collaborative relationships and negate the perhaps sometimes excessive concern with power and its related notions. On the basis of the analysis of the data, we conclude that power is more important to nursing than it is to other disciplines. A higher level of understanding of power and its ramifications for the scope of nursing practice in a collaborative practice would likely improve nursing's ability to collaborate comfortably with medicine.

Are there any shortcuts to establishing a full-blown collaborative partnership? Philosophical and theoretical or conceptual analyses of past, current, and prospective approaches and models of practice and their antecedents may provide some beginning answers to this important question. How can coalitions and consortiums develop strong collaborative partnerships in a situation in which the relationship may only be temporary and may be dismantled when the immediate problem is addressed or the pace of change no longer mandates that a particular problem be addressed? Because the need for collaboration is so great, the specter of failure to collaborate so real, and the consequences of such failure so grave, these become very important research questions.

Further analysis of related concepts and surrogate terms is another important area of study. Increased clarity of understanding of concepts such as collegial and cooperative or shared governance and coalition will assist our clear and consistent usage of the terms. This clarity will also help to clarify meaning and clear usage of the main term, collaboration.

Policy and Policy-Related Research

The mandating of collaborative practice by state legislatures and the implementation of legislation through action by regulatory boards across the United States are a recent and significant trend (see Chapter 11). The analyses of these rules and regulations and their impact on collaborative practices in the various states are a major policy research topic. The concept analysis documents that the process of building a collaborative relationship works best when the collaborators themselves determine a need and a desire to practice collaboratively. The other necessary ingredient is a supportive environment. Successful collaboration cannot be legislatively mandated or forced by external pressures. What, then, happens when legislators and government officials attempt to legislatively mandate collaboration? Despite the assumed discomfort of these external pressures to health care providers and organizations, are society and health care providers better off in an environment in which collaboration is forced, rather than in one in which collaborative practice is absent?

Legislators and other policymakers have a need to know about collaboration. They are subject to misinformation as various stakeholders pursue their agendas. An opponent of collaborative practice might, for example, tell legislators that collaborative practice is an error-filled practice because more than one person is involved in making patient care decisions. Designing a protocol to share the findings of this concept analysis and other similar work with policymakers is one way to counterbalance such false information. Likewise, professional health care providers who have a stake in advancing collaborative practice need to be educated about collaboration, particularly regarding the strategies that advance collaboration and those that do not. The development and wide discussion of model collaborative practice and partnership guidelines might advance the utility of the regulatory and legislative processes to the development of functional collaborative practices.

Another avenue for policy research lies in the design of databases to gather information about collaborative practices and collaborating practitioners. How many collaborative practices are in place? How large are the practices? Are they meeting the needs of the people in their practice catchment areas? If not, why not? Are their practices well received by the clientele? How is the workload decided and divided? The questions to be asked are numerous. Virtually none of these data are available. They are needed for policy analyses for workforce planning, health care financing, and support for models of collaborative practice. Directly or indirectly, this concept analysis provides a foundation and a stimulus for the continued development of our understanding of collaboration and our ability to achieve collaborative practices. Hegyvary (1991), in extolling the virtues of collaboration, states that "[a]chieving these goals [of collaborative relationships in service, education, and research] requires the commitment of time, energy, and resources. The results could be astounding for nursing, health care, and the people we serve" (p. 148).

Acknowledgment

The author wishes to acknowledge Lyons et al. (1992), for their fine presentation of their birthing center, Coluccio and Kelley (1994), for the fine example of interorganizational collaboration presented in their article and Iseminger (1996) for sharing the heartwarming, multidisciplinary, rural practice AHEC model.

References

Arcangelo, V. P. (1994). The myth of independent practice. *Nursing Forum*, 29, 3–4.

Baggs, J. G. and Schmidt, M. H. (1988). Collaboration between nurses and physicians. *Image: Journal of Nursing Scholarship*, 20, 145–149.

Baker, C., and Diekelmann, N. (1994). Connecting conversations of caring: Recalling the narrative to clinical practice. *Nursing Outlook*, 42, 65–70.

Burchell, R., Thomas, D., and Smith, H. (1983). Some considerations for implementing collaborative practice. *The American Journal of Medicine*, 74, 9–13.

Butterfoss, F. D., Goodman, R. M., and Wandersman, A. (1993). Community coalitions for prevention and health promotion. *Health Education Research*, 8, 315–330.

Clifford (1994). Clifford, J. C. (1994). Collaboration (Beth Israel Hospital). *Nursing Administration Quarterly*, 18(4), 10–11.

Coluccio, M. and Kelley, L. K. (1994). Transformational partnership for delivery of RN baccalaureate education: A service/education leadership model. *Nursing Administration Quarterly*, 18, 65–71.

Coluccio and Maguire (1983). Coluccio, M. and Maguire, P. (1983, Summer). Collaborative practice: Becoming a reality through primary nursing. *Nursing Administration Quarterly*, 59–63.

Copp, L. A. (1994). Faculty behavior: collegiality or conflict? *Journal of Professional Nursing*, 10, 195–196.

Devereux, P. M. (1981) Essential elements of nurse–physician collaboration. *Journal of Nursing Administration*, 1(5) 19–23.

Dumont, J., and Niziolek, C. (1991). The Cornerstones of Collaboration. *Journal of Professional Nursing*, 7, 331.

Evans, J. A. (1994). The role of the nurse manager in creating an environment for collaborative practice. *Holistic Nursing Practice*, 8, 22–31.

Giardino (1994). Giardino, A. P., Giardino, E. R., and Burns, K. M. (1994). Same place, different experience: Nurses and residents on pediatric emergency transport. *Holistic Nurse Practitioner*, 8(3), 54–63.

Gibbons, K. B., Salter, J. P., Pierce, L. L., and Govoni, A. L. (1995). A model of professional rehabilitation nursing practice. *Rehabilitation Nursing*, 20, 23–28.

Hegyvary, S. T. (1991). Collaborative relationships for education and practice. *Journal of Professional Nursing*, 7, 148.

Henneman, E. A. (1995). Nurse–physician collaboration: A poststructuralist view. *Journal of Nursing Administration*, 22, 359–363.

Henry, V., Schmitz, K., Reif, LuA., and Rudie, P. (1992). Collaboration: Integrating practice and research in public health nursing. *Public Health Nursing*, 9, 218–222.

Iseminger, J. (1996) Going the distance. *On Wisconsin, March / April*, 26–30.

Jones, P. K. (1994). Developing a collaborative professional role for the staff nurse in a shared governance model. *Holistic Nursing Practice*, 8, 32–37.

Katzman (1989). Katzman, E. M. (1989). Nurses' and physicians' perceptions of nursing authority. *Journal of Professional Nursing*, 5(4), 208–214.

Kilman and Thomas (1977). Kilmann, R., and Thomas, K. (1977). Developing a forced-choice measure of conflict handling behavior: the mode instrument. *Educational Psychology Measures*, 37, 309–325.

King, M. B. (1990). Clinical nurse specialist collaboration with physicians. *Clinical Nurse Specialist*, 4, 172–177.

Knaus, W. A., Draper, E. A., Wagner, D. P., and Zimmerman, J. E. (1986). An evaluations of outcome from intensive care in major medical centers. *Annuals of Internal Medicine*, 104, 410–418.

Lyons, N., Reinke, C., Sutherland, K., Zelenkov, K. (1992) The ultimate birth center: A collaborative model for innovation. Nursing Clinic of North America, 27(1), 99–106.

McMahon, J. M. (1992). Shared governance: The leadership challenge. *Nursing Administration Quarterly*, 17, 55–59.

Mechanic, D. and Aiken, L. H. (1982). A cooperative agenda for medicine and nursing. *New England Journal of Medicine*, 307, 747–750.

Miccolo, M. A. and Spanier, A. H. (1993). Critical care management in the 1990s: Making collaborative practice work. *Critical Care Clinics*, 9, 443–453.

Notkin, M. S. (1983). Collaboration and communication. *Nursing Administration Quarterly*, 8, 1–7.

Pellegrino (1966). Pellegrino, E. (1966). What's wrong with the nurse-physician relationship in today's hospitals?: A physician's view. *Hospitals*, 40:70, 77–8, 80.

Prescott, P. A., and Bowen, S. A. (1985). Physician–nurse relationships. *Annuals of Internal Medicine*, 103, 127–133.

Ritter, H. A. (1983). Collaborative practice: What's in it for medicine? *Nursing Administration Quarterly*, 7, 31–36.

Rubenstein, L. Z., Josephson, K. R., Wieland, G. D., English, P. A., Sayre, J. A., and Kane, R. L. (1984). Effectiveness of a geriatric evaluation unit. *New England Journal of Medicine*, 311, 1664–1670.

Styles, M. M. (1984). Reflections on collaboration and unification. Image: Journal of Nursing Scholarship, 16, 21–23.

Warner, M., Ford–Gilboe, M., Laforet–Fliesser, Y., Olson, J., and Ward–Griffin, C. (1994). The teamwork project: A collaborative approach to learning to nurse families. *Journal of Nursing Education*, 33, 5–13.

Webster's Ninth New World College Dictionary, 3rd edition (1996). MacMmillan, New York.

Weiss, S. J. (1983). Role differentiation between nurse and physician: Implications for nursing. *Nursing Research, 32(3)*, 133–139.

Weiss, S. J. (1985). The influence of discourse on collaboration among nurses, physicians, and consumers. *Research in Nursing and Health*, 8, 49–59.

Weiss, S. J., and Davis, H. P. (1985). Validity and reliability of the collaborative practice scales. *Nursing Research, 34*, 299–305.

Theoretical and Contextual Analyses

3

Toni J. Sullivan

To understand collaboration as it is evolving at the end of the 20th century, not only is a discussion of its conceptual analysis necessary (see Chapters 1 and 2), but the contextual analyses and the theoretical underpinnings, used by scholars and scientists to shape discussion, analyses, or research designs for study of all or some of its components is also necessary. This chapter explores and describes why they approached the topics as they did, the utility of the conceptual tools selected, and the contributions made. In order to obtain a proper perspective, it is important to review collaboration's past triumphs and failures, its values, its challenges and opportunities, and its role in health care in particular and society as a whole.

An overview of events since the 1970s in nursing and health care within the framework of the larger society provides much of the necessary context for collaboration in health care. Change—dynamic, constant, and transforming—is the major thread that is woven throughout this notion of health care in a rapidly changing society. This theoretical model is based on the definition of collaboration proposed in Chapter 1: *collaboration is defined as a dynamic, transforming process of creating a power-sharing partnership for pervasive application in health care practice, education, research, and organizational settings for purposeful attention to needs and problems and in order to achieve likely successful outcomes.* A further foundation for the theoretical model is the work of the myriad scholars and practitioners who have led the way to greater understanding of collaboration.

This presentation of the theoretical model includes recommendations for further development, application, and study. In addition to the 81

65

articles and books that comprised the database for the concept analysis, several articles and books have been purposefully selected and added to the database for this theory analysis. These additional materials are mainly on the topic of theory development and theory analysis, in general, and systems and role theory, in particular.

CONCEPTUAL OR THEORY MODELS IN THE LITERATURE

Many, if not most, of the articles in the database were influenced overall by some philosophical, conceptual, or theoretical approach to meaning. The influence of either role theory or systems theory was especially present. A level of analysis whereby clues were identified and the overall conceptual approach of each article in the body of literature was categorized was not undertaken. Only when conceptual or theoretical perspectives were named or frameworks or models presented, was the conceptual approach in a particular article selected out for inclusion. The conceptual or theoretical entities identified are, therefore, very obvious in the literature.

The labeling of conceptual frameworks and models has been done here in such a manner as to show the body of work in the literature from the many perspectives presented. Changes in the level of sophistication of the work over time can teach us much about what stage we are at with respect to knowledge development and what work remains to be done. The nursing literature itself is unsettled with respect to definitive definitions of theories, models, and conceptual frameworks for nursing and health care. For the purpose of this chapter, these have been identified as follows:

Conceptual Frameworks may be described as *taxonomies*—classification or categorization of phenomena; *paradigms*—patterns or schemes that attempt to describe a process; and *models*—symbolic representations of perceptual phenomena, which are classified as pictorial (lowest level), descriptive and focused on relationships among phenomena (middle level), and mathematical (highest level) (McKay 1969, p. 326).

Theory may be defined as "a set of interrelated constructs (concepts), definitions, propositions that present a systematic view of phenomena by specifying relations among variables" (Kerlinger 1973, p. 9, cited by Fawcett 1980, p. 426). For the purpose of presenting the conceptual or theoretical models from the literature, little or no distinction is made between descriptive models or theory.

Concepts may be classified as *nonvariable*—referring to classes or categories of phenomena, such as women or plants; or *variable*—resulting from observations falling on a continuum, such as weight or age. Variable conceptualizations are said to facilitate theory development (Hardy 1973, p. 374). Nonvariable or variable concepts are discussed by Dickoff et al. (1968, p. 476) as the tools of factor-isolating or level-one theory. Systematically naming factors or attributes and subfactors is the first step in theory building.

Twenty-nine articles were identified as articulating a conceptual or theoretical framework either as a basis of the article or as an outcome of the work reported. These articles were sorted and categorized according to whether they were pre-1991 (early) or post-1991 (later), by focus of education, research, practice, education–practice, or organizational practice and by type of conceptual or theoretical framework—taxonomies (continua, lists), models (pictorial), or models (descriptive) or theories. A three-dimensional matrix was thus formed, with 15 articles placing early—from 1981 to 1990—and 14 articles placing later—from 1991 to 1995. In the early literature, 13 of 15 articles focused in direct practice; 1 focused in organizational practice; and 1, in education-service. Nine of the early articles present two conceptual taxonomies and a pictorial model; 4 use role theory; and 1 presents a systems model.

In the post-1991 articles, 9 of 14 focused in direct practice; 3 focused in organizational practice; 1, in research; and 1, in education–service. The greatest indication of growth and change is in the type of conceptual or theoretical designs. Four of the designs, as compared with 9 in the earlier set of articles, are distinct conceptual taxonomies, whereas the remainder of articles use more complex and higher-level conceptual or theoretical schema. Of the remainder of articles, 2 are steeped in role theory and 8 are from a systems theory perspective. This proportional use of these 2 approaches can be contrasted with the early set, which is just the opposite—1 systems approach to 4 role approaches. It represents a paradigm shift from a particularistic to a holistic perspective. Role theory focuses upon boundaries and rules; conflict occurs when people or disciplines overstep their boundaries or break the rules.

Systems models and ways of thinking, on the other hand, focus upon wholes. "It is a framework for seeing interrelationships rather than things, for seeing patterns of change rather than static snapshots" (Senge

1990, p. 68). This type of approach to meaning is precisely what is needed in the present and future, according to Senge (1990, p. 69) and many others. As the world has become exceedingly complex, systems thinking offers the antidote to the feelings of being overwhelmed and helpless that we are prone to experiencing in the face of such complexity. Systems models and their application provide us with the conceptual and theoretical tools needed for understanding the structures present in our society and institutions and for navigating them with much success.

EARLY LITERATURE

National Joint Practice Commission Model

The first conceptual work identified in the literature was as a result of the work and stated requirements of the National Joint Practice Commission (NJPC). At least five authors list and name the elements that were required before a hospital would be considered as a participating hospital in the W. K. Kellogg–funded NJPC demonstration project (Baggs and Schmitt 1988, Devereux 1981, Koerner et al. 1985, Prescott and Bowen 1985, Ritter 1983).

The five elements under the rubric joint practice were the following:

(1) primary nursing [only primary nurses could participate in collaborative practice], (2) clinical decision making by nurses within the scope of nursing practice as defined within the hospital, (3) the integrated patient record as a formal means of nurse–physician communication in the care of patients, (4) joint patient care review and (5) a joint practice committee to monitor this relationship and recommend appropriate actions supporting joint practice (Ritter 1983, p. 33).

These five subfactors make up an early conceptual framework for joint practice, later defined as collaborative practice. The authors report very favorable outcomes with implementing this framework of collaboration. Ritter states in 1983, although the demonstration projects had ended in 1980, that:

The spirit of the NJPC is alive and well. Nurses on the leading edge have not forgotten; physicians who were involved in the demonstration projects have become disciples. Without exception, in every hospital where the five elements of joint practice were demonstrated, the concept is alive, well and spreading throughout the institution and to neighboring or related facilities (pp. 33–34).

In fact, in a 1985 article, Koerner et al. describe establishing collaborative practice at Hartford Hospital, Hartford, Connecticut, according to the NJPC model. They report being counseled by several of the original NJPC participants to incorporate all of the model elements *at the same time,* an action that elevates the level of this categorization scheme to a middle-range descriptive model or paradigm. Failure to incorporate all elements at the same time, they say, could doom the project. Little more than a decade ago, therefore, this model comprised of these specific five elements provided the formula for successful collaboration.

Ritter (1983) and others also provided a list of factors that spelled out an organization's readiness for collaboration. Paraphrasing the list of essential elements, they are the following:

1. Are the present working relationships of physicians and nurses compatible? Do they accept each other as professionals with a common goal and unique competencies?
2. Is hospital administration committed to collaborative practice and to quality care? Will it support making the necessary organizational changes to support collaborative practice?
3. Is the nursing staff clinically competent?
4. Does the medical staff communicate and consult with the nursing staff and accept a collegial relationship with the clinically competent nurses?
5. Is the hospital committed to primary nursing? Can the physicians identify who are the patients' nurses?
6. Is clinical excellence of nurses rewarded?

This listing of attributes that constitutes readiness provided a template, or checklist, against which organizations could compare themselves when considering developing collaborative practice. Some developed a shorthand list to refer to these: communications, administrative support, competence, accountability, and trust (Baggs and Schmitt 1988, Prescott and Bowen 1985). There seems to be a clear inference that all these elements need to be present in order for an organization to predict a level of success in collaborative practice. Although the work of the NJPC seems simplistic just a few short years later, it is also very evident that this work has had a great deal of influence on the development of approaches to collaborative practice and to collaborative practice itself.

The Unity Continuum

Styles (1984) provided the only education–service conceptual model identified in this body of early literature. The *unity continuum* is a device for imaging and analyzing stages or degrees of unity between entities within or across education and/or service settings. It ranges from no relationship to a middle-range collaborative relationship to a unified structure. In the collaborative mode, two parties representing two organizations agree to join forces to work toward common goals they could not meet on their own. In the unified structure, a lead organization assumes ownership of another organization. Goals and resources are joined, and leadership is singular. At that time (1984), unification was a much-discussed approach to the rejoining of nursing education and nursing service. A unification model was in effect at the University of Rochester, Rochester, New York, and at Rush University, Chicago, Illinois. Styles, however, verifies that within this continuum, collaboration is more palatable to nurse educators and administrators than unification. She describes the continuum as having either stages or degrees of unity. Stages, of course, depict movement or progress in a linear fashion, whereas degrees depict a fixed position somewhere along the line.

In a companion continuum, Styles presents the skeletal forms of conceptual models (to use her phrase) presenting elements necessary to achieve various levels of unity. For example, a middle-range (collaborative) relationship requires communication, consultation, unified policy, and consent of all parties.

Styles's intent was that the continuum be useful prospectively to study situations, plan relationships, and develop proposals. She expected that it would be useful retrospectively to study professional trends. Moreover, she predicted that the approach of choice for joining education–service endeavors would prove to be collaboration. In this prediction, Styles has proved to be correct.

This continuum model of the variable concept, unity, was widely used by nurse educators and executives for many years. It is not broadly quoted in this body of literature; however, it is thought to have been cited by many. Although there is no indication of any education–service typologies or classifications that were created later, a newer conceptualization that takes into account many more complexities of today's health care education and service organizations is needed. See Chapter 10 for the foundaton of a proposed new conceptual model for interorganizational collaboration including education–service collaborating entities.

Two-Dimensional Grid of Collaboration

Without shared decision making, collaboration arguably is absent, regardless of the presence of other attributes. Shared decision making is apparently the sine qua non of collaboration, especially to nurses. It is not surprising, therefore, that early in the modern era, several nurse researchers studied the topic of decision making between physicians and registered nurses (RNs).

A two-dimensional grid originally formulated by Blake and Mouton (1970) and adapted by Kilmann and Thomas (1977) was used as the paradigmatic conceptual framework to study decision making and related variables by at least three research teams. Baggs and Schmitt (1988), in an essay about collaboration, also report extensively on the use of the model by the three research teams. The two interrelating elements are assertiveness, placed on a vertical axis, and cooperativeness, placed on the horizontal. Five modes of functioning are formed by the interaction of the two elements along the continuum formed. The modes, ordered from the highest and most desirable level of functioning (from the perspective of collaboration) to the lowest level, are as follows:

High assertiveness + high cooperation = Collaboration
Moderate assertiveness + high cooperation = Compromise
Low assertiveness + low cooperation = Avoidance
High assertiveness + low cooperation = Competition
Low assertiveness + high cooperation = Accommodation

Although the results of four studies using the two-dimensional grid are reported in Chapter 5, findings are briefly shared here for the purpose of judging the contribution to conceptual or theory development made by this paradigm. Weiss and Davis (1985) used the grid to develop two collaborative practice scales (CPSs)—one to measure physicians' collaborative behaviors and one to measure nurses'—and geared their study to determining the reliability and validity of the CPSs. Their instruments each include 30 forced-choice items that operationalize and measure the five modes of interpersonal problem solving: accommodation, competition, avoidance, compromise, and collaboration. They report that the dominant construct measured by both scales is synergistic interaction between nurses and physicians, a type of patient care theoretically linked to the features of collaboration espoused by Blake and Mouton (1970).

Weiss and Davis found, in general, that nurses had difficulty engaging in problem-solving behaviors at the highest level. They found that much of the difficulty was attributable to nurses' intrapersonal weaknesses, such as discomfort accepting responsibility, having low regard for one's professional expertise and, indeed, having low regard for the profession itself. The RNs also had difficulty because of perceptions of physicians' lack of valuing of RN communications.

In another study, also reported in 1985, Prescott and Bowen use Thomas and Kilmann's work to develop a model for handling disagreements. Physicians and nurses from 15 general hospitals participated in the study, completing a brief questionnaire and also participating in semi-structured interviews. Extensive data were gathered on disagreements that nurses and physicians had in decision making about patient care as one component of data gathered in this massive database.

Using the two-dimensional grid, data were plotted into the five modes. Competition was shown to be the most common mode for managing disagreements, followed by accommodation. The researchers judged competition to be a more desirable mode than accommodation for dealing with disputes, but found it to be less desirable than collaboration. Their rationale for preferring competition to accommodation as a mode of dispute resolution was that the former encompasses advocating for patients' welfare. Nurses disagreed with physicians most often regarding plan of care, specific orders, and patient disposition such as discharge from the hospital. The researchers noted: "Most disagreements are settled rather than resolved. Settling relies on compromise and imposed authority; resolutions are more integrative solutions that view disagreements more as problems to be solved" (Prescott and Bowen 1985, p. 132).

In a later study, published in 1990, Baggs and Ryan used the two-dimensional grid to study nurse satisfaction with collaborative practice in intensive care units (ICUs). Their sample consisted of the 68-member staff of one ICU. All completed the Weiss and Davis CPSs, as well as several other measures. Their hypotheses that "when ICU nurses perceive the decision-making process associated with patient transfer to be more collaborative, they are more satisfied" (p. 390) was supported by the data. A significant positive correlation was found between collaboration and satisfaction in the specific decision-making situation for nurses (p. 390).

Clearly, this paradigm was extremely useful as an operational tool for the early study of problem solving and the decision-making process. It is not, of course, a continuum of levels of collaboration. It is, however, a continuum of methods of dispute resolution. As such, it proved to be very useful for gaining insights into how and why nurses and physicians in interactive practice settings, as well as in formally labeled collaborative practices, act as they do in settling disagreements over patient care. Baggs and Schmitt (1988), after analysis of early research using the two-dimensional grid, recommend that any instrument developed to study collaboration must measure "openness of communication, coordination, cooperation and sharing during planning, and implementation of care. It should also examine administrative support for collaboration" (p. 148). They go on to say that the instrument "should not be limited to conflict resolution or interactions that result in the formulation of new plans" (p. 148).

Role Theory or Concepts

Katzman (1989) reports on a study using a sample of 110 nurses and 53 physicians from one southwestern hospital to compare perception of the current and ideal status of decision-making authority of the nurses. To undertake the task, Katzman designed and used the Authority in Nursing Roles Inventory (ANRI). The tool consisted of 25 items derived from the literature that were critiqued and refined by an expert panel. The items concerned areas of decision making by RNs. By asking physicians and nurses to respond on a Likert scale to both current and ideal positions, the underlying question of power and authority for decision-making was addressed. "The findings support the premise that in spite of expanded nursing roles emphasizing nursing authority, there are differences between nurses' and physicians' perceptions of the current and ideal authority of nurses" (p. 208).

This study is yet one more study that focuses on decision-making. Its role theory perspective and the use of the ANRI also bring into focus the subject of power—its meaning and its usage in collaborative practice. The subject of power is of great interest to the scholars who use role theory in their work.

Katzman found that because of either actual or perceived lack of decision-making authority, both staff nurses and nurse practitioners frequently were unable to carry out their legal and ethical roles in nursing and health care. Furthermore, the nurses and physicians frequently disagreed on what the nurses' legitimate roles were or ought to be (p. 208). Katzman also notes that the idea of nurse power connotes negative images and that for some nurses, the concept of authority rather than power is more acceptable. In fact, she asserts that not all health professionals, indeed not all nurses, are supportive of full professional status for nurses.

McClain (1988) used a conceptual or theoretical framework of critical theory for a phenomenological and participant observation study of the collaboration of nine physicians and nine family nurse practitioners. "The problem studied by critical theory is power, the major interest is emancipation, and the primary methodological approach is self-reflection. The goal of critical theory is thus transformation and emancipation from the constraints of unequal power relationships" (p. 392).

Methodologically critical theory focuses on patterns of communication that distort "ideal speech," which is speech that promotes understanding, truth, sincerity, and the legitimacy of the speaker (p. 392).

This study was categorized by this researcher as a role theory study because of its focus on power and on power from a status perspective rather than from a competency-based perspective. Clearly, this approach is normative. It contains value-laden goals of emancipation from power struggles and speech that is less than ideal. Normative theory is the type of theory needed within practice disciplines such as nursing and medicine in which the goal is to produce desired changes or outcomes (Dickoff et al. 1968; Chinn and Jacobs 1978). One might question, however, the application of critical theory with its sharp focus on breaking down the stature of MDs' roles and reflective communication patterns to the processes of building and studying collaborative practice between MDs and RNs.

The data in the McClain study demonstrate significant barriers to, and significant possibilities for, collaborative practice. The data document that both nurses and MDs participate in distorted communication. McClain indicates that in the sample studied, collaborative practice was not the norm but, rather, practice patterns were competitive or even hostile.

Weiss (1985) reported using concepts of role theory in a study that brought together 72 professionals and consumers in small multidisciplinary groups for monthly meetings over 2 years. The underlying value was that "[c]ollaboration requires a dynamic, flexible distribution of status and authority whereby responsibilities and influence vary from point to point, depending on which individual or group has the superior competence required for a particular task in a particular situation" (p. 50). Weiss hypothesized that bringing actors together away from the practice setting would facilitate developing collaborative attitudes and behaviors. "Exposure to one another in a less role-prescribed context, with opportunity for egalitarian discussion regarding shared responsibility, could positively influence nurse, MD, and consumer dispositions toward collaboration in health care" (p. 50).

The design of the study was pretest–posttest, with the discussion groups as the intervention. Three instruments were completed by the participants: The Health Professional Locus Of Control Scales, scales that measure specific measures of internal and external locus of control beliefs; The Health Role Expectations Index, a scale designed to measure attitudes toward the amount of shared responsibility that should exist in relationships between nurse, MD, and consumer; and The Management of Differences Exercise, the two-dimensional grid of Kilmann and Thomas (1977), already presented.

Not surprisingly, the discussion groups did little or nothing to change attitudes, beliefs, and values of MDs, nurses, and consumers. In fact, previously held attitudes and role stereotypes may have been reinforced. Collaboration, it appears, must be planned for, prepared for, and practiced, in order for it to be present. Although the conceptual background of choice for engaging in collaboration may not be role theory, the implementation of collaborative practice is necessary for developing true collaboration. Weiss's study did contribute to the understanding of patterns of behavior that prevent or promote collaboration by RNs and by MDs. She found that uneven nurse competence was central to poor interdisciplinary relationships between RNs and MDs as there followed a lack of trust and mutual respect. Greater exploration of this finding can be found in Chapter 5.

Leonard I. Stein published "The Doctor–Nurse Game" in 1967. A role theory approach to understanding MD–nurse relations, with a basis in game theory, it struck a sharp chord within nursing circles, where there was a loud chorus of agreement with its tenets. Looking back on the doctor–nurse game in 1990, Stein and two MD coauthors describe the original game as follows:

> In 1967 there was clear agreement between doctors and nurses that their relationship was hierarchical, with doctors being superior to nurses. All their interactions were carefully managed so as not to disturb the hierarchy. Nurses were to be bold, have initiative, and be responsible for making important recommendations, while at the same time they had to seem passive. In short, nurses were to make recommendations, but their recommendations had to appear to be initiated by the physician. . . . The cardinal rule of the game was that open disagreement between the players had to be avoided at all costs" (p. 549).

Four nurse scholars write with hindsight about the doctor–nurse game in the literature of the 1990s. (There was no explicit mention of the doctor–nurse game in the earlier literature in this database.) All agree that the game is changing, as do Stein et al. (1990). Eubanks (1991), in a discussion of the mandate hospitals have from their accrediting body, discusses the centrality of nurse–physician collaboration to hospital-based quality of care. She paints an optimistic picture: "The nature of the RN–MD relationship is changing from the old stereotype of nurse-as-handmaiden and doctor-as-deity to a collaboration of two different, valuable professionals" (p. 29).

In a general essay about the challenges and accomplishments of collaboration between nurses and physicians, Fagin (1992) notes that nurses have stopped playing the game because of their interest in autonomy, changes in women's status, improved education, and their desire to improve the satisfaction of nursing. "The stubborn rebel replaces the willing supplicant in the game" (p. 295). Fagin in 1992 continued to describe a role theory approach to collaboration by discussing role overlap. She stated, "If we envision the knowledge and activities of nurses and the knowledge and activities of physicians as occupying two partly intersecting spheres, we can see that much is shared. . . . The present and future are placing great pressure upon the ways these spheres intersect" (p. 302).

In a random mail survey of 59 nurses and 67 physicians, R. A. P. Jones (1994) used an adaptation of the Weiss CPS scales to study power control, practice spheres, concerns, and goals of physicians and nurses.

This tool was supplemented by practice spheres and goals checklists. The changing doctor–nurse game is the conceptual basis for the study. "Today RN–MD interactions are shaped by high technology, consumer awareness, and cost consciousness. Today's nurses are autonomous, independent, assertive, and collaborative" (pp. 38–39). The differences in the ways nurses and physicians rated the variables of competition, compromise, and accommodation that might have been predicted in the past when the doctor–nurse game was fully engaged did not materialize, according to Jones. Nurses were much like their physician counterparts—equally as assertive and competitive. Jones briefly recommends a team approach to achieving collaboration based on an integration of four elements: vision and shared objectives, participative safety, commitment to team excellence, and support for innovation (p. 255).

A Swiss nurse educator, in a 1995 paper on the state of interprofessional cooperation in hospitals from the perspective of nurses, stated, "It is high time and possible to revise the doctor–nurse game from one based on power to one based on professionalism and personality—for the patient's sake" (p. 254). Kappeli's notion of revision is a lot more than simply changing the rules of the game. She wants to abandon the game and rebuild the social, cultural, psychological, and intellectual structures undergirding nurse–physician relationships and the whole of health care delivery. "Changing society without changing its structures is not possible" (p. 255).

In the doctor–nurse game, there were winners and losers, with physicians the winners and nurses the losers. Stein et al. stated in 1990, "The traditional doctor–nurse game exerts a stifling, anti-intellectual effect on nurses, and the resultant dissatisfaction with professional roles and interprofessional relationships contributes substantially to the nursing shortage" (p. 549). Kerfoot (1994) recommends changing the games played by health care providers from games that have win–lose rules to games that have zero-sum or win–win rules.

The articulation of the doctor–nurse game, the warmth with which it was embraced by the nursing community, and the subsequent distancing from the game by the nursing community parallel the larger changes in nursing and health care and society as a whole. The study of the utilization of the game as a framework for describing physician–nurse relations by nurse and physician scholars was at one time extremely instructive; it is no longer. At the very least, a new game is needed; at most, a whole new paradigm is preferred.

Systems Paradigm

The final conceptual or theoretical framework found in the early literature and presented in this section was an extension of the work of the
NJPC into a very simple systems model. Koerner et al. (1985) describe
how several years after the four NJPC demonstration projects had
ended, they implemented collaborative practice on a model unit at Hartford Hospital. Several features described certify their approach as a
systems approach. First, they describe the patient care system they were
designing as comprised of organizational factors, workload factors, and
environmental factors, and they speak of this approach as useful for
addressing the interrelatedness of all these variables to patient care outcomes. Second, they describe a planning process occurring over several
months and integrating education, communication, and planning. Finally,
following the unanimous recommendation of participants in the original
NJPC model, the implementers at Hartford Hospital executed all five
elements of the NJPC model *at once*.

Koerner et al. (1985) reported that they had defined collaboration as
"[a] planned system through which members of the medical and nursing
professions, together with other related health care disciplines, work to
assure consistent, quality patient and family care" (p. 40). Following
implementation of the collaborative practice model, evaluation was conducted. Findings are reported as very positive. "In the collaborative practice system, patients see an environment of mutual respect that enhances
communication, coordination, and continuity between nurses, MDs, and
patients. The result of this is more knowledgeable care providers, improved quality of care delivered to patients, and increased family involvement in the process" (p. 320).

LATER LITERATURE

Integrative Research Taxonomy

In urging new integrative models of interdisciplinary research because
simply "combining research concepts and approaches is not sufficient,"
Rosenfield (1992, p. 1345) proposes a simple taxonomy of cross-disciplinary research in three levels. Level one (lowest level) has researchers
working in parallel or sequentially from their specific disciplinary bases

to address common problems. Level two (mid-level) has researchers working jointly but still from their disciplinary bases to address common problems. Level three (highest level on the continuum) has researchers working together from shared conceptual or theoretical frameworks to address common problems jointly described.

Rosenfield also describes implications and opportunities (actual or projected) from the implementation of these various levels, asserting that the mid-level needs strengthening and that the highest level does not exist. Positive outcomes of mid-level approaches could be problem solving and creative new programs, whereas outcomes at the top level could be broadly based programs and long-range problem solving; new concepts, methods, and policies can be inferred (pp. 1351–1353).

If interdisciplinary research is accepted as a collaborative model, a tentative idea, this taxonomy then, perhaps, represents a continuum of collaboration. The issue could become a determining factor in deciding which approach to disciplinary integrative research is most desirable for exploring a particular topic and resolving specific problems. Approaching a particular problem from two or more disciplinary perspectives such as occurs in an interdisciplinary approach might be the most fruitful way to proceed. It also might be best to approach a topic from both interdisciplinary and transdisciplinary perspectives.

This assertion that the integrative research continuum is a continuum of collaboration is a most interesting one, particularly if this means that collaboration occurs in stages or that one can move from a lower level of collaboration to a higher level. In other words, using this example, can the interdisciplinary researcher or research team advance from the level of interdisciplinary research to that of transdisciplinary research as a result of engaging in the former? The idea of a typology, which means kinds or types of collaboration, usually occurring at a different place on a continuum (often and in this case, vertical), also is of some interest.

The findings of the concept analysis presented in Chapters 1 and 2 support the notion that one cannot have a little bit of collaboration. It seems that either a relationship is collaborative or it is not. Also, the concept analysis demonstrated repeatedly that nonsupportive environments, poor relationships, minimal effort, or absence of shared goals did not and could not lead to collaboration. In other words, negative positions on a conceived continuum are not starting points in collaborative models that either have been written about or are actually occurring. What seems then to be possible is that there could be two kinds of collaboration here—interdisciplinary and transdisciplinary. Both are collaborative; they share the same or almost identical attributes but are configured somewhat differently. This still leaves us with the problem of levels of collaboration, unless these two kinds are equal in strength and potential effectiveness of both process and outcome. If that is the case, however, the idea of levels ceases to be of concern. This is an important issue because we are seeing that the literature contains myriad continua even though the concept analysis would seem to negate their conceptual validity.

It should be noted that all other continua considered thus far were of a concept other than collaboration, such as assertiveness and cooperation. Even the conceptual framework put forward by Styles to study education–service continua is of one of unity not of collaboration. The following are suggested propositions concerning continua of collaboration:

> One cannot progress from an oppositional or negative position on collaboration to collaboration in a linear pattern of progression. (Such a continuum would be one of other than collaboration to collaboration.)
>
> One may move from a neutral position on collaboration to a positive position, but the neutral position is not a necessary starting point of or for collaboration.
>
> A continuum of collaboration, connoting levels of strength or growth, might be used relative to configuring young to mature collaborative relationships. A new relationship might still be fragile with respect to decision making or trust, as examples.

Miccolo and Spanier (1993) in their report of developing collaborative practices in ICUs describe a paradigm of contracting along a continuum. They seem to be proposing that a process of developing and refining a contract is parallel and essential to the development of a collaborative practice. This is a continuum that occurs in three stages, or levels. In the beginning, the would-be collaborators form a contract. This is the stage at which the nature of the collaboration is decided; roles, along with performance expectations, are outlined. Questions of who, where, why, and of what the attributes of the relationship will be are addressed. Stage 1, thus, is contract development.

Stage 2 is contract execution. Individuals begin to be comfortable working together; a feeling of partnership begins to be present. "Constant testing occurs throughout [this phase] and serves to keep the process dynamic" (p. 445). Protocols for the practice are designed during this period.

Stage 3 is contract refinement. Negotiation skills develop; the team works together to solve problems. The true strength of the relationship begins to be manifest. At this stage, the relationship usually becomes self-correcting and self-generating.

This paradigm starts out as a linear continuum of contracting for collaboration but develops more of a systems approach as the evaluation and refinement of the paradigm plays out in the actual situation. This continuum represents the type of continuum whereby the maturity of a collaborative model can be either plotted or tested. The idea of contracting, so long as it is broadly and informally defined, could prove to be a useful way to define operationally the development and implementation of a collaborative practice.

The concept of contracting, in a very formal sense, to establish a collaborative practice arrangement is widespread in the United States in connection with implementing collaborative practices mandated by state legislatures and monitored by regulatory agencies. Chapter 11 explores the efficacy of such mandates. In the meantime, Miccolo and Spanier (1993) take pains to point out that they are not talking about externally forced relationships when they speak of contracting. This seems to be an important difference as compared with forced or induced collaboration. "Collaboration or partnership arose . . . out of a defined need and was not legislated. It required nurturing, fostering, and development" (p. 444).

Integrative Practice Continuum

Shawler et al. (1990), followed later by Kopser et al. (1994), describe an integrated practice model for collaboration among nurses. The model itself is of interest here because it is presented as part of a so-called continuum of collaborative models clearly described by Schroeder (1992). The continuum describes four approaches to collaboration: the parallel approach, the antagonistic approach, the avoidance approach, and the integrated approach. The integrated approach is described as involving group problem solving and open communication. The model is used in these cases by teams of collaborating nurses—clinical nurse specialist, nurse manager, and staff development instructor. Based on our prior discussion and a simple review of the terms, it is readily apparent that this is not a continuum of collaboration. It is, perhaps, a typology of kinds of relationships that nurses in practice develop with each other over time.

Course Outline

Only one content-based curriculum model was found in the database of 81 articles. Although not presented as a conceptual framework, the list of topics intends to encompass a comprehensive package of cognitive and affective knowledge required for entering and sustaining a MD–RN collaborative practice. Reynolds et al. (1994) developed their course to be taught by an interdisciplinary faculty to an interdisciplinary student body. They suggest that the course work be supplemented by clinical experiences and culminate in actual collaborative practices. The course content outline is as follows:

- "Systems barriers to interprofessional collaboration,
- "Delivery models that enhance collaboration and interdisciplinary care,
- "Examination of successful collaborative practice case studies,
- "Differing vocabularies and clinical perspectives of various disciplines,
- "Principles of team building and team leadership, and
- "Communication, negotiation, and conflict resolution skills" (p. 561)

Poststructuralist View

Henneman (1995) urges adoption of a poststructuralist view of the nursing disciplinary world, particularly one that steeps the discipline in the views of Michel Foucault, poststructuralist philosopher. Henneman apparently strongly believes that this philosophical perspective provides nursing with a firm foundation for then entering into collaborative relationships in practice and research with MDs and other colleagues in the health sciences.

Poststructuralism holds that the ultimate way to understand, the ultimate way to approach a practice challenge, is to have no methodological or sociological structures imposed. In conducting research and scholarship, theories and methodologies are considered restrictive if they limit the possibilities of discovery. Foucault (cited in Henneman 1995, p. 361) holds that knowledge is power, and that dominant groups (such as medicine) have controlled knowledge and used it to advance their own ends.

Henneman's principal concern is with research and scholarship, rather than practice, although the thesis of *power is knowledge* very directly impacts practice. She discusses, for example, nursing being forced into a logical positivist view of science that has retarded nursing's development as a distinct discipline able to make its special contribution to patient care, to the detriment of people in need of care. Three themes clearly emerge in Foucault's work: power or knowledge, discipline, and theory. Henneman presents the following several assumptions, derived from Foucault, and relates them to nursing knowledge or science and collaboration:

"Assumption 1. Power or knowledge relations are not fixed." (Henneman 1995, p. 362). Shared power, therefore, through collaboration, is possible for nursing despite hierarchies that might reinforce traditional power relations.

"Assumption 2. Meaning is not stable." (Henneman 1995, p. 362). Meaning is always related to time and social context. Our task is to describe the present and ourselves in the present. The present requires a reevaluation of the independent and interdependent roles of health professionals.

"Assumption 3. The 'official' discourse is not the 'real' discourse." (Henneman 1995, p. 362). To study power or knowledge relations, one must get beyond the official rules and dialogue to the underlying real rules in order to get beyond institutional control of thought and action.

"Assumption 4. Theory is practice. The poststructuralist believes theories to be oppressive in that they are limiting" (Henneman 1995, p. 363). The energies of the investigator or theorist or scientist of collaboration would best be directed toward reexamination of the rules that at present guide the way nurses work with other disciplines.

"Assumption 5. Truth is not the goal of science. Our goal should be to never stop inquiring" (Henneman 1995, p. 363). There are multiple truths and multiple ways of knowing the truth. The goal of inquiry is to find resolutions for problems we are facing. The goal of nursing in a practice discipline is to affect patient care outcomes positively (Henneman, p. 363).

Role Theory

Only one article in the later literature uses a clear role theory framework, although the language and many of the concepts of role theory seem to be ingrained in the health care lexicon. For example, Henneman (1995), who espouses approaching collaboration from no prior perspective, still speaks of negotiating roles.

A new kind of game, briefly discussed in the early literature section, is proposed by Kerfoot (1994) to promote health care workers changing from a we-versus-they perspective to a perspective that focuses on the organization, working with teams, being patient focused, and empowering employees (p. 100). The game is a non–zero-sum or win–win game instead of a win–lose game. In a non–zero-sum game, "the concept of an opponent is inappropriate, the players are not envious of each other, and the interests of the participants partially coincide and partially conflict" (p. 100).

Unfortunately, most of us have been brought up to play zero-sum games. We need to work hard to overcome the conditioning that propels us to keep on playing win–lose games. Kerfoot urges that "[i]n an era of health care that values partnerships, coalitions, mergers, and alliances, we must unlearn our zero-sum, win–lose games and rethink a paradigm of non–zero-sum games in which cooperation, collaboration, and win–win is the norm" (p. 100). The game model, which is of course a role theory approach, is then encompassed by Kerfoot within a systems approach for its implementation. The theory of cooperation, a systems-type model, is briefly described in the next section.

Systems Models

Kerfoot (1994) uses Axelrod's (1984) theory of cooperation as the framework for motivating transforming behaviors from win–lose to win–win gamesmanship. Although Kerfoot does not describe the theory of cooperation fully, some interesting concepts emerge: 1) Cooperation can occur among workers without strong central authority. Democratic models of sharing authority within synergistic, high-performing teams facilitate the development of cooperation. 2) "By developing close associations over time, a degree of relatedness ensues" (Kerfoot 1994, p. 100). Those wanting to work in a cooperative mode must be in close and frequent association over time. 3) The higher and more frequent the degree of association, the more positive the degree of altruism. People reciprocate altruism that is directed toward them. 4) "An important new type of cooperation in this era of health care reform is *reciprocal altruism* . . . trading of altruistic acts in which benefit is larger than cost so that over a period of time both enjoy a net gain" (p. 100).

This conceptual model or theory of cooperation is clearly useful for adapting to a complex health care environment, such as a hospital or an interorganizational coalition, and for developing cooperative and, likely, collaborative relationships. Within the hospital setting, nurse managers, for example, must closely associate with a wide variety of workers across many disciplines in order to achieve transdisciplinary care delivery that is beneficial to patients and families. Close connections must also be developed and maintained with social workers, home care workers, payors and so forth in the integrated health care networks of the present and the future. The theory of collaboration promotes these close and continuous associations. It is also noted that as a part of applying the theory of cooperation, people should "be taught caring and reciprocity so that we have the cultures within which to cooperate" (p. 101).

Several continua are put forward in the later literature from a systems perspective. The first presented here is a continuum model of interprofessional communication, as proposed by Mailick and Jordan (1977) and used by Miccolo and Spanier (1993) as a component of their work in developing a collaborative practice model in an ICU. The model asserts three levels of interprofessional communication. From the least to the most collaborative, these are authoritative, consensus, and true collaboration. "The effectiveness of the communication is contingent on the congruency between the expectations and the needs of the individual, the task to be performed, and the goals of the practice" (p. 446). The highest level of interprofessional communication is the level of true collaboration. At this level, there is mutual goal setting and a partnership. This is, of course, not a continuum of collaboration. It is, rather, a continuum of interprofessional communication with only one level, the highest level, being one of collaboration.

In 1994, Murphy and Stern published the results of a grounded theory study. They interviewed 14 staff nurses and 2 staff MDs in a small ICU. In addition, they used participant observation techniques. They were seeking insights from these practitioners about successful strategies for collaboration. The set of strategies they discovered are expert interpersonal skills, professional accountability, competence, trust, and equal contribution to health care. From their data they described a nascent conceptual framework for collaboration: joining forces.

Joining forces is defined as the process whereby RNs and MDs come together and work together; it influences the quality of care (p. 18). Two categories, *relating* and *accountability,* are the conditions that enable the joining of forces in critical care. Respecting, valuing, and risk taking are elements of relating; advocating, coordinating, and liaisoning are elements of accountability (p. 18). Murphy and Stern suggest that this framework represents a beginning for capturing the rich data gathered. Although the authors do not describe it as such, it appears that the connections or link-ages of these elements to each other and their integration and interrelation among collaborators justifies labeling this framework as a systems type.

Bruiniks et al. (1994) write at length about the problems of fragmen-tation of social and health services for children in the United States. As outcomes of a multidisciplinary conference about children at the Univer-sity of Minnesota, two models were created to address reform of services for children and ways to structure community approaches to children's services. It is noteworthy that the problems have been those of both frag-mentation and ignorance. The solutions addressed require linking com-munity organizations, and developing common knowledge bases for understanding and action. The inclusion of this article in the database and the two continuum models put forward add substantially to the depth and breadth of our conceptualizations of interorganizational collaboration.

The mission being addressed is "To insure a healthy future for chil-dren, systems of support must evolve a more holistic focus on individual and family needs through practices that maximize collaboration among education, health, social, and economic support services" (Bruiniks et al. 1994, p. 242). The conceptual framework designed to respond to this mission has four linked components:

"1. Reform services for children and youth by linking social, health, and economic support services more closely to schools and related educational institutions . . .

"2. Policy coherence and values. These are the foundation of any reform initiative. Integrated services must be grounded in clear and explicit beliefs, values, goals, outcomes, and standards. These beliefs and values become the underlying policy guidelines upon which just and ethical decisions are based.

"3.   Leadership. Leadership in service integration reform is needed to clarify the values and benefits of collaboration and the limits of authority. It is needed at every level—federal government to family—to create the vision and reality of coherent policies and to construct principles to guide legislation, policy, and service strategies. (The point is also made that to achieve true collaboration, leadership should be shared broadly and many people empowered with decision-making capabilities.)

"4.   Structure. The collaborative work to achieve service integration must address the issues of structure. Collaboration, cooperation, and coordination differ in structure from each other [and the organizational designs should strengthen the selected approach]" (pp. 244–245).

These four features—reform services linked to schools and to each other, policy coherence and values, leadership that is empowering and promotes collaboration, and facilitative organizational structure—constitute a system for designing and succeeding in the provision of comprehensive services for children and youth. It seems that they could also be very useful in designing other health and social services or in the analysis and evaluation of existing social services. The model design is comprehensive in its reach and offers a framework for holistic approaches to children within a multidisciplinary and collaborative perspective. It is depicted as a pictorial model (p. 244) in a diamond shape with structure, leadership, resources (services), and policy coherence each occupying one of the angles in an unbroken symbol.

Bruiniks et al. (1994) proceed to articulate a typology of structures. They defined these types after analyzing structures of extant models throughout the United States. The desired structure, they say, is one that supports collaboration, not merely cooperation or coordination. It shares responsibility, resources, and rewards and assumes mutual authority and accountability. Three distinct structures have emerged around the country. They present on a continuum with three levels of collaborative strength:

Lowest level: Ring Model—cooperative. Multiple agencies have a common mission. Each maintains separate identity and autonomy. The model is usually voluntary.

Middle level: Spoke Model—coordination. A primary agency is at the hub with links to other agencies. All agencies share broadly based goals.

Many collaborating agencies are functioning at the local level providing direct services while linked to the central agency, which is coordinating services and facilitating them.

Highest level: Spiral Model—collaboration. A single agency grows by acquiring and administering previously separately owned and administered agencies. This model has the strength of one administration but the weakness of other organizations lacking a sense of buy-in or ownership (p. 245).

The model can be contrasted with Styles's (1984) unity continuum for education–service organizations. The highest level of Styles's model, unification, is much like this highest model, spiral. As discussed earlier, neither continuum is a continuum of collaboration. This continuum, especially, seems conceptually flawed. The so-called highest level of structure, labeled *collaboration,* is not collaboration at all. The middle level, labeled *coordination,* seems to be the most integrated model and, therefore, contains many attributes of collaboration. Yet, the authors tell us that both "the ring model and the spoke model encompass some principles of successful collaboration, but do not cement relationships because funding and resources are not shared or the sharing is limited" (p. 245).

Systems Vignettes

Several systems models are briefly presented to complete this presentation of the conceptual or theoretical frameworks in the literature. Similarities are recognizable as all make use of systems approaches and concepts.

Using storytelling and narrative as conversational tools, Baker and Diekelmann (1994) call for *connecting conversations* among nurses, MDs, and all members of the health care team, as well as patients and families, to recall the narrative to our shared practice, to collaborate in the story of healing. The premise this activity is based on is that "[c]entral to building collegial, collaborative relationships within the health care disciplines is an understanding of the lived experience of the other within her or his caregiving practices" (p. 66). From a systems perspective, connecting the systems loops or closing the openings between the loops is a central task. The system cannot become or remain whole without connectedness. Storytelling appears to offer much promise in facilitating the development of collaborative systems of care.

Transformational leadership and its important role in an organization's or group's task of creating a *shared vision* is described in an essay by McMahon (1992). Both strategies are connecting tools for creating, sustaining, and developing collaborative systems. Transformational leadership pulls the group toward a shared vision, which is recognized as profoundly different than pushing toward a goal (Evans 1994, McMahon 1992). It is a defining characteristic of transformational leadership that it engage the group in the process of developing a shared vision.

"Vision has two fundamental elements. One is to provide people a conceptual framework or paradigm for understanding the organization's purpose . . . the second important element is the emotional appeal: the part of the vision that has a motivational pull with which people can identify" (Tichy and Devanna 1986, p. 1). "The vision rarely tends to be one person's dream but rather the expressed commitment of the group" (Tichy and Devanna, p. 128). McMahon (1992) advocates integrating the processes of transformational leadership and shared visioning within a shared governance model, which is a systems framework in and of itself.

Evans (1994) describes *transformational leadership* as a paradigm of empowerment and as a facilitator of collaboration within an organization or group. Evans hypothesizes that it is *the* leadership model needed to foster collaboration in health care organizations. Transformational leaders have charisma, vision, self-confidence, and inner strength. They treat workers as individuals, raise subordinates to higher levels of awareness of issues of importance, and generally create a *capacitating environment*, a feature of which is a "fit" between the individual worker and the environment as well as the resources in the environment (Evans, pp. 28–29).

Capacitating Environments

- Empower workers
- Stimulate creativity of workers
- Promote teamwork and learning
- Promote comfort with implementing change
- Motivate staff to accept increased responsibility
- Develop workers' potential
- Facilitate staff understanding of organizational goals
- Leaders delegate responsibility appropriately
- Enable workers to communicate openly and directly
- Foster collaboration with peers (Evans 1994, p. 29)

The elements of a capacitating environment all constitute implicit relational statements that could form premises of a conceptual or theoretical framework or could form hypotheses that could be used in research designs to indeed test the validity of these claims for a capacitating environment. Evans offers the model as a speculative act. She believes in the assertions she makes, but admits these to be her speculations. The model offers a useful systems conceptualization to the literature and adds greatly to our understanding of the environment and the leadership required to facilitate collaboration.

Case management, P. K. Jones (1994) asserts, is but the latest nursing service delivery model imposed on nursing by external forces, the earlier ones being functional nursing, team nursing, and primary nursing. These were forced, respectively, by the industrial society, a nursing shortage, consumer demand, and cost containment (p. 32). Case management came about because of the demand for cost containment. It also requires a focus on quality. These two seemingly disparate demands—do good, but do it with less—have given rise to concerted efforts to achieve high-quality care in cost-beneficial ways. Case management, by definition, contends Jones, requires collaboration. The various providers and disciplines must work together to avoid costly duplication of care and to bring to the patient and his or her family the collective expertise of all necessary providers.

Jones then suggests that teamwork and collaborative decision making enable systems to improve their case management strategies and their total quality management (TQM). The obvious conclusion Jones reached was that the entire multi-institutional system with which she was concerned needed to be transformed from one of other practice models to collaborative practice. Peter Senge's (1990) model of *systems thinking* was utilized by Jones and co-workers to design a leadership curriculum for the entire Franciscan health care system. The goal is to transform all of the system's facilities into shared governance, collaborative practice models. The model combines Senge's five disciplines of personal mastery, mental models, team learning, shared vision, and systems thinking with quality improvement tools and an implicit conceptualization of transformational leadership into an integrated curriculum entitled "Planning For Future Leadership."

Unfortunately, reports of outcomes of the curriculum design, as well as the implementation, are anecdotal and brief. One recommendation

P. K. Jones did make was that *all* departments and disciplines at *all* levels in the organization needed to participate in both design and implementation activities. Although not expounded upon here, Senge's model of systems thinking has much to offer to the topic of collaboration by health care practitioners within health care education and practice organizations. It is shared at length in the next chapter on theory development for collaboration. Overall, Jones's model presents a fairly comprehensive systems model for approaching a huge task of transforming a large, complex system. Certainly, her work would be useful to another organization contemplating similar changes. It would have been helpful to have a stronger focus on implementation and the processes of promoting the change over time, including the inputs to the systems, the reinforcements, the connections, and the balancing mechanisms.

As an outgrowth of mentoring of doctoral students over the years, Meleis et al. (1994) proposed a conceptual framework of *collaborative mentorship*. It is defined as an "active, dynamic approach that demonstrates solidarity in the pursuit of scholarship, incorporating principles of feminist pedagogy" (p. 179). The features of collaborative mentorship, we are told, are negotiated relations, mutual interactions, facilitative strategies, and empowerment.

Negotiated relations imply that the student may legitimately seek different mentors depending on the student's substantive learning need. It also means that the student may modify mentoring relationships through "mutual negotiation to accommodate changing academic needs" (Meleis et al. 1994, p. 179). "Mutual interactions are horizontal communications, not paternalistic or unidirectional. Collaborative mentoring is an ongoing dialogue among and between colleagues characterized by reciprocity. Feminism emphasizes mutual give and take" (p. 179).

Facilitative strategies demonstrate "solidarity" (p. 179) in celebrating academic accomplishments. Participants, regardless of rank or position, support the scholarly work of the other(s). Colleagues join together to assist with scholarly papers, projects, presentations, pursuit of funding, and all the various work—exalted and mundane—of scholarship.

Empowerment is demonstrated through collectivity, consciousness-raising, and change. Collectivity refers to the student not being confined to a single mentor, but rather able to benefit from the aggregate wisdom of several; empowerment involves consciousness-raising by systematically questioning unquestioned assumptions that keep nursing from growing toward its full potentials; and change is an outcome of the empowering mentorship. The intellectual, sociocultural, and political competencies of the mentees are all greatly enhanced (Meleis et al. 1994, pp. 179–180).

Although the particulars of the subject may change in topics of orga-nization, education, research, or practice, it is apparent that in all foci, the dynamics and principles of collaboration form recognizable patterns and interrelationships. The attributes of collaboration are present from setting to setting and from partnership to partnership. Also apparent is the conceptual or theoretical mandate for a holistic view of collaboration, rather than a fragmented image. Collaboration does not seem to occur in fragments; it is or it is not. Systems approaches to knowing and doing collaboration, therefore, seem to be the way to proceed. They offer the tools for holistic and comprehensive treatment of the subject within a dynamic context.

While the earlier conceptualizations of collaboration were dispropor-tionately couched in role theory models, later conceptualizations are dis-proportionately weighted in favor of systems models. The reason for this could be that the pace and direction of the larger society is propelling health care practice and service and collaboration in the direction of sys-tems approaches as a desired way to deal with and manage ever-increas-ing complexity. Or there may be another explanation. The next section ventures to answer to these questions as collaboration in health care is placed into the larger societal context.

SOCIETAL CONTEXT OR COLLABORATION

Enlightened Problem Solving

During the 1970s and early 1980s, health care educators and practition-ers and policy influentials utilized collaboration to overcome serious and persistent, but clearly defined, problems. Registered nurses voiced widespread dissatisfaction with their practices in hospitals arising out of their powerlessness to influence the direction of patient care. This was the major impetus for the NJPC and the subsequent establishment of the model demonstration projects. At the same time, there was acknowl-edged concern with the fragmentation of patient care in hospitals.

Collaborative practice could improve nurse satisfaction with hospital-based practice while also providing better coordination of patient care. The idea was to give nurses more control over their practice, to give them a greater and shared role in decision making about patient care and to empower them. The reasoning was sound, but the problem was deep-seated and widespread.

The dissatisfaction of RNs with hospital practice led to a decline in interest in nursing as a career choice. Coupled with the openness to women of fields such as management that had not traditionally welcomed them, the sharp drop in applications to schools of nursing by the mid-1980s was recognized as a very serious potential problem for the future of health care. Educational institutions were immediately affected, and they were recognized as also being part of the problem. Educational reform in response to enrollment decline was rampant. Of interest to our subject of collaboration is the attention shown to collaboration between education and service to enrich the education of the students.

Collaborative arrangements as outlined in Styles's (1984) unity continuum were enacted. Faculty practice, staff appointments as faculty, and student preceptorships are but some of the strategies that were developed. The long-standing and persistent separation of education and service was perceived as contributing to the sense of powerlessness in the field along with a persistent sense of lack of credibility with peers in the health sciences. The practice discipline of nursing was peopled by faculty who did not practice nursing and by staff nurses who did not teach nursing. The joining of nursing education and nursing service facilitated an increased sense of control over nursing in both the education and service arenas. The resulting growing sense of legitimacy of nursing as a peer practice discipline increased the sense of empowerment of nurse educators and clinicians. In turn, students likely received a higher-quality, more energetic education.

Another early problem addressed was the federally defined shortage of primary care physicians. The nascent nurse practitioner educational programs aimed to prepare a provider who, practicing with a physician collaborator, could offer most of the services that would be offered by a physician, if one were available. Nurse practitioner education received tremendous support from the Surgeon General's report *Toward Quality In Nursing* (1963), which strongly recommended that nurses be given authority to use independent judgment in meeting their responsibilities. It was recognized that with increased education, nurses could provide much of the primary care offered by MDs. Within much of the nursing community, it was also recognized that nurse practitioners practicing from their nursing discipline could provide a unique and desirable blend of nursing and medical care.

Empowerment Movements

The loud and clear messages transmitted by hospital staff nurses about their dissatisfaction with practice signaled a new assertiveness—an unwillingness to endure any longer conditions unacceptable to them. Their behavior was illustrative of the societal empowerment movement for women's rights. Nursing, primarily a field of work peopled by women and doing work labeled as mainly women's work, strengthened its activities to advance the field to both professional and academic disciplinary status. The focus on achieving college education for nursing at the entry level intensified. The pursuit of master's and doctoral degrees in nursing and the correlative explosive growth of new master's programs to prepare nurses for specialty practice in advanced roles, as well as the growth of doctoral programs to prepare nurse scientists and academicians, spread across the nation. New graduates at both entry and advanced levels were socialized as patient advocates; they were expected to pursue autonomous nursing practice for the patient's sake.

At the same time that nurses were seeking a greater voice in health care, so were consumers. Their expectations of receiving information about their health and their bodies pressured MDs, in particular, and other health care providers to change the doctor–patient relationship. Patients—called consumers of health care—demanded a greater voice in their own care. Interest groups, performing in unison, demanded and gained a greater voice in health care policy making. Who can forget Maggie Kuhn, founder of the Gray Panthers and tireless advocate on behalf of the elderly, educating, persuading, and cajoling government officials, insurance companies, and fellow citizens to provide for the rights of the elderly, especially their right to decent health care? She taught us all about advocacy and, indeed, set a new standard for self-advocacy by an organized interest group in the United States. It is common at present to define the seriousness of the problems of a given population group by the presence or absence of effective advocacy. "Who will advocate on behalf of children?" we say, or "No one cares enough about the poor to advocate on their behalf."

With their newfound sense of empowerment, consumers began to question the decisions and behaviors of their physicians. There was growing recognition that MDs did not have all the answers, nor were they as concerned about patients as consumers thought they ought to be. Doctors began to be perceived by consumers as interested mainly in their incomes and status to the detriment of their concern for their patients. As Gillick stated in her 1992 analysis of the changed attitudes toward MDs: "Doctors are criticized for not spending enough time with patients, for being insufficiently caring, for an excessive reliance on technology, and generally for inadequate attention to the whole person" (p. 83).

Nurses started to refuse to play the doctor–nurse game. Their newfound sense of professional self-esteem emboldened them to join forces with consumers to let it be known that the biomedical model, with its major focus on curing disease to the exclusion of a more integrative focus that would also include psychosocial and behavioral processes, was not providing people with high-quality health care (Weiss 1985). A multidisciplinary team-oriented approach to health care was needed to provide this more comprehensive focus. Perhaps a new era in health care was at hand. A new balance of power and resulting new relationships were occurring between and among nurses, patients, and MDs.

Weiss wrote in 1985:

It is increasingly apparent that physicians have neither the education nor experience to deal with those aspects of health care involving human needs and behavior. Physician expertise, as a norm, is limited to a thorough, scientific understanding and use of these areas of competence which underlie collaboration in health care: for collaboration assumes that the strengths and skills of all individuals are recognized and used to their greatest potential. Collaboration also assumes that tasks are negotiated, in light of conflicting interests and goals, rather than coercively prescribed; and that inputs and actions of the collaborative team build upon one another in a mutual problem-solving fashion, rather than via strict hierarchies established by a unilateral source (p. 49).

Hospital-Based Illness Care Is Changing

Traditional definitions of patients, nurses, and physicians were changing by the early to mid-'80s. The work of the NJPC had had an impact. Even though relationships among these groups were the same as they always had been, in most places there was a new sense of what was possible, which likely caused *dis-ease* among those who preferred the traditional mode of operating. To add to the discomfort caused by these changes was the universal realization that hospital-based practice was changing dramatically.

Hospitals increasingly were places of high-technology care; patients were sicker than ever; the numbers of specialties and subspecialties proliferated along with the numbers of professional or technical providers and assistive workers. (The author noted at least 22 different uniforms signifying the various types of workers at a single community hospital in 1974.) Attending MDs, however, spent noticeably less time with their patients as highly skilled intensive care nurses and salaried house doctors cared for the patients while in the extremely complex hospital setting.

By 1982 or 1983, the chorus of calls for cost containment became loud and persistent. The implementation of diagnostic-related groups (DRGs) and other cost-containment methods accelerated the challenges of complexity that hospitals and providers were facing. These prospective payment models paid so much and no more for patient care in a given diagnostic category. The idea of keeping people at home for as much of their illness episode as possible came into vogue. Patients were entering the hospital later in their course of illness and were discharged sooner. *Sicker and quicker* became the shorthand phrase for this universal reality. The idea of empty hospital beds, which had been anathema in the old, retrospective payment model, was welcomed in the new cost-containment model of payment as long as the hospital entity had the person registered as a patient. Same-day surgery centers, 23-hour admissions, home care units, and other arrangements aimed at minimizing time spent in the hospital thus came into being. The notion of a hospital without walls was born.

After struggling for a few years with this increasingly complex world of the hospital, the chorus began to shout for quality control in hospitals and, in order to promote quality, renewed vigor in employing collaborative practice. In the cover story of *Hospitals,* April 20, 1991, Eubanks states:

> Improving nurse–physician relations has long been tagged as a top concern by nurse and physician executives, as well as by many hospital CEOs. But only recently has this concern become an action item on many hospitals' agendas. The time is ripe for change, hospital executives say. They cite a confluence of factors that have forged opportunity in this area: the effects of cost containment, the rising acuity of patients, expanded use of high-technology treatments, chronic labor shortages, the

impact of the consumer and feminist movements, and society's shifting values regarding work. . . .

[P]erhaps the strongest stimulus for change in nurse–physician relations is the quest for quality. Hospital administrators say that efforts to improve quality may serve as a vehicle for transforming the relationship between the two professions. The success of individual hospitals will be linked to the ability of each institution to facilitate the nurse–physician relationship, executives say. Nurse–physician relations have to be the highest priority now (p. 26).

The focus on TQM and the related requirement of physician–nurse collaborative practice was codified in the Joint Commission on Accreditation of Health Care Organizations (JCAHO). Standards and criteria requiring that quality control systems be in place have been incorporated into guidelines for accreditation (Dumont and Niziolek 1991, Eubanks 1991).

Enlightened Professionalism

There is evidence in the literature that by the 1990s, many health care organizations and providers were passionately committed to interdisciplinary and collaborative practice in their settings as a result of the previously discussed environmental and societal changes (Cowley 1994, Evans 1994, Kerfoot 1994, McEwen 1994, Miccolo and Spanier 1994). As early as 1990, myriad professional associations created and put forward policy or position statements endorsing collaboration within and between disciplines for both practice and education. The American Hospital Association, the American Academy of Pediatrics, the National Perinatal Association, The Nurses Association of The American College of Obstetricians and Gynecologists, and the American Association of Colleges of Nursing are but a few of the many endorsing organizations.

Movement was away from turfism and toward shared practices as a way to ensure the very survival of a good health care system in the United States and even internationally. Cowley (1994), speaking of health care in Great Britain, asserts: "It is highly unlikely a single practitioner could maintain sufficient expertise to cover all the health needs in a given area or caseload" (p. 14). McEwen (1994), speaking of health care in the United States, asserts: "The human service professions are facing problems so complex that no single discipline can possibly respond to them effectively. . . . [E]ach crisis] requires a comprehensive approach and necessitates that professionals relate to many clients and institutional systems and collaborate with many professions" (p. 307).

Health Care Reform

With the hindsight of time passing and the insights gained from this analysis, we are neither surprised by, nor do we believe it was unexpected that, the chorus reached a crescendo of demand for health care reform by 1992. In the political election for the U.S. Senate in the fall of 1991, however, it was a shock to the country and to the politicians when unknown educator Harrison Wofford of Pennsylvania was elected to complete the term of an incumbent who had died in office. He had run on a platform of health care reform. In winning, he defeated a well-known, well-regarded former U.S. Attorney General, Richard Thornburgh. Presidential candidate Bill Clinton took notice. Health care reform at the federal level became a cornerstone of his campaign for the presidency. Access to health care, affordability of health care, and quality health care became, and largely still are, the three foci of health care reform.

Terms to describe U.S. health care were, and are, high-technology, specialist-oriented, hospital-based, illness-oriented, emergency-oriented, expensive, and wasteful. A new paradigm of health care, it was and is argued by some policymakers, health care providers, insurors, and foundations, should encompass a health care system that shifts from treatment to prevention, illness to wellness, hospital to community, episodic care to primary care, costly to cost containment, specialist to generalist, disease-centered to person- and family- and community-centered, MD-driven to consumer-driven, individual providers to teams of providers, and fragmented to networked. The nation seemed poised to adopt a major health care system that would address the major shifts outlined. The thrust toward collaborative practice to provide high-quality, cost-effective care seemed inexorable. The need was sharply defined, the efficacy of collaborative practice well documented, and the background of experience in establishing collaborative practice available to draw upon. It seemed that the nation was going to achieve massive health care reform and that collaborative practice was going to be a centerpiece.

Such was not to be the case. The moment came and went. The debate in Congress became very acrimonious and partisan. The reforms Congress called for were largely financial despite the ambitious health care reform plans put forward by the President and others. Congress aimed to overcome such economically based issues as insurance inequities, maldistribution of providers, and wastefulness and administrative bloat. Reforms such as management of care, integration of care, and waste reduction were called for. Current federal policy discussions concerning health care focus on substantially slowing the growth of Medicare and shifting Medicaid responsibilities exclusively to the states in block grants. (In 1996, a modest reform bill was enacted into law. It protects workers who can afford to pay the premiums from losing their health insurance when they are between employment.)

Despite federal failure to enact health care reform legislation and the federal shift in foci, major changes are occurring in the financing of health care in the United States that are largely being initiated by the private sector. Managed care as a way to finance health care is rapidly replacing fee-for-service care. The focus of managed care is on keeping people out of costly hospital beds and away from high-technology illness care. The most cost-effective hospital bed in a managed care model is, indeed, an empty bed.

Those with limited access to health care in the traditional health care system are at increasing risk for lack of access in a managed care environment. Those who lack health insurance because they are between jobs (unless they can pay costly premiums) or because they are poor and cannot afford insurance, or those who reside in poor inner city or remote rural areas with a shortage of providers, will have a high likelihood of being excluded from managed care. Yet these very populations often represent those at highest risk for using costly acute care. Primary health care including health promotion, disease prevention, health education, case finding, and primary care increasingly came to be recognized as essential for those at risk in society by policymakers in state governments and other influentials concerned with having to foot the bills.

It was reasoned that high-risk populations had to be brought into managed care networks and that they had to have access to primary health care. Obviously, this care also had to be cost-effective. Who better to provide such care than advanced practice nurses (APNs) who are educated to provide such care—and who earn only a fraction of the income earned by MDs who are educated to provide only a portion of the needed primary health care? State legislatures in state after state have broadened the authority of APNs, especially nurse practitioners and certified nurse midwives, to receive direct payment for their services and to write prescriptions. Even though some type of working arrangement with MD colleagues is usually required, many MDs have been threatened by these privileges for nurses, whereas others have welcomed the new possibilities (Mundinger 1994).

In addition, managed care is discounted care. In a competitive marketplace, providers band together to bid for the contract to provide care to the populations of persons who are purchasers of care through an intermediary such as employers and or insurors. In most instances, it is an employer who is purchasing a package of services for employees. Those providers who are in the network participate in the plan and receive a share of the negotiated revenues. Those outside the plan are not reimbursed for their services. Unless patients choose to pay out-of-pocket, they therefore do not have access to those out-of-plan providers. This reality has become clear and has impacted the behaviors of health care providers. Clearly, it is advantageous to be in the network and to keep competitors out. Moreover, as revenues are limited, it is perceived to be desirable to have fewer providers with whom to share the revenues.

Many MDs, acutely aware of the dynamics of health care in a managed care environment and fearful of a loss of income and of patient caseload, have become negative about working in collaborative practice with APNs. (A long-term view, however, leads to opposite conclusions: 1) The larger the network of providers, the wider its scope and the more successful it will be in contract negotiations. 2) The inclusion of APNs in provider practices will increase the cost-effectiveness of the practices, as well as offer more choices to patients, again increasing the competitiveness of the network.)

Health care reform, therefore, has been a mixed blessing to collaborative practice as well as to nurse and physician providers. Arcangelo (1994) states: "In this era of healthcare reform, a conflict has arisen between medicine and nursing concerning the market share of primary care and about the practice of advanced practice nurses" (p. 3). The American Medical Association (AMA), in an aggressive and protectionist action, published a position paper in 1993 urging that MDs proceed with great caution in forming collaborative practices with APNs. Of particular concern to the AMA House of Delegates, apparently, was the idea of nurses practicing in settings where the MD may not be on site. The model espoused for practice was supervisory, rather than the partnership model that is collaboration.

In the AMA position paper, remote practice is likened to independent practice and treated with disdain. Selected quotes illustrate these points: "The delivery of care by nonMDs, in the context of the health care team, where the MD retains the responsibility for the supervision of patient care, is the traditional model in which nonMDs act as extensions of the MD. Until recently, scope of advanced nurse practice has successfully taken place in practice paradigms where the MD has full responsibility, oversight, and supervision of patient care. . . . Most nurses, especially those practicing in remote areas, do not consider independent practice to be professionally responsible and believe that care is best delivered by doctors and nurses together [working side by side]."

In 1994 (a full 25 years after the modern beginnings of collaborative practice), Felton, clearly angered and frustrated by the AMA position paper, asks how to get beyond this negative stance and the bad feelings engendered by it. She suggests perseverance and wisdom: "The challenge is to nurture closer ties between the profession of nursing and the profession of medicine. . . . Our task now is to assess and keep the good and effective parts [of collaboration], change what has outlived its time and purpose . . . and participate in creating the emerging world of tomorrow by using sound and sustainable argument" (p. 86).

Felton's statements are wise, especially the reference to "the emerging world of tomorrow." The world is changing and calls for new ways of thinking and behaving in health care and in all of society. If collaborative practice is *the* paradigm for health care delivery, education, and practice in the world of tomorrow, as this author believes, we had best get on with this work.

The World Is Changing

While each segment of society sees itself as uniquely impacted by the rapidly changing world, there are generic changes impacting all segments of society. Myriad scholars (Bruiniks et al. 1994, Fagin 1992, Porter–O'Grady 1994, Wheatley 1992) speak of the extraordinary dynamics that are changing the world we live in as we approach the millennium: 1) the spread of technology, especially communication systems; 2) international trade linking nations into new economic coalitions thus altering global competition; 3) national and international debt that has driven nations and societies to redefine their level of wealth and the abilities of their bureaucratic structures to resolve problems; 4) the complexity and interrelatedness of problems and issues; and 5) the emergence of health, rather than illness, as a national and international concern along with the growing realization that health is a personal, family, and community concern.

Perhaps the most disconcerting perceptions that countless millions of us share, regardless of cultural, national, or socioeconomic background, are feelings of powerlessness and bewilderment fueled by both a lack of understanding of the dynamics occurring and loss of confidence in our institutions to resolve the problems. Society is not working anymore. It is chaotic and out of control. Our traditional solutions to political and social problems have failed, and they have left us bankrupt. Despite all the hard work and diligent and well-meaning efforts, our politicians, our organizations, and our institutions have all failed us. The integration of economic concerns (everything is so costly and we cannot afford to pay for needed solutions, even if we knew what to do) with profound demographic shifts in the United States and worldwide are perhaps leading to a greater sense of urgency to do something about these major problems. If not, the next century may be drastically different for our children and our children's children.

Bruiniks et al. 1994 describe our service systems—public and private—as discontinuous, inefficient, and fragmented in terms of their ability to provide services to children. They speak of a concept of *antergism* as opposed to synergism. Antergism represents a concept whereby the whole is less than the sum of the parts. Thus, programs assess problems, which is good, but fail to address how the problems will be resolved. Or solutions are only partial, such as providing money to hire more elementary school teachers but failing to take into account the critical shortage of classroom space. Every one of us can think of examples of antergism.

Holistic ways of addressing the needs, concerns, and problems of communities, nations, and the world must be found. Overcoming antergism and achieving synergism whereby the whole is greater than the sum of its parts must be achieved. Connections, not fragments, are desperately needed. Systems thinking rather than linear thinking is needed. The model of mechanistic or linear thinking that flourished in the heyday of the bureaucracy or the assembly line needs to give way to a model that functions in a state of change and fluidity. Change and fragments cannot be controlled as in bureaucratic thinking; they can be ordered and influenced as in systems thinking.

People are yearning for connections. Within health care, connections are essential within and between disciplines. Certainly, no one discipline can deal with the entire gamut of health needs of an individual, a family, a community, a population, or a nation. Within health care, connections are needed between health and illness. Societies can no longer afford to provide costly illness care when health care is so much more cost-beneficial. Nor can societies continue to squander the health of their youth and their productive citizens by ignoring such health-promoting measures as health education and case finding. Societal institutions that have been places of illness care need to learn about health care and make connections with systems that have traditionally focused on health care. Maintaining health and minimizing illness is a lifelong process. An illness episode is not an isolated event. This recognition requires a dramatic shift from an episodic cure orientation for illness care to a continuum of health-illness care that requires an integrated approach to health-illness as a lifelong process.

The needs for synergism, connections, integration, process, and community in health care are worldwide and ongoing. In order for health care to respond to the needs of the people, and societies of the world to be healthy, health care institutions and providers must transition into integrated, collaborative delivery systems. In the United States, the current shift in health care financing from a retrospective costly approach to a cost-contained managed care approach to health care will inevitably focus more and more on providing interdisciplinary collaborative approaches to care. This sharpened focus will occur as payors and consumers increasingly realize that fundamental transformation of provider behaviors represents a long-term solution to achieving high-quality, cost-effective care, as opposed to the short-term solution of merely negotiating deeper discounts in a medically dominated model. Managed care and the emergence of a more mature approach to managed care, however, is only the beginning of a process of transformation of health care to a new paradigm that will contain the features discussed. Central to the new paradigm will be collaborative, interdisciplinary teams of peer providers functioning within supportive and enabling integrated delivery systems. If not, some of our worst fears about the future may be realized.

Senge (1990) captures our need best:

Today, systems thinking is needed more than ever because we are becoming overwhelmed by complexity. Perhaps for the first time in history, humankind has the capacity to create far more information than anyone can absorb, to foster far greater interdependency than anyone can manage, and to accelerate change far faster than anyone's ability to keep pace. Certainly the scale of complexity is without precedent. All around us are examples of "systemic" breakdowns—problems such as global warming, ozone depletion, the international drug trade, and the U.S. trade and budget deficits—problems that have no simple local cause. . . . Systems thinking is the antidote to the sense of helplessness that many feel as we enter the *age of interdependence*" (p. 69; emphasis added).

References

American Medical Association, House of Delegates. (1993, Fall). *Economic and quality of care issues with implications on scopes of practice—physicians, and nurses.* (B of T Rep. I-93-35). Author.

Arcangelo, V. P. (1994). The myth of independent practice. *Nursing Forum, 29,* 3–4.

Axelrod, R. (1984). The evolution of cooperation. New York: Basic Books.

Baggs, J. G. and Ryan, S. A. (1990). ICU nurse-physician collaboration and nursing satisfaction. *Nursing Economics, 8,* 386–392.

Baggs, J. G. and Schmitt, M. H. (1988). Collaboration between nurses and physicians. *Image: Journal of Nursing Scholarship, 20,* 145–149.

Baker, C. and Diekelmann, N. (1994). Connecting conversations of caring: Recalling the narrative to clinical practice. *Nursing Outlook, 42*(2), 65–70.

Blake, R. R., and Mouton, J. S. (1970). The fifth achievement. *Journal of Behavioral Science, 6,* 413–426.

Bruiniks, R. H., Frenzel, M., and Kelly, A. (1994). Integrating services: The case for better links to schools. *Journal of School Health, 64,* 242–248.

Chinn, P. L., and Jacobs, M. K. (1978, October). A model for theory development in nursing. *Advances in Nursing Science, 1*(1), 1–11.

Cowley, S. (1994). Collaboration in health care: The education link. *Health Visitor, 67,* 13–15.

Devereux, P. M. (1981). Essential elements of nurse–physician collaboration. *Journal of Nursing Administration, 1*(5), 19–23.

Dickoff, J., James, P., Wiedenbach, E. (1968). Theory in a practice discipline part 1: Practice oriented theory. In L. Nicoll (Ed.) (1992). *Perspectives in Nursing Theory*, 2nd edition. Philadelphia, PA: J.B. Lippincott Company, pp. 468–500.

Eubanks, P. (1991). Quality improvement key to changing nurse–MD relations. *Hospitals, 65*(8), 26–30.

Evans, J. A. (1994). The role of the nurse manager in creating an environment for collaborative practice. *Holistic Nursing Practice, 8,* 22–31.

Fagin, C. M. (1992). Collaboration between nurse and physicians: No longer a choice. *Academic Medicine, 67,* 295–303.

Fawcett, J. (1980). A framework for analysis and evaluation of conceptual models of nursing. In L. Nicoll (Ed.) (1992). *Perspectives on Nursing Theory*, 2nd edition. Philadelphia, PA: J.B. Lippincott Company, pp. 424–431.

Felton, G. (1994). Guest editorial: A response to the AMA. *Nursing Outlook, 42,* 84–87.

Foucault, M. (1980). In C. Gordon (Ed.) *Power/Knowledge: Selected interviews and other writings 1972–1977* (C. Gordon, L. Marshall, J. Mephan & K. Soper, Trans.). New York: Pantheon.

Gillick, M. R. (1992). From confrontation to cooperation in the doctor–patient relationship. *Journal of General Internal Medicine, 7,* 83–86.

Hardy, M. E. (1973). Theories: Components, development, evaluation. In L. Nicoll (Ed.) (1992). *Perspectives on Nursing Theory*, 2nd edition. Philadelphia, PA: J.B. Lippincott Company, pp. 372–384.

Henneman, E. A. (1995). Nurse–physician collaboration: A poststructuralist view. *Journal of Nursing Administration, 22,* 359–363.

Jones, P. K. (1994). Developing a collaborative professional role for the staff nurse in a shared governance model. *Holistic Nursing Practice, 8,* 32–37.

Jones, R. A. P. (1994). Nurse–physician collaboration: A descriptive study. *Holistic Nursing Practice, 8*(Suppl. 3), 38–53.

Kappeli, S. (1995). Interprofessional cooperation: Why is partnership so difficult. *Patient Education and Counseling, 26,* 251–256.

Katzman, E. M. (1989). Nurses and physicians perceptions of nursing authority. *Journal of Professional Nursing, 5,* 208–214.

Kerfoot, K. (1994). The theory of cooperation and the nurse manager's challenge. *Nursing Economics, 12,* 100–101.

Kerlinger. F. (1973). *Foundations of behavioral research.* New York: Holt, Rinehart, and Winston.

Kilmann, R. and Thomas, K. (1977). Developing a forced-choice measure of conflict handling behavior: The mode instrument. *Educational Psychology Measures, 37,* 309–325.

Koerner, B. L., Cohen, J. R., and Armstrong, D. M. (1985). Collaborative practice and patient satisfaction: Impact and selected outcomes. *Evaluation and the Health Professions, 8,* 299–321.

Kopser, K. G., Horner, P. B., and Carpenter, A. D. (1994). Successful collaboration within an integrative practice model. *Clinical Nurse Specialist, 8,* 330–333.

Mailick, M., and Jordan, P. (1977). A multi-model approach to collaborative practice in health settings. *Social Work Health Care, 2,* 445–454.

McClain, B. R. (1988). Collaborative practice: A critical theory perspective. *Research in Nursing and Health, 11,* 391–398.

McEwen, M. (1994). Promoting interdisciplinary collaboration. *Nursing and Health Care, 15,* 304–307.

McKay, R. (1969). Theories, models, and systems for nursing. In L. Nicoll (Ed.) (1992). *Perspectives on Nursing Theory,* 2nd Edition. Philadelphia, PA: J.B. Lippincott Company, pp. 325–334.

McMahon, J. M. (1992). Shared governance: The leadership challenge. *Nursing Administration Quarterly, 17*(1), 55–59.

Meleis, A. I., Hall, J. M., and Stevens, P. E. (1994). Scholarly caring in doctoral nursing education: Promoting diversity and collaborative mentorship. *Image: Journal of Nursing Scholarship, 26,* 177–180.

Miccolo, M. A. and Spanier, A. H. (1993). Critical care management in the 1990s: Making collaborative practice work. *Critical Care Clinics, 9,* 443–453.

Mundinger, M. O. (1994). Advanced practice nurse—good medicine for physicians? *Nursing Forum, 330,* 211–213.

Murphy, G. T. and Stern, P. N. (1994). Joining forces to collaborate: The essence of critical care nursing practice. *Canadian Association of Critical Care Nurses, 5,* 17–21.

Porter–O'Grady, T. (1994). Building partnerships in health care: Creating whole systems change. *Nursing and Health Care, 15,* 34–38.

Prescott, P. A. and Bowen, S. A. (1985). Physician–nurse relationships. *Annals of Internal Medicine, 103,* 127–133.

Reynolds, P. P., Giardino, A., Onady, G. M., and Siegler, E. L. (1994). Collaboration in the preparation of the generalist physician. *Journal of General Internal Medicine, 9*(Suppl. 1), S55–S63.

Ritter, H. A. (1983). Collaborative practice: What's in it for medicine? *Nursing Administration Quarterly, 7,* 31–36.

Rosenfield, P. L. (1992). The potential of transdisciplinary research for sustaining and extending linkages between the health and social sciences. *Social Science Medicine, 35,* 1343–1357.

Schroeder, P. (1992). Collaboration is considered one of the central tenets of quality improvement philosophies [Editorial]. *Journal of Nursing Care Quality, 6*(3), viii.

Senge, P. M. (1990). *The Fifth Discipline.* New York, NY: Doubleday.

Shawler, C., Stepler, H., and Kinnaird, S. (1990). Model for integration of CNS with nursing management and staff development. *Clinical Nurse Specialist, 4,* 98–102.

Stein, L. I. (1967). The doctor–nurse game. *Archives of General Psychiatrics, 16,* 699–703.

Stein, L. I., Watts, D. T., and Howell, T. (1990). The doctor–nurse game revisited. *New England Journal of Medicine, 322,* 546–549.

Styles, M. M. (1984). Reflections on collaboration and unification. *Image: Journal of Nursing Scholarship, 16,* 21–23.

Thomas, K., and Kilmann, R. (1978). Comparison of four instruments measuring conflict behavior. *Psychological Report, 42,* 1139–1145.

Tichy, N. M., and Devanna, M. A. (1986). *The transformational leader.* New York: Wiley.

U.S. Department of Health, Education, and Welfare, Report of the Surgeon General (1963). *Toward Quality in Nursing* (Public Health Service Publication No. 992). Washington, DC: U.S. Government Printing Office.

Weiss, S. J. (1985). The influence of discourse on collaboration among nurses, physicians, and consumers. *Research in Nursing and Health, 8,* 49–59.

Weiss, S. J. and Davis, H. P. (1985). Validity and reliability of the collaborative practice scales. *Nursing Research, 34,* 299–305.

Wheatley, M. J. (1992). *Leadership and the New Science.* San Francisco, CA: Berrett–Koehler Publishers, Inc.

A Systems Theory 4
or Model

Toni J. Sullivan

Initially presented in this chapter is an overview of relevant systems concepts. Experts in the field of systems theory are cited. Next presented is a beginning systems model for thinking about collaboration. Premises, symbolic representations of collaboration, and propositions for collaboration as a whole or for component parts are described. This skeletal model, however, is far from a complete depiction of collaboration from a systems perspective.

THEORY

Systems Concepts

"A whole which functions as a whole by virtue of the interdependence of parts is called a system" (Rapoport 1968, p. 17, cited by McKay 1969, p. 328). Originating in the natural sciences, systems theory is a multidisciplinary way to discover and study systems occurring in nature. The study of a wide variety of systems became known as the general systems theory, and the concepts came to be applied in the social and human as well as natural sciences.

Systems may be classified as open or closed. Closed systems, such as a chemical reaction occurring in a test tube or even an isolated, withdrawn person, do not exchange energy, material, or anything else with

109

the environment. Open systems exchange matter, energy, information, and the like with the environment. Closed systems tend toward entropy or disorder, equilibrium or homogeneity, and finally maximum disorganization and decay.

In open systems, another force is at work: negative entropy, which acts as a countervailing force tending toward the achievement of more complex order and heterogeneity. The open system also tends toward balance, but it is a steady state, rather than equilibrium. The steady state allows for the continual exchange and flow of component materials (McKay 1969).

Other properties of systems as named by McKay (1969) are as follows: 1) Every order of system except the smallest has subsystems. 2) All but the largest systems have suprasystems consisting of the system and its environment. 3) Every system has a boundary that distinguishes it from its environment. 4) The environment of a system is everything external to it, including suprasystems or higher order systems.

Systems Thinking

Collaboration is an open system. To further our understanding of collaboration, its dynamics as an open system, and our abilities to collaborate effectively within it, the work of Peter Senge and his conceptual model of systems thinking is instructive. In articulating the learning organization in his classic work *The Fifth Dimension* (1990), Senge applies the concepts of systems theory to human endeavors and organizations in an understandable way not before undertaken. He also articulates principles and guidelines that serve as intellectual tools for creating and sustaining human systems.

"Systems thinking is a discipline for seeing wholes. It is a framework for seeing interrelationships rather than things, for seeing patterns of change rather than static snapshots" (p. 68). Discipline is defined by Senge as "a body of theory and techniques that must be studied and mastered to be put into practice. . . . To practice a discipline is to be a lifelong learner" (p. 10). In his learning organization, Senge articulates five disciplines: systems thinking, mental images, shared visioning, team learning, and personal mastery. All these disciplines are, in fact, very relevant for the systems model of collaboration.

Circle of Causality

Senge describes the basic ideas of systems theory by articulating a systems language in everyday terms. It is nonetheless profound in that it aims to change the way we think about reality. To start with, reality is made up of circles, whereas we only see straight lines. Our language, with its subject–verb–object structure, directs toward linear thinking. If we are to see systemic interrelationships, we need a language that is more circular in its structure. As an example, consider first the attributes of the process of developing a collaborative relationship in a linear fashion (see Figure 4-1A) and then in a circular fashion (see Figure 4-1B).

Systems thinking requires that we think in circular patterns. Notice that in the circular presentation of the attributes of the process of establishing a collaborative relationship there is no starting point. In systems thinking, all information, actions, energy (feedback) is a flow of influence and every influence is both cause and effect. Nothing is ever influenced in just one direction. In analyzing situations that occur in systems, it is necessary, therefore, to analyze processes, rather than snapshots or static events. Problems, too, are usually a product of processes occurring in the system, rather than attributable to poor performance of individuals or singular events.

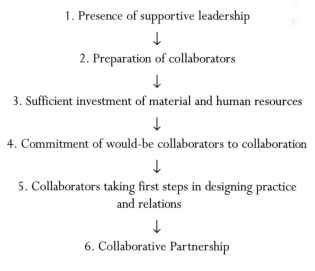

1. Presence of supportive leadership

↓

2. Preparation of collaborators

↓

3. Sufficient investment of material and human resources

↓

4. Commitment of would-be collaborators to collaboration

↓

5. Collaborators taking first steps in designing practice
and relations

↓

6. Collaborative Partnership

Figure 4-1.   **(A)** *Linear listing of attributes of process of developing collaboration.*

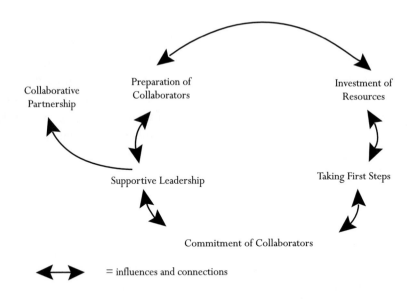

Figure 4-1.   **(B)** *Circular presentation of attributes of process developing collaboration.*

Complexity

Systems, especially open systems, are highly complex entities. Complexity, Senge (1990) asserts, is of two types: detail complexity—myriad variables are components of the system—and dynamic complexity—situations in which cause and effect are subtle and the effects of interventions over time are not obvious. Effects of dynamic complexity may be different in the short term and long term and in different parts of the system. Also with dynamic complexity, doing the obvious thing does not necessarily produce the obvious desired outcome.

All of us can think of people who are extremely attentive to details and very hard working but are ineffective in terms of solving the problem or meeting the goals. They are likely focused on detail complexity only and not on attending to dynamic complexity. It is not necessarily simple to identify dynamic complexity occurring in a system, but Senge tells us that the real leverage (opportunity to improve a system) lies in understanding dynamic complexity, not detail complexity.

Feedback

The feedback process is a circle, or loop, of cause–effect relationships brought about by inputs to the system and by the connections and inter-relationships within it. Feedback is any reciprocal flow of influence, and every influence is both cause and effect. There are two types of feedback. *Reinforcing feedback* is the engine of growth (and analogous to entropy). Reinforcing loops either accelerate growth, or if out of control, they accelerate decline.

Many everyday expressions capture the meaning of reinforcing feedback. We speak of the "snowball effect" when an activity or innovation gathers momentum seemingly of its own accord. When we prejudge a performance or set a positive expectation of outcome, we may create a "self-fulfilling prophecy." When we underfund an effort, such as recruiting students, we may fail in our efforts to meet our recruitment goals. In turn, we underfund our next round of recruitment efforts and fail even more dismally. We have thus set up a "vicious circle." These effects, understood and managed, can be turned into positives; the vicious circle can be the "virtuous circle."

Balancing feedback is feedback that operates whenever goal-directed behavior is present. Analogous to negative entropy, it is the steering wheel or the brakes within the system. Myriad expressions are used to speak of balancing feedback. We "put on the brakes," "take time out," "steer a steady course," and "keep our eyes on the prize.'" In addition, we "stay the course," "take our time," and "take it easy," knowing that "slow and steady wins the race."

These two types of feedback can operate in a complementary manner to keep the system in a steady state, or they can impede each other and create havoc. Growth has its limits and does not go unchecked. It can be said that the system has its own agenda. Balancing feedback mechanisms are everywhere in nature. They enable organisms to maintain conditions for survival in a changing environment. Balancing mechanisms prompt us to seek food when we are hungry and shelter when we are tired and to cover ourselves when chilly. Reinforcing mechanisms, on the other hand, enable growth, for example, from adolescence to adulthood and eventual death, despite the balancing efforts to forestall death.

In human systems, balancing processes underlie all goal-directed behavior . . . implicit as well as explicit.

Whenever there is resistance to change you can bet on there being one or more hidden balancing processes. Resistance to change is neither capricious nor mysterious. It almost always arises from threats to traditional norms and ways of doing things. Often the norms are woven into the fabric of established power relationships. Rather than pushing harder to overcome resistance to change, artful leaders discern the source of the resistance [and try to remove or neutralize it] (Senge, p. 88).

Much of the success in sustaining and promoting vigorous systems lies in discerning the balancing influences and counteracting or nurturing them as appropriate in the given situation or system.

Delays

Delays, when the effect of one variable on another takes time, are everywhere in human systems; virtually all feedback processes have some form of delay. Consider, for example, recruiting a brilliant new graduate to your collaborative partnership. Although your goals and expectations are for a very successful partnership, you recognize that there will be a long span of time, perhaps months, before the partnership flourishes. This is also true of developing junior faculty or educating new MDs or nurses for entry into practice. An endless list of other examples of delays could be cited.

Unrecognized delays can lead to instability and breakdown of the system. Determining how much time it takes to achieve the goals driving the behaviors is most challenging. People, it must be remembered, are not outside the system; they are the system and/or major system components. Time and resources are essential to create and sustain any system. Senge asserts that when efforts are made to overcome system delays by aggressively taking reinforcing actions, the system will respond by increasing instability and oscillation. When recruiting students to an academic program, for example, if the recruiter only acts by persistently contacting and aggressively selling the program to the few potential students who have expressed interest, these prospects may be "turned off" from formally applying to the program, perhaps because the recruiter seems too anxious. If, on the other hand, the recruiter focuses on learning what needs the potential students have that need to be responded to before they can enroll in the program, such as financial aid or course scheduling, the system might well be able to progress toward balance.

Systems Archetypes

Senge speaks of systems archetypes—the kinds of systems issues and actions that occur over and over again. Understanding them can facilitate acting effectively in many situations to prevent, reduce, or correct many systemic problems. *Limits to growth* and *passing the blame* are two systems archetypes commonly encountered. First, remember that the system is generally oriented toward a long-term view. This is certainly so in human organizational systems. Generally, it is far better to remove the limits to growth than it is to push growth directly. In the long term, the system will likely support additional growth. The limiting factors may be found in the balancing feedback loop.

In one example, a school of nursing has a goal of developing faculty as researchers. A second goal is to quadruple the external funding. Ideally, the external funding will come from faculty research projects, and this is very likely to occur in the long run. In the short run, however, the school is generating several million dollars of funding for training grants (which is also responsive to the school's other goals).

The reality here is that several of the faculty who are expected to devote their time to generating funded research projects are spending time administering these grants. This success, paradoxically, has limited the growth of the school. One option to address this situation could be to force the faculty to work longer hours and take on a larger assignment and to admonish them to quit complaining. Another possibility could be simply to recognize the necessity of the current situation toward meeting the overall goals and be thankful for the level of success attained. A third method could be to take action to reduce the time spent on these projects by the faculty to the extent possible. The first action constitutes pressure on the reinforcing feedback mechanism and is a choice that would have unsettling consequences. The second and third choices are viable, as they act on the balancing feedback mechanisms. Perhaps a combination of the second and third would have the most beneficial influence on the system.

Another very common type of behavior in systems is to shift the blame. Attention is shifted from the underlying problem to another problem; a quick fix is used and the symptoms go away. The underlying problem is, therefore, never addressed and usually comes back worse than ever, or the system deteriorates toward further decay and a new set of problems reflective of decay. Senge exhorts us to "beware the sympto-matic solution. People come to rely on them" (1990, p. 104). Chronic underinvestment, it would appear, could be one negative outcome of the quick fix; eroding goals could be another undesirable outcome.

The drug problem in the United States offers a good example of the quick fix. During the Reagan administration, Nancy Reagan achieved much attention for her "Just Say No!" campaign. At the same time, little or nothing was done to address underlying problems of poverty, family breakdown, decaying cities, and so forth. (Failure to address underlying problems is true of both major political parties.) The burden is shifted from the underlying problem to the symptoms that present.

The "Just Say No!" campaign achieved some success, as so often hap-pens with symptomatic treatment. Statistics for teen-aged drug use showed some improvement. Mrs. Reagan was praised by many, especially members of the Republican Party, as having conducted a wonderful pro-gram. Perhaps, the drug problem in the United States was going away or was at least under control. In 1992, a new administration came into office. "Just Say No!" ceased to exist. Those reading this example know what happened: the drug problem reasserted itself in 1996 with a vengeance. It is about as bad as ever; the teen-age usage statistics are shocking.

President Clinton, in his effort to cut costs and reinvent government, had cut the budget for fighting drug abuse in the United States. Perhaps, he, too, thought the problem was resolving. The paltry dollars being expended were cut even further. The mistake of the quick fix was, not surprisingly, compounded by the mistake of underinvestment. As of this writing, the only action being taken is that the Republicans are blaming the Democrats for the increase in the drug problem in the United States. President Clinton and the Democrats do not present a high standard for drug-free living, Republicans say. This is a classic case of passing the blame to symptoms and using the quick fix. The underlying problems worsened; decay is increasing. Such negative outcomes are predictable; regrettably, they are also highly undesirable.

Leverage

The foregoing discussion is really about leverage. Leverage is seeing situa-tions in which actions and changes in system *structure* can lead to significant, enduring improvements. In human systems, structures are the system components of people, problems, programs, goals, and resources. People do not usually see the structure; rather they see the symptoms or the reinforcing feedback processes. They do not think in circles at all; they see a linear image captured in time.

Leverage lies with the balancing feedback processes. It is necessary to figure out what is going on with the balancing mechanisms. In the case of the drug problem in the United States, realistic actions would have to be taken in the structural components of the system in order to achieve any level of lasting success. Goal-directed actions might include allocation of resources to school-based educational programs and community-based jobs-training programs for teens and their parents. All such actions would best be incorporated into public policy that makes explicit a level of societal commitment to resolving the problem.

Another more manageable example might be a so-called collaborative practice wherein one party is refusing to collaborate with the other party (in a practice dyad). The reason stated for this change in behavior is the noncommunicative and even nasty attitude of the other collaborator. This definition of the problem is a classic case of passing the blame. The approach with the most leverage for addressing this situation would be to recognize the symptoms as indicative of an underlying problem in the system structure and to work openly and honestly with both partners to address it in the structure. It would be a mistake to decide the partnership was not worthy of continued support without making an effort to repair the relationship. It would be a mistake to find these behaviors to be acceptable, albeit not the most desirable. The first mistake represents underinvestment; and the second represents eroding goals. These are negative outcomes of passing the blame, and all are to be avoided. Hopefully, the collaborative partnership can be repaired and sustained. The leverage lies in the balancing feedback mechanisms, not the reinforcing. One's goals should be for a structural fix, not a quick symptomatic fix.

> The art of systems thinking lies in seeing through complexity to the underlying structures generating change. . . . What we most need are ways to know what is and what isn't important, what variables to focus on and which to pay less attention to and we need ways to do this which can help groups or teams develop shared understanding (Senge 1990, p. 128).

PREMISES OF A SYSTEMS MODEL
OF COLLABORATION

1. Collaboration is a whole, a system, the attributes of which are all connected within a pattern of interrelations and actions that influence each other in predictable ways.
2. Collaboration can be understood as a whole only by studying patterns occurring among and between the attributes and their connections, rather than static images.
3. Collaboration, as defined, is comprised of four major attributes or systems components: process, partnership, practice, and outcomes; each system component is a component of a subsystem of the larger system of collaboration. (See Figures 4-2, 4-3, and 4-4 for symbolic presentations of subsystems.)
4. The attributes of collaboration, as defined, are generalizable within health care situations regardless of setting or focus.
5. Health care professionals desire to provide high-quality care to people in need of their services; they desire to do their best.
6. In the dynamically complex health care world of the present and foreseen future, collaborative systems of health care practice, education, research, and organizational management are the preferred paradigmatic approach to resolving problems, meeting needs, and accomplishing the work to be done; there is no known health care situation that would not benefit from a collaborative approach.

Model

Collaboration is a

Dynamic, transforming *process*

of creating a power-sharing *partnership*

for pervasive application in health care practice,
education, research, and organizational settings for
purposeful attention to needs and problems (*practice*)

In order to achieve likely successful *outcomes*.

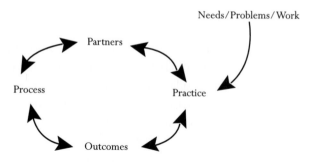

Figure 4-2. *The collaboration system.*

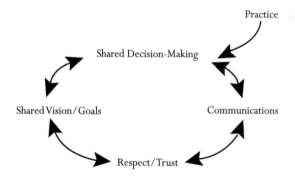

Figure 4-3. *The collaborative partnership subsystem.*

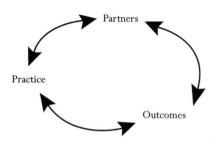

Figure 4-4. *The collaborative practice subsystem.*

PROPOSITIONS

The System and Process of Establishing

1.A. If the leadership of the larger system(s) (organization[s], environment) is supportive of collaboration, if the designated collaborators are prepared for their collaborative work, if sufficient material and human resources are invested in the collaborative practice, if the designated collaborators are committed to collaboration, and if the larger system(s) and collaborators are investing time and energy in taking first steps in developing the collaborative practice, then the collaborative practice(s) is highly likely to be successful.

1.B. Would-be-collaborators who fail to incorporate all five attributes of the process of collaboration in developing and sustaining a collaborating partnership will probably not succeed in developing or sustaining a collaborative partnership and practice.

1.C. If all the attributes of the collaborative process and partnership are present and supported on an ongoing basis, then collaborative system(s) will likely function successfully on an ongoing basis.

2.   As defined, an activated collaborative partnership, in the presence of a need or problem seemingly requiring collaboration, is highly likely to achieve successful outcomes.

3.A. Assuming that the other attributes of collaboration are actually or potentially present, would-be-collaborators who themselves choose to develop a collaborative partnership are highly likely to succeed.

3.B. Even if the other attributes of collaboration are actually or potentially present, would-be-collaborators who have collaborative practice arrangements externally imposed on them are highly unlikely to succeed in becoming collaborating partners.

4.   Collaborators engaged in a collaborative practice system may interrelate with other health care and health-related entities in order to fulfill the mission and meet the goals of the collaborative practice; in the process of doing so, they may form new systems.

5.   Collaborative practice systems that are subsystems of larger collaborative practice systems are highly likely to be strong and long-lasting.

The Partnership and the Practice

1.   Collaborators who approach their partnership and activities from a systems perspective by engaging in systems thinking

and actions are likely to achieve successful outcomes on an ongoing basis.

2. Collaborators who describe their partners as competent or highly competent are likely to accord them a high level of trust and a high level of professional respect.

3. Collaborators who accord their collaborating partners a high level of trust and a high level of professional respect are highly likely to have a strong commitment to the professional welfare of their collaborating partners.

4. Collaborators who describe their partnership as strongly or truly collaborative are highly likely to articulate a shared vision and goals for their practice.

5. Collaborators who describe their partnership as strongly or truly collaborative are highly likely to share responsibility for their practice and share decision making for practice decisions.

6. Collaborators who spend time working together and communicating openly regarding work-related matters are highly likely to maintain a professionally satisfying partnership.

7. Collaborators in a collaborative practice arrangement who are having difficulty agreeing on practice guidelines and practice decisions are highly likely to be having difficulty agreeing on other aspects of collaboration.

8. In the absence of shared decision making, collaborative partnerships are likely to fracture or terminate.

9. Collaborators who are dissatisfied with the quality of the relationship with their partners are likely to withdraw from the relationship over time.

10. Collaborators who describe their collaborative practices as highly satisfactory are likely to refuse to return to a traditional practice model, if given a choice.

The Outcomes: Patient Care

1. Collaboration, as defined, operationalized in collaborative practice arrangements, improves the quality of patient care.

2. Collaboration, as defined, operationalized in collaborative practice arrangements, increases patients' satisfaction with their care and their care providers.

3. Collaboration, as defined, operationalized in collaborative practice arrangements, leads to fewer errors in patient care than occurs in traditional practice arrangements.
4. Collaboration, as defined, operationalized in collaborative practice arrangements, results in lower patient mortality rates.

The Outcomes: Providers

1. Collaboration, as defined, operationalized in collaborative practice arrangements, results in all participating members of disciplines and subdisciplines reporting a high degree of sharing of responsibility.
2. Collaboration, as defined, operationalized in collaborative practice arrangements, results in all participating members of disciplines and subdisciplines reporting a high degree of sharing of expertise.
3. Collaboration, as defined, operationalized in collaborative practice arrangements, results in all participating members of disciplines and subdisciplines reporting a high degree of mutually satisfying problem solving.
4. Collaboration, as defined, operationalized in collaborative practice arrangements, results in all participating members of disciplines and subdisciplines reporting that excellent communications are occurring.
5. Collaboration, as defined, operationalized in collaborative practice arrangements, results in participating nurses and physicians reporting a high degree of job satisfaction.
6. Collaboration, as defined, operationalized in collaborative practice arrangements, results in participating nurses and physicians reporting a high degree of professional growth.
7. Collaboration, as defined, operationalized in collaborative practice arrangements, results in participating nurses and physicians reporting a high degree of nurse involvement in decision making.

The Outcomes: Organization

1. Collaboration, as defined, operationalized in collaborative practice arrangements, results in more cost-effective care than occurs in

traditional practices when comprehensive data concerning both expenses and cost savings are projected over a period of time.

2. Collaboration, as defined, operationalized in collaborative practice arrangements, results in highly satisfactory job performance and productivity indicators as rated by employers.

3. Collaboration, as defined, operationalized in collaborative practice arrangements, results in improved retention of professional staff as compared with staff retention in traditional models of practice.

CONCLUSION

This undoubtedly skeletal presentation is only the beginning of development of a systems theory or model for application by practitioners, educators, researchers, and organizational leaders. The interrelation of the research findings as organized in the concept analysis found in Chapters 1 and 2, the prior work in collaboration from theoretical perspectives as well as the contextual analysis found in Chapter 3, all provide the foundations and core conceptualizations of this systems model. A companion systems model on "coalition" may be found in Chapter 9.

The propositions presented can guide research, stimulate educational models or curricula, offer a backdrop for developing a blueprint for organizational collaboration, and provide a clear framework for designing patient care delivery models. Propositions may need testing and subsequent refinement. Obviously, myriad additional propositions concerning each of the attributes of the collaboration system still need to be articulated. The finest tribute to this work would be the active participation by many colleagues to furthering this work.

References

Hardy, M. E. (1973). Theories: Components, development, evaluation. In L. Nicoll (Ed.) (1992). *Perspectives on Nursing Theory*, 2nd edition. Philadelphia, PA: J.B. Lippincott Company, pp. 372–384.

McKay, R. (1969). Theories, models, and systems for nursing. In L. Nicoll (Ed.) (1992). *Perspectives on Nursing Theory*, 2nd edition. Philadelphia, PA: J.B. Lippincott Company, pp. 325–334.

Rapoport, A. (1968). Foreword. In W. Buckley (Ed.), *Modem Systems Research for the Behavioral Scientist*. Chicago: Aldine.

Senge, P. M. (1990). *The Fifth Discipline*. New York, NY: Doubleday.

Research Review and Analysis
5

Toni J. Sullivan

INTRODUCTION AND RESEARCH QUESTIONS

What research on collaboration has been accomplished? Specifically what questions have been studied? How have they been studied? What are the research findings? Do they support the assertions made in this book and elsewhere of the positive outcomes of collaboration? Is the research itself supportable in terms of its quality? What, if any, are the notable trends in this body of research that give direction for future research?

Because a major aim of this book on collaboration is concept and theory building for the 21st century, a second set of questions proceeds from the work presented in the first four chapters. How does the research that has been reported on in this database fit the systems theory or model of collaboration? What dimensions of the theory have been studied? What new questions emerge for study?

PRIOR REVIEWS

The 327 pieces of literature in the database compiled for this book include three prior reviews of research relating to collaboration. Two of these (Baggs and Schmitt 1988 and Fagin 1992) are bundled within larger literature reviews. Both focus on collaboration in patient care delivery exclusively, and the subjects studied focus almost solely on registered nurse (RN)–MD collaboration. Baggs and Schmitt state that they are reporting only on studies of collaboration in intensive care units

(ICUs), whereas Fagin indicates a focus on all practice venues. In fact, both reviews report on collaboration in multiple settings. The third research review (Brown and Grimes 1995) is a meta-analysis of nurse practitioners and nurse-midwives in primary care. Brown and Grimes, however, do not define *primary care*. This review (Brown and Grimes 1995) focuses on comparing the quality of nurse provider care with physician provider care in terms of outcomes. This interdisciplinary comparative focus varies sharply from the research directly addressing collaboration, which compares collaborative care provided by intradisciplinary or interdisciplinary teams with noncollaborative care. It also must be said that in both instances (interdisciplinary and collaboration-noncollaboration comparisons), the focus on outcomes is neither as prevalent nor as strong as it ought to be.

All three reviews (Baggs and Schmitt 1988, Fagin 1992, Brown and Grimes 1995) are informative about the research done on collaboration or related topics. Using the quality indicators that are shared in the methodology section of the chapter, the Brown and Grimes meta-analysis is an outstanding research report. It should prove to be an indispensable aid to those wishing to study differences in outcomes of primary care provided by nurse practitioners or nurse-midwives compared with that provided by MDs.

Four of the 10 studies reported on by Baggs and Schmitt are also reported on here and will, therefore, only be mentioned in passing. They are Knaus et al. (1986), Temkin-Greener (1983), Weiss (1983), Weiss and Remen (1983), and Prescott and Bowen (1985).

Baggs and Schmitt state that their impetus for doing a literature review was the Knaus et al. (1986) landmark study that linked the quality of the RN–MD relationship in ICU practice settings with patient mortality data (using APACHE II acuity ratings). Knaus et al. documented that the higher the coordination of care, the lower the mortality rates. Baggs and Schmitt divide their review of the research studies into three groups: 1) those that focus on the interdisciplinary team, 2) those that study nurse–physician interaction, and 3) those that examine collaboration between nurses and physicians in caregiving.

The first group emphasizes teamwork and the roles of team members. Temkin-Greener (1983) interviewed nurse and MD department chairs and found disparate perspectives on the roles and expectations of nurses and MDs on so-called collaborative teams. They also found that teams lacking administrative support were hindered in their efforts to be collaborative. Lamb and Napadano (1984) interviewed nurse and physician collaborating primary care partners. They defined collaboration as face-to-face interchange, sharing of problem solving, integration of ideas, and formulation of a new plan. The researchers found little of the concept they sought.

Feiger and Schmitt (1979) conducted a quasiexperimental study at a long-term care facility. They randomly assigned diabetic patients to team care or usual care. A model of collegial interaction was used to compare actual behavior at team meetings with the ideal behavior expressed in the model. "Over a year's time the team care versus usual care resulted in less decline in functional status and more positive change with less decline across a variety of physiological, physical, social and emotional health outcomes" (cited in Baggs and Schmitt 1988, p. 146). Rubenstein et al. (1984) also conducted a quasiexperimental study at a geriatric facility. Patients were randomly assigned to a newly designed geriatric evaluation unit (GEU) or to a regular floor. The GEU provided a team form of care. The patients on the experimental unit had

> lower mortality, fewer acute care days, fewer nursing home placements [the facility was a Veterans Administration hospital], fewer nursing home days, fewer hospital readmissions, improved functional status and morale and lower 12 month direct costs for institutional care than did the usual care patients (cited in Baggs and Schmitt 1988, p. 147).

The next cluster of studies focuses upon nurse–physician interaction. The study by Weiss (1983) and reported in the literature by Weiss (1983) and Weiss and Remen (1983) analyzes data from structured dialogue sessions held over 20 months by RNs, MDs, and consumers. They focused on the nature of the interactions and posited that dialogue might facilitate the development of collaborative interactions. The results suggested that physicians and nurses were very far apart in their perceptions of the roles and behaviors of the other. Dialogue did not facilitate collaborative interactions; rather, it enhanced traditional beliefs.

In two other studies briefly mentioned by Baggs and Schmitt (1988), Spoth and Konwecko (1987) found that a lack of respectful consideration from MDs and poor MD–RN communication were the most frequent and severe stressors faced by ICU staff nurses. Speedling et al. (1981) reported that newly hired nurses perceive nurses and physicians working as a team to be correlated with quality care and a positive work environment. Prescott and Bowman (1985), using the two-dimensional model of affiliation and control of Kilmann and Thomas (1977), investigate how disagreements are handled between physicians and nurses. They found that most resolutions to disputes were handled competitively.

Collaboration in caregiving is the third way in which Baggs and Schmitt (1988) categorize their research review. They report on two studies that did not set out to look at collaboration but found that it was important as a cause of the outcome they were investigating. Gavett et al. (1985) concluded from their study investigating high-cost patients in a teaching hospital that "lack of communication and coordination among health care providers was an important cause of unnecessarily high-cost stays" (cited in Baggs and Schmitt 1988, p. 148). They propose the use of a case manager. Baggs and Schmitt then discuss for a second time the Knaus et al. (1986) study, focusing on the assertion that coordination and interaction of the nurse–physician staff influenced significantly the effectiveness of care, including the patient mortality rates.

Baggs and Schmitt conclude that the tools used in these studies and their analysis of them are sufficient to begin to identify an instrument to measure collaboration in the ICU. They specify that "the tool should measure openness of communication, coordination, cooperation and sharing during planning, and implementation of care" (cited in Baggs and Schmitt 1988, p.148). They recommend that the instrument need not measure face-to-face interactions nor hierarchical relations and that it should not be limited to either conflict resolution or planning only (p.148). (It also became apparent after the extensive study of collaboration done in preparation of this book that there is no substitute for face-to-face interaction in developing and sustaining a strong collaborative partnership. Experience in practice situations, as well, validates this premise.)

Fagin (1992) divides her review of research studies into hospital care, elder care, and barriers to collaboration. She includes both studies on collaboration and studies that relate to collaboration. Five studies of hospital care are reported on. Aiken et al. (1991) documented the positive outcomes of care including a lower inpatient mortality rate for patients with human immunodeficiency virus (HIV) and pneumonia who were treated in hospitals with large volumes of HIV patients. Many, if not most, of these hospitals have model nursing units where nurses "are the primary providers of care and where collaboration with physicians is exemplary" (cited in Fagin 1992, p. 296). In a comparative study of 30 hospital emergency departments, Georgopoulos (1985) reports that the findings link patient outcomes with the quality of both medical and nursing care. Fagin infers that the quality of the nurse–physician relationships played an important part in the quality of care.

Two studies, both focused on administration of analgesia, assert that the therapeutic interventions involved require collaborative behavior. They also call for interdisciplinary education (DeFede et al. 1989, Kitz et al. 1989). Fagin also reports on the Knaus study, calling it "perhaps the most important study concerning the effect of collaboration and coordination between nurses and physicians in hospitals. . . ." (p. 297).

Although Fagin (1992) cites several articles and documents concerning long-term care, she describes only one study of collaboration in long-term care. Williams et al. (1987) conducted a randomized controlled clinical trial to evaluate the effectiveness of a team approach to outpatient geriatric care. In the experimental group, a multidisciplinary team assessed the patients' physical, mental, and social functioning and provided counseling and family support. In the control group, each patient was cared for by a general internist. Fagin provides no other information about care provided to the patients in the control group. Hospital lengths of stay showed a 39.8% difference over a 1-year period. A 25% net reduction in costs of care was also documented. No reduction in patient satisfaction or patient functional status occurred (p. 297).

In her discussion on barriers to collaboration, Fagin (1992) cites and briefly describes four studies, two of which were also discussed by Baggs and Schmitt (Weiss 1983, Prescott and Bowen 1985). Three of the four (Weiss 1983, Prescott and Bowen 1985, Katzman 1989) are included in this chapter's review. With respect to Weiss's study, Fagin notes that the blurring of role distinctions between RNs and MDs, as well as the lack of a clearly defined nursing domain, were related to the lack of collaboration between nurses and physicians. Fagin also notes that despite nurses and physicians describing their relationships as mostly positive (Prescott and Bowen 1985), they differed markedly in their descriptions of a good relationship. Also, the collaborative relationship was shown to be ego building for nurses, but merely ego enhancing for MDs.

In 1980, a study by Kurtz reports that MDs would prefer not to be interactive. Under conditions of stress or conflict, MDs tend to withdraw from group process and become authoritarian and confrontational. In a 1989 study, Katzman reports that when studying nurses and physicians' perceptions of nursing authority, MDs reported (in the strongest finding) that they perceive nurses in collaboration to be assistive to MDs. These latter two studies seem to focus mainly on the process of creating a collaborative relationship. It would be useful to have a way to code or rate collaborative relationships, such as a maturity index or a strength index. It also would be helpful to specify which system component of collaboration is being studied. In many instances, the so-called collaboration may be less than collaboration or the relationship may be very new or undersupported or lacking some other fundamental factor. Also, as became very apparent in the concept analysis, there do not seem to be any shortcuts to collaboration; it, too, is hard work.

Neither the Baggs and Schmitt (1988) review nor the Fagin (1992) review can be categorized as bona fide integrative reviews of research. Nevertheless, they pull together a comprehensive, if not universal, report of the research on collaboration pertinent to that time. Both report on ten studies, three of which overlap. Whereas Baggs and Schmitt offer research-related suggestions, Fagin (1992) poses the following:

> The challenge for physicians and nurses to work together to address the very real health care problems of our present and future has never been greater. A single discipline, self-centered view of the future will be destructive to both professions, to the newly emerging health care system, and most of all, to those who must be healed (p. 302).

The quality of care provided by nurse practitioners and nurse-midwives, with MD care serving as the standard of care, is the topic of the meta-analysis conducted by Brown and Grimes (1995). They inferred quality of care from patient outcomes. Using exemplary methodology, they selected from the literature and reviewed and analyzed 38 nurse practitioner (NP) and 15 nurse-midwife (NM) studies. Thirty-three outcomes were analyzed. Twelve of the 28 NP studies and only one of the NM studies used random assignment of NPs or NMs and MDs to patients. A variety of methods of assignment composed the other studies, such as patient self-selection or assignment by provider. Outcomes related to care varied from one diagnosis to multiple diagnoses to case finding to well patients. The only outcome that was consistent through a minimum of three experimental studies was patient compliance.

Brown and Grimes (1995) used effect size and a simple test of statistical significance to calculate the findings. Nurse practitioners and nurse midwives (NMs) fared very well in this analysis. Nurse practitioners offered slightly more laboratory tests than did MDs ($P < .0001$). Nurse practitioners scored higher than MDs on resolution of pathological conditions. They also received higher patient satisfaction scores. Nurse practitioners and MDs were equivalent on quality of care, prescription of drugs, functional status, number of visits per patient, and use of the emergency room (pp. 336–337). With respect to nurse midwives, "With low-risk patients, . . . NM patients received significantly less analgesia, anesthesia, fetal monitoring, fewer episiotomies, amniotomies, forceps deliveries, and intravenous fluids. . . . Rates of cesarean sections were equivalent between nurse midwife and MD patients" (p. 337). In addition, NMs' patients experienced more spontaneous vaginal deliveries and more perineal lacerations (mostly first degree) than did MD patients. Nurse-midwife and MD patients were equivalent on fetal distress and Apgar scores, although NMs delivered fewer low birth weight babies than did MDs.

Brown and Grimes urge more research designs that randomize patients in order to increase research rigor and thus increase confidence in the findings. None of the studies described the care activities of the provider, whether nurse or physician. The meta-analysis could not, therefore, relate the activities of the provider to any of the outcomes. Nevertheless, Brown and Grimes conclude:

> Results of this meta-analysis represent the extant research on NP and NM care, compared with physician care. Trends in these data are more important than any individual statistical finding and suggest that NP/NM care is equivalent to, or sometimes better than, physician care. The lack of . . . rigor, however . . . leaves many unanswered questions about NP/NM practice. These questions must be answered so that nurses are not in the position of arguing their value on moral principle, right to practice, or naked power (pp. 337–338).

This meta-analysis contributes to the literature on collaboration by providing valuable knowledge of competent practice by two categories of advanced practice nurses (APNs). As some studies point out (Weiss 1983, Prescott and Bowen 1985), neither nurses nor physicians take the competence of all nurses for granted. In addition, documentation of the practice strengths and practice approaches each discipline brings to the collaborative partnership can only facilitate the development of strong team practices.

SEARCH PROCESS

As previously described in Chapter 1, the literature used to compile this database included articles and books from the Cumulative Index of Nursing and Allied Health Literature (CINAHL) articles dating from 1982 to 1995, articles and books from MEDLINE from 1992 to March 1996, and six articles from the *New England Journal of Medicine*, all published from 1992 to July 1995.

These were searched using the key words in each database that would yield the work on collaboration. Using the criteria outlined in Chapter 1, articles were selected. In addition, as articles were reviewed, citations were noted. Articles cited over and over again were added to the database. These procedures yielded 310 articles. Subsequently 17 more references were added, mainly on theory development and systems theory, as well as on leadership and change. The current database contains 327 listings on collaboration or topics relevant to collaboration.

The term *research-based* was assigned to any article that boasted a research design as foundational to its presentation. No judgments were made about the validity of the assertion, and the article was duly coded as research-based. Forty-nine of 327 were so coded.

Next, all 49 articles' abstracts were reviewed. If there was a question about the research design basis of the article, the article itself was reviewed to determine whether indeed the article was a report of accomplished research on collaboration, in whole or in part. No judgments were made about the quality of the work when making the decision to include or exclude articles from the list selected for review. Of the 49 articles, 26 appeared to be bona fide reports of completed research on the broad topic of collaboration; 1 was a meta-analysis on nurse-midwives and nurse practitioner practice as compared with MD practice (Brown and Grimes 1995) and is reported on in the section of this chapter on prior reviews; 22 were not research-based articles and were thus excluded. When the 26 articles were reviewed and coded, 1 was deleted because it was not, in fact, the report of a research study. Thus a .96 intrarater reliability and a .96 interrater reliability were achieved on the decision of whether the article was indeed a research report and with the help of a research assistant.

The 25 articles in this integrated review database are all reports on the general topic of collaboration in the health sciences, regardless of collaborating subjects or settings or areas of practice. Patient care, research, education, administration, and combinations of these areas of focus are all meant to be included. The process of developing a collaborative relationship or practice, focusing on the collaborative relationship, or focusing on the outcomes of collaborative practice are all topics of articles contained in the research review.

From the perspective of the systems theory or model of collaboration (presented in Chapter 4), the four elements of the theory are used as categorizers for themes or foci of the research reports. These elements are 1) dynamic transforming *process* of creating; 2) a power-sharing *partnership;* 3) pervasive application in health care practice, education, research, and organizational settings for purposeful attention to needs and problems *(practice)*; and 4) likely successful *outcomes.* In short, the four systems elements of collaboration are process, partnership, practice, and outcomes.

The sample has at least two limitations. Research articles are limited to this database, which, although large and comprehensive, is not exhaustive. The entire universe of published reports of research on collaboration in the health sciences involving nursing alone or nursing and other health sciences disciplines is not included. In addition, this review is limited to published reports of research. Scholarly presentations, master's theses, and doctoral dissertations are excluded. The listing, therefore, is biased toward published reports of research.

METHODOLOGY

A code book was designed for gathering and storing the data from the 25 research articles (22 studies). Coding was divided into three broad categories: bibliographic data, methodological data, and substantive data. Author(s), year of publication, and journal constitute the bibliographic data; sample numbers and procedures, research type and method, and quality assessment constitute the methodological data; setting and practice area, purpose or questions or hypotheses constitute design including statistics used; and outcomes reported constitute the substantive data.

Using the coding system, each research article was systematically reviewed by the researcher and a research assistant, each working independently. Differences in interpretation were discussed and consensus reached. Coding was adjusted accordingly. Each reviewer independently completed the quality assessment. Scores were then compared and differences of 0.3 or greater—a difference of 10%—were noted. If the difference was 10% or greater, articles were rereviewed and rerated. In the few instances where this occurred, the quality assessment scores came within a less than 10% differential on the second review.

The quality assessment tool used to rate the quality of these research reports is from Smith and Stullenbarger (1992) as presented by Broome (1993). The Quality of Study Instrument includes four broad categories: introduction, methodology, data analysis and results, and conclusions or recommendations. Each section of the tool contains a listing of comprehensive indicators. Such items as statement of problem or purpose, design described, control of validity threats, statistical treatment, results related to problem and/or hypotheses, and conclusions logically derived from findings are judged.

Each statement is scored low (1), medium (2), high (3), or absent (3). Scores are summed in each category and divided by the total number of scores. All four scores so derived are then divided by 4. The achieved scores can range from 1 to 3. The researcher has chosen to report the quality assessment scores as low (1.0–1.9), medium (2.0–2.7), and high (2.8–3.0). The inference is that the validity of the findings of the research may be judged in relation to the overall quality rating. One caveat is necessary, however: The quality score may be more a rating of the article than it is of the actual research project. In some instances, the research may be very complete, whereas the article presenting the research is incomplete. The reader may also cautiously infer from this comment that low ratings may be attributed to incomplete presentation of research elements as well as to less-than-adequate design quality.

RESULTS

Table 5-1 charts bibliographic and methodological characteristics of the sample of 25 published research reports of 22 studies. It also includes the substantive variable of the collaborative component(s) studied, and it incorporates the quality rating. Table 5-2 presents three broad categories of substantive variables for the 25 reports: purpose or research questions or research hypotheses, study design and procedures, and study findings. Considering the two tables side by side provides the reader with a comprehensive picture of the 25 publications.

(Text resumes on page 152)

Table 5-1. Bibliographic and Methodological Characteristics of 22 Studies on Collaboration

Study no. (First author, Journal, year)	Sample/Selection	Type of study Collaborative Practice Area/Setting	Focus within Systems Theory	Quality rating
1 Huckabay, L., MD J Nurs Admin, 1979	46 RNs/Convenience	Descriptive correlational Service/hospital ICUs	Process partnership	Medium
2[a] Weiss, S.J. & Remen, N. West J Nurs Res, 1983	24 RNs, 24 MDs, 24 consumers/Stratified random	Descriptive, prospective, quasiexperimental/service/mixed setting	Process partnership	Medium
3[a] Weiss, S.J. Nurs Res, 1983	24 RNs, 24 MDs, 24 consumers/Stratified random	Descriptive, prospective, quasiexperimental/service/mixed setting	Process Partnership Practice	High
4[a] Weiss, S.J. Res Nurs Health, 1985	24 RNs, 24 MDs, 24 consumers/Stratified random. Adds matched and control groups of 24 RNs, 24 MDs, 24 consumers each	Descriptive, prospective, quasiexperimental/service/mixed setting	Partnership	High
5 Temkin-Greener, H. Millbank Mem Fund Q, 1983	6 RN Department chairs, 6 MD Department chairs/convenience	Qualitative Education–service Academic health center	Process Partnership	Low
6 Davidson, R.A. Res Nurs Health, 1984	15 pairs of NP/MD/ 10 pairs convenience, 5 pairs random	Descriptive Service/outpatient practices	Practice	High
7 Weiss, S. Nurs Res, 1985	95 RNs, 95 MDs/Convenience	Descriptive correlational, tool developmental Service/academic health center	Process Partnership	High

(continued)

135

Table 5-1. Bibliographic and Methodological Characteristics of 22 Studies on Collaboration (*cont.*)

Study no. (First author, Journal, year)	Sample/Selection	Type of study Collaborative Practice Area/Setting	Focus within Systems Theory	Quality rating
8 Prescott, P.A. *Ann Int Med*, 1985	3 RNs, 2 MDs, 1 RN supervisor, 1RN head nurse from 90 hospital units in 15 hospitals/12 of 15 hospitals purposive/3 random Other RNs and MDs interviewed or completed questionnaires by both convenience and random selection	Descriptive correlational Service/tertiary hospital/ICUs	Process Partnership	Medium
9 Knaus, W.A. *Ann Int Med*, 1986	5030 patients from ICUs/Purposive	Descriptive correlational retrospective	Process Partnership Practice Outcomes	High
10 Hinshaw A.S. *J Nurs Admin*, 1987	1597 RNs/Convenience rural RNs; random, urban RNs	Causal modeling Service/hospitals	Process	Medium
11 Baldwin, A. *West J Nurs Res*, 1987	422 RNs, 318 MDs, 7 administrators/ Convenience	Descriptive correlational Service/academic health center	Process Partnership	Low
12 McClain, B.R. *Res Nurs Health*, 1988	9 FNPs, 9 MDs/Stratified random	Qualitative/critical theory Service/outpatient practices	Partnership	Medium
13 Anderson, M. *Dimensions Crit Care Nurs*, 1988	544 ICU and medical–surgical RNs/Convenience	Descriptive comparative Service/ICUs	Partnership Practice	Medium

Source	Sample/Sampling	Design/Setting	Concepts	Rating
14 Katzman, M.E. *J Pediatr Nurs*, 1989	110 RNs, 53 MDs/Convenience	Descriptive correlational Service/hospitals	Partnership Practice	Medium
15 Campbell, J.D., Neikirk, H.J., et al. *Fam Prac*, 1990	412 Patient provider clinic visits (132 with NPs, 276 with MDs/Convenience	Descriptive correlational retrospective Practice, outpatient settings	Practice Outcomes	High
16[b] Campbell, J.D., Mauksch, H.O., et al. *Soc Sci Med*, 1990	412 Patient provider clinic visits (132 with NPs, 276 with MDs/Convenience	Descriptive correlational retrospective Practice, outpatient settings	Practice	High
17 Pennebaker, D.F. *J Nurs Ed*, 1991	46 students/Convenience	Descriptive retrospective, evaluation, research, education Practice–education setting	Process Partneship Practice Outcomes	Medium
18 Salsberry, P.A. *Public Health Nurs*, 1991	1 case study/Purposive	Descriptive research Health dept. and home setting	Practice	Not rated as incomplete
19 Baggs, J.G. *Heart Lung*, 1992	286 consecutive transferred patients, 56 RNs, 31 MD residents/Purposive	Descriptive correlational Service/ICUs (academic health center)	Partnership Practice Outcomes	High
20 Clark, N.M. *Health Ed Res*, 1993	7 case studies/purposive	Descriptive Service/organizational	Process Partnership Practice	High
21 Coeling, H.V. *Nurs Admin Q*, 1994	180 RNs, 90 MDs/Convenience	Descriptive comparative Education service/hospitals and ICUs (3)	Partnership	Medium

(continued)

Table 5-1. Bibliographic and Methodological Characteristics of 22 Studies on Collaboration (*cont.*)

Study no. (First author, Journal, year)	Sample/Selection	Type of study Collaborative Practice Area/Setting	Focus within Systems Theory	Quality rating
22 Langridge, M. *ACORN J*[c] 1994	12 OR RNs/Purposive	Qualitative/phenomenological Service, hospitals	Process Partnership	High
23 Giardino, A.P. *Holistic Nurs Prac*, 1994	22 RN coordinators, 56 MD chief residents/purposive	Qualitative/phenomenological Service, emergency transport teams	Partnership Practice	Medium
24 Jones, R.A.P. *Holistic Nurs Prac*, 1994	59 RNs, 67 MDs/Random	Descriptive correlational Service, varied settings	Partnership Practice	Medium
25 Goode, C.J. *Nurs Econ*, 1995	107 patient treatment group; 107 control group/Purposive Also, 31 RNs, 6 MD residents, 5 MDs, 1 each SW, pharmacists, pathologist, dietician in treatment group; 21 multidisciplinary providers in control group	Quasi-experimental/case study Service/hospital (academic health center)	Practice Outcomes	Medium

[a] Studies 2, 3, and 4 are reports on the same study.

[b] Studies 15 and 16 are reports on the same study.

[c] *Austalian Council of Operating Room Nurses Journal.*

FNP, family nurse practitioner; ICU, intensive care unit; MD, physician; RN, registered nurse.

Table 5-2. Substantive Characteristics of 22 Studies on Collaboration

Study no.	(P) Purpose/(RQ) Research Question(s)/(H) Hypotheses	Design Questionnaires	Findings (Outcomes)
1	(P) Identify, verify, measure and rank order factors in the ICU that the nurse perceives as stressful.	Knowledge of stressors and degree of control over stressors are the two variables used. Two questionnaires were used: identification and rank ordering of stressors and demographic	• 16 Component stressors in ICU directed into 4 categories: patient care, IPR, environment, and knowledge base • Most stressful: patient care • The more years of experience in ICU the less stressed ($P = <.05$)
2	(P) Determine whether dialogue sessions among RNs, MDs, consumers could result in their consensual development of a behavioral model for more effective allocation of responsibility in health care relationships. (P) Examine nature of interactions.	Multidisciplinary dialogue groups over 20 months; divided into four subgroups meeting 1mo. for 2.5 hrs. in comfortable environment; began with nominal group process and developed 13 areas for structured discussion; verbatim transcribing using a court reporter. Grounded theory approach with constant comparative analysis.	• 23 of 44 catagories defined reflected a state of nursing powerlessness; 7 of the 23 stem from RNs. Four fit three patterns: 1) lack of identification with nursing profession, 2) invalidation of professional expertise, and 3) reluctance to assume greater responsibility.

ANOVA, analysis of variance; BSN, Bachelor of Science in Nursing; ICU, intensive care unit; IPR, interpersonal relations; IRR, interrater reliability; MANOVA, multivariate analysis of variance; MD, physician; NP, nurse practitioner; RN, registered nurse; SW, social worker.

(continued)

Table 5-2. Substantive Characteristics of 22 Studies on Collaboration (cont.)

Study no.	(P) Purpose/(RQ) Research Question(s)/(H) Hypotheses	Design Questionnaires	Findings (Outcomes)
3	(P) Determine whether a series of dialogue sessions among RNs–MDs–consumers would result in consensus regarding a) unique areas of nursing practice as different from MD practice and b) areas of common practice	Perceived areas of role differentiation between RNs and MDs identified through analysis of verbatim transcripts from dialogue sessions. Also, all completed Collaborative Behavior Inventory (CBI), a Likert-like tool with 22 categories ranking nurse role responsibilities and MD role responsibilities. In addition, 417 behaviors from the CBI were rated by RNs–MDs–consumers regarding whether these behaviors were appropriate to RN role or MD role or both.	• 22-item scale: 9 of 22 items were rated as within the nursing domain; 12 of 22 rated as areas of common practice; 20 of 22 rated as within the medical domain. MDs were seen as more responsible for all aspects of health care planning and decision making. ($P = <.02$) • Of the 417 behaviors, 342, or 82%, consumers recorded as overlapping RN–MD functions. No behavior of the 417 was identified by the total group as unique to nursing. The nursing subgroup also failed to reach consensus that any behavior belonged uniquely within the nursing domain.
4	(P) Identify major problems in relationships among RNs–MDs–consumers; identify specific role responsibilities and behavioral approaches that would alleviate these problems. (H) Exposure in less role prescribed context with egalitarian discussion would positively influence RNs, MDs,	Pretest–posttest design; experimental group met in daily sessions over 20 months; matched and random control groups did not meet. All groups completed 3 questionnaires pre and post: Health Locus of Control Scales (HLCS), Health Role Expectations Index (HREI), Management of Differences Exercise (MODE).	• The random sample believed there should be less shared responsibility in health care relationships than either the matched sample or the experimental sample. ($P = <.001$) • Although RNs in the experimental group scored higher than MDs on orientation toward collaboration, the differences lessened after 2 years of dialogue, that is,

(continued)

#	Purpose/Question	Method	Results
	consumers toward collaboration in health care.		RN commitment to collaboration declined. • Consumers in experimental group believed RNs should assume less responsibility than RNs believed. This held for 2 years.
5	(P) Explore ways in which leaders in nursing and medicine understand and define the team concept and its purposes and goals; i.e., its structural and normative aspects. (RQ) What is teamwork? Does it work as well as it could or should?	Two-part structured interview questionnaire: a) concept of team, involvement in team; b) structure of team. All tape recorded and transcribed verbatim.	• 4 structured failures identified: 1) teams not identifiable with goals and objectives; rather are ad hoc, 2) individuals are not designated as team members, 3) conflict noted over decision making and leadership, and 4) teams are not evaluated; individuals are.
6	(P) To describe role complementary and similarity. (H) Given vignettes NPs and MDs would choose: subset best cared for by NPs, subset best cared for by MDs, subset to be cared for by either provider.	Care–cure dichotomy is the framework. Panel of expert judges selected vignettes developed by researchers and classified as NP–MD–both for care. Vignettes totaled 9. Each provider responded to two scales (1 MD, 1 NP) on 1–9 ranging from highly inappropriate to highly appropriate.	The 3 hypotheses were partially supported. NPs chose vignettes with high psychosocial and educational components. MDs chose those with high-risk physical situations. Role disagreement was great for two vignettes where both felt they could best care for patients. (On study no. 8, $P=.01$) These were acute episodic vignettes.
7	(P) Determine the validity and reliability of the Collaborative Practice Scales (CPS), 2 distinct self-report measures that assess the degree to which the interactions of nurses (Scale 1) and physicians (Scale 2) enable synergistic influence of patient care.	Theoretical basis of scales is Kilmann and Thomas's two-dimensional model of assertiveness and cooperation. Also used expert observers to document theoretical elements in practice. Administered CPS scales to sample along with Health Role Expectations Index (HREI), and Management of Differences Exercise (MODE). All were administered in test–retest procedure.	• Some correlations between tools (HREI, MODE, CPS) were statistically significant. Also, some items on CPS were statistically significant between RNs and MDs. Results support reliability (alpha coefficient .83 and .85 at retest) and validity of CPS. • Dominant construct measured appears to be synergistic interaction.

Table 5-2. Substantive Characteristics of 22 Studies on Collaboration (*cont.*)

Study no.	(P) Purpose/(RQ) Research Question(s)/(H) Hypotheses	Design Questionnaires	Findings (Outcomes)
		Used myriad statistics for reliability and validity and reductive validity. (Predictive validity weak.)	• RNs lacking BSN scored lower on assertion of professional expertise. • An important feature of collaboration is constructing and operationalizing a framework for practice. • MDs want to achieve consensus with RNs but do not want to share responsibility (no correlation).
8	(P) To examine how administrative, organizational, and practice factors in hospitals are related to staffing problems with RNs	MDs and RNs completed self-report questionnaires using Likert-type scoring regarding four categories: nursing practice, working conditions, relationships, and demographics. Also in interviews asked to describe: RN–MD relationships, example of RN–MD disagreement, and how disagreement was resolved. Independent raters were used for content analysis (IRR = 90%, catagorizing responses pairwise = 80%)	• Four elements of positive relationships emerged: 1) mutual trust and respect, 2) open communication, 3) willingness to cooperate with each other, and 4) competence in performance of one's role. RNs emphasized respect most: MDs emphasized the other three factors most. • 2 statistically significant predictors explained 39% of variance in MD–RN valuations of competence and respect: 1) administrative adequacy of the unit and 2) average job satisfaction of RNs. • Disagreement does not have adverse impact on relationship; most disagreements were settled competitively.
9	(H) The degree of coordination of intensive care significantly influences its effectiveness.	5030 patients from ICUs in 13 tertiary care hospitals purposively selected were prospectively studied. Each hospital's patients were	Rates at Hospital I significantly better than predicted ($P<0.001$); rates at Hospital 13 significantly worse than predicted

	Purpose / Hypotheses	Methods	Results
		stratified by individual risk of death using diagnosis, indication for treatment, and APACHE II Score. In addition, participants fromeach ICU completed a questionnaire concerning care delivery and administration of the ICUs. Research team members visited each ICU to validate reports. Researchers compared actual with predicted death rates using group results as the standard. Units were classified as Level I, II, III.	$(P<.01)$. Hospital 1 had notable more and better MD–RN coordination of care, shared decision-making, and clinical staff authority. (RNs, e.g., could cancel surgery.) Hospitals 3 and 4 also had excellent (unpredicted) mortality records and excellent MD–RN coordination and preparation. Hospital 13, with poorest record, had no dedicated MD or RN staff; poor communications also noted.
10	(P) Identification of retention issues so that innovative retention strategies can be created. (H) 1) Actual turnover predicted to be influenced by anticipated turnover. 2) Organizational and professional job satisfaction would influence anticipated turnover. 3) Control over nursing practice and individual autonomy predicted to increase both job and professional satisfaction. 4) Demographics would influence turnover.	Non experimental causal modeling. Used a 5-stage theoretical design of anticipated turnover among nursing staff. Used several statistics, including factor analysis and multiple regression analysis.	• Actual turnover weakly predicted by anticipated turnover. • Job satisfaction buffers job stress, whereas job stress had no direct impact on anticipated turnover. • Three factors influenced anticipated turnover: 1) organizational job satisfaction, 2) group cohesion, and 3) control over practice in terms of personal resources. • 72.61% of stayers can be predicted.
11	(P) To investigate relationship between nurses self-esteem and their views and willingness to collaborate with MDs and health administrators. (H) 1) RNs with high self-esteem will express more positive views of other nurses.	Administered: Self-Esteem Scales (SES), Semantic Differential, Collaborative Practice Scales (CPS). All with reported acceptable reliability and validity scores.	Likert scoring of the SES produced most of the significant results. Hypothesis 1 supported. Hypotheses 2, 3 and 4 partially supported. Hypotheses 5 mainly supported.

(continued)

143

Table 5-2. Substantive Characteristics of 22 Studies on Collaboration (*cont.*)

Study no.	(P) Purpose/(RQ) Research Question(s)/(H) Hypotheses	Design Questionnaires	Findings (Outcomes)
	2 and 3) RNs with high self-esteem will report more positive views of administrators; of MDs. 4) RNs with high self-esteem will increase collaboration with MDs. 5) Demographic factors, such as position, education, will have no relationship to RN self-esteem.		
12	(P) Critically analyze essence of the joint practice relationship in the primary care setting between NPs and MDs.	Critical theory basis, also dialogic retrospection—a form of participatory action research which engages its subjects as active partners in order to facilitate self-reflection and subsequent critique. Used structure interviews with five categories: 1) interaction, 2) decision-making, 3) critique of health care system, 4) issues in health care delivery, and 5) relationship between education and practice. Focused in this report is interaction.	• Picture was both negative and positive regarding ideal versus real interactions. • MDs too often hierarchical and powerful. • 4 of 9 RNs describe excellent interactions with MDs and toward mutuality. • MD interactions showed medicocentricity and/or mutuality. • 6 of 9 MDs not interested in improving relations; 6 of 9 RNs were interested. • RNs participate in distorted communications.
13	(P) Compare the stressors reported by nurses on general med–surg units with those in ICUs. (H) 1) Overall stress exposure of RNs will be 2 times higher than Bailey surveys of ICU nurses in 1977–1978. 2) Ranking of stressful categories will differ from 1970s.	Cross-sectional survey using Nursing Stress Project Questionnaire (NSPQ), The Stress Audit (uses critical incident techniques), and Bibliographic Questionnaire. Six categories of stressors questioned: 1) patient care, 2) management of unit, 3) IPR, 4) role instability, 5) knowledge and skills, and 6) physical work environment.	• Hypothesis 1: Not supported. Hypothesis 2: Partially supported. Hypothesis 3: Supported. Hypothesis 4: Partially supported. • The top 3 1977–1978 stressors are still the same, but ranking differs. • 2 1977–78 categories did not appear (life events and administrative rewards)

(continued)

3) Medical–surgical nurses will also report occupational stress.

4) Stressor categories will be ranked differently by ICU and medical–surgical nurses.

- ICU nurses ranked IPR #1, patient care #2, management of unit #3; medical–surgical RNs ranked unit management #1, patient care #2, and IPR #3.

14

(P) 1) Identify and quantify the conflict areas between nurses and physicians. 2) Evaluate programs and strategies to resolve conflicts.

Administer the Authority in Nursing Roles Inventory (ANRI), a Likert-type questionnaire with 25 items. Power and roles underlie questions. Tool seeks both current and ideal scores. (Valid and reliable tool.)

- The differences using MANOVA and ANOVA are highly significant between RNs and MDS for both the current and the ideal.
- Both RNs and MDs have highly significant total scores between the current and the ideal. The RNs desired more authority for nurses than did physicians.
- Nurses having a say in health policy making is the most significant ideal difference.

Nurses being perceived as physicians assistants by MDs is the most significant current difference.

15

(P) Examine providers actions with patients, and describe factors associated with pursuing psychosocial issues.

412 visits by patients to NPs or MDs in outpatient settings were videotaped and analyzed. Patients were interviewed on exit. MDs also rated skill of NPs. NPs rated skills of MDs.

Interactional analysis focused on clinical activities; a coding method was developed (50 visits served as a pilot). From the verbal behaviors, a 5-indice construct of practice was developed (see study 16), plus a Psychosocial Concern Index, which was used to score providers. (Tool reliable, 0.75, and valid.)

- Psychosocial concern scores higher for well care and chronic illness visits by both MD and NP providers.
- NPs had higher psychosocial concern scores than MDs consistently for all types of visits.
- Statistically significant correlation between patient satisfaction and high psychosocial concern by provider.
- Correlation between: patient recall of self-care, prevention, compliance and high perception of providers psychosocial

Table 5-2. Substantive Characteristics of 22 Studies on Collaboration *(cont.)*

Study no.	(P) Purpose/(RQ) Research Question(s)/(H) Hypotheses	Design Questionnaires	Findings (Outcomes)
			concern or more psychosocial content during visit. • NPs expressed more satisfaction in doing psychosocial care than MDs. • Both MDs and NPs believe NPs are more proficient than MDs in psychosocial care. • NPs believe psychosocial care more important to quality care than MDs.
16	(P) Examine providers style of interaction with patients and compare the styles of NPs and MDs in joint practice. (H) 1) High affiliation associated with positive patient evaluation of care. 2) High dominance (control) associated with negative patient evaluation of care.	412 visits by patients to NPs or MDs in outpatient settings were videotaped and analyzed. Patients were interviewed on exit. MDs also rated skill of NPs. NPs rated skills of MDs. Interactional analysis focused on clinical activities; a coding method was developed (50 visits served as a pilot). From the verbal behaviors, a 5-indice construct of practice was developed (see study 16), plus a Psychosocial Concern Index, which was used to score providers. (Tool reliable, 0.75, and valid.) Plus a two-dimensional interpersonal grid designed by Argyle of affiliation and control and a model of clinical tasks integrated yielded the five Indices of practice activities/style dimensions:	• Little differences between NP and MD style of interaction. • As length of time together in practice increases, the more similar the styles of partners becomes. • NPs showed more concern with psychosocial care than MDs ($P = <.01$) • There is logical progression from problem-oriented approach in initial visit to relationship or interpersonal approach in later visits. • There is logic in type of style used, i.e. patient education in chronic care. Typology of practice types developed using cluster analysis: • curative style • patient education style

146

- general approach style
- general approach style
(⅔ of visits are general approach style)

- Affiliation
- Control
- Somatic diagnosis and treatment
- Information
- Psychosocial diagnosis and treatment (reliability and validity data provided)

17	(P) Present findings about costs and benefits derived from a collaborative approach to teaching undergraduate nursing research.	Used a modified 26-item scale developed by Jackson and Driever on the costs and benefits of collaboration in research. Identifies variables of time spent, and valuing of outcomes. Items are rated using a 1–4 Likert-type scale and then ranked. This is a post course evaluation research study. Internal consistency scores of .88 on costs items and .92 on benefits items using Cronbach's alpha.	Mean for the benefit items (2.82) was greater than mean for the cost items (2.08). Statis. significant ratings: • Greatest cost = time spent in meetings, followed by time for maintaining long-term involvement • Greatest benefit = intellectual stimulation, followed by support from student peers, followed by opportunities to clarify ideas.
18	(P) Determine service needs and evaluate effectiveness of protocol for persons who are positive for HIV virus and in need of home care.	Collaboration between nurse researchers and clinicians to design and test a case management protocol. Study is being reported in stages: initiating contact, generating ideas, generating the proposal, process problems, problems of content, implementing proposal, analyzing data, and disseminating findings.	Project incomplete but presentation suggested strategies for improving effectiveness and efficiency of each stage. Helpful. Notes the importance of time to develop trusting relationships and group ownership.
19	(P) Examine the relationship between amount of interdisciplinary collaboration involved in making a patient care decision and ICU patient outcomes. (H) RNs and MD (residents) reports of	Studied potentially collaborative act: the decision to transfer from ICU to area of less intense care, and studied the decision context as this could increase or decrease alternatives (e.g., the bed needed). Used APACHE II to control for sever-	• Amount of interdisciplinary collaboration reported by RNs a significant predictor of risk of negative outcome; residents report not a significant predictor. • Hypothesis supported with respect to

(continued)

Table 5-2. Substantive Characteristics of 22 Studies on Collaboration (*cont.*)

Study no.	(P) Purpose/(RQ) Research Question(s)/(H) Hypotheses	Design Questionnaires	Findings (Outcomes)
	collaboration would be positively associated with patient outcomes (controlling for severity of illness) and the relationship would be stronger when more alternative choices were available.	ity of illness. Subjects completed: Decision About Transfer (DAT), a new tool that defines collaboration and has a 7-point scale of no collaboration—(1), to complete collaboration—(7); Collaborative Practice Scales (CPS); and Index of Work Satisfaction (IWS) by RNs only. Content and foci reliable and valid. Negative outcome: readmit to ICU or death during same admission. Weakness: attending MD role in transfer decision not assessed.	nurses. • When RNs reported no interdisciplinary collaboration, risk of negative outcome to patients was 16%; when the transfer decision was reported by RNs to be fully collaborative, the predictive risk of a negative outcome was 5%.
20	(P) What strategies are used in collaborative problem solving (in large scale interorganizational projects) to sustain the cooperative effort and achieve the common goal?	Two stages: 1) Case studies were developed; a team of 7 international experts developed criteria for selecting cases representative of collaborative problem-solving. Ultimately, 7 were selected—1 from each of 7 nations. Team developed protocol for gathering data; hired writers and trained them in use of the protocol. 2) The data gathered were analyzed by the team and by independent reviewers using in vivo coding and constant comparison. Four main categories emerged: —initiation —obstacles —strategies	Community empowerment did occur in several cases. Obstacles included (in order presented): —Lack of financing —Dearth of leadership —Procedural problems —Little prior experience working together —Lost momentum or energy —Difficulty convincing community members of need —Issues of power —Lack of government support (sometimes) —Costliness of cooperation Strategies categorized as:

—Cooperative
—Maintenance
—Pressure
Subcategories also listed

21

(P) Utilize the pragmatic communication perspective to begin to identify specific aspects of communication and specific communicative relationship styles that facilitate or hinder collaboration, thus developing a blueprint for collaboration in health care settings.

Four small studies clustered; use pragmatic perspective as conceptual frame work. Studies three elements:
—Communication content
—Relationship styles
—Element of time
Used interviews and questionnaire compiled from Verbal Aggressiveness Scale, Norton's Communication Style Scale, Free Speech Scale, and newly devised and open-ended questions. Original tools reliability and validity data reported.
Four styles of relationship dimension:
—Disconfirmation (worst)
—Aggression
—Affirmation
—Collaboration (best)
Percentiles used to rank order and report data.

- RNs identified greatest barrier to communication as lack of time.
- RNs placed greater value on relationship dimension than MDs who placed greater value on content dimension.
- RNs emphasized need for MDs to develop collaborative style, including joint effort and courteous treatment.
- Residents more concerned with relationship dimension than attendings.

22

(P) Identify a common definition of collaboration and increase awareness of collaboration as requirement for nursing practice.

Phenomenological study using a Heideggarian Hermeneutics method of case analysis.
Audiotaped, open-ended interviews conducted, transcribe verbatim and coded. Ethnographic computer program searched for commonly coded segments, and a thematic analysis done.

- Operating room RNs perceive collaboration as multidisciplinary health care providers working together as a team to achieve goals. (Longer definition in article.)
- Collaborative behavior is reported to

(continued)

Table 5-2. Substantive Characteristics of 22 Studies on Collaboration (*cont.*)

Study no.	(P) Purpose/(RQ) Research Question(s)/(H) Hypotheses	Design Questionnaires	Findings (Outcomes)
			have a positive impact on the standards of care.
			• A list of prerequisites or preconditions emerged: #1 is ability to have mutual respect.
			• A list of barriers to collaboration also emerged: #1 is unpredictable or difficult personalities—compounded when staff are overworked or tired.
23	(P) Survey transport nurse coordinators and chief residents to ascertain how each views the others on five collaborative practice dimensions.	Comparative analysis using Colaizzi's approach to content analysis (phenomenological) of survey questionnaires using forced choice and open-ended questions. Responses to questions thematically organized into percentage rankings.	• Open-ended responses were all in positive direction. • Large differences: RN is: RN View MD View Assistant to resident 24% 47% Consultant to resident 52% 27% Co-equal partner to resident 95% 67% Evaluation of resident 48% 6%
24	(P) Investigate the nature of RN–MD collaboration using four indicators:	Random mail survey of licensed RNs and MDs in Midwestern county (low return). The four	• Findings do not seem to be generally significant.

(RQ/P/H)	Methods	Findings
power-control, practice spheres, mutual concerns, goals. (RQ) 1) Are there any differences in the perceptions of independent groups of nurses or physicians for each of the four collaborative indicators? 2) Are there any relationships between demographic variables and collaboration indicators for independent groups of nurses or physicians?	indicators are from ANA Social Policy Statement (1980). Used the Feiger and Schmitt Communication Scale for RNs and similar form of it for MDs; and an adaptation of the Collaborative Practice Scales (CPS). Both tools are reliable and valid and both use Likert-type scoring. In addition, participants completed a Practice Spheres Checklist and a Goals Checklist. Descriptive statistics used.	• RN–MD are homogeneous on ratings of power-control, mutual concerns. • RN–MD are homogeneous on practice spheres using CPS scales, and agree on 6 of 10 spheres using Practice Spheres Checklist. • RN–MD agreed on goals for only 4 of 24 items.
25 (P) Evaluate the effect of a care map and nursing case management on patient satisfaction, staff job satisfaction, collaboration and autonomy. (H) Patient satisfaction, staff job satisfaction, collaboration, and autonomy will increase with use of the new care delivery model (care map and case management).	Cohort study design control group with care as usual with total patient care; experimental group had multidisciplinary plan of care outlined in care map with coordination by case manager. Patient satisfaction measured by Blegen and Goode Quality of Multidisciplinary Care Scale, 31 items with 7 subscales (reliability r = .94 with Cronbach's alpha). Job satisfaction measured by Atwood and Hinshaw modified scale. Collaboration measured by Collaborative Practice Scales (CPS). Staff autonomy measured by Dempster Practice Behavior Scales. All instruments have acceptable reliability and validity scores; all use Likert-type scoring.	• Patient satisfaction increased, hypothesis supported, statis significant. • Job satisfaction increased, hypothesis supported, statis significant. • Collaboration did not increase, hypothesis not supported. • Autonomy did not increase, hypothesis not supported. It is posited that case managers were already collaborative and autonomous and these ratings would not, therefore, increase. • The hypothesis that the mutlidisciplinary team would increase job satisfaction, collaboration, and autonomy was partially supported.

All the studies are nonexperimental. The largest design by far is descriptive–correlational; 12 of the studies (13 publications) fit this category. Two of the studies (4 publications) are prospective or quasi-experimental designs; 2 are retrospective or ex post facto designs; 1 is a causal modeling design; and 1 is a tool development study. Three of the studies are case studies, 2 of the studies use a phenomenological qualitative design, and 1 is a critical theory qualitative design. (The numbers total 23 because 1 case study design [Goode 1995] is also counted as quasiexperimental.)

The sample populations in the studies are very diverse. Five of the study populations are intradisciplinary within nursing; four samples are comprised of RNs, and one is a group of RN students. Eight of the sample populations are interdisciplinary between nursing and medicine: two are NP–MD pairs and six are RN–MD samples. Seven studies (10 publications) use multidisciplinary samples. These complex samples are composed of one RN–MD–consumer sample (three publications), one NP–MD–patient population (two publications), two RN–MD–patient samples, two RN–MD–administrator populations, and one population that includes RNs, MDs, MD residents, a social worker, a pharmacist, a pathologist, and a dietician in two matched multidisciplinary teams. Two of the samples are interorganizational—six collaborative ventures in six nations, and a home care program for HIV patients designed jointly by nurse clinicians and nurse researchers. To add to this diversity, clinic visits were studied, as were decisions to transfer patients from an ICU to less intensive care units.

Convenience sampling (12 of the 22 studies) was easily the most common type of sampling procedure used. In several instances, studies could have been strengthened had a more rigorous sampling procedure been used. In other instances, such as the Campbell et al. (1990) study, convenience sampling seems very appropriate. Purposive sampling was used, as well, in 7 studies. Only 1 study (3 publications) employed a random sample, and 2 others a stratified random sample.

The study designs using the random-type samples are quasiexperimental, qualitative (critical theory), and descriptive–correlational. Several of the studies using primarily convenience or purposive sampling also used a partial random sampling to select their very complex study populations. Davidson and Lauver (1984), for example, selected 10 NP–MD pairs by convenience sampling and 5 by random sampling. Their intent is to strengthen the design by so doing.

The hospital setting is the predominant locale for these studies. Of the 22 studies, 15 take place in hospitals: 5 are on general patient care units, 5 are in ICUs and/or general care units, and 5 are in academic health center–type hospitals on varied units. Four outpatient practices (5 publications), 2 neutral/non–health care settings (4 publications), and 1 each of a practice–education setting, home setting, interorganizational setting, and emergency transport setting complete the practice sites.

Although the database intends to accommodate patient care, education, research, and organizational leadership and management, 21 of the studies (22 publications) concern direct patient care providers or patient care. Three studies have education–service as their practice focus, whereas only 1 concerns collaboration in research. Although 2 of the studies investigate interorganizational collaboration, they have been categorized as patient care because their focus is on programs for care delivery.

Four components of collaboration, as developed in the systems theory or model of collaboration, were used to categorize the collaborative component(s) addressed in each study. These components are *process* of developing a collaborative relationship or partnership, collaborative *relationship or partnership*, collaborative *practice*, and *outcomes* of collaborative practice. The categories of collaborative components are shown in Table 5-1, and the research questions asked and research findings that are indicative of these categories can be found in Table 5-2. Most of the studies deal with more than one collaborative component, although usually one component is dominant.

Partnership

The relationship or partnership is a major focus in 14 publications, either alone (4) or coupled with the process component (6) or with practice (4). Two studies include all 4 components. Study topics included registered nurses and physicians perceptions of practice roles, abilities, and expectations of each other; their attitudes, beliefs, and values about and for each other; the nature of their communications; and the nature of their relationship.

This set of studies is, in fact, preoccupied with nurse–physician interaction. The studies examine the nature of interaction (Weiss 1983), question whether dialogue would result in greater understanding and acceptance of RN and MD roles by the other and by consumers (Weiss and Remen

1983), ask what are the major problems in the RN–MD relationship (Weiss 1985), perform a critical analysis of RN and MD interview data to learn what is the essence of the joint practice relationship between NPs and MDs (McClain 1988), identify and quantify conflict areas between nurses and physicians (Katzman 1989), and begin to identify specific communication patterns and survey how nurses and medical residents each views the other on five collaborative practice dimensions Giardino (1994).

Two of the studies (McClain 1988, Coeling and Wilcox 1994) use different conceptual frameworks to analyze the nurse–physician relationship: critical theory and pragmatic perspective, respectively. These frameworks enable one to see relationship dimensions through new lenses. For the most part, however, the same set of issues was addressed in 1994 that had been addressed in 1983.

We have learned a great deal about the nurse–physician relationship from these studies and do not necessarily like what we have learned. In these studies, we find that RNs feel powerless in many relationship and practice areas and that they themselves are responsible for most of their powerlessness (Weiss and Remen 1983); that RNs, consumers, and MDs believe MDs to be more responsible than nurses for health care planning and decision making (Weiss 1983); that RNs are unable to identify any unique roles, functions, and behaviors for themselves (Weiss 1983); that dialogue away from the practice setting about collaboration not only does not improve collaborative relationships but, in fact, serves to entrench traditional views (Weiss 1985); and that the picture of RN–MD relationships is both positive and negative (McClain 1988).

Additionally, these studies focused on relationships and found that MDs are not especially interested in improving relationships, whereas RNs are interested in doing so (McClain 1988); that RNs participate in distorted communications with MDs (McClain 1988); that RNs desire more authority for nursing than MDs desire for nursing, specifically that MDs disagree with nurses about nurses having a say in health policy and that MDs perceive nurses as MD assistants far more often than nurses do (Campbell and Mauksch 1990); that RNs perceive lack of time as the greatest barrier to developing collaborative relationships (Coeling and Wilcox 1994); that RNs value the relationship dimension of collaboration most, whereas MDs value most the content dimension (Coeling and Wilcox 1994); and that nurse coordinators and resident physician members of an emergency transport team had very different perspectives on the nurses' role: the residents viewed the nurse coordinators as physician assistants far more often than did the nurses and viewed the nurse as a consultant far less often than did the nurses (Giardino 1994). Clearly, in these studies, a different world view of the collaborative relationship emerges as being held by physicians and nurses. Each discipline appears to value the other and to value collaboration, but the perspective on collaboration and on the expectations held for the other and for the collaborative partnership vary greatly. We have also learned again that collaboration is not automatic and it is not easy. Both or all parties to collaboration are responsible for the relationship.

Practice

Of the 22 studies, 13 report on practice topics. Only 3 are exclusively practice, and the rest are combined with process and/or partnership; 3 concern all facets of collaboration: process, partnership, practice, and outcomes. The practice focus in these studies is not especially clear. Practice seems to be secondary to the other components. Sample research topics include the care–cure dichotomy and role complementarity and role similarity between RNs and MDs (Davidson and Lauver 1984), the validity and reliability of the Collaborative Practice Scales (Weiss 1985), examination of NP and MD actions with patients and description of factors associated with pursuing psychosocial issues (Campbell, Neikirk et al. 1990), examination of NP and MD providers' styles of interactions with patients and comparison of their styles in joint practice (Campbell and Mauksch 1990), and determination of service needs and evaluation of effectiveness of case management model for persons with HIV (Salsberry et al. 1991).

Practice findings (as separate from outcomes of practice) include that NPs and MDs have a great deal of role complementarity and similarity, as well as disagreements over who is the best caregiver for selected vignettes in which the patients have acute episodic illness (Davidson 1984); that the Collaborative Practice Scales have demonstrated reliability and validity, and the dominant construct measured appears to be synergistic interaction (Weiss 1985); and that an important feature of collaborative practice is the need for collaborators to build and operate from an integrated model of collaborative practice (Weiss 1985).

Additionally, nurse practitioners are consistently rated as having higher psychosocial concern for all types of patients in all types of visits (Campbell, Neikirk et al. 1990); NPs and MDs working together, in practice demonstrate very little difference in their practice styles—in fact, the longer they work together the more alike their practice becomes (Campbell and Mauksch 1990); the exception to NP and MD comparable practice styles is that NPs attend more to psychosocial care (Campbell, Neikirk et al. 1990); the importance of time is noted for developing trusting relationships and group ownership of the practice (Salsberry et al. 1991). Given the mixed nature of the relationship findings, one might expect more negative or mixed practice findings. The few studies available present quite positive findings. (This is also true of those studies that link practice with outcomes.)

Process

About a dozen studies focus in whole, or in part, on process. Only two focus solely on process, whereas the rest combine with one or more other components. Process questions concern how to do, or what strategies to use, or the ways in which related elements in the practice environment relate to collaboration. Some of the process-type studies or questions concern readiness of RNs for collaborative practice, either directly or indirectly.

Representative process questions asked in these studies are what are stressors in the ICU for RNs (Huckabay 1979); what is teamwork and how do leaders in nursing and medicine understand and define teamwork (Davidson and Lauver 1984); how are administrative, organizational, and practice factors in hospitals as related to staffing problems with RNs (Prescott and Bowen 1985); the identification of retention issues for RNs (Hinshaw 1987); what is the relationship between nurses' self-esteem and their views and willingness to collaborate with MDs and health care administrators (Baldwin et al. 1987); and what strategies are used in collaborative problem solving to sustain the cooperative effort and achieve the common goal (Clark et al. 1993).

Findings are informative: patient care is the greatest stressor faced by nurses in the ICU (Huckabay 1979); the greatest stressor faced by nurses in intensive care is in interpersonal relations with MDs, and the second-greatest stressor is patient care (Anderson et al. 1988); four structural failures of teams, and by inference ways to structure teams successfully, are articulated (Temkin-Greener 1983); four elements of a positive relationship between RNs and other coworkers and interdisciplinary colleagues emerge (Prescott and Bowen 1985); three factors influence retention of RNs in hospital settings led by group cohesion and control over practice (Hinshaw 1987); nurses with a high measure of self-esteem report more positive views of colleague MDs and health care administrators and report more positive relationships (Baldwin et al. 1987); a framework for designing, conducting, and evaluating collaborative problem solving is presented containing a wealth of material about obstacles to and strategies for collaboration (Clark et al. 1993).

Outcomes

All five of the studies that address outcomes are, not surprisingly, complex studies in that they link outcomes with one to three other components of collaboration. Practice is the one consistent linkage to outcomes. In every case, outcomes represent a dependent variable in the study. Four of these studies deal with patient outcomes; one with costs and benefits of a teaching intervention for students. All are powerful and more studies with a focus on outcomes would certainly prove useful.

Knaus et al. (1986) ask, What is the degree to which coordination of intensive care will significantly influence its effectiveness? In a well-designed study, they learn that hospitals with more and better coordination of care, shared decision making, and RN clinical staff authority will achieve significantly better actual mortality rates than predicted mortality rates. Coordination of care, although not explicitly defined, is operationalized by factors such as full-time nurse and physician heads of service, staff education, and dedicated staff. The Knaus et al. findings are duplicated somewhat by the findings by Baggs et al. (1992).

Baggs et al. ask, What is the relationship between the amount of interdisciplinary collaboration involved in making the patient care decision to transfer a patient from the ICU to a less intense care setting and ICU patient outcomes? A negative outcome was defined as readmission to the ICU or death during the same admission. When RNs reported no interdisciplinary collaboration, the risk of a negative outcome to patients was 16%. When RNs reported that the transfer decision was fully collaborative, the risk of negative outcomes to patients was 5%. This is a very substantial and statistically significant difference.

Campbell et al., in their 1990 study of providers' actions with patients and descriptions of psychosocial concerns, note (as already reported) that

RNs consistently show more psychosocial concern for patients. Campbell et al. also document a statistically significant relationship between the providers' psychosocial concern and the patients' satisfaction with care. They also document that patients who had received more psychosocial care, usually from a nurse, recalled more self-care and prevention content 1 month after the visit. Perhaps most important, they documented that these patients were significantly more compliant with their plan of care. The researchers note the importance of research linking practice and outcomes to assessment of quality of care. They suggest that their content-based analysis does this and serves to show that it can be done.

In a simple study design that would certainly be replicable, Pennebaker (1991) derives data about costs and benefits of teaching research to undergraduate students from an education–service collaborative approach. The benefits of the approach substantially outweighed the costs. The greatest cost was time spent in meetings, followed by time required for maintaining long-term involvement; the greatest benefit was intellectual stimulation, followed by support from student peers.

Finally, Goode (1995) evaluates the effects of a care map and nursing case management model (a model with definite collaborative features) on patient satisfaction, staff job satisfaction, collaboration, and autonomy. This creative research design combines a quasiexperimental cohort study with evaluation research and achieved strong and impressive findings. Patient satisfaction with care increased, as compared with the control group. Staff job satisfaction increased for the case manager and all staff involved. Autonomy and collaboration did not increase significantly, most likely because the case managers were autonomous and collaborative prior to assuming the case manager position.

DISCUSSION

Several observations are offered here concerning this body of research. The most important finding (and one that was quite surprising) is that the vast majority of these studies of collaboration or a related topic are using study subjects who are not necessarily collaborators, from settings that are either unknown or traditional. Of the 25 reports of research, only 8 either use collaborators as subjects or are case studies about collaborative practices or projects in which the participants are in various stages of maturity as collaborators. The remaining 17 publications (15 studies) are mainly in hospital settings in largely undescribed practices.

Of the 15 remaining studies, 5 concern RNs and related practice issues, all of which are directly or indirectly germane to their ability to enter into collaborative practice with nurses, MDs, or other colleagues. Stress, self-esteem, and job retention are the topics of these studies and we learned from them that RNs desire and flourish in a congenial and supportive environment. Of the 12 remaining reports, 7 are set in locales that by the close proximity of workers or by the complexity and intensity of patient care problems may foster collaborative behaviors. In any event, these settings and the people working in them have been studied as if they were collaborating. The 5 remaining reports (3 studies) have drawn their samples from widespread advertisement to receive applications from mailings to licensed RNs and MDs in a particular legal jurisdiction and from many and varied patient care units in hospitals.

Given the selection of settings and subjects that are not assuredly collaborating and the backdrop of a systems theory or model of collaboration, it is perhaps surprising that the findings in these studies are as positive as they are regarding collaboration and collaborative partnerships. There is, after all, no evidence in any of these studies, with the exception of Knaus et al. (1986), that any preparation, education, or planning for collaboration had occurred. The eight studies that use distinctly collaborative practices report notably more positive findings; only two of these report any negative findings. Davidson and Lauver (1984) found that NPs and MDs had conflict over two of nine vignettes. Each believed they could best care for these acutely ill patients. McClain (1988), in a study using critical theory, found that both nurses and MDs engaged frequently in distorted communications.

One recommendation is to select settings and subjects for study that meet stated criteria for collaboration when collaboration is being studied. Noncollaborating settings and subjects would serve very well as control groups or matched pairs in comparative and/or quasiexperimental studies. The settings and the subjects, in addition to being collaborative, also need to be more tightly controlled. Instead of convenience sampling, researchers need to use more random sampling; instead of descriptive correlational studies, researchers need to use more quasiexperimental research designs. The lack of rigor in some of these research designs opens them to criticism about their quality and the integrity of their findings.

Another finding about this body of work is that the study designs did not explicitly evidence any systems thinking in their approach to the topic of collaboration, despite the fact that it is a system. The study designs were quite fragmented, the majority focusing sharply on relationships and secondly, on practice. Only two of the studies were judged as encompassing all four components of collaboration, and three studies related three collaborative components. In no case, however, was there an explicit mention of collaboration as a system.

Because collaboration is a system, it is not surprising that elements of systems asserted themselves in the study findings. We noted that dialogue in a setting removed from practice does not facilitate the development of a collaborative set of attitudes, beliefs, and values. We learned that an important feature of collaboration is constructing and operationalizing a framework for practice. We learned that teams could be better structured to facilitate teamwork. Strategies were extrapolated from two case studies to enable development of more effective and stronger collaborative programs. Several of the studies noted the great importance of time to developing and sustaining collaboration. Finally, Knaus et al. (1986) documented explicitly the relationship between patient mortality and several features of a collaborative practice system (not explicitly defined as such).

A recommendation is to design studies that utilize explicit systems frameworks in order to learn far more about collaborative systems with all of their interrelating systems elements. Three of these studies (which did use collaborative settings) used the case study method, which could prove to be an effective way to incorporate a systems process with one or more system elements. The case study method, incorporated in varied research designs, is recommended.

Time is an independent variable that presented in several of the studies. We learned that time in meetings was the greatest cost in collaborative student–faculty–staff research. We learned that time or lack of it was the greatest barrier to RN–MD interaction in one ICU. We learned that it is crucial to spend time together in order to develop a trusting relationship. We learned from a pragmatic perspective that time is one of the critical elements of communication. Inferences about time could be teased out of several more studies, as well.

Time is an intriguing topic. First, time is an element of systems and points us toward a long view when making change or judgments about success or failure. Also, with many of the dramatic changes occurring in health care delivery such as prospective payment (managed care) and downsizing and downgrading staff, one cannot help but wonder what will be the impact on time to practice collaboratively in both the short and long term. The explicit incorporation of the variable of time into systems-type study designs will prove useful.

There is some evidence of change in the characteristics of more recent studies as compared with the older studies. Ten studies (11 publications) are dated 1990 through 1995. Of the 10 studies, 6 are actually of collaborative practices. Three of the 6 are case studies. Three of the 4 studies that consider 3 or 4 components of collaboration are post-1990 publications. These are encouraging numbers. It is also of interest that the last study included in the review, Goode (1995) is of care mapping and nursing case management. In the future, far more studies of new models of collaborative care delivery need to be incorporated into research designs so that we learn about their costs and benefits and how best to do them.

Another observation about this set of studies is that only one (Clark et al. 1993) is an international study, despite the database including several international journals and many international articles. Clearly, international research on collaboration is needed. Such research should include all types of collaboration—intradisciplinary, interdisciplinary, and multidisciplinary—as well as research in patient care, education, and research in organizational, national, and international ventures. Comparisons of similarities and differences between and among nations would undoubtedly enrich our understanding of collaboration and the contexts in which it flourishes or languishes.

This analysis implies a research agenda for the future. Tighter and more controlled research designs and studies focused on collaboration from a systems perspective are priorities for future research. Also a priority are studies that link collaboration to current and projected health care delivery, such as managed care, case management, health promotion and health maintenance, and patient self-care. The studies ought to demonstrate their relatedness to the dynamically complex environments in which health care and collaboration is occurring.

Because many studies have documented the high-quality care provided by APNs in collaborative practice (Brown and Grimes 1995, Campbell, Neikirk et al. 1990a, Campbell, Mauksch et al. 1990, Coeling et al. 1994), further focus on such related studies might be on the complementary aspects of APN care to MD care, as well as on the costs and benefits of collaborative practice as compared with more traditional practice. Far more research attention needs to be paid to collaboration in education, research, education–service, organizational, and interorganizational settings. Finally, this integrated research review ought to be repeated every 3 to 5 years using a sample that overcomes the limitations of this sample. Despite the limitations of this sample, however, this review does provide a comprehensive presentation of the last 15 years of published literature on collaboration in health care in which nursing is a participant.

References

Aiken, L., Smith, H., and Lake, E. (1991, August). *Effects of organizational innovations in AIDS care on 'burnout' among hospital nurses.* Paper presented at the annual meeting of the American Sociological Association, Cincinnati, Ohio.

Anderson, M., Chiroga, D. A., Bailey, J. T. (1988). Changes in management stressors on ICU nurses. *Dimensions of Critical Care Nursing, 7*(2), 111–117.

Baggs, J. G. and Schmitt, M. H. (1988). Collaboration between nurses and physicians. *Image: Journal of Nursing Scholarship, 20,* 145–149.

Baggs, J. G., Ryan, S. A., Phelps, C. E., Richeson, F., and Johnson, J. E. (1992). The association between interdisciplinary collaboration and patient outcomes in a medical intensive care unit. *Heart and Lung, 21,* 18–24.

Baldwin, A., Welches, L., Walker, D. D., and Eliastam, M. (1987). Nurse self-esteem and collaboration with physicians. *Western Journal of Nursing Research, 9,* 107–114.

Bennis, W. (1984). The four competencies of leadership. *Training and Development Journal, August,* 145–149.

Broome, M. (1993). Integrative literature reviews in the development of concepts. In B. L. Rodgers & K. A. Knafl *Concept development in Nursing.* Philadelphia: W.B. Saunders Company.

Brown, S.A., Grimes D. E. (1995). A meta-analysis of nurse practitioners and nurse-midwives in primary care. *Journal of Nursing Research, 44*(6), 332–339.

Campbell, J. D., Neikirk, H. J., and Hosokawa, M. C. (1990a). Development of a psychosocial concern index from videotaped interviews of nurse practitioners and family physicians. *Journal of Family Practice, 30,* 321–326.

Campbell, J. D., Mauksch, H. O., Neikirk, H. J., and Hosokawa, M. C. (1990b). Collaborative practice and provider styles of delivery health care. *Social Science Medicine, 30,* 1359–1365.

Clark, N. M., Baker, E. A., and Maru, M. (1993). Sustaining collaborative problem solving: Strategies from a study in six Asian countries. *Health Education Research, 8,* 385–402.

Coeling, H. V. and Wilcox, J. R. (1994). Steps to collaboration. *Nursing Administration Quarterly, 18,* 44–55.

Davidson, R. A. and Lauver, D. (1984). Nurse practitioner and physician roles: Delineation and complementarity of practice. *Research in Nursing and Health, 7,* 3–9.

DeFede, J. P., Dhanens, B. E., and Keltner, N. L. (1989). Cost benefits of patient-controlled analgesia. *Nursing Management, 20,* 34–35.

Fagin, C. M. (1992). Collaboration between nurse and physicians: No longer a choice. *Academic Medicine, 67,* 295–303.

Feiger, S. M., and Schmitt, M. H. (1979). Collegiality in interdisciplinary health teams: Its measurement and its effects. *Social Science and Medicine, 13*(A), 217–229.

Garett, J. W., Drucker, W. R., McCrum, M. S., and Dickinson, J. C. (1985). *A study of high cost in patients in Strong Memorial Hospital.* Rochester, New York: Area Hospital Corporation and University of Rochester.

Georgopoulos, B. S. (1985). Organizational structure and the performance of hospital emergency services. *Annals of Emergency Medicine, 14,* 677–684.

Giardino, A. P., Giardino, E. R., and Burns, K. M. (1994). Same place, different experience: Nurses and residents on pediatric emergency transport. *Holistic Nursing Practice, 8,* 54–63.

Goode, C. J. (1995). Impact of a CAREMAP and case management on patient satisfaction and staff satisfaction, collaboration, and autonomy. *Nursing Economics, 13*(6), 337–348, 361.

Hinshaw, A. S., Smeltzer, C. H., and Atwood, J. R. (1987). Innovative Retention Strategies for Nursing Staff. *Journal of Nursing Administration, 17,* 8–16.

Huckabay, L., and Jagla, B. (1979). Nurses' stress factors in the intensive care unit. *Journal of Nursing Administration, 9*(2), 21–26.

Jones, R. A. P. (1994). Nurse–physician collaboration: A descriptive study. *Holistic Nursing Practice, 8*(Suppl. 3), 38–53.

Katzman, E. M. (1989). Nurses and physicians' perceptions of nursing authority. *Journal of Professional Nursing, 5,* 208–214.

Kilmann, R. H., and Thomas, K. W. (1977). Developing a forced-choice measure of conflict-handling behavior: The mode instrument. *Educational and Psychological Measurement, 37,* 309–325.

Kitz, D. S., McCartney, M., Kissick, J. F., and Townsend, R. J. (1989). Examining nursing personnel costs: Controlled versus non-controlled oral analgesic agents. *Journal of Nursing Administration, 19,* 13–14.

Knaus, W. A., Draper, E. A., Wagner, D. P., and Zimmerman, J. E. (1986). An evaluations of outcome from intensive care in major medical centers. *Annals of Internal Medicine, 104,* 410–418.

Kurtz, M. E. (1980). A behavioral profile of physicians in management roles. In R. Schenke (Ed.), *Physicians in management* (pp. 33–34). Tampa, FL: American Academy of Medical Directors.

Lamb, G. S., and Napadano, R. J. (1984). Physician-nurse practitioner interaction patterns in primary care practices. *American Journal of Public Health, 74,* 26–29.

Langridge, M. (1994). Exploration of OR nurses' reported patterns of collaboration practice behavior during the delivery of patient care. *ACORN Journal, 7,* 25–27.

McClain, B. R. (1988). Collaborative practice: A critical theory perspective. *Research in Nursing and Health, 11,* 391–398.

Notkin, M. S. (1983). Collaboration and communication. *Nursing Administration Quarterly, 8,* 1–7.

Pennenbaker, D. F. (1991). Teaching nursing research through collaboration: Cost and benefits. *Journal of Nursing Education, 30,* 102–108.

Prescott, P. A., and Bowen, S. A. (1985). Physician–nurse relationships. *Annals of Internal Medicine, 103,* 127–133.

Salsberry, P. J., Nickel, J. T., and O'Connell, M. (1991). AIDS Research in the community: A case study in collaboration between researchers and clinicians. *Public Health Nursing, 8,* 201–207.

Smith, M. C., and Stullenbarger, E. (1992). A prototype for integrative review and meta-analyses of nursing research. *Journal of Advanced Nursing, 16*(11), 1272–1283.

Speedling, E. J., Ahmadi, K., and Kuhn-Weissman, G. (1981). Encountering reality. *International Journal of Nursing Studies, 18,* 217–225.

Spoth, R., and Konewko, P. (1987). Intensive care staff stressors and life event changes across multiple settings and work units. *Heart and Lung, 16,* 278–284.

Statham, D. (1994). Working together in community care. *Health Visitor, 67,* 16–18.

Temkin–Greener, H. (1983). Interprofessional perspectives on teamwork in health care: A case study. *Health and Society, 61*(4), 641–658.

Weiss, S. J. (1983). Role differentiation between nurse and physicians: Implications for nursing. *Nursing Research, 32,* 133–139.

Weiss, S. J. (1985). The influence of discourse on collaboration among nurses, physicians, and consumers. *Research in Nursing and Health, 8,* 49–59.

Weiss, S. J. and Davis, H. P. (1985). Validity and reliability of the collaborative practice scales. *Nursing Research, 34,* 299–305.

Weiss, S. and Remen, N. (1983). Self-limiting patterns of nursing behavior within a tripartite context involving consumers and physicians. *Western Journal of Nursing Research, 5,* 77–89.

Williams, M. E., Williams, T. F., Zimmer, J. G., Hall, W. J., and Podgorski, M. S. (1987). How does the team approach to outpatient geriatric evaluation compare with traditional care: A report of a randomized, controlled trial. *Journal of American Geriatrics Society, 35,* 1071–1078.

Interdisciplinary Collaboration

Collaborative Practice in the 1980s

James D. Campbell

Historically, medicine and nursing represent distinct professional systems with different approaches to practice. By tradition, socialization and education, medicine has been cure related, whereas nursing has been care related (Mauksch and Campbell 1985). Advanced practice nurses, however, are playing a more important role in the delivery of health care, especially in managed-care settings where the quality of service needs to be improved and the expenses related to them need to be decreased (Mezey and McGovern 1993). Given these changes, collaborative practice between nurses and physicians is becoming more essential for good health care (Fagin 1992). There is a pressing need to work together.

To provide a perspective on current advanced practice nurse or nurse practitioner (NP)–MD collaboration, presented here is a review of a large-scale evaluation, or research project, conducted during the 1980s and designed to answer the question: Is there a difference between what nurse practitioners (NPs) do and what MDs do in collaborative practice settings? From the perspective of the systems model of collaboration presented in Chapter 4, the foci of the several study components of this project are on both process and outcomes. The collaborative practice issues addressed in this study, such as regulation, status, attitudes, gender, and education, are similar to those being addressed in the current decade (Coeling and Wilcox 1994). In this context, the results of this earlier work remain topical; as well, it represents one of the few empirical investigations of RN–MD collaborative practice.

In 1981, the author, along with the late Hans Mauksch from the University of Missouri–Columbia, embarked on what was to become a 7-year project designed to evaluate joint or collaborative practice between NPs and MDs delivering primary care. Funded by the W.K. Kellogg Foundation, the project evaluated collaborative practice in a variety of settings in the United States, including the Midwest, West, East, and South. At the time, there was considerable debate regarding the role of the NP in primary care.

Much of the debate centered on establishing the practice of the NP. The nurse practitioner was intended to play a nursing role, incorporating an emphasis on health assessment and promotion, accountability of practice, management of common health problems, and support of clients in coping with the problems of daily living. The NP was supposed to complement the MD by helping patients adjust to changes in health status while MDs kept responsibility for disease-related problems. Originally, the NP was not regarded as an MD substitute or assistant. Rather, the NP was to augment and complement MD services. Nurse practitioner services were to be based on a nursing care model in which biological, psychological, interpersonal, organizational, and environmental factors converge to produce a quality outcome (Unpublished manuscript of WR Scott, cited in Lysaught 1981).

Regarding the nurse practitioner as physician substitute prevents a full exploration of the nursing presence in collaborative practice. Although this evaluation project might have found that nurse practitioners are primarily agents of physician care, such a finding would be valid only if the research design had not predetermined the results. Instead, the careful methodology employed in the evaluation, or research project, revealed that notwithstanding tradition and power, some nursing priorities are indeed distinct from those of medicine. The potentially complementary relationship between nurse practitioners and physicians became a central theme of the project.

The thrust of the findings, as well as many facets of the two professional subcultures, could have been anticipated. Nevertheless, the prejudice and stereotyping of collaborative practice by both professions were a surprise. Leaders in both professions showed resistance when those in the nursing field categorically stated that there was no way in which a nurse could work closely with a physician without surrendering the essence of nursing. In some ways, it appeared as if a battle had been declared lost before ever raising an engagement. Likewise, a number of

MDs, some in leadership positions, asserted that there was absolutely no way to provide first-class care if a nurse practitioner were included as a caregiver. Nurse practitioners, by definition, provide second-class care, according to these MDs.

The most uncompromisingly negative statements always came from individuals who either held professional offices that they felt represented their respective professions or were in practice settings involving no present or past contact with collaborative opportunities. Those engaged in collaborative practice, who formed the focal population for this study, rarely made such statements. Negative comments in this group came only from those who were working through the first months of collaborative practice and, thus, were in a period of experimentation and adaptation. The majority of NPs and MDs who were observed, whose stories were recorded, and whose behaviors were videotaped consistently acknowledged the value of cooperation to themselves and to their clients. They conveyed a sense of convention that collaborative practice rests on preconditions of cooperation such as mutual respect and acceptance of the validity of different approaches to patient care. For example, MDs in collaborative practice acknowledged that NPs were more proficient than they were in educating patients, dealing with psychosocial issues, and providing information about nutrition and illness prevention.

The findings of the project were consistently that collaborative practice teams were aware of the negative attitudes of their respective peers and that their collaboration frequently conflicted with professional pressures, formal procedures, and general expectations. Thus, collaborative practice arrangements have to be evaluated cautiously because most of them do not operate under unfettered and unconstrained circumstances. Rather, they should be viewed as functioning under conditions of relative obscurity. Only when they could not be overheard would some MDs in collaborative practice confide to the researchers that after having worked several years with an NP, they would again choose collaborative practice with an NP over a partnership with another MD.

Likewise, nurse practitioners, particularly in certain regions, found their most serious obstacle to be the reluctance or refusal by nursing service administrators to accord them practice privileges in local hospitals. The administrators said there was no "protocol for supervising" NPs. Many NPs in those regions resorted to obtaining licensing as physician's assistants in order to gain privileges through the medical staff. In so doing, however, several departments of nursing essentially chased one of its own into an association and identification with the very profession from which nursing wishes to maintain a distinct identity.

The experiential and subcultural context of the study is crucial because it sheds light on the origin and meaning of the data. Even though both members of the collaborative practice team function under constraints, the impact of these constraints is not the same for physicians as it is for nurses. Although the MDs understood medical norms and expectations, their identity as medical doctors carries with it a sense of autonomy and self-assurance that serves to reduce their susceptibility to restraining messages.

With these caveats in mind, the balance of this chapter presents information regarding the methods employed by the project and demographics of the samples, followed by a summary of the major findings of the evaluation project, only parts of which have been published elsewhere (Campbell et al. 1990a; Campbell et al. 1990b). The findings are organized by the following topical themes: patterns of collaborative practice, working arrangements, styles of practice, outcomes, and gender.

METHODS AND SAMPLES

Our initial evaluative question was, Who does what? Using observation, interview, and questionnaire methods, data were gathered from 60 ambulatory clinic sites that were identified by nurse practitioner training programs. Four hundred twelve provider–patient clinic visits were videotaped, including 276 with MDs and 136 with nurse practitioners. As a comparative sample, 92 of the 412 provider–patient clinic visits were with MDs in solo practice.

The mean age of providers in the sample was 37 years, with the average for NPs being 35,and for MDs, 38 years. Two hundred thirty-five clinic visits were with male providers (including 14 with male NPs) and 136 were with female providers (including 55 with female MDs). Eighty percent of the MDs had trained in a residency program in family medicine. The NPs had been in practice for an average of 6 years, whereas the MDs' average length of practice was 9 years.

The mean age of patients was 26 years, with 176 (43%) male and 236 (57%) female patients. The type of visit was categorized as acute, chronic, well care, or follow-up. Acute visits were those in which the patient's problem had a sudden onset and short course demanding immediate attention. Chronic visits were those in which the problem was of long duration or frequent recurrence. In well-care or health-maintenance visits, the reason for the consultation was not related to disease. Well-care visits included normal pregnancy checks, well-child examinations, and yearly physical examinations. Follow-up visits were for monitoring an acute problem. There were 155 (38%) acute visits, 118 (29%) chronic visits, 74 (18%) well care visits and 65 (16%) follow-up visits.

To learn more about the structure of collaborative practice from a larger sample, a survey was sent to 915 collaborative practice providers throughout the United States. A directory of providers, compiled as part of the project, served as the source for this mailing, and 481 (53%) providers responded. Of those responding to the mailed survey, 302 were nurse practitioners and 179 were physicians.

FINDINGS

Patterns of Collaborative Practice

Given the restrictions on nurse practitioners and the potential for legal challenge to them, how did collaborative practitioners interpret and react to their legal situation in the 1980s? This project's national survey of collaborative practice providers included legal issues and provides information on their perceptions and attitudes regarding regulations for nurse practitioners and collaborative practice.

With respect to practice settings, Sultz et al. (1984) found graduates employed in a variety of settings. Other studies of collaborative practice also show that collaborative practice can be found in a variety of settings and that it may work in others. Private group practice was the most common setting for collaborative practice in this study and two thirds of the respondents were practicing in urban areas.

Occupational and geographic mobility was common among the providers surveyed. Nearly 60% of the providers were practicing in states other than those where they had trained. This trend was more pronounced for physicians than for nurse practitioners. Thirty-five percent of the providers had changed practice location within the past 5 years. This tendency was stronger for female MDs and younger providers than for male MDs and older providers. Among respondents who had changed their practice, three in five moved from another collaborative practice into their current collaborative practice. The remainder moved from a noncollaborative practice into collaborative practice. The median length of time in their current collaborative practice was 7 years for physicians and 4 years for nurse practitioners.

Concerning issues involving NP regulation, respondents were asked whether these practices were currently permitted in their state and whether the practices should be permitted. For all the issues, the MDs were less likely than NPs to know or to have an opinion.

A majority of physician and nurse practitioner respondents (62%) preferred that the state nursing board regulate nursing practice, although NPs were more likely than MDs to prefer this. One in four MDs, but virtually no NPs, preferred the state medical board. Conversely, the nursing boards were preferred by one in six NPs, but by very few MDs.

Nurse practitioners strongly supported legal authorization of independent solo practice, prescription of medications, and medical diagnosis by nurse practitioners, whether they practiced in states allowing those activities or not. Among nurse practitioners who lived in states where they could practice without a special license, about 60% supported continuation of that status, whereas an overwhelming majority (90%) of nurse practitioners living in states requiring a special license supported the requirement. A very strong majority of NPs (89%) opposed the ability to practice without certification. This opinion was held equally in states where certification was, and was not, required.

MD respondents opposed practice by NPs without special license (87%) or certification (91%), but they supported the right of NPs to diagnose patient problems (94%). This was true regardless of the MD's perception of the legal status of these rights. Concerning independent solo practice and prescriptive authority, however, MDs tended to support the status quo. A majority of MDs (67%) who recognized that NPs now possessed those rights supported continuation, but 80% who indicated that NPs did not have those rights were opposed.

The results of the survey show that legal restrictions did not seem to significantly influence providers' practice choices. Many providers, in fact, were unaware that restrictions existed. Eighty-two percent of the nurse practitioners, but only 50% of the physicians, had been aware, before establishing their practices, of state legal restrictions on nurse practitioners.

The arguments over statutory restrictions and regulations, judicial challenges to unfair trade practices, and medical control over health care seem to transpire primarily at the level of professional associations. Individual case law and the establishment of precedence in law, however, are the most fruitful means of challenging unfair restrictions and regulations that affect collaborative practice. These maneuvers require awareness and action by individual practices and providers. If nurse practitioners in collaborative practice are functioning in a complementary and collaborative role, both they and their physician partners are vulnerable to litigation in many states. Conversely, when NPs perform in a completely dependent capacity, they do not fulfill the ideal of complementarity between medicine and nursing. There would seem, then, to be disparities between the legal status of collaborative practice, as idealized and perceived at the level of the professions of medicine and nursing, and the reality of collaborative practice at the level of individual practice. To understand these apparent discrepancies, we needed to examine the variety of collaborative practice arrangements that exist. (Our attention to regulatory matters in the 1980s presages the preoccupation with both legislation and regulation in the 1990s to foster collaborative RN–MD practice.)

Working Arrangements

The allocation of specific tasks and functions are an important part of every professional relationship, and this is particularly crucial to a collaborative practice. Among the providers we surveyed, the recognition of distinct areas of interest and competency between physicians and nurse practitioners was a defining feature of a collaborative practice. Despite this recognition, the configuration in actual practice was fairly uniform, with a modest complementarity of working arrangements between MDs and NPs being evident. In addition, differing MD and NP perceptions of collaborative practice structure seemed primarily related to NP autonomy.

Because the experience of collaborative practice is linked to the rise of the NP, special emphasis is placed on how the role is defined. Where it is more structured and clearly defined, implementation is enhanced (Zammuto et al. 1979). Large institutions, for example, that have written job descriptions, policies, and procedures tend to formalize and employ the NP more quickly than do MDs in private practice. In private practice, there are few formal guidelines, which can make this process slower or nonexistent. Some NPs leave such practices because of poor implementation.

Little (1980) came to the conclusion that NP–MD relationships are often shaped by the structure of the setting and the methods of social control used by MDs. The two major controls that MDs exert are 1) structural, whereby institutional policies and procedures mandate the division of labor, and 2) personal, in which the MD personally places sanctions on the NP. Practice setting characteristics determining the type of social control used and the forms of professional relationships are ownership and size of the organization, continuity of patient care, number of MDs, and MD investment in the work of the agency controlling the practice.

In private practices, structural control is usually low, and personal control can be either high or low. When personal control is high, NPs are treated as assistants to MDs and probably will not have their own caseload. When personal and structural controls are both low, NPs are treated as colleagues. In large institutions, such as medical centers and prepaid practices, personal control is usually low and structural control is usually high. MDs in these practices rotate through the clinics and NPs provide the continuity of care. NPs become gatekeepers for the clinic.

Ambulatory care clinics supported by county and city funds also may have medical students and residents rotating through the clinic; however, because structural control is usually low in these clinics, NPs, while providing continuity of care, are expected to assume a supportive role for the MDs. These NPs act as managers and occasionally colleagues, depending on how much MDs are involved in the agency.

With respect to the evaluation project, there were few differences between the descriptions and reported preferences for practice arrangements of the two provider groups (observed providers and surveyed providers), which seems to indicate that collaborative practice in the United States has a fairly uniform configuration. The data also suggest that collaborative practitioners have consistent intra-professional similarities and inter-professional differences regarding preferences and perceptions about practice arrangements.

In the study, each provider rank ordered a list of activities according to the relative amount of time spent doing them. Comparisons revealed that the MDs spent a greater proportion of their time treating physical illness, whereas the NPs spent more time doing well-health assessment and patient education.

There was a difference between the group that was observed and the group responding to the mail survey, with regard to treatment of emotional problems. In the observed sample, MDs spent more time than NPs on this activity; however, the mail survey NPs reported spending more time treating emotional problems than the MDs in that group.

These findings indicate that there is some degree of complementarity of functions between MDs and NPs in these groups. The extent of complementarity, however, may be modest. On average, MDs reported seeing only two to three more patients per day than the NPs. Although this finding casts doubt on the argument that NPs are not cost-effective because they spend much more time with each patient, it also raises questions about the complementarity of their role. Activities such as patient education and counseling tend to take more time to do well than traditional diagnosis and treatment of acute illness. The fact that NPs do not seem to spend much more time with patients than MDs could indicate that the division of labor in collaborative practice does not allow NPs to use all of their skills regularly. The lack of opportunity to use nursing skills is, thus, a potential source of dissatisfaction for NPs.

Provider satisfaction

Nurse practitioners reported receiving significantly more satisfaction than MDs from psychosocial care, patient education, prevention discussion, and counseling (see Table 6-1). MDs reported higher satisfaction from using sophisticated technology and from diagnosing complex medical problems. These results were found in both provider groups.

Proficiency

Proficiency is another factor affecting NP activities. Jelinek (1978) states that NP independence in performing various functions depends on demonstrating competence. Levine et al. (1976) write that the degree of NP autonomy varies with expertise, the nature of the task, and the type of medical problem that the patient presents.

Both collaborative practice evaluation study groups consider NPs to be more proficient than MDs in psychosocial assessment, counseling, well-child exams, patient education, information provision about prevention and nutrition, health history taking, and giving telephone advice for routine problems. MDs were considered more proficient in performing physical examination, ordering prescription drugs, and performing minor surgery.

The results shown in Table 6-2 indicate awareness by providers of the special areas of competency of both MDs and NPs. The areas of interest

Table 6-1. Comparison of Physician and Nurse Practitioner Ratings for Satisfaction with Activities

Activity		Mean Rating*	N	df	T value	P
Dealing with social and	NP	4.13	303	533	6.12	.000†
psychological aspects	MD	3.67	232			
of patient care						
Diagnosing complex	NP	3.63	298	527	−7.26	.000†
medical problems	MD	4.25		231		
Maintaining control	NP	3.36	294	482	.94	.35
of all aspects of	MD	3.27	228			
patient care						
Educating patients	NP	4.65	306	536	9.34	.000†
about their illness	MD	4.13	232			
or condition						
Discussing prevention	NP	4.57	306	536	10.06	.000†
of health problems	MD	3.92	232			
with patients						
Counseling patients	NP	4.32	306	536	9.12	.000†
and families	MD	3.68	232			
Using sophisticated	NP	2.61	295	483	−3.46	.000†
medical technology	MD	2.92	229			
Deciding what is best	NP	3.37	295	490	.27	.78
for patients regarding	MD	3.35	228			
their health						
Implementing treatments	NP	3.79	296	497	.81	.42
to reduce patient	MD	3.73	224			
complaints						

df, degrees of freedom; MD, physician; N, population; NP, nurse practitioner;
P, probability; T, statistic comparing differences in means.
p value less than .00.
*Rating scale was 1 equals minimum satisfaction to 5 equals maximum satisfaction.
†Significant difference.

Table 6-2. Comparison of Provider Ratings of Physicians and Nurse Practitioner Proficiency for Various Activities

Activity		Mean Rating*	N	df	T value	P
Obtaining health history	MD	3.52	540	539	−5.10	.000†
	NP	3.67				
Instructing patients about prevention of future health problems	MD	2.90	540	539	−26.06	.000†
	NP	3.77				
Performing physical examinaton	MD	3.70	545	544	6.54	.000†
	NP	3.49				
Assessing results of laboratory tests and x-rays	MD	3.84	545	544	.00	1.000
	NP	3.84				
Counseling patients and families	MD	3.08	541	540	−18.26	.000†
	NP	3.66				
Prescribing drugs	MD	3.80	539	538	25.26	.000†
	NP	2.96				
Giving telephone advice for routine problems	MD	3.37	536	535	−10.11	.000†
	NP	3.72				
Performing minor surgery	MD	3.62	507	506	27.45	.000†
	NP	2.17				
Performing well-child exams	MD	3.38	485	484	−9.34	.000†
	NP	3.70				
Advising patients about nutrition	MD	2.65	542	541	−26.72	.000†
	NP	3.63				
Providing patient education	MD	2.86	543	542	−28.63	.000†
	NP	3.81				

df, degrees of freedom; MD, physician; N, population; NP, nurse practitioner;
P, probability; T, statistic comparing differences in means.
p value less than .00.
*Rating scale was 1 equals no proficiency to 4 equals high proficiency.
†Significant difference.

and competency of both professions seem well delineated, suggesting an optimal division of labor for collaborative practice that capitalizes on the complementary differences between the two professional orientations.

Ideal practice components

The providers also indicated which of a list of characteristics were present in their practice and which would be present in an ideal practice. For all the providers, the most common characteristics of collaborative practice are the following:

1. Independence of the MD and NP in patient visits
2. Negotiation of disagreements between providers
3. Determination of patients seen by provider availability and convenience
4. Independent referral by NPs
5. Referral to nonMD consultants by NPs
6. Prescription of medications for common problems by NPs
7. Nurse practitioner initiation of problem- and prevention-oriented teaching or counseling
8. Management of common problems by NPs
9. Ordering of common laboratory tests and procedures by NPs
10. Compensation by salary for both MDs and NPs

With regard to providers' perceptions of an ideal collaborative practice, the tendency was for all providers to desire 1) independence and autonomy for NPs, 2) negotiation and collaborative decision-making, written contracts and/or employment agreements between providers, and 3) partnership arrangements, wherein providers receive a percentage of the practice revenues. There were differences, however, between MDs and NPs. MDs tended to prefer less autonomy for NPs and more authority for MDs; NPs preferred the opposite and also desired direct third-party reimbursement for their services, although MDs did not feel strongly about this. For MDs, the primary discrepancy between their current and their ideal collaborative practice was in the areas of written contracts and compensation for services. Although MDs desired written contracts and partnerships, they were salaried and had no contracts. The primary discrepancy between current and ideal collaborative practice for NPs also involved remuneration. They desired but did not have partnerships and direct third-party reimbursement for services.

Providers were also asked to describe their current practices in terms of the autonomy, authority, and independence of their own position and to indicate their satisfaction with this situation. Both the MDs and NPs desired more autonomy, authority, and independence. Nurse practitioners, however, generally perceived there to be more, and were more satisfied with the level of, autonomy and authority in their positions than the MDs did.

These findings suggest that NPs perceive themselves as more independent and autonomous than MDs believe them to be. This difference in perception may be the result of a lack of communication between collaborative practitioners. With little day-to-day communication with their NPs, MDs might be unaware of the amount of independence and autonomy exercised by NPs. Observations and interviews with providers concerning their interactions, however, did not support this explanation.

A more likely explanation is based on the relationship between experience and expectations. Most MDs and NPs in collaborative practice arrangements have had experience as health care providers. On the one hand, MDs have been socialized to believe that they are ultimately responsible for all aspects of patient care. For most MDs, nurses are seen as a non-independent, non-autonomous adjunct to medicine. Nurse practitioners, on the other hand, have been socialized first as traditional nurses (at least in this study), which accustoms them to functioning in a relatively dependent way.

The conditioning of both professions creates relatively low expectations of autonomy for the nursing role. In addition, MDs in collaborative practice are still ultimately responsible, in a legal sense, for the care delivered in the practice. For NPs, however, collaborative practice offers a much higher level of autonomy than traditional nurses expect. The increased independence and autonomy of the NP could result in a heightened perception of the actual amount of autonomy that they currently exercise.

This reasoning suggests that MDs and NPs in collaborative practice are reasonably satisfied with their positions and with the organization of their practices. Although perceptions differ between the two professions, these differences have not led to extreme dissatisfaction. The histories of nursing and medicine, plus the personal histories of the professionals involved, have created expectations that collaborative practice can satisfy.

The chief discontent for NPs in this sample is financial remuneration. They desire direct third-party reimbursement and partnerships rather than salaried-employee status. MDs are primarily concerned with being the final authority in decision-making. Although the financial concerns of NPs are important, the MDs' concern for authority is key. Conflict over decision-making authority can forestall the realization of collaborative practice as a partnership of professionals, with equal and complementary roles, who work together to provide health care.

Differing patterns, orientations, conceptions, and work arrangements, which constitute the structural dimension of collaborative practice, have been discussed. Although these elements are important at the professional and organizational levels, a complete understanding of collaborative practice must also include a process dimension.

Styles of Practice

The clinical encounter is a complex, interactive process between provider and patient that is based on communication. As a fundamental element of patient care, communication between the provider and patient serves several basic functions, including diagnosis, cooperation, counsel, and education (Cassell 1985, Costello 1977). In this context, a description of providers' interaction styles with patients is presented, along with a comparison of the styles of nurse practitioners with those of MDs.

Observation of videotaped clinic visits was used to study interactive behavior during provider–patient encounters. Because collaborative practice offers the opportunity for increasing the scope of primary health care delivery by integrating nursing and medicine approaches to patient care, comparing nurse practitioner and physician styles of clinical interaction provides a way of examining this integration.

Interpersonal style has been addressed by several authors, including Michael Argyle (1972), who has described the interpersonal behavior style as the set of characteristic techniques an actor employs to achieve certain goals or to solve problems. These techniques have both biological and cultural origins. They are developed, adapted, and displayed according to the personal and interpersonal needs and experiences of the actors.

The characteristic behavior that a provider displays in dealing with patients can be viewed as a combination of these personal and cultural qualities that are in some ways unique, and in other ways typical, of other providers in similar situations. The basic model of interpersonal style that emerges from the literature is a two-dimensional model as represented in Figure 6-1.

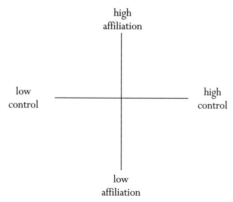

Figure 6-1. *Model of interpersonal style.*

The interpersonal style of an individual may be measured by exhibiting behaviors along two dimensions: affiliation and control. The affiliative dimension of interpersonal style includes many of the elements that have been called the "art" of medicine. These include empathy, warmth, and friendliness at one end of the continuum and rejection, aggression, hostility, and coldness at the other extreme. The end points of the control dimension can be called dominance and submission.

When Buller and Buller (1987) used these dimensions to study how provider styles affect patient evaluations of their care, affiliation was found to be associated with more positive impressions. Dominance was associated with negative evaluations. Provider style was found to be more important in determining patient evaluations for less severely ill patients and for patients who had seen the provider less often before the evaluation.

New patients relied on interpersonal style when forming first impressions of providers. Affiliative styles were found to put new patients at ease and to facilitate disclosure, whereas dominant styles increased patient anxiety and reduced disclosure. Provider interpersonal style is, therefore, an important dimension of medical competence and a major factor in patient evaluations of health care.

Similar to the conceptualization of interpersonal style, the task-related behaviors of a provider can be measured along several dimensions (Hall et al. 1988). These dimensions are specific to the diagnostic or therapeutic tasks that define patient care in the clinical setting and include somatic, psychosocial, and information tasks.

Somatic tasks refer to physical diagnosis and treatment-related activities, which are the primary focus of medical education and practice.

Psychosocial tasks refer to diagnosis and treatment activities that involve the assessment of social and emotional factors affecting patients. These factors affect physical illness and are affected by it. Holistic patient care is largely based on an awareness of the importance of psychosocial influences on the patient. Although medicine—most notably the relatively new specialty of family medicine—increasingly recognizes the importance of psychosocial diagnosis and treatment, this area is still somewhat neglected in relation to somatic diagnosis and treatment. The nursing profession, however, emphasizes psychosocial implications of care and has made that a major focus of university-based nursing education (Lysaught 1981).

The third dimension, information provision, has been shown to be one of the primary determinants of patients' evaluations of their care (Buller and Buller 1987, Donabedian 1985, DiMatteo and DiNicola 1982, Powers et al. 1984). Patient satisfaction, compliance, and recall of information have been found to depend substantially on the amount and type of information provided, as well as the manner in which providers present the information to the patients.

Table 6-3 illustrates three diagnostic or therapeutic styles of provider interaction. Figure 6-2 represents the conceptual relationship between the dimensions of interpersonal and diagnostic or therapeutic style. Because the evaluation project was designed to evaluate nurse practitioners practicing with MDs in primary care, these dimensions are relevant to the clinical performance of both providers.

Different approaches to measuring interaction were used and have been described in detail elsewhere (Campbell et al. 1990a). The first of these analyses, the form analysis, was a detailed, utterance-by-utterance analysis based on a modified form of Stiles Response Modes System (Stiles 1978). This analysis yielded six provider communication strategies consisting of combinations of individual communicative acts:

Table 6-3. Model of Diagnostic or Therapeutic Provider Style

Provider Style	Somatic diagnosis or treatment	Psychosocial diagnosis or treatment	Information provision
Curative	X		
Caring		X	
Educator			X

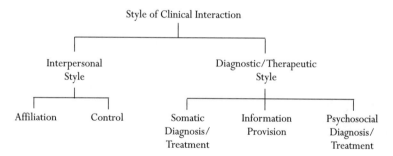

Figure 6-2. *Model of style of clinical interaction.*

- An interview–intervention strategy consisting of diagnostic and therapeutic communications
- A patient disclosure strategy in which patient feelings and thoughts were addressed
- A provider conversation strategy involving provider disclosure and social interaction
- An immediate physical problem strategy focusing on the diagnosis, treatment, and follow-up of the present problem
- An exploratory strategy focusing on past medical history, family medical history, system review, and physical examination without a current illness focus
- A psychosocial strategy involving concern with present and past psychosocial issues and informal or social talk

Nurse practitioners were found to use the interview–intervention, exploratory and psychosocial strategies more frequently than were MDs. These three strategies are weighted heavily in favor of detailed history taking and physical examination. The complete health history and physical examination are areas that are stressed very heavily in NP education programs because they involve skills that are new to nurses. The impact of this stress is, thus, seen in the use of these strategies by NPs. This finding also reinforces anecdotal comments by patients and MDs that were recorded in research field notes: "NPs are more thorough than MDs" and "the NP does a better history than most MDs."

The second type of analysis of videotaped provider–patient encounters was a content analysis. On average, 35% of all providers' behaviors involved medical diagnosis and treatment, 27% involved giving information to the patient, and 7% consisted of activities associated with psychosocial issues. The remaining 31% of the activities were unrelated to these areas and included introductory remarks, plans for the current visit, and casual conversation.

Examination of provider activities associated with psychosocial issues showed that 60% of this activity pertained to patients' current life situation and 31% pertained to health beliefs and behavior. Very little time was spent on patients' past development, mental health history and examination, counseling, therapeutic listening, and intervention associated with changing a lifestyle.

From the content analysis, indices of the components of provider style were developed. The content analysis resulted in proportional scores for indices of affiliation, provider control, patient control, somatic and psychosocial diagnosis or treatment, and information provision.

In addition to the videotaped patient encounters, post-observation patient interviews were conducted. From these interviews, indices of patient-perceived provider affiliation and control, patient control, and information provision and psychosocial concern by providers were developed. By using a combination of videotape- and interview-derived indices of provider style, it was possible to determine whether there were any differences between objective measures of provider behavior and patients' subjective impressions of this behavior. As is discussed in the section on outcomes, this also made it possible to compare the effects of objectively measured behavior and patient perceptions of that behavior on outcome.

The relative emphasis placed by providers on each of the components of style of clinical interaction is shown in Table 6-4. The mean percentage out of all possible activities for each index is shown for all episodes and all providers, for MDs in all episodes, for NPs in all episodes, for each of the types of visit for both providers, and for each of the categories of visit history for both providers in the table. The type of the visit categories are acute, chronic, well-care, and follow-up. These categories refer to the primary reason for the visit. Visit history is a measure of provider–patient familiarity with each other. Visit history category "1" indicates that the episode was the first time the patient had seen the provider, category "2" refers to the patient's second visit with the provider, and "3" indicates that the patient was seeing the provider for at least the third time. The affiliation and somatic diagnosis or treatment components of interaction style shown in the table are composite indices. Several sub-indices of different

Table 6-4. Mean Percentage of Activities for Clinical Interaction Style Dimensions as Measured by Content Analysis of Videotaped Observations*

Style Component	All Episodes/ All Providers (N=412)	MDs/ All Episodes (N=276)	NPs/ All Episodes (N=136)	Acute Visits/ All Providers (N=155)	Chronic Visits/ All Providers (N=118)	Well-care Visits/ All Providers (N=74)	Follow-up Visits/ All Providers (N=65)	1st Visit/ All Providers (N=122)	2nd Visit/ All Providers (N=21)	3rd or more Visits/ All Providers (N=240)
Psychosocial diagnosis										
Treatment	7	6	8	5	7	10	6	7	9	6
Information provision	27	27	26	27	27	25	27	25	29	27
Control										
Provider control	4	4	4	4	4	3	4	4	4	4
Patient control	5	5	5	5	6	3	5	4	5	5
Affiliation	19	19	19	17	18	23	20	18	17	20
Sensitivity	12	12	12	11	11	15	13	11	12	13
Physical examination sensitivity	4	4	4	4	3	5	3	4	3	3
Support or comfort	3	3	3	2	3	4	4	3	2	4
Somatic diagnosis or treatment	35	35	35	38	35	29	35	39	33	33
History taking	28	28	28	30	29	20	27	31	27	26
Physical examination	5	5	5	5	4	8	5	6	4	5
Intervention	2	2	2	2	2	1	2	2	2	2

*Activities are reported as an average percentage out of all possible provider activities coded across the episodes.

aspects of these components were constructed, and mean values for each of the indices are shown indented.

As the table shows, somatic diagnosis or treatment received the most attention in visits regardless of the type of visit or provider. Information provision and affiliation were heavily emphasized also. Statistical analyses of mean differences in percentage of total activities were done for various comparison groups.

Nurse practitioners were found to exhibit more concern with psychosocial issues than were MDs both in general and especially in visits for acute problems. Their differences were statistically significant. There were no differences between MDs and NPs for any of the interview-derived indices of clinical style. This indicates that patients do not perceive and/or report differences between the two provider types.

Both types of visit and visit history were found to influence providers' styles of clinical interaction to a somewhat greater extent than their professional affiliation. Acute visits are characterized primarily by diagnostic or treatment behaviors. Chronic and follow-up visits reveal high levels of patient-perceived psychosocial concern. Well-care visits are differentiated by increased provider sensitivity, psychosocial concern, and physical examination activity.

When MDs and NPs were compared in different types of visits, it was found that MDs seem to vary their behavior with regard to type of visit more than NPs. The MDs 1) concentrated on history taking and patient-perceived psychosocial concern in chronic visits; 2) emphasized physical examination, psychosocial issues, and sensitivity in well-care visits; and 3) concentrated on information provision in follow up visits. The behavior of the NPs, however, was found to be similar regardless of the visit type, with two exceptions: increased diagnostic activity in acute visits and increased sensitivity in well care visits. Because the NPs generally concentrated more on psychosocial issues than did the MDs, the lack of variance of this aspect of clinical style with visit type merely could be a function of higher overall levels of psychosocial concern by the NPs.

The findings for visit history showed a logical progression from a problem-oriented approach in first visits to an interpersonal or relationship-oriented approach in later visits. Providers concentrated on somatic diagnosis and treatment and exerted more control in initial visits with patients. In later visits, the emphasis changed to include psychosocial issues and information provision to patients. Providers in later visits also tended to relinquish control to patients and to be more affiliative. Thus, the provider–patient relationship in primary care can be described as one that begins with identifying somatic or physical problems and then proceeds to exploration of psychosocial factors and provision of information to the patient. Over time, this relationship also becomes more affiliative and egalitarian and less problem-oriented.

In addition to considering each of the clinical interaction style indices separately, a typology of provider style using a cluster analysis on the summary indices was developed. The result of this analysis was a four-cluster solution revealing four distinct clinical styles that correspond to the diagnostic or therapeutic styles shown in Table 6-5.

The most common style used by the providers in the study was the general approach style. This is not surprising, as this style is designed to cover as much territory as possible without emphasizing any single aspect of care. Its prevalence, however, does not necessarily imply that it is the best style for all purposes.

Exclusive use of the general approach style could create in patients a sense of being on an assembly line where one's special needs and desires are not being met. This homogeneous approach is easier for the provider because it does not require one to adapt one's approach for each encounter. The general approach style also fails to use the special competencies of individual providers.

Providers tended to use the patient education style in visits for chronic problems such as diabetes and hypertension and in third or greater visits where the patient and provider knew each other. The curative style was used more in first visits, during which providers needed to become acquainted with the patient's physical condition. There were no differences by the type of visit or visit history in the use of the caring style.

Table 6-5. Clinical Styles

A curative style characterized by somatic diagnosis and treatment (*n*=67)

A patient education style characterized by information provision (*n*=45)

A caring style involving psychosocial diagnosis and treatment and high levels of both affiliation and control (*n*=10)

A general approach style characterized by average levels of all the style components (*n*=253)

There were also no differences in the proportions of MDs and NPs, male and female providers, male and female patients, or combinations of patient and provider gender characteristics of the four types of style.

Similarity of partner styles

Do partners' styles become more similar over time, or is there self-selection of partners with similar styles when a collaborative practice arrangement is created? To investigate this question, all collaborative practice partnerships for which all the necessary data were available were examined.

Twenty-four partnerships with varying lengths of practice together were considered. For these partnerships, a total of 105 patient encounters were available for style comparisons. Distance matrices (extent of style variance) were calculated for the encounters of each partnership, based on the six summary indices. From these distance matrices, an average distance between partners was calculated and a correlation between length of practice and average distance was performed.

The result of this analysis was a correlation coefficient of -0.44 which was significant at $P = .001$. Thus, as the length of practice increases, the average distance between partners decreases, and the more similar the styles of the partners become.

As the NPs and MDs in collaborative practice interact over time, they will mutually influence each other. The extent of influence on each partner will depend on factors such as differences in power and status. The evidence from this study shows that NPs change most in a collaborative practice relationship. Their unique and complementary role tends to be suppressed. This increasing homogeneity of clinical style is probably, at least in part, a function of the greater power and status accorded to MDs by the social and legal systems. Although NPs do seem to maintain a certain degree of distinctiveness through the use of different communication strategies, their differences alone are not likely to impact noticeably on the quality and scope of care offered by collaborative practice. More current research, however, is needed to investigate this hypothesis further.

Interaction style and personality

The relationship between provider interaction style and personality was investigated. The question of interest was: Do personality traits influence the clinical behaviors of primary care providers and/or the ways in which these providers are perceived by patients? We administered seven scales from California Psychological Inventory (CPI) (Goldberg 1977) and cor-related these scores with clinical style index scores.

The most revealing personality scales were tolerance, psychological mindedness, and achievement via independence. Providers whose personalities were permissive, accepting, nonjudgmental (tolerance), and responsive to and accepting of the inner needs and experiences of others (psychological mindedness) tended to have clinical styles higher in affiliation and lower in diagnosis or treatment activities and provider control. The relationship between tolerance and psychological mindedness versus affiliation and control in clinical style was stronger for MDs than for NPs; however, this relationship was not significant.

The effect of the tolerance personality trait in providers is most important not only for objectively appraised clinical style and communication strategy use, but also in terms of patient perceptions of providers. Providers whose personalities were described as more tolerant—accepting and non-judgmental—were perceived by patients to be more affiliative and less controlling. Tolerance as a personality trait in providers was also associated with higher patient-perceived information provision by those providers.

Two other provider personality traits were also associated with increased patient perception of information provision. Patients thought they received more information from providers who could be described as adaptable in thinking and social behavior (flexibility) as well as independent and self-reliant (achievement via independence).

The effect of a more dominant personality varied among providers. MDs who were high in dominance exhibited less psychosocial concern but had no other differences in clinical style or patient reaction. Nurse practitioners described as more dominant in terms of personality, however, exhibited styles of clinical interaction that were lower in patient control and had patients who were less satisfied.

The attitude survey portion of the provider questionnaire also contained questions regarding attributes of providers who would do well in a collaborative practice. Providers listed three attributes and indicated which was the most important for successful collaborative practice. The most often selected attributes were competence, cooperativeness, flexibility, compassion, confidence, and good communication skills. Table 6-6 lists the frequencies for each of these attributes. Competence, cooperativeness, and flexibility were selected as most important by 44% of the respondents.

Table 6-6. Frequencies for Most Important Attributes for Collaborative Practice

Attribute	Frequency
Competent, knowledgeable, thorough, has good clinical skills	17
Cooperative, nonauthoritarian, uses team approach, democratic, fair minded	15
Flexible	11
Honest, trustworthy, has integrity	9
Has good communication skills	6
Confident, assertive	6
Open-minded, willing to learn, willing to take risks	6
Humanistic, caring, compassionate, sensitive	5
Other	5
Humble, knows own limitations	4
Intelligent, exercises good judgment	4
Committed, dedicated, conscientious	3
Congenial, affable, has sense of humor, accommodating	3
Pleasant personality	1
Adaptable	1
Independent, self-directed	1
Creative	0
Patient	0

Outcomes

"Outcomes are those changes, either favorable or adverse, in the actual or potential health status of persons, groups, or communities that can be attributed to prior or concurrent care" (Donabedian 1985, p. 256). Donabedian's definition of outcome encompasses a variety of specific outcome measures. These include economic indicators such as cost containment, health status indices, patient compliance, patient understanding and recall of information given by providers, and patient satisfaction. In our evaluation project, two outcome measures were particularly consequential: patient satisfaction and provider psychosocial concern.

Patient satisfaction has emerged as a prominent topic for research at a time when the social and psychological aspects of illness are receiving more attention and when patients are assuming greater responsibility for their own health (Koerner et al. 1985). Patient responses to the exit interview were used to construct an index of patient satisfaction.

As is true of most studies of patient satisfaction, the evaluation project found that patients were generally satisfied with their care. None of the type of practice (academic or private practice), the provider (NP or MD), number of providers seen during the clinic visit (single provider or NP–MD team), type of visit (acute, chronic, well-care, or follow-up), or age of the patient were found to affect patient satisfaction.

Two other structural variables did show differences in patient satisfaction, however. Patients seen in private practices were more satisfied than those seen in academically based practices. Also, longer term patients—those being seen for at least the third time by the provider or at the practice—were more satisfied than patients who were new to the provider or practice.

Although structural variables do not seem to be strongly related to patient satisfaction, patients' perception of the care process is related to satisfaction. Patients were significantly more satisfied when 1) they believed that the provider was sensitive and gave them information, 2) they believed they had some control over the interaction, 3) they actually received more information from the provider. The "patient education" provider style was associated with higher levels of patient satisfaction also.

These results emphasize the importance of information and the interpersonal component of care for patient satisfaction. Patient satisfaction was not, however, related to whether a provider used or did not use any of the six communication strategies.

To learn about how patients evaluate their health care, they were asked to indicate what they liked most and liked least about the clinic visit and about the provider(s) they saw. Patients appeared to be very content with both the clinic and their provider(s). Most stated that there was nothing they disliked. The few patients who mentioned a disliked aspect most often mentioned waiting time, cost, and the nature of the interpersonal interaction with the provider. The most frequently mentioned likes were the quality of the interpersonal relationship(s), proficiency of providers, provision of information by providers, and short waiting or visit time.

Patients were also asked to indicate the reasons why they felt comfortable or uncomfortable asking questions and why they were satisfied or dissatisfied with the answers they received. Again, the quality of the interpersonal interaction and the proficiency or professional attitude of the provider(s) were very important. Patients were satisfied with the answers given to their questions when the information itself was reassuring and when the answers were complete.

These findings indicate the importance of psychosocial issues during the patient–provider encounter. As many as 50% of patient visits to primary care providers include psychosocial complaints (Ashworth et al. 1984). Also, primary care training increasingly emphasizes psychosocial assessment skills, therapy, and intervention.

Psychosocial concern

A psychosocial concern index was constructed from the subset of coding categories used in the content analysis (Campbell et al. 1990b). The psychosocial concern index score for each provider was calculated by coding the number of times each MD or NP engaged in an activity corresponding to each category and then adding the frequencies for all categories in the index. Each provider's absolute score was affected by the length of the patient encounter. Thus, psychosocial concern index scores were expressed as a proportion of the total number of behaviors coded for the encounter. It was possible, therefore, to determine the relative emphasis providers placed on different types of activities.

The patient exit interview provided information on the patients' perceptions of provider concern with psychosocial issues. For patients younger than 10 years of age, the parent or guardian was interviewed. Responses were recorded and later coded for a patient-perceived psychosocial index. The total number of issues mentioned formed the index of patient-perceived psychosocial concern.

When comparing differences by type of visit for all providers combined, psychosocial concern index scores were highest in well-care and chronic-illness visits and lowest in follow-up and acute care visits, whereas patient perceived psychosocial concern index scores were highest in chronic-illness visits followed by follow-up, well-care, and acute-care visits.

Nurse practitioners and physicians engaged in significantly different amounts of psychosocial activity. Nurse practitioners had higher mean psychosocial concern index and patient-perceived psychosocial concern index scores than physicians for all types of visits combined. When controlling for type of visit, the differences in mean scores failed to reach significance. The NPs' scores on the psychosocial concern index and the patient-perceived psychosocial concern index, however, were consistently higher than MDs' scores for each of the four types of visit.

The number of times a patient had seen a provider (visit history) was less important than type of visit in determining the provider concern with psychosocial issues. Although there were no significant differences between nurse practitioners and physicians on either observed provider psychosocial concern or patient-perceived psychosocial concern, they both displayed more psychosocial concern during second visits than during initial or later visits.

These findings appear understandable given the need for providing comprehensive care in chronic- and well-care visits. Patients, however, perceived more psychosocial concern in chronic and follow-up visits than in well-care or acute care visits. From the patient's perspective, the greater perception of psychosocial concern in chronic and follow-up visits may reflect their recognition of continuity of care. It is also possible that patients who were more compliant in terms of returning for scheduled visits were more likely to be sensitive to provider activities that were psychosocially oriented. Although the possibility of a case mix bias may confound these results, another possible explanation for this finding may be that providers focus primarily on the chief complaint that prompted a first visit. After the initial visit, providers may then focus on psychosocial issues.

Female providers showed more psychosocial concern than male providers, particularly with female patients. Observed exploration of psychosocial issues and patient perceptions of provider psychosocial concern were greatest for female provider–female patient interactions and lowest for male provider–male patient pairs.

There was a significant correlation between scores on the provider psychosocial concern index and patient satisfaction index scores. So, as the amount of provider psychosocial concern in a clinic visit increases, the patient's level of satisfaction with the visit also increases.

In general, NPs exhibited more psychosocial concern than MDs, when interacting with patients. Patients also perceived more psychosocial concern by NPs. Provider psychosocial concern, however, was not found to be related to patient-reported medical outcome measures such as recovery from a problem, relief of current symptoms, or number of days to recover.

The findings on patient satisfaction, psychosocial concern, proficiency, and information provision indicate that patients want providers to be friendly, to show sensitivity and concern, and to create a comfortable atmosphere for asking questions. Patients also want to have confidence in the knowledge and skills of their providers. With regard to information, patients want providers to provide information voluntarily and in an understandable, complete, and reassuring manner.

Patient satisfaction was, to a moderate degree, influenced by practice type (academically-based versus private practice) and length of acquaintance with the provider. The most important determinants of patient satisfaction, however, were patient perceptions of certain characteristics of provider style. Patients were more satisfied when they believed that their provider was sensitive, when they felt a sense of personal control over the interaction, and when they believed they had received information from the provider.

Information recall

The amount and type of information given to patients also affect another frequently studied outcome measure, patient compliance. Effective communication with regard to the nature of the patient's illness and treatment, including explanations in terms the patient can understand and accept, is essential for patient compliance. Patients cannot comply with regimens that they do not understand. While the nature of the information given to patients, that is, its clarity and intelligibility, is important for compliance, there is evidence that the amount of information given is equally important. Patients must recall the instructions they are given about treatment regimens in order to comply with them.

For this reason, the evaluation project investigated the recall of health information by patients. During the 1-month phone follow-up interview of videotaped patients, they were asked whether they recalled information given to them in two areas—self-care for the current problem and prevention of future problems. Recall of this information differed depending on the type of practice in which the patients were seen. Patients from solo practices recalled more information related to self-care, whereas recall of prevention information was better for collaborative practice patients.

Recall of both self-care and prevention information was associated with higher levels of patient-perceived psychosocial concern. Also, patients were more likely to indicate that they had followed the provider's suggestions for prevention. Comparison of the observed information given during the initial visit with information recalled on follow-up interviews showed that patients who recalled information did so with 70% accuracy.

Patients who reported following the self-care suggestions had perceived higher provider control and received less support or comfort-related behaviors from their providers. Patients who thought that the self-care suggestions were helpful were more satisfied at the time of the initial clinic visit. Patients who saw another provider for their problem perceived themselves to have had less control during the original clinic visit and were less satisfied at the time of the visit. These patients also had lower observed levels of physical examination activity and provider control.

In summary, the data show that patients who perceived more psychosocial concern were more likely to recall provider information and follow suggestions for prevention. But the medical outcome measures— recovery from the original problem, current symptom status, and number of days to recovery— incorporated in the follow-up interview showed no relationship to provider concern with psychosocial issues in the clinic visit. The ability to generalize these findings to other patient populations, however, is limited in this study by the subjective nature of the outcome measures and the mix of patient diagnosis and illness severity. Even so, these findings suggest possible process–outcome relationships that merit further exploration.

Gender

In addition to differences in professional orientation, medicine and nursing are segregated by gender. As a result, medicine and nursing are invested with gender-linked stereotypes. The image of the nursing profession, for example, is pervasively linked to females (Mauksch and Campbell 1985). As individuals, nurses (RNs) are described as warm, loving, compassionate, and emotional. Their primary professional duties are perceived as stereotypically feminine rather than masculine.

The image of MDs is also influenced by gender-linked stereotypes. The medical profession has been overwhelmingly male, although this is certainly changing, and performance of the MD role has been stereotypically male. The physician has been designated leader of the health-care team—a practitioner trained to make decisions. MDs have had considerable functional autonomy and have managed the resources of the health-care agency—material, human, and temporal—and controlled the division of labor between them and other health-care workers.

Given the influences of gender and professional socialization, how does gender affect the way providers behave and the way others perceive them? To help answer this question, providers viewed four videotapes of NPs and MDs in actual patient encounters (Horman et al. 1987). The viewers, NPs and MDs, responded to an open-ended questionnaire about what they had seen. They were not told which of the professionals on tape were MDs and which were NPs. The professional status and gender of the provider were varied, so that a male and female MD and a male and female NP were shown.

In the tapes, the two representatives of each profession behaved similarly to each other but differently from the representatives of the other profession. To learn whether the clinical performance of these providers was representative of their professions, we proportionally scored their performance with the same observation-based instrument used for measuring provider clinical interaction style. After viewing each taped clinic visit, respondents completed a questionnaire containing, among other items, the following questions:

Was, in your judgment, the provider a: (a) MD or (b) NP?
Was the provider typical of his/her profession?
Was the provider's behavior influenced by the provider's sex?

A χ^2 analysis found a statistically significant relationship between taped providers' gender and the status they were assigned ($\chi^2 = 65.82$, $P = .00$). As Table 6-7 shows, male providers tended to be identified as MDs and females were identified as NPs. Viewers were very confident that the taped providers typified their respective professions. They cor-

6-7.   Accuracy of Status Identification per Episode

Episode No.	Identification assigned	Accurate		Inaccurate		Total	
		%	N	%	N	%	N
1	Female NP	84.4	38	15.6	7	100.0	45
2	Male MD		98.0	45	2.0	1	100.0	46
1	Female NP	32.0	9	68.0	19		100.0	28
1	Male MD		25.6	11	74.4	32	100.0	43

MD, physician; N, population; NP, nurse practitioner.

rectly identified the male physician and female nurse practitioner more than 84% of the time. However, the respondents correctly identified the female MD and male NP only 32% of the time. This occurred despite objective evidence showing that the female MD and the male NP displayed clinical behavior more like their professional than their gender counterparts.

Respondents' reasons for assigning a professional status to a taped provider, as well as their reasons for believing that that provider was typical of this profession, provide clues to the images each profession held of the MD and the NP. The distinctions between medical and nursing approaches to health care were recognized by these respondents and stereotypically associated with the two professional roles on the basis of gender.

Those assigned the NP status were perceived more often to have emphasized prevention, done extensive client education, and informed clients in a commendable manner. The inability of NPs to prescribe without consultation was also noted. Those assigned the MD status were characterized by fewer teaching or prevention activities but also by the ability to prescribe medications freely and to provide extensive information to the client.

When comparing the assessment between male and female providers, it was apparent that all the respondents, including NPs, were familiar with conventional sex-role stereotypes. Both male and female respondents cited stereotypical characteristics that distinguished male providers from female providers. Male providers were described in terms consistent with male stereotypes *(assertive, directive, cocky, non-empathetic)* and in terms reflecting complaints patients have expressed about the impersonal nature of health care *(tactless, patronizing, routine, uncomfortable in interpersonal interaction)*. Male providers were also distinguished by substandard methods of handling "intimate" health matters, or those unique to female clients.

Respondents described female providers with stereotypical feminine traits such as empathy, nonassertiveness, and interpersonal comfort. Their clinical behavior was characterized by those things that patients sometimes believe MDs often ignore—exploring the impact of a patient's lifestyle on illness.

More respondents believed that gender influenced clinical performance when the taped provider's status was incongruent with gender-role stereotypes than when it was congruent. But belief in gender influence was unrelated to how accurately respondents identified status. Respondents were significantly more willing to concede that gender influenced behavior after viewing the later episodes than the earlier ones. Because episodes three and four were both gender-role incongruent; these results on belief in gender influence are confounded by the repeated asking of respondents if provider gender affected behavior, which may suggest to them that it could.

It is impossible to ascertain from this study whether episode-by-episode differences in reported belief in gender influence is due to characteristics of the taped providers, to order effects, or to interview sensitization. Randomizing the order of presentation of taped episodes in future research would, at least, eliminate presentation-order effects and reveal the extent to which respondents become sensitized to the gender influence question.

Patients' perceptions of providers are also influenced by gender. As was previously mentioned, the female provider–female patient interaction received the highest scores on both provider psychosocial concern and patient-perceived psychosocial concern, whereas the male provider–male patient combination received the lowest scores.

Gender can affect the content of provider-patient interaction in several ways. Female providers could be conforming to the feminine stereotype that women are more interpersonally oriented than men. This orientation would predispose female providers to be more concerned with the social and psychological factors in patients' lives. The expectations of patients and providers could also affect provider behavior—patients may expect female providers to be more interested in psychosocial issues than are male providers. Female providers, likewise, could expect their female patients to be more concerned about social and psychological issues than are their male patients. A third possibility is that same-sex provider–patient dyads enhance communication, resulting in discussion of issues beyond the scope of purely physical problems.

Similar results were found for patient satisfaction—female patients were more satisfied than male patients with both female and male providers, but both male and female patients had higher satisfaction scores for female than for male providers.

A fundamental question arises from this investigation: Are the perceived differences between male and female providers and patients based on gender-related stereotypes or on behavioral and attitudinal differences?

Several studies of MDs have found that on entering medical school, female medical students are more interpersonally and psychosocially oriented than male students (Burkett and Kurz 1987, Potts et al. 1986,

Maheux et al. 1988). These studies found that the differences between male and female medical students attenuated or disappeared during medical training and were not as evident in practicing MDs. Thus, the effects of professional socialization for MDs tend to temper the effects of gender socialization on attitudes toward patient care.

For NPs, however, one would expect the relative effects of professional and gender socialization to be somewhat different. Nursing education stresses an interpersonal orientation, communication skills, concern with psychosocial influences on health and illness, and a more "humanistic" approach to patients. Female NPs would be expected to possess these characteristics when they enter nursing school and to emerge from the training period with these attitudes intact. Male NPs would also be expected to begin their education with higher levels of these attributes than male medical students and upon entering practice, to have retained these nontraditional attitudes.

The evaluation project found no difference between male and female NPs with regard to preferences for dealing with psychosocial issues, counseling, and educating patients. Both male and female NPs valued these aspects of patient care more than MDs did.

When NPs attempt to enter practice as colleagues of MDs, they find that feminine characteristics are viewed as "inferior" by MDs. Nurse practitioners soon become aware of the need to develop more traditionally "masculine" traits, such as assertiveness, self-reliance, aggressiveness, and competitiveness. This realization does not erase all the differences that might be expected based on the influences of gender socialization. But fewer differences than might be expected are actually found. More recently, Fagin (1992) noted that, "For some reason the women's movement did not penetrate into hospitals to homogenize role expectations and behaviors" (p. 299).

As evidenced in this study, NPs exhibited more psychosocial concern than MDs when interacting with patients. Patients also perceived more psychosocial concern by NPs. Because of the potential confounding effects of provider gender, an analysis of variance examining the separate and combined effects of gender and profession on the observation- and interview-based indices of psychosocial concern was performed. The results show that gender was not a significant influence on observed provider actions or patient perceptions of providers' actions. This suggests that the differences between these two types of providers may be the result of differing professional orientations. A more recent survey of nurses supported this premise. It indicated that more than 55% found their working relationships with women MDs to be no better or worse than those with men MDs (Editors of Nursing 91 1991).

As with perceptions, the behaviors of providers are influenced by patient gender. This investigation found that both male and female providers exhibited more psychosocial concern and affiliative behavior with female than with male patients. Female patients, in turn, also displayed more affiliation than male patients with both male and female providers.

All the evidence suggests that gender plays an important part in provider–patient interaction and, perhaps, in the professional roles of both MDs and NPs. The relative contributions of gender and professional socialization, however, to the attitudes, values, and behaviors of providers have yet to be definitively determined. Indeed, the continual interaction of these two forces throughout the professional lives of providers is probably more important than a static evaluation at any given point in time. If this is true, the future of NPs, as part of a "female occupation" in the male-dominated medical world has yet to be determined and can be affected by changes in professional attitudes, political climates, and gender composition of the professions.

SUMMARY

The findings of the evaluation project emphasize the complexity of the factors that affect collaborative practice between MDs and NPs. The results of health care given by a MD–NP team were in some ways different from the care given in a non-collaborative practice setting. At the same time, these findings were equivocal and, in detailed analyses, yielded fewer clear distinctions between NPs and MDs than might have been expected. Although stereotypes of gender and occupation and inequalities of status and power were factors in analyzing the structure, process, and outcome of collaborative practice arrangements, they were less powerful variables than anticipated.

This project started with the evaluative question, Who does what? From allocation of tasks, this study moved to clinical styles and processes and to considering priorities and assumptions that underlie the provider–patient relationship. The data suggest that within the framework of identical goals there can be variations in collaborative arrangements. The emergence of a wider repertoire of health care approaches may indeed be a significant step toward improvement of health care and enhancement of the sensitivity and capability of front-line practitioners.

Many factors are currently shaping the health care marketplace, including the pressure for cost containment and the efficient use of resources, the recognition of nursing services as reimbursable, the need for accessible and affordable care for all, and the increasingly complex care problems (Koch et al. 1992). These factors will favor collaboration among nurses and physicians and help create new models of working together to help meet the present-day challenges (Mezey and McGovern 1993).

The findings of this study also suggest that an evaluation of professional performance must explore the relationship of tasks to the objectives of the practitioner, the orientations of all participants, and the styles of performance. The experience of this study demonstrates the simultaneous importance of institutional arrangements, occupational traditions, and individual approaches and relationships. Although common patterns and generalized categories of behavior were searched for, the influence of individual situations proved an important factor. Collaborative practice teams are the result of interpersonal negotiations, accommodation, and preconditions as much as they are the byproducts of professional norms, areas of competence, and institutional structures.

The factor that emerged as a major force in the functioning of collaborative practice teams turned out to be the persistence of the traditional medical model. This model not only restrained NPs from practicing or recording behaviors derived from a nursing model, but it also influenced the behavior of MDs, who seemed to feel pressures against expanding into broader approaches to patient care. Thus, while in some instances the complementarity of NP and MD approaches ran into problems stemming from unequal power, both team members were more typically affected by the weight of medical tradition.

These findings evoke a number of responses. Foremost, the importance and implications of the subtlety of these data have to be emphasized. Neither assumptions of normal distribution nor assumptions of free and unskewed reporting of information can be applied to this harvest of observations, self-reports, and questionnaire responses. No matter how slight the differences, attention should be paid to the indicators that show that regardless of gender, MDs and NPs reflect their respective occupations when their actual behavior is examined. The perceptions of them either by professional peers or by the public is, however, dominated in part by gender stereotypes. This has far reaching implications for practice, for professional education, and for media management.

At the same time, one can respond to the findings as largely anticipated. Most difficult to document, and yet significant in the long term, are the accumulated cues that something occurs in collaborative practice that may not be identified fully by evaluative methods. The suggestion that MDs and NPs in collaborative practice seem to absorb some of each other's style and behaviors appears to contradict the impression that the collaborative arrangement actually frees both partners to be more a MD or NP, respectively. Nevertheless, both observations seem appropriate. The collaborative model may offer the NP a better opportunity to demonstrate a nursing presence and to implement a nursing model of care than the nurse in traditional, institutional settings. Similarly, the MD may feel enabled, or even encouraged, to move into dimensions of care that medical tradition has downplayed and that are appealing to MDs in primary care.

Another dimension not immediately identifiable was the relationship within the team. Observations, casual remarks, and the physical and social context of the clinics visited provided a fairly adequate picture of the degree to which the term *collaborative practice* was an operational reality rather than merely a label. We did find many settings in which complementary and colleague-like relationships were the prevailing pattern, but we also found settings where strong remnants of traditional MD–nurse structures persisted. The importance of not only mutual respect but also of the acceptance of different priorities and styles emerged as a key ingredient of a successful collaborative practice team. It was under these conditions that learning from each other was a free exchange between colleagues. The findings that acceptance, respect, and partnership serve as the lubricant for adaptive behavior and for learning have far-reaching meaning for education and team development. MDs in collaborative practice not only manifested changes due to the nursing presence, but they actually acknowledged them.

Considering the time and context in which this evaluation project was conducted, it is interesting that many of the issues identified by the project are still present. For example, Stein et al. (1990), in an article that revisits the doctor–nurse game, believe that the nurses' role of "stubborn rebel" has replaced, more often than not, "willing supplicant." Kassirer (1994, p. 204), in an editorial in the *New England Journal of Medicine* stated that, "The claim that nurse practitioners provide primary care equal in quality to that provided by MDs is based on weak data." In that same issue of the journal, Mundinger (1994, p. 214) declared that, "The best model—one that reduces costs while enhancing quality and comprehensiveness—is collaborative practice." The editorial by Kassirer and the article by Mundinger created a flurry of letters, both positive and negative, to the journal. As one exasperated MD replied, "in the words of Rodney King, 'Can't we get along?'" (Bloom 1994).

In many ways, collaborative practice is no longer a choice (Fagin 1992). With the increase in managed care settings there will be more opportunities for NPs to form group practices and to increase innovative roles in the health care industry. Achieving true complementarity of roles and functions in primary care collaborative practice is the responsibility of both NPs and MDs. It requires negotiation as well as commitment to the ideals that gave birth to the concept of collaborative practice. Success should result in benefits for both providers and patients.

References

Argyle, M. (1972). *The psychology of interpersonal behavior* (2nd ed.). London, England; Cox and Wyman, Ltd.

Ashworth, C.D., Williamson, P., and Montano, D. (1984) A scale to measure MD beliefs about psychosocial aspects of patient care, *Social Science and Medicine, 19*(11), 1235–1238.

Bloom, J.M. (1994, May) Letter. *New England Journal of Medicine, 330*(21), 1539.

Buller, M. K. and Buller, D.B. (1987, December). MDs' communication style and patient satisfaction. *Journal of Health and Social Behavior, 28*(4), 375–388.

Burkett, G. and Kurz, D. (1981). A comparison of the professional values and career orientations of male and female medical students: some unintended consequences of U.S. public policy. *Health Policy and Education, 3*, 33–45.

Campbell, J.D., Mauksch, H.O., Neikirk, H.J., and Hosokawa, M.C. (1990a) Collaborative practice and provider styles of delivering health care. *Social Science and Medicine, 30*(12), 1359–1365.

Campbell, J.D., Neikirk, H.J., and Hosokawa, M.C. (1990b) Development of a psychosocial concern index from videotaped interviews of nurse practitioners and family MDs., *Journal of Family Practice, 30*(3), 32–326.

Cassell, E. (1985). *Talking with patients: Vol. 1. The theory of doctor–patient communication.* Cambridge, MA: MIT Press.

Coeling, H.V. and Wilcox, J.R. (1994, Summer) Steps to collaboration. *Nursing Administration Quarterly, 18*(4):44–55

Costello, D. E. (1977). Health communication theory and research: An overview. In B. Ruben (Ed.), *Communication yearbook 1.* New Brunswick, N.J.: Transaction, Inc.

DiMatteo, M. R. and DiNicola, D. D. (1982). Social science and the art of medicine: From Hippocrates to holism. In H. Friedman and M. DiMatteo (Eds.), *Interpersonal issues in health care* (pp. 9–31). New York: Academic Press.

Donabedian, A. (1985). *Explorations in quality assessment and monitoring. Vol. III: The methods and findings of quality assessment and monitoring: An illustrated analysis* (p. 256). Ann Arbor, MI: Health Administration Press.

Editors of Nursing 91 (1991, June) The nurse–doctor game. *Nursing 91*, 21:60–64.

Fagin, C. (1992, May) Collaboration between nurses and MDs; no longer a choice. *Academic Medicine, 67*(5), 295–303.

Goldberg, L. (1977) What if we administered the "wrong" inventory? The prediction of scores on personality research form scales from those on the California psychological inventory, and vice versa. *Applied Psychological Measurement, 1*(3), 339–354.

Hall, J. A., Roter, D. L., and Katz N. R. (1988, July). Meta-analysis of correlates of provider behavior in medical encounters. *Medical Care, 26* (7), 657–675.

Horman, D.J., Campbell, J.D., and DeGregory, J.L. (1987, September) Gender and the attribution of the nurse practitioner and MD status. *Medical Care, 25*(9), 847–855.

Jelinek, D. (1978, January–February). The longitudinal study of nurse practitioners: Report of phase II. *Nurse Practitioner, 3,* 17–19.

Kassirer, J.P. (1994, January) What role for nurse practitioners in primary care? *New England Journal of Medicine, 330*(3), 204–205.

Koch, L., Pazaki-Palashi, H., and Campbell, J.D. (1992, February) A review of nurse practitioner literature in the first 20 years: an evaluation of joint practice issues. *Nurse Practitioner, 17*(2): 62–71.

Koerner, B.L., Cohen, J.R., and Armstrong, D.M. (1985, September) Collaborative practice and patient satisfaction. *Evaluation and the Health Professions, 8*(3), 299–321.

Levine, D. M., Morlock, L. L., Mushlin, A. I., Shapiro, S., and Malitz F. E. (1976, April). The role of new health practitioners in a prepaid group practice: Provider differences in process and outcomes of medical care. *Medical Care, 14* (4), 326–347.

Little, M. (1980, September) Nurse Practitioner–MD Relationships. *American Journal of Nursing, 80*(9), 1642–1645.

Lysaught, J. P. (1981). *Action in affirmation towards an unambiguous progression of nursing.* New York: McGraw-Hill, Inc.

Maheux, B., Defort, F., and Beland, F. (1988) Professional and sociopolitical attitudes of medical students: Gender differences reconsidered. *Journal of the American Medical Women's Association, 43,* 73–76.

Mauksch, H.O. and Campbell, J.D. (1985, September) Political imperatives for nursing in a stereotyping world. In *Perspectives in Nursing, 1985–1987.* NLN Publications, 41-1985, pp. 222–229.

Mezey, M.D. and McGovern, D.O.(1993) *Nurses, nurse practitioners: Evolution to advanced practice.* New York: Springer Publishing Company, Inc.

Mundinger, M. (1994, January) Advanced-oractice nursing: good medicine for MDs? *New England Journal of Medicine, 330*(3), 211–214.

Potts, M.K., Katz, B.P., and Brandt, P.H. (1986). Sex differences in medical student and housestaff attitudes toward the handicapped. *Journal of American Medical Women's Association, 41*, 156–60.

Powers, M., Jalowiec, H., and Reichelt, P. (1984, February). Nurse practitioner and MD care compared for nonurgent emergency room patients. *Nurse Practitioner, 9* (2), 39, 42, 44–45.

Scott, W. Richard. "Professional Work and Professional Power: Some Implications for Nursing," unpublished paper, Rush University, Chicago, March 1976, p. 11.

Stein, L.I., Watts, D.T., and Howell, T. (1990, February) The doctor–nurse game revisited. *New England Journal of Medicine, 322*(8), 546–549.

Stiles, W. B. (1978). Verbal response modes and dimensions of interpersonal roles: A method of discourse analysis. *Journal of Personality and Social Psychology, 36* (7), 693–703.

Sultz, H. A., Henry, O. M., Bullough, B., Buck, G. M., and Kinyon L. J. (1984, May–June) Nurse practitioners: A decade of change. Part IV. *Nursing Outlook, 32* (3), 158–163.

Zammuto, R. F., Turner, I. R., Miller, S., Shannon, I., and Christian J. (1979, March–April). Effect of clinical settings on the utilization of nurse practitioners. *Nursing Research, 28*, 98–102.

Clinical Management by Family Nurse Practitioners and Physicians in Collaborative Practice: A Comparative Analysis

7

Marcia Flesner and Julie Clawson

INTRODUCTION

Differences in the clinical management of patients by family nurse practitioners and physicians are often implied or explicit in the literature (Brodie et al. 1982, Campbell et al. 1990, Feldman et al. 1987, McGrath 1990, U.S. Office of Technology Assessment 1986, Ramsey et al. 1982, Rosenaur et al. 1984). Research has revealed that the quality of clinical management by nurse practitioners may, in some areas of health care, be equal to or better than that of physicians (Moscovice 1977, Ramsey et al. 1982, Salkever et al. 1982, Spitzer et al. 1976 , Watkins and Wagner 1982). To help minimize the occurrence of costly illness in light of the current movement toward cost-containment approaches to health care and concerns related to access to care, services of nurse practitioners are being used widely in ambulatory sites.

Organized medicine provides ambivalent support for the role of the nurse practitioner, and in the constrained and volatile environment of the 1990s, the need for an evaluation of the differences in clinical management styles of physicians as compared with those of nurse practitioners is a priority. An early study (Brown et al. 1979) comparing 12 behaviors of nurse practitioners and physicians in a preventive medicine program, as described by their patients, reported the nurse practitioner receiving significantly more favorable evaluations for 8 of the 12 behaviors. Of the sample (26%) who had a new health problem discovered during their visits, nurse practitioners found new problems in 31.8% of their patients, as compared with the physicians, who reported new problems in 19.7% of their patients. Comparing processes of care employed by nurse practitioners and physicians in the overall clinical management in primary care practices, Bibb (1982) found that the differences between nurse practitioners' and physicians' management of commonly occurring problems were "almost entirely in the NP's more frequent inclusion of expressive 'caring' functions which have been traditionally the focus of nursing" (p. 29).

In the 1980s, cost comparisons were a priority topic in the research concerning nurse practitioners and physicians. Although not a precise measure, reductions in costs to patients in ambulatory patient care sites seem to indicate that behavioral differences were occurring at the practice sites. Thompson et al. (1982) found total costs per general examination in a health maintenance organization (HMO) clinic staffed by nurse practitioners, as compared with those performed in an HMO clinic staffed by physicians, to be comparatively more cost-effective. The fiscal data showed a substantial savings compared with the physician-run clinic, even though the duration of the examinations was longer for nurse practitioners than for physicians. The U.S. Congressional Office of Technology Assessment report (1986) validated that nurse practitioners had a positive impact on the reduction of costs and identified a component of the savings to be a result of the salary differential between nurse practitioners and physicians. The report found that several nurse practitioners could be trained for the same cost as educating one physician, which had cost implications for taxpayers who subsidize educational programs through government support, as well as for patients.

Examination of the process of clinical judgment making in nursing has been a goal of nurse educators. Tanner (1987), in a review of clinical judgment research studies, counseled the reader that nursing practice was more than the analytic problem solving suggested by application of the nursing process with its assessment, planning, diagnosis, intervention, and evaluation steps. Benner's (1984) classic book *From Novice to Expert* introduced a qualitative data-gathering method whereby "the intentions, expectations, meaning, and outcomes of expert practice can be described, and aspects of clinical know-how can be captured by interpretive descriptions of actual practice" (p. 4). Brykczynski (1989) used a hermeneutic phenomenological approach, modeled after Benner's (1983, 1984) research, to describe the clinical judgment practices of nurse practitioners, with an emphasis on how nurse practitioners use aspects of the discipline of nursing in their practice. Her findings indicated that nurse practitioners were holistic, supportive, and participatory and provided health maintenance and promotion activities along with illness treatment. This chapter reports on a qualitative research project examining the differences in the clinical management styles of collaborative nurse practitioner–physician pairs, using a phenomenological approach.

METHODOLOGY

Research Questions

The following research questions were posed:

1. Are the clinical management decisions and approaches of the nurse practitioner different from the decisions and approaches of the physician in a collaborative arrangement?
2. Does the nurse practitioner in a collaborative arrangement use a body of knowledge that is recognized as the discipline of nursing?

Research Design

Phenomenology is a qualitative research method that has been influential in the social sciences (Boyd 1993). A particular phenomenological methodology as outlined by Patterson and Zderad (1976) was used for this research project. The aim of this method is to describe the experience as it is and give an account of the pertinent facts via a reflective activity that allows the data to be thematically sorted and classified. The approach used by Patterson and Zderad (1976) for conceptualizing nursing phenomena consists of three phases: intuitive grasp, analytic examination, and description and synthesis. All phases were completed in this study and their conduct is described in the Method of Analysis section.

The research project was approved by the Health Sciences Institutional Review Board of the University of Missouri–Columbia.

Setting

The settings were ambulatory primary care practices in the state of Missouri. The context of the research setting is essential when using a qualitative phenomenological approach to a research endeavor. During the interview time frame, new legislation had been approved by the Missouri legislature, and guidelines for recognition as an advanced practice nurse (APN) within the state and for the APN–physician collaborative practice had been approved via the regulatory process. The 3-year struggle to create the rules was fresh in the memories of the APNs, with many of the interviewed nurse practitioners anxiously awaiting advanced practice nurse recognition. (See Chapter 11 for details of the experience.) This climate had the potential for creating an intervening variable, but the researchers do not believe the collaborative relationships were impacted negatively.

Sample

Ten collaborative pairs were recruited from central Missouri via a mail recruitment. A collaborative pair was defined as a licensed physician (medical doctor or doctor of osteopathy) and a nurse practitioner who was a graduate of an advanced practice nursing educational program and certified by the American Nurses Credentialing Center (ANCC). The recruitment criterion for the pair was that they be a nurse practitioner and physician who had been practicing together in a collaborative arrangement for at least 6 months.

Names for the nurse practitioner sample were obtained from a database maintained at the Sinclair School of Nursing, University of Missouri–Columbia. A purposive convenience sample of nurse practitioners located within a 120-mile radius of Columbia, Missouri, was obtained. Nurse practitioners were mailed a recruitment letter, signed by the authors, outlining the purpose of the study. The nurse practitioner member of the dyad was asked to recruit his or her collaborative physician to participate in the study. One of two preprinted forms was then to be completed and returned in a self-addressed, postage prepaid envelope included in the packet, indicating whether the collaborative pair were willing to participate and be interviewed. Mail recruitment continued until 10 collaborative pairs were obtained. A total of 20 recruitment letters were mailed, resulting in the final sample of 10 pairs who indicated a willingness to participate (50% positive response rate). A phone contact then was made by the researchers to arrange for an appointment for the interviews.

Instrument

After a review of the nursing and medical literature, researchers designed a semistructured survey instrument. The questionnaire documented demographic data, including the length of time as a practitioner, the time frame of the collaborative arrangement, and the motivation of each individual in selecting their current practice setting. The participants were asked to describe the method that they used when making clinical decisions in their practice setting. The questionnaire also inquired about the respondent's viewpoint as to which behaviors are essential for a successful collaborative practice. Finally, a proposed treatment plan was elicited from the physician and the nurse practitioner based on a case vignette concerning abdominal pain, used in a previous research study (Avorn et al. 1991). A pilot questionnaire was administered to nurse practitioners with active practices and who were faculty at the Sinclair School of Nursing, University of Missouri–Columbia; alterations were made to the questionnaire to clarify the intent of the questions.

Procedure

The interviews took place within a 5-month time frame at the work site of the collaborative pairs and were conducted by one of the two authors. Before administration of the questionnaire, the purpose of the study again was reviewed with each individual and questions concerning it were answered. Consent had been obtained via return of a Willingness to Participate form. The physician and nurse practitioner each were interviewed separately, and their responses were tape recorded. The interviews lasted between 45 minutes and 1 hour and 30 minutes.

The taped interviews were transcribed, resulting in 60 double-spaced pages of dialogue.

Method of Analysis

Phase one of the phenomenological method, as outlined as by Patterson and Zderad (1976), consists of intuitive behaviors, defined as preparation of the researcher and primary data collection. The goal of the behaviors described in this phase is for the researcher to be open to the phenomena of study and immersed in the topic. Both interviewers approached the project with the goal of setting aside any preconceived ideas. A second behavior essential to the intuitive phase is the immersion of the researcher in the phenomena of interest. The interviewers were doctoral candidates at the time of the interviews. One interviewer was a graduate of a university master's level nurse practitioner program, certified by ANCC, and was a faculty member at a baccalaureate program. The second interviewer managed a primary care practice staffed by nurse practitioners and was active in the research of collaboration and the historical evolution of the nurse practitioner role. An extensive search of the literature in the area of nurse practitioner studies was performed as an additional step toward immersing the authors in the field.

Phase two of the method, analytic examination, was performed by repetitive review of the typed interview contents by each of the researchers separately. The unit of analysis was the sentence. As meanings emerged from the sentences, the sentence was highlighted and the meaning written in the margin of the transcript. The sentences then were clustered using the MARTIIN computer program. Reflection on the themes of the clusters by the reviewers led to the identification of common themes. Phase three consisted of description and synthesis of the phenomena of interest, which is reviewed here.

Interrater reliability was evaluated by the authors when, independent of each other, they compared the thematic categorizations they had interpreted from the data. Full agreement was reached between the authors as to the main themes. Intrarater reliability was evaluated by reanalysis of the same unmarked transcripts by both authors. The results were an intrarater reliability of 100% for one author and 97% for the other (the unmarked segments contained 28 references).

Analysis of the Data

The length of time the collaborative pairs had been in practice together varied from a minimum of 6 months to a maximum of 8 years, with the average being 2.5 years. Five of the 10 physicians had worked with nurse practitioners previous to their current arrangement. The gender breakdown consisted of 10 female nurse practitioners, 5 female physicians, and 5 male physicians. The practice sites of the 10 pairs were seven private practice offices in rural communities, a practice located in an urban setting that served a predominantly rural population, a county health department clinic for indigent care in a city of 70,000 people, and rural hospital outpatient clinics. All the work sites identified their specialty as family practice.

The physicians' ages ranged from 31 to 68 years, with an average age of 42 years. The nurse practitioners' ages ranged from 34 to 63 years, with an average age of 47 years. The majority of the practitioners were master's-prepared graduates of a nursing school. Six of the nurse practitioners had been immersed in a particular nursing theory in their master's programs. Their specialties were in family practice, with two individuals jointly certified in family practice and gerontology. The duration of experience as a nurse practitioner ranged from 6 months to 20 years, with an average of 9 years practicing in a collaborative arrangement with their existing partner or in previous partnerships.

FINDINGS

Research Question No. 1

To elicit information concerning the differences between the clinical management decisions of physicians and those of nurse practitioners, two approaches were used. First, the individual being interviewed was asked the following question: "What method or methods do you use to process clinical decisions?" Initially, both physicians and nurse practitioners struggled to explain their processes. Two physicians identified the medical model as their framework. Two physicians described their approach as problem-based, whereby they would begin with the broad options and then, as information was gained, narrow the diagnosis through the process of elimination.

One physician, who had been in a private practice over 30 years, related his ability to understand a patient's problems instinctively, owing to his years of diagnostic experience. He described the mental protocols used to start the process of elimination while gathering data during patient examinations. One physician insisted that she did not use a process, but then described her deductive approach to gathering as much data as possible to determine a plan of action. One physician succinctly responded, "Hopefully, rationally."

Nurse practitioners described their clinical decision making as based on the goal of determining a diagnosis after obtaining as much information as possible from a patient interview, a physical examination, and past medical records, if available. The nurse practitioners mentioned behaviors such as "listening to the patient for clues," "asking the patient to describe what their basic health pattern has been like in the past," "observing the affect of the patient," "looking for patterns," and "assessing the patients' lifestyle behaviors and living arrangements." One practitioner, whose clientele was faced with a multitude of physical, emotional, and financial challenges and restraints, discussed the need to focus on "the problem of the day." In her setting, consideration of psychosocial issues were just as important as determining a diagnosis and a plan of care.

One practitioner discussed developing treatment options from the perspective of a "blending the medical and nursing points of view." Once a diagnosis was selected by the nurse, the plan of treatment was structured around the patient's abilities, resources, and willingness to participate in the plan of care. One nurse practitioner advised, "My practice is more instinctive as I gain experience and a routine that you develop as you practice."

Evidence of inductive reasoning was present in comments by three practitioners whose perspective is displayed by the following comment:

> I always try to start treatment from the simplest of treatment to the more complex, and always try to take cost into account, particularly when it comes to medication or how complicated the medication really is. My goal is trying to keep medication to a minimum as you get a whole lot better compliance if you do.

The viewpoint of awareness of the patient's psychosocial resources was discussed by the majority of the nurse practitioners when describing the variables to consider when choosing a treatment modality. Twenty-three comments addressing the psychosocial domain by the nurse practitioners were identified. Examples of the comments included "I would like to know what is going on in his life," "I would like to know about his personal situation," "I look at the support systems with the family and what do we need to do (to help patients) to take care of themselves," and "You have to deal with the psychosocial before you can deal with the medical problem." The importance of affect and of an assessment of the patient for depression was discussed by two practitioners.

For the second approach to elicit information on clinical management differences, a simulation using a clinical vignette from a prior research study (Avorn et al. 1991) was used. The following scenario of a patient with abdominal pain was presented to the nurse practitioners and physicians:

> A man you have never seen before comes to your office seeking help for intermittent sharp epigastric pains that are relieved by meals, but are worse on an empty stomach. The man is in his late 70's. The patient has just moved from out of state and brings along a report of an endoscopy performed a month ago showing diffuse gastritis of moderate severity, but no ulcer (p. 695).

The following question was then asked: "Is there a particular therapy you would choose at this point or would you need additional information?" Additional clinical data about the clinical vignette patient was available to the interviewee if requested. The additional information, slightly revised from the original research by the researchers, provided data on the patient's social and psychological history (death of a son 2 months ago in car accident, widower 4 years, moved to town to be near daughter, retired factory worker), diet (no restrictions, drinks five cups of coffee per day, eats out at restaurants, does not eat when home alone), medication usage (two aspirins as needed for stomach pain, daily vitamin every morning), smoking (two packs per day for 30 years), and past history (no chronic disease, no living brothers or sisters, parents died in their 80s of cardiac disease).

Both groups were identical in their final recommendations related to medication management, recommending treatment of possible peptic ulcer disease with a variety of prescription or over-the-counter medications, and a follow-up visit. The variations in the steps taken to reach the treatment plan are identified as follows.

Physicians. Requests for additional information averaged three questions (range, 0 to 8) before offering a recommended plan of care. Two of the physicians requested no additional information, recommending a trial administration of medication. The questions posed by the other eight physicians related to obtaining as much clinical information as possible via a physical examination, obtaining the past history of the patient via a patient interview or old medical records, and performing diagnostic laboratory tests. The activities were categorized as data gathering. Before proceeding to a recommended medication regimen, two physicians inquired as to the history of past successful methods of symptom relief. None of the physicians inquired about the patient's living arrangements or the support systems available to the patient.

Two physicians expressed an appreciation of the need to determine the cost of medications before prescribing them. Three physicians requested additional information related to the lifestyle behaviors of the patient, including information on smoking and diet. When advised that the patient was a long-term smoker with a two-pack-a-day habit, the physicians indicated that they would instruct the patient to stop smoking but did not comment on how they would assist the patient with accomplishing the goal. Dietary habits were addressed by two physicians who advised that they would provide information on a diet regimen for the patient to follow. Educational material related to lifestyle behaviors was not mentioned by any of the other physicians as an option to offer the patient. One physician explained that before planning a course of treatment, he would make an effort "to determine if the patient wants to get better." This comment was the only one made by any member of the physician group that appeared to be in a consultative mode, involving the patient in determining a plan of care.

Nurse practitioners. Requests for additional information averaged 10 questions (range, 4 to 19), and their questions covered a broader array of topics than the physicians'. The nurse practitioners described data-gathering activities similar to those of the physicians, such as additional past history information, copies of old medical records, and the desire to check laboratory values, that would provide essential information to assist them in determining a treatment plan. Twenty-eight comments were made by the nurse practitioners related to the activity of data gathering. An area of particular importance to the nurse practitioners was asking the patient to describe any successful prior methods of treatment of the pain.

A key intervention that was recommended by the nurse practitioners but absent from the physician recommendations was concern for the immediate relief of the patient's pain while in the office, if possible. This empathetic response was offered by five of the 10 nurse practitioners who were interested in a more detailed picture of the patient's pain than was the physician.

Regarding lifestyle behaviors, such as smoking, dietary intake, and alcohol consumption, the nurse practitioners asked 10 questions about these habits and commented on the importance of explaining to the patient their possible role in causing the abdominal pain being experienced. Their educational and consultative role was an evident theme in 23 comments made by the nurses. The phrases used by the nurse practitioners consistently started with "We would talk about. . ." or "I would discuss with the patient the. . ." or "I would consult with the patient about. . .," followed by a lifestyle habit that had the potential of contributing to the patient's discomfort. The nurse practitioners discussed educational materials such as videotapes or written literature that could be made available if the patient appeared interested.

The living arrangements and the support systems of the patient were additional areas of concern for the nurse practitioner group. All of the nurse practitioners requested information about the patient's family and the family's availability to the patient. Financial resources, in the form of 14 questions (concerning matters such as insurance availability, the patient's ability to pay for medications, and a possible return visit) was a consideration of the nurse practitioners. One method to assist the patient with their financial situation was by offering office samples to the patient to reduce the cost of the initial therapy.

Life stressors were a theme discussed by eight nurse practitioners. Ten comments concerning stress were offered such as ". . . [I] wonder if there is some grief going on," " I usually ask them if they are experiencing more stress than normal," "I would discuss the role of stress and how it can contribute to the abdominal pain," "We need to talk about stress and life changes," and "I would talk with the patient about stress and how it can influence his body."

The importance of negotiating with the patient for changes in the patient's behavior was a theme apparent in the nurse practitioners' responses. They verbalized that the "plan of treatment could only be implemented if the patient was willing to alter his lifestyle," in addition to complying with a medication regimen. One comment that explained the purpose of the consultation was "I would consult with the patient as to what habits he feels he can change at this point in his life." Four nurse practitioners discussed the importance of starting with a "simple and realistic treatment plan" that "doesn't overwhelm the patient" and that has a better chance of compliance in the long term.

Consultation among health care providers was a theme that emerged during discussion of the management of the case vignette. None of the physicians mentioned consultation with their collaborative nurse practitioner as a part of the clinical management process, although four physicians did mention referral to another physician as an option for difficult or complex cases. Four nurse practitioners indicated that they would consult with their collaborating physician to evaluate if they had considered all the treatment possibilities.

Both groups were asked how often they collaborated with each other concerning patient management decisions. The perceptions of eight of the physicians were that their nurse practitioner consulted with them daily; one physician recalled the consultation as occurring frequently, and one physician perceived the consultation as occurring occasionally. The nurse practitioners' perceptions were different, with five reporting daily consultation with their collaborative physician, one reporting weekly consultations, three reporting occasional consultations, and one reporting frequent consultations. The physicians were also asked their perception of how often they consulted with their nurse practitioners about clinical management issues. Five of the physicians reported that they consulted with their nurse practitioner on a daily or weekly basis, with the rest of the sample reporting doing so occasionally or rarely.

Table 7-1 reflects a comparison of the comments of the nurse practitioners and those of physicians, categorized by the themes identified in the transcripts.

Research Question No. 2

Brykczynski (1989) identified four commonly recognized aspects of the discipline of nursing as holistic personalized assessment; involvement of the patient and family in care; incorporation of health maintenance and promotion into care, along with illness treatment and detection; and inclusion of teaching, counseling, and supportive interventions (p. 79). Throughout the transcripts, evidence of these aspects of the nursing discipline by the sample of nurse practitioners can be seen.

Table 7-1. Comment Comparisons Between Nurse Practitioners' and Physicians' Clinical Management Styles

	No. of Comments by Physician	No. of Comments by Nurse Practitioner
Data gathering	1 2	28
Education role	7	23
Consultative role	1	17
Psychosocial	1	27
Role of stress	1	10
Financial considerations	2	14
Empathy (relief of pain)	0	6

Six nurse practitioners had been exposed to a nursing theory during their educational experience. Three of the 10 nurse practitioners advised that they used components of the nursing theory when assessing the patients' ability to manage their care. An example of such use of nursing knowledge is evidenced by the comment, "I try to figure out a medical diagnosis, and then look at how I can help the patient from the viewpoint of nursing." One nurse practitioner reported using a "blended approach" when using nursing theory, using pieces from different nursing theorists to assist her in planning the care of the patient. None of the nurse practitioners used the terminology of nursing diagnosis, such as is contained in the NANDA classification system during the interviews. (Nursing diagnoses tend to focus on human responses to health and illness. They usually combine a verb with a human response or symptom. *Alterations in comfort* is one example.)

Five nurse practitioners discussed the value of using the medical model, in addition to their nursing perspective, in their decision-making process. The importance of developing consistent habits in the collection of patient data was stressed by three practitioners. One nurse practitioner discussed how the use of a protocol for a physical assessment, learned from her collaborating physician using the medical model, assists her in patient care.

A revealing comment was offered by an experienced nurse practitioner who commented, "My style of practice is very much through a medical model type approach with an emphasis on nursing. We (nurse practitioners) take the medical model, and nurse practitioners modify it with the sweet taste of nursing." Following is a representative example of comments offered by the two nurse practitioners addressing the holistic perspective in their practice:

> I think nurses are good at holistic stuff. I am not treating you for your peptic ulcer disease exclusively. I am treating you as a whole person and I want to know what your track record is. I want to know if you have been getting a yearly exam, a prostate check, when is your next physical due, rather than saying I'll see you in six weeks.

Additional Findings

Two of the physicians discussed their difficulties in maintaining practice arrangements with physicians who had not worked out in their practice and how pleased they were with their decision to recruit a nurse practitioner.

The interviewers asked the following question: "If your collaborative partner disagreed on a method of treatment for a patient, how would the conflict be resolved?" Almost all the respondents verbalized that they rarely had disagreements over a recommended plan of treatment. The physicians discussed how there were a variety of modalities to consider with any diagnosis. Physicians were willing to allow their nurse practitioners to offer alternative therapy as long as the nurse practitioners advised the patients that the treatment was an alternative method. The nurse practitioners were open to deferring to their collaborative physician if necessary, but all the nurses reported never having experienced a situation of that type. Open disagreement was experienced by three of the collaborative pairs, but no treatment-decision overrides had resulted as a result of the willingness to debate the merits of different treatment protocols.

The collaborative pairs were asked the following question: "What behaviors do you believe are essential to a collaborative arrangement between a physician and an advanced practice nurse?" Trust and respect of each other were the most frequently offered response by both nurse practitioners and physicians. Common practice styles by the collaborative pair were also viewed by both groups as a key variable contributing to a successful practice. Physicians and nurse practitioners who had worked previously in unsuccessful collaborative arrangements were vocal about the need to have a strong work ethic evident in both partners. The ability to communicate in an open and easy manner was a key variable affecting collaboration that was mentioned by both groups.

Physicians identified different attitudes, skills, and behaviors to be essential to collaboration. Their discussions centered on the need of both partners to have confidence and strong personalities while placing their egos in the background. Proficient diagnostic skills were observed by the physicians to be possessed by their practitioners. The physicians viewed themselves as broad-minded individuals who were able to promote the cause of the nurse practitioners, especially in the rural locations.

The two groups differed in terms of the importance each placed on the various attitudes, skills, and behaviors. Nurse practitioners valued the physician's intelligence, their clinical and diagnostic skills, their willingness to share their expertise, the knowledge they possessed as a result of their experience, and their open style of communication both with their patients and with the nurse practitioners. The availability of the physician for consultation was a behavior also stressed by a majority of the nurse practitioners. Three nurse practitioners expressed an appreciation of their physician's ability to develop rapport with their patients.

Physicians valued behaviors they labeled "people skills" in their collaborating partners. The accommodating personalities of the nurse practitioners was a factor mentioned by over half the physicians. A repeated observation was of the nurse practitioner's ability to spend adequate time with the patients, their ability to negotiate with the patients about the patient's willingness to alter lifestyle behaviors, and their ability to use cost-effective modalities. Functional abilities, such as thorough physical examinations, assessment skills, and organized and complete documentation skills, were also valued by the physicians. This finding is similar to that of Prescott and Bowen (1985), wherein physicians defined a positive relationship as occurring when the hospital nurses they worked with were competent and willing to help. Finally, the collaborating physicians who were in isolated practice settings, identified the value of the practitioner as a support in terms of maintaining their knowledge of clinical topics and the comradeship of another professional.

CONCLUSIONS

The physicians in the study were supporters of the role of the nurse practitioner, and they verbalized the positive benefits to the practice and the patients attributable to the nurse practitioner's presence. Although the final medication treatment recommendations were identical between the two groups, the process used to reach the decision varied between the groups. The decision making by the nurse practitioners for the simulated scenario was accomplished within the context of the patient's environment and available resources. Resource management was evident in the many comments and questions offered by the nurse practitioners. Physicians were more directive, targeting their instructions to what the patient needed to do to improve his status, but not how the patient was to accomplish the changes.

Nurse practitioners interviewed in this study evidenced a holistic approach to the management of patient care. As one nurse commented, "I would discuss with the patient how I cared whether he got well or not, and that I was available to work with him on the problem." The authors viewed this comment as indicating a desire to create an "intimacy" with the lived experience of the patient and their experiences on the road to achieving health.

Benner (1984) advised the nursing community not to ignore knowledge gained from clinical experience. Clinical decision making occurring within collaborative pairs is an area ripe for continued qualitative exploration by nurse researchers. The limitation of a simulated case vignette needs to be replaced with participant observation in the practice sites of collaborative pairs. Collaboration by physicians and nurse practitioners, along with other health care providers, continues to be touted as a major solution to many of health care's problems. Understanding the interactions that occur within collaborative pairs, as well as the strengths each partner brings to the clinical management of the patients' health care, can contribute to a future in which health care professionals actively influence the design of new health care systems that provide high-quality, cost-beneficial care.

References

Avorn, J., Everitt, D. E., and Baker, M. W. (1991). *Archives of Internal Medicine, 151,* 694–698.

Bibb, B. A. (1982). Comparing nurse practitioners and physicians: A simulation study on processes of care. *Evaluation & the Health Professions, 5*(1), 29–42.

Benner, P.E. (1983). Uncovering the knowledge embedded in clinical practice. *Image: Journal of Nursing Scholarship, 25*(2),36–41.

Benner, P.E. (1984). *From novice to expert: Excellence and power in clinical nursing practice.* Menlo Park: Addison-Wesley.

Boyd, C. O. (1993). Phenomenology: The method. In P. L. Munhall & C. O. Boyd (Eds.), *Nursing research: A qualitative perspective* (pp. 99–132). New York: National League for Nursing Press.

Brodie, B., Bancroft, B., Rowell, P., and Wolf, W. (1982). A comparison of nurse practitioner and physician costs in a military out-patient facility. *Military Medicine, 147,* 1051–1053.

Brown, J. D., Brown, M. I., and Jones, F. (1979). Evaluation of a nurse practitioner practitioner-staffed preventative medicine program in a fee-for-service multi specialty clinic. *Preventive Medicine, 8,* 53–64.

Brykczynski, K. A. (1989). An interpretive study describing the clinical judgement of nurse practitioners. *Scholarly Inquiry for Nursing Practice: An International Journal, 3*(2), 75–104.

Campbell, J. D., Mauksch, H. O., and Hosokawa, M. C. (1990). Collaborative practice and provider styles of delivering health care. *Social Science & Medicine, 30*(12), 1359–1365.

Feldman, M. J., Ventura, M. R., and Crosby, F. (1987). Studies of nurse practitioner effectiveness. *Nursing Research, 36*(5), 303–308.

McFarland, G. K. and McFarland, E. A. (Eds.) (1993). *Nursing diagnosis & intervention: Planning for patient care.* Mosby: St. Louis.

McGrath, S. (1990). The cost-effectiveness of nurse practitioners. *Nurse Practitioners, 15*(7), 40–42.

Moscovice, I. (1977). A method for analyzing resource use in ambulatory care settings. *Medical Care, 15,* 1024–1040.

Patterson, J. G. and Zderad, L. T. (1976). *Humanistic nursing.* Wiley: New York.

Prescott, P.A. and Bowen, S.A. (1985). Physician–nurse practitioner relationships. *Annals of Internal Medicine. 103*(1), 127–133.

Ramsay, J. A., McKenzie, J. K., and Fish, D. G. (1982). Physicians and nurse practitioners: Do they provide equivalent health care. *American Journal of Public Health, 72*(1), 55–57.

Rosenaur, J., Stanford, D., Morgan, W., and Curtin, B. (1984). Prescribing behaviors of primary care nurse practitioners. *American Journal of Public Health, 74*(1), 10–13.

Salkever, D. S., Skinner, E. A., Steinwachs, D. M., and Katz, H. (1982). Episode-based efficiency comparisons for physicians and nurse practitioners. *Medical Care, 20*(2), 143–153.

Spitzer, W. O., Roberts, R. S., and Delmore, T. (1976). Nurse practitioners in primary care. VI. Assessment of their deployment with the utilization and financial index. *Canadian Medical Association Journal. 114,* 1103–1106, 1108.

Tanner, C. A. (1987). Teaching clinical judgement. In J. J. Fitzpatrick and R. L. Taunton (Eds.), *Annual Review of Nursing Research* (pp. 153–173). Springer Publishing Company: New York.

Thompson, R. S., Basden, P., and Howell, L. J. (1982). Evaluation of initial implementation of an organized adults health program employing family nurse practitioners. *Medical Care, 20*(11), 1109–1127.

U.S. Office of Technology Assessment (1986). *Nurse practitioners, physician assistants, and certified nurse-midwives: A policy analysis.* Washington D.C.: U. S. Government Printing Office.

Watkins, L. and Wagner, E. (1982). Nurse practitioner and physician adherence to standing orders criteria for consultation or referral. *American Journal of Public Health, 72,* 22–29.

Registered Nurse– Physician Collaborative Practice: Success Stories

Julie Bailey and Jane M. Armer

Collaborative practice is widely espoused as the preferred approach to health care delivery (Buchanan 1996, Lamb and Napodano 1984, McLain 1988b, Norsen et al. 1995, Steel 1986). Registered nurse–physician practice teams are referred to as the "ideal model toward which all nurse–physician relationships should strive" (McLain 1988a, p. 31). The basic premise underlying collaboration in health care is that the provision of quality patient care is dependent on the successful integration of the expertise, skills, and unique perspectives of professionals from different disciplines (Lamb and Napodano 1984; Norsen et al. 1995). The dilemma for many practitioners, however, seems to be how best to accomplish this integration.

The purpose of this qualitative study by Bailey was to identify, through personal interviews, the characteristics and conditions present in successful collaborative practices, as well as the individual attributes of advanced practice nurses (APNs) and physicians that contribute to success. Sharing the stories of practitioners who have realized success in their collaborative ventures offers guidance to those pursuing collaborative endeavors. *Success* is defined lexicographically as "the favorable or prosperous termination of attempts or endeavors" (*Random House College Dictionary* 1982, p. 1312). For the purpose of this study, however, *success* was defined subjectively by the participants; those who agreed to participate viewed their collaborative practice to be an example of a successful one.

Traditionally, health care in the United States was based on a hierarchical relationship between nurses and physicians. The physician was

225

viewed as the dominant leader or as "captain of the ship," whereas the nurse was socialized to be a deferent follower of the physician's "orders" (Jones 1994). This interactional pattern was labeled the "doctor–nurse game" by Stein (cited in Will 1995), who noted in 1967 that nurses learned to offer recommendations and seek advice in ways that maintained the hierarchy and avoided conflict.

Changes in the health care climate have provided multiple opportunities for nurses to achieve greater autonomy and independence in their roles (Hilderley 1995). One of the most significant changes has been the growth and development of several categories of APNs. Nurse practitioners (NPs), one category of APN, have been associated with primary care since the inception of the role in 1965 as articulated by Loretta Ford and Dr. Henry Silver at the University of Colorado (Briggs 1990). This new nursing role, which prepares nurses to perform many acts traditionally performed only by physicians, challenged the traditional hierarchical relationships between nurses and physicians and has forced the disciplines to redefine roles and responsibilities. Additionally, sweeping changes in the regulation and delivery of health care, coupled with increasing consumer demand for coordinated, quality care have opened the door for a new model of health care practice: collaborative practice (Norsen et al. 1995).

REVIEW OF THE LITERATURE

Several authors have emphasized the potential benefits of collaboration among health care team members. Knaus et al. (1986, cited in Baggs and Schmitt 1988) found a positive relationship between collaboration and patient outcomes in the intensive care unit setting. Blickensderfer (1996) noted that nurses express a greater sense of job satisfaction when working in collaborative environments. Steel (1986) asserts that practitioners engaged in collaborative practice benefit from a "richer sense of professionalism, achievement, and feelings of success" (p. 5). She adds that the very nature of this type of relationship has the potential for improving the status of health care in general.

Some studies, however, reveal that the traditional hierarchical relationship between nurses and physicians, characterized by limited collaborative efforts, continues to exist. In a phenomenological study of nine nurse practitioner (NP)–physician dyads in separate collaborative practices, McLain (1988a) discovered that interactions between the two disciplines were primarily for the purpose of basic information exchange and were not collaborative in nature. Nurses sought advice, clarification, and help from the physicians, and the physicians instructed and/or corrected the NPs. In Lamb and Napodano's 1984 study of two primary care teams (each consisting of one physician and one NP), the data revealed that the practitioners interacted very little, with the physician team members rarely initiating the interactions.

Simborg et al. (1978) conducted chart reviews of patients seen by physicians and nonphysician practitioners in six different primary care practices. They investigated how the disciplines perceived patient problems, assigned priorities to those problems, and responded to information documented by another practitioner. The authors concluded that the complementary potential of collaboration was not fully realized by the practitioners. These reports appear to support McLain's (1988a) conclusion that although, theoretically, collaborative practice is viewed as the ideal model of provider organization for health care delivery, it remains difficult to isolate true collaboration in actual practice relationships.

In contrast, there are many anecdotal examples in the literature of successful collaborative ventures between nurses and physicians. *Together: A Casebook of Joint Practices in Primary Care* (National Joint Practice Commission 1977) is an early compilation of several examples of collaboration in action. Almost 20 years later, Hall and McHugh (1995) describe a collaborative project between two NPs and two family practice physicians in New York that was created to meet the needs of an underserved community. The NPs in this setting were viewed as full partners, with admitting privileges to the area hospital and shared call responsibility with the physicians. The authors describe a model in which patient care discussions and consultations flow equally between providers. Dontje et al. (1996) report on the establishment of a comprehensive breast care clinic in Michigan that initially paired two NPs and one surgeon in a collaborative arrangement. Continuous role definition and clarification was viewed as an important factor in the success of this endeavor. The NPs expressed the importance of maintaining independent roles within the collaborative practice model, as opposed to being viewed as "physician extenders" (p. 98). The idea of being conceptualized as a mere extension of the physician is generally viewed negatively by APNs (Baggs and Schmitt 1988, Johnson 1993).

As changes continue to occur in health care at a dizzying speed, collaborative or joint practice has been increasingly embraced as the most appropriate approach to providing health care. In reviewing the recent literature, four major themes became evident in the definition of collaboration. First, the terms *joint effort, working together,* and *joint responsibility* are commonly seen in discussions about collaboration (Anderson and Finn 1983, Avery 1995, Buchanan 1996, Henneman 1995, Hughes and Mackenzie 1990, Jones 1994, Lamb and Napodano 1984, Norsen et al. 1995, Sebas 1994, Weiss and Davis 1985, Will 1995). In fact, the word *collaboration* comes from the Latin words *col*, meaning "with or together," and *laborare*, meaning "to work" (cited in Blickensderfer 1996). Lamb and Napodano (1984) emphasize the element of integration as follows "Collaboration implies the generation and evaluation of *new* problems and plans which result directly from the integration of individual contributions rather than simply the coordination of individual ideas" (p. 26).

Second, the purpose of this joint venture is the attainment of mutually satisfying goals to include the provision of quality, coordinated, and comprehensive patient care. Third, respecting and utilizing the unique abilities and qualities of each professional within their respective scopes of practice is emphasized. Fourth, a collegial and equal relationship is stressed as opposed to a hierarchical, supervisory one. With these themes in mind, *collaborative practice* could be defined as a practice in which the partners espouse and value the major themes inherent in the concept of collaboration.

Numerous authors have documented the elements or characteristics that are basic to the concept of collaboration (Baggs and Schmitt 1988, Gardner and Fiske 1981, Hall and McHugh, 1995, Henneman 1995, Hughes and Mackenzie 1990, Koerner et al. 1986, Lamb and Napodano 1984, Norsen et al. 1995, Steel 1981 and 1986, Weiss and Davis 1985). Norsen et al. (1995) lists six critical attributes of collaboration that define the concept and ensure its success when integrated successfully by collaborators. The attributes—cooperation, assertiveness, responsibility, communication, autonomy, and coordination—are united by the common element of trust.

Cooperation involves mutual acknowledgment of and respect for each professional's views and opinions. Collegiality and equality are emphasized. As Henneman (1995) points out, "The traditionally hierarchical, and hence competitive relationship which typifies nurse–physician interactions does not exist in a collaborative environment. Instead, power is shared; it is based on knowledge and expertise rather than on title or role" (p. 360). Cooperation is achieved when collaborators recognize and acknowledge the unique talents and contributions of each discipline to the collaborative effort. Additionally, individuals within the collaborative practice must recognize and be able to articulate their personal strengths and weaknesses. In knowing this information, collaborators may improve the complementary nature of their relationship by utilizing strengths and augmenting weaknesses (Steel 1986).

Assertiveness ensures that individuals within the team are capable of expressing their views with confidence. Confidence has been emphasized as an important feature in successful collaborations (Davidhizer 1993, Steel 1986). Weiss and Davis (1985) propose that both assertiveness and cooperativeness are necessary in order to achieve the ultimate goal of collaboration, forming integrative solutions that capitalize on each professional's perspectives. Assertiveness also aids the important task of continuous negotiation to alter the course of the collaboration in response to the spiraling changes in health care. Flexibility is a complementary skill to assertiveness that allows the collaborators to embrace change as both an opportunity and a challenge (Norsen et al. 1995).

Responsibility refers to accepting accountability for views expressed and, ultimately, for the decisions made. Steel (1986) asserts that decisions that are made through consensus must be equally supported regardless of the outcome. Accompanying this attribute is the explicit understanding that the focus of collaboration is improved patient care; hence, the primary responsibility of the professional is to the patient.

The inherent nature of collaboration requires that communication be an ongoing process. This attribute implies not only accessibility on the part of each collaborator, but an environment in which a free flow of ideas is valued and nurtured (Hughes and Mackenzie 1990).

Autonomy ensures that individuals are empowered to carry out the plan of care within their respective scopes of practice. Implicit in this attribute is the need for clear understanding of each disciplines' mission, defined boundaries, and competencies.

The organization of care efforts is enhanced through coordination, which reduces duplication or misunderstandings and ensures that issues are addressed by the person most qualified to do so. Successful coordination establishes complementary merging of the disciplines and avoids the temptation to view partners as mere substitutes for each other.

The characteristics noted in the previous paragraphs are ones that have been isolated by the many authors cited as being crucial to the establishment and maintenance of successful collaboration. However, the conclusions of these authors are primarily based on anecdotal evidence of their observations of, or participation in, successful collaborative ventures. There is a paucity of research that queries collaborators regarding their perception of the essential elements of collaboration. One study, conducted by Prescott and Bowen (1985) questioned physicians and generalist nurses about the factors they believed enhanced the working relationship between the two disciplines. The elements identified most often were mutual trust and respect, open communication, cooperation, and competence.

METHODS OF PROCEDURE

Design

The methodological approach for this qualitative study was phenomenology. According to Polit and Hungler (1995), the focus of phenomenological inquiry is "what people experience regarding some phenomena and how they interpret those experiences" (p. 197). The phenomenon under investigation was successful collaboration between APNs and physicians. Non-experimental methods of data collection were used to elicit participants' definition of collaboration, views regarding the components of collaboration, and identifying information about the individual and the clinical site in which each participant collaborates.

Sample

Because the intent of this study was to interview APNs and physicians in successful collaborative partnerships, random sampling was not used to elicit participation. Additionally, because many APNs have collaborative agreements with more than one physician, the investigator chose initially to invite participation from the APNs in designated successful collaborative practices and then to allow the APN to choose the physician partner to be approached. Successful collaborative practices were identified through discussions with APN faculty at the University of Missouri–Columbia. Additional inclusion criteria for the APNs included current participation in a full-time collaborative practice with a physician partner, practicing within a 60-mile radius of the researcher, and ability to designate one physician partner who would also agree to participate in the study.

Procedure

The APNs were approached first via a mailed invitation to participate. In the mailing, the nurses were asked to return the name, address, and phone number of the physician partner whom they preferred to be interviewed. A follow-up call was made 3 to 4 weeks after the mailing to those APNs who had not returned the information in the enclosed self-addressed, stamped envelope. The named physicians were sent a similar invitation to participate in the study, and follow-up calls were made 1 to 2 weeks after the mailing. Participation was thus elicited on a voluntary basis by response to the written request and/or telephone call. Confidentiality was ensured by using code numbers for each individual within the dyad. Participants were advised that the raw data would not be shared with their partners.

The APN and physician dyads who agreed to participate in the study were interviewed separately over a period of 3 months. The audiotaped interview was conducted in an environment chosen by the participant and at a time he or she deemed convenient. All but four interviews were conducted in the participants' office or clinic site. One interview was conducted in a private office at the university where the participant had an academic appointment. Two others were completed at that university in private conference rooms; one participant dictated responses to the interview guide prior to leaving the country for several weeks during the data collection period. In addition to taping the face-to-face interviews, the researcher took detailed notes to compare with the completed transcription.

Questions asked during the scheduled, semi-structured interviews were open-ended in form to allow respondents to express their views fully. The participants were provided with a list of questions that would be asked during the meeting; however, the interview deviated from the script whenever the participant chose or when comments were made that required clarification or expansion. The purpose of many of the questions was to elicit each participant's views regarding the essential components of successful collaboration, the personal and professional attributes of collaborators that contribute to success, and conditions that enhance the collaborative effort. Additional questions probed the working relationship between the two disciplines; how conflict is resolved, how responsibilities for patient care and administrative details are allocated, and how decisions are made. Detailed demographic information was solicited, as well, for the purpose of description only. Transcripts of the interviews were returned to the participants to ensure accuracy; only one corrected transcript was returned.

As is common in qualitative research, additional questions became evident during early interviews that required the researcher to reconnect with seven of the participants. These individuals were sent a list of between one and five questions to respond to in writing. All but one participant returned this additional information.

Analysis

Thematic analysis of the qualitative data was conducted with the respondents' complete thought as the unit of analysis. Manual analysis of the data was carried out by initially reading all transcripts, first in their entirety, then across individual questions. Conceptual files were maintained for each of the themes that emerged from the data. A search for concurrent themes among the partners of each dyad was conducted to investigate commonalities and variations in the subjects' responses. Last, a template approach to content analysis was used to examine the existence of the six critical attributes of collaborative practice, as proposed by Norsen et al. (1995).

Sample Characteristics

The sample for this study consisted of seven APN and MD dyads (n = 14) practicing in collaborative arrangements in the mid-Missouri area. Sixteen APNs were approached. Reasons for nonparticipation included the following: changed position and terminated previous collaborative agreement before the initiation of the data collection period (n = 2), preferred not to participate with no reason expressed (n = 1), unable to participate because of busy schedule (n = 2), physician did not respond to mailings or calls by researcher (n = 3), and APN did not respond to mailings or calls (n = 1).

The APN sample consisted of one male and six female NPs; all were master's prepared, except one who lacked master's preparation but was certified in women's health. The age range was 31- to 46-years old, with a mean age of 38 years. All but one was an established APN prior to engaging in the current collaborative practice; one had worked at the same site as an RN before becoming an APN. Four of the partnerships knew their collaborating partner in advance. Participating APNs had been certified between 1 and 16 years, with a mean of 8.7 years, and the majority had worked in other collaborative arrangements before the current one. The amount of time spent in the current collaborative arrangement ranged from 1 to 4 years (mean = 2 years). The average number of patients seen per week varied widely between APNs, with one professional seeing only 15–25 patients and another seeing 100 patients on a weekly basis.

Among the physician sample, three males and four females participated. All were medical doctors; one physician had a master's degree in public health and another had received additional education in both family practice and geriatrics. The age range was 30–44 years, with a mean age of 39 years. The physicians in this sample had been practicing for between 3 and 14 years, with a mean of 6 years. All but one had worked in a collaborative practice prior to the current arrangement. The number of patients seen weekly by the physician sample varied widely as well (mean = 80 patients per week), although some of the physicians interviewed worked part time at the clinical site.

The sites represented by the APN–physician dyads included three rural satellite clinics operated by two different hospital systems, one public health clinic, one county health department, one hospital outpatient service, and another hospital long-term care unit. The written collaborative agreement for two of the dyads was provided by the Missouri State Nurses' Association (MONA). Three dyads used agreements similar to the MONA document or used a formal agency agreement, and two utilized written protocols.

RESULTS

Rationale for Collaborative Practice

Because Missouri statute mandates that APNs practice within a collaborative arrangement, the stated rationale for entering and maintaining a collaborative practice was obvious for the APN sample and was stated frequently. The majority of NPs (n = 6), however, had been in collaborative practice before the legislative mandate and expressed positive views regarding collaboration, many articulating the complementary nature of such an arrangement. The overwhelming theme emerging from the data was that the NPs did not desire a solo practice. One NP stated:

> My experience over 10 years has been that very few NPs want to be solo providers. [In my opinion] they either have no interest in it or don't feel very adequately prepared for it. I never entertained the thought of hanging up my own shingle and being a solo provider and working independently. After doing this as long as I have, I would feel competent in being able to do that but am not interested in doing that. I think that working collaboratively, I can enhance a physician's practice and he can enhance my practice because we have different skills, different experiences.

Another NP stated that she found it necessary to enter a more formalized collaborative arrangement because of problems in receiving third-party reimbursement when she practiced in a more independent role.

For the majority of physicians (n = 4) in the sample, the collaborative practice was in place prior to their joining the practice. Two of the physicians, however, stated that they chose their present practice site because it afforded them the opportunity to practice in collaboration with APNs. In one practice, the physicians realized that they needed to add an additional partner to the clinic, and they actively recruited an NP for the position. Three physicians made statements that illuminated the value they place on the complementary nature of collaboration. For example, one physician stated, "My feeling about nurse practitioners is that they're important, they're essential. They add so much that physicians don't have." Another physician's comments described the collegiality she felt with her partner: "[I]t gives me a colleague to discuss things with, bounce things off of, . . . interact with."

Two of the physicians described the nurse practitioner role largely as an extension of the physician. One stated:

> [S]he [the APN] lightens my work load and allows me to get more done. She does some of the more mundane stuff and I get a chance to do some of the research, like if we're not sure what to do next with a patient and I need to go read up on it.

Subsequent comments made by this physician also implied that a hierarchical, albeit supportive, relationship existed within this dyad.

Overall, the rationales for collaboration expressed by the participants emphasized the value of collegiality in improving patient care. This finding is in contrast to McLain's (1988b) investigation, which concluded that reasons for entering collaborative practice relationships were shaped more by political and economic forces than the value placed on the collaborative model.

Many of the respondents (four APNs and six physicians) commented that their previous exposure to, and experiences in, collaborative efforts helped them define to some degree how they would like to approach future endeavors. Two physicians stated that effective collaboration was modeled for them during their training. Many of the participants provided specific examples of the type of person and practice situations they had sought out.

Definition of Collaboration

The practitioners' definitions of the term *collaboration* mirrored the themes found in the literature. The descriptive theme expressed most often by both disciplines was that of "working together" with mutually-defined goals. The majority of respondents also offered the complementary nature of collaboration in improving patient care as an identifying benchmark. One physician commented on the integrative problem-solving potential of collaboration.

Elements of a Successful Collaborative Practice

The physicians and APNs in this study offered similar opinions when asked to name the characteristics of a successful collaborative practice. Communication was discussed as an important component by all of the physicians and four of the APNs. Words used to describe the type of communication deemed necessary in a collaborative practice included *frequent, open, honest, easy,* and *strong.* One APN identified that communication is enhanced in a collegial type of relationship:

> There's no room for a collaborative practice situation with partners who don't really consider themselves to be partners. There's no room for a hierarchical chain of command because that really inhibits communication. Both partners need to be safe confronting each other when necessary and be able to stand up for each other when necessary. That's more difficult to do in a hierarchical position.

All dyads stated that they communicated via phone or in person on a daily basis, primarily regarding patient care issues, and six of the seven dyads schedule formal meeting times. According to the physicians in the sample (n = 6), the majority of interactions are initiated by the APN. Only four of the APNs agreed; two felt that the interactions are initiated equally. One dyad agreed that such interactions are equally initiated. Previous reports (Jones 1994, Lamb and Napodano 1984, McLain 1988a) in the literature support the contention that the majority of physician–nurse interactions are initiated by the nurse for the purpose of consultation and clarification.

Trust and respect were mentioned equally by respondents. As one physician commented, "If you don't trust your nurse practitioner, I don't know how you can ever utilize her to the full extent. If you're going to have to be looking over her shoulder all the time—why bother?" The identification of mutual trust and respect mirrors the findings of Prescott and Bowen (1985). Stressing the importance of these two elements, one physician stated, "I think basically if you have a relationship that's built upon respect and trust, all the rest falls into place."

The majority of APNs (n = 5) named acknowledged personal strengths and weaknesses and knowing the boundaries of one's scope of practice as being essential to successful practice. Three physicians agreed on the importance of these characteristics, with one physician adding that the ability to acknowledge one's limits is "very critical for a relation-ship with doctors, probably even more so than with nurse practitioners." Three APNs clearly defined the theme of knowing the boundaries or scope of practice for understanding and defining each partner's role within the collaborative practice. As one APN stated:

> [Y]ou need to have a good understanding of what your role is and you need to know that there is a difference between a physician and a nurse. . . . you need to know that you are not trying to be a junior doctor. You are trying to be a nurse and you do come at it from a different perspec-tive and you meet in the middle and that's where the patient is.

Other themes that emerged were the mix or fit of the individuals involved in the collaboration; their availability and approachability; the taking of equal responsibility for patient care; the personal attributes of flexibility, integrity, and honesty; the designation of adequate time in the practice for the provision of quality patient care; and the establishment of a true partnership without a sense of hierarchy.

Conditions Identified as Necessary or Conducive to a Successful Collaborative Practice

Articulating the conditions necessary for, or conducive to, a successful collaborative practice proved to be a difficult question for some of the participants to answer; however, many similar themes appeared in the data. "Having enough space to provide care efficiently" was mentioned by four of the physicians and two of the APNs. Implied in the comments describing space and the physical layout of the clinical site was the concept of parity between providers. Parity in the relationship was mentioned directly by three of the APNs. As one APN stated:

> . . . [I]t should be mutual. It shouldn't be, well because you're the physician or because you're a nurse practitioner you get a secretary or you don't get a secretary. . . . [W]e're practice partners and it should be even. You need to break down the external barriers that are for the hierarchical system.

Supportive legislation was identified as an important condition by three physicians and an equal number of APNs. One physician commented that legislation requiring physicians to sign APN documentation is "unhealthy to the nurse practitioner and it's a deterrent to physicians to enter an agreement." Another physician commented on the continuous negotiations that have taken place in Missouri between the governing boards of various professions

> [T]he Nurses' Association and the Missouri State Medical Association and the Pharmacy Board need to figure out exactly how they're going to deal with this issue. I think that the Missouri State Medical Association needs to stop being so threatened by nurse practitioners. I think the nursing board needs to understand that it's absolutely essential that nurse practitioners work alongside of physicians and not remotely from them.

Although the concept of geographic proximity in practice sites has become a controversial issue in Missouri, the vast majority of respondents in this study felt that working in close physical proximity with their partner was a positive and beneficial aspect of their practice. There were, however, obvious variations between the disciplines in the importance ascribed to this condition. The majority of physicians (n = 4) found close proximity to be very important, whereas the majority of APNs (n = 4) believed it was "nice but not necessary." Similar results were found among Prescott and Bowen's (1985) sample of physicians and generalist nurses. Participants in that study expressed that familiarity between providers, defined in terms of amount and longevity of contact, was an important factor in positive working relationships. In the current study, two APNs and one MD felt it was of no importance. As one APN stated, "It is not a matter of miles, but a matter of mind-set." (See Chapter 11 for a presentation of the Missouri experience.)

Third-party reimbursement for APN services was identified by two of the physicians and one APN as being an important condition in collaborative practices. In all the practices, charges for primary care services were the same, whether the service was provided by the APN or the MD.

Two APNs and one physician commented on the important role institutional administrations play in fostering successful collaborations. Previous authors (Koerner et al. 1986, Norsen et al. 1995) have proposed that administrative support consists of providing an environment that promotes and nurtures collaboration. Two themes emerged from the data that described the influence of administrative support: ensuring a complementary mesh of individual personalities and seeking input from providers for administrative decisions. The majority of providers expressed that personality mix is a vital feature in successful collaborations. One physician stated:

> Personality is extremely important. Not only is it important because of the need to develop a relationship between the physician and the nurse practitioner, but also because of the need to have a comfort level with each partner's style with patients. They will be seeing each other's patients, and if their personalities are so different that patients routinely are not satisfied with the partner, it makes it difficult to work together.

Respondents believed that the administration at the clinical site has a responsibility to ensure that providers mesh well. As one stated, "You just can't hire somebody in and say you two are going to work together. It's kind of like a marriage. You have to know each other and like each other and be able to express yourself honestly." Another APN explained that the administration of the institution she works in has become more supportive of her role and of the concept of collaboration largely because she educated them. Early in her career as an APN, the hospital chose a collaborating physician for this APN without consulting her or even allowing her to meet him before the agreement. She stated:

. . . [W]hen I get discouraged and I think I haven't made progress with educating about how I am and what I do and why my opinion counts, I look at things . . . and now I really do have a lot more say in my practice.

The amount of influence each of the dyads believed they had in administrative decision making varied widely. In one of the dyads, decisions were made internally through consensus. In three of the dyads, administrative decisions were made externally, but providers sensed that their input was valued. As one APN described, "It's very unique . . . in that every person, whether the janitor, the secretary, the nurse, the nurse practitioner, the physician, you all are on equal grounds in regards to voicing opinions. Opinions are actively sought out." The remaining dyads described environments in which decisions were generally made without their input. One APN expressed that this pattern was a "frustration in our office." While seen as a significant source of frustration, the providers believed that they were still able to collaborate successfully by using each other as "sounding boards" and aligning themselves as a united front on issues important to them. (See Chapter 15 for a discussion of transformational leadership as a facilitator of successful collaboration.)

Other conditions mentioned by the respondents were understanding of the APN role by support staff, acceptance of APNs by consumers, flexible policies and procedures that maximize the APNs' ability to provide care, access to computer technology for isolating resources and information, reduced paperwork, and a positive reaction by physician colleagues to the APN role.

Partner and Personal Attributes Identified

All respondents were asked to define what personal or professional attributes of each individual contributed to success within a collaboration. The attributes identified by the APN sample for their own discipline were diverse, with no dominant theme identified. Those attributes identified most often (n = 3 each) were assertiveness and confidence, understanding one's role and the boundaries inherent in the role, and the ability to get along well with others. Other attributes named by two physicians and two APNs were clinical competence, being a life-long learner, and a commitment to the profession. In contrast, all of the physicians in the sample believed that good communication skills were an important attribute for successful APNs to have. This attribute was identified by only one of the APNs, although many in the sample had discussed the importance of communication more globally as a characteristic of successful collaboration.

Physicians also identified clinical competence (n = 5) and understanding role (n = 3) as additional attributes. Steel (1986) emphasizes that APNs must not only understand their role in terms of the discipline and the specific collaboration, but they must also be able to articulate what their role is. "Nurses need to be able to draw distinct parameters around their own practice so they will know what to bring to the practice arrangement . . . Each nurse needs to find his/her own unique contribution within the scope of nursing practice" (p. 12). One APN echoed Steel's remarks regarding the individuality of scope of practice: "I don't think you can lump us all together and say all nurse practitioners do this or all nurse practitioners do that. . . . When you're negotiating, it's very individualized."

When asked to identify attributes of the physician that contribute to success, several of the physicians (n = 3) voiced that the attributes are the same for each discipline. Communication was stressed by two of the physicians. Two physicians commented that physicians must avoid the temptation of being "paternalistic" and must be comfortable not being in charge. As one physician stated, "I think a lot of physicians are not willing to treat other practitioners as colleagues and they like to treat them as employees and I think that's a problem." This theme was mentioned by three of the APNs as well. The majority of APNs (n = 5) identified respecting and understanding the APN's role and contribution as being significant. Also mentioned by APNs were trust and confidence in the APN, as well as the physician partner exhibiting flexibility, honesty, availability, and approachability.

Concurrent Themes Within The Partnerships

The raw data provided by members of each dyad were also analyzed for the purpose of uncovering concurrent themes between the partners. In all the relationships, the perceptions expressed by the physician and the APN of how each believed their role to be perceived by the other were accurate when compared with that partner's responses. It appeared that this understanding was fostered informally, not through direct communication of role or other issues. The majority of providers expressed that discussions about role or scope of practice either never occurred, occurred rarely, or took place only in the early phase of the relationship.

The overwhelming majority (n = 12) expressed positive feelings about how their role was perceived. For example, one APN stated:

> I feel they perceive my role accurately, that they understand what my role is all about, that they understand me personally, in terms of my competencies and my contribution to the practice. I feel accepted, acknowledged. I really can't think of any negative connotations or feelings, which is a little different from some of the feelings I had with some of the providers I collaborated with in the past.

The APN and physician members of one dyad expressed beliefs that demonstrated inaccurate perceptions by the physician regarding the APN role. The APN stated:

> I think there's still a little bit of that predominant belief of what a physician extender is. We've had discussions along this line. . . . I think [the physician] has a hard time seeing that piece [difference between APNs and physician assistants]. But at the same time I think [the physician] does know and understand that I have an ability of bringing the whole environment together and that's definitely my nursing.

Comments made throughout the interview by the physician member of this dyad revealed that the physician did harbor a more hierarchical view of the relationship, which was perceived accurately by the nurse partner. The APN's comments suggested that she felt the relationship was a successful collaboration, in spite of the obvious dominance by the physician. It is important to review this evaluation in the context of the dyad's environment, which was a more restrictive government-controlled agency.

In contrast, the relationship and working environments described by the other six dyads were devoid of a sense of hierarchy between the physicians and APNs. Themes of complementary independence, equality, collegiality, and partnership were expressed by both members of the dyad. In one dyad, the physician described the APN as a "full partner in the practice." The APN, in turn stated, "They [the collaborating physicians in the practice] accept me as a colleague and equal, and treat me that way and relate to me that way both when we're working together with patients and when we're discussing patients separately." Another physician commented: "It's not like it's my practice and [the APN] helps me. It's like we're equal."

In one dyad, the nurse's comments implied deference to the physician, which was perceived and expressed by the physician, even though both members of the dyad described a nonhierarchical relationship. The physician stated:

> Sometimes I think she purposely acts more deferential than she needs to because I think she may be afraid to offend me or to step on toes or something like that. I think it may be from previous experiences, I'm not sure. I think now, though, after working together for two years, we're pretty comfortable with each other and I think she realizes that there's no need for that. But I think, periodically, she does reassert, "I'm the nurse practitioner" just to kind of at least make me aware that she understands that, which, to be perfectly honest, I don't think is necessary. I think a lot of physicians have accused nurse practitioners in the past of kind of stepping on their turf or trying to take over their jobs. I think maybe she's doing that just to reassure that's not the case. Although, I've never had even the slightest worry that that is the case.

The physician explained that she has not discussed her perceptions with the nurse practitioner and described it as "more subtle than anything else." She also added that she did not believe it was an issue of confidence, in that she viewed the APN as a confident person. Instead, she stated, "I think it's just more our stereotypical roles." The APN member of this dyad expressed several comments throughout the interview that intimated that the physician's perceptions were accurate. It appeared, however, that she viewed her approach as both a personality trait and a necessity in order to be accepted by the medical community of the small town in which she practiced. She told of her initial experiences in this community, where the last nurse practitioner was reportedly "run out of town" 10 years earlier. She described, in detail, the hostility she initially endured from the medical community and the process she went through to prove herself. Her comments revealed that she viewed her approach, which she described as nonthreatening, as both an effective method for introducing the community to nurse practitioners and a way to gain acceptance for her role. Statements made regarding the working relationship in her current collaboration were synonymous with the physician's: democracy as opposed to hierarchy was the basis of the relationship, and integrative, patient-centered problem-solving was consistently used. The

APN commented on how she valued the approach her physician partner uses to respond to the APN's consultation requests: ". . . This dear lady will say to me, 'now this is not what you have to do, this is what I'd recommend. But the final decision is yours, because it's your patient.'"

Existence of Critical Attributes

As has already been discussed here, collaboration has been identified by Norsen et al. (1995) as having six critical attributes: cooperation, assertiveness, responsibility, communication, autonomy, and coordination, all of which are linked by the common element of trust. The data were analyzed to determine the existence of these critical attributes in the dyads' collaborations. It appeared that varying degrees of these attributes existed in all of the relationships.

Cooperation

Cooperation was a primary theme in all of the collaborative partnerships, as demonstrated by several variables. In all of the relationships, the interdependence of the professions was expressed by the utilization of each practitioner's identified area(s) of expertise. As one APN stated:

> There's many times that [the physician will] say to me, "This is a nurse practitioner patient," and it's somebody that has all kinds of sociological problems. Problems that I could coordinate, get everybody in that could possibly help this patient. And that's good; that's a compliment to nursing. He actually has learned what we do.

Mutual respect for each professional's views, opinions, and contributions—another benchmark for cooperation—was both identified as an important characteristic in successful collaborations by a majority of the respondents and perceived as existing, to some degree, in all of the relationships. One APN described how her physician partner expressed her beliefs about the value of nurse practitioners:

> She's the one, when I first got here, who brought an article in to me . . . it was talking about nurse practitioners' treatment of patients with arthritis, and it was saying that nurse practitioners did a better job. She brought it in to me and she said, "I want you to know that I do believe this is true." That is why I'm willing to drive 48 miles one way. Because she is absolutely wonderful to work with and I've learned so much.

The dyads' approach to decision-making demonstrated another feature of cooperation. In all but one dyad, decisions regarding patient care and internal practice issues were determined through consensus by negotiation and discussion. Last, one physician's comments demonstrated her willingness to examine and change her personal beliefs and perspectives, noting that "there's more than one way to do something correctly."

Assertiveness

Assertiveness, defined by Norsen et al. (1995) as "self-advocacy," was slightly more elusive to uncover in the raw data. One APN identified this concept as an essential attribute in a successful APN's armamentarium. Many of the APNs articulated examples of situations in which they asserted themselves, either to air their views or to advocate for a patient. The fact that decisions in six of the seven dyads were made through negotiation and discussion implies that these professionals were imbued with a certain level of assertiveness.

Responsibility

Responsibility, identified as mutual accountability and shared acceptance for decisions made through consensus, was discussed by many of the providers as key features of their practices. Additionally, all of the providers' comments either directly identified or indirectly implied that responsibility for patient outcomes was the driving force behind their collaborations. This concept was demonstrated in one APN's comments:

> If there's a patient who calls in and has a question about my treatment or she sees a patient when I'm not there, they call and say "I'm just not better," she'll say things like "If I had treated you, I would have given you the same thing." It just sets the patient at ease because they realize that we're working together. When I see a patient and it's someone that she's seen in the past and they're not better, I do the same thing for her.

Communication

The premium importance of communication among collaborators has already been presented. Many of the respondents described factors in the relationship that foster communication, including accessibility. As one APN noted:

> [O]ne thing that totally amazes me is that no matter how busy the clinic day can be and no matter how far behind he can be, if I need him, he stops and he listens with undivided attention without being rushed. . . .

He listens clearly. He respects what I'm saying to him. . . . He is approachable regardless of how bad his day may be going. . . . He's committed himself to realizing that this is the relationship that I have and he's very easy to communicate with and very easy to talk to.

Autonomy

Autonomy was discussed in much more detail by the APNs in the sample than by their physician partners. Several of the APNs identified acknowledging one's scope of practice and personal limitations as important characteristics of successful collaborations. As one stated, "You must be willing to expand your boundaries but know your limitations and where you feel comfortable in your practice." Inherent in the concept of autonomy is the bestowing of trust on individual members of the team to practice independently within the defined scope of practice. Autonomy was demonstrated in all of the relationships by the independent provision of patient care by all providers based on mutually defined goals of the practice.

Coordination

Last, coordination efforts were demonstrated in a variety of ways in the practice settings. Most obvious was the formal and informal direction provided to office staff for the purpose of triaging patients so that the most qualified provider could address the problem. As exemplified in the comments by one physician:

[The APN] really enjoys the kids and I do too, but she winds up doing a lot more pediatrics than I do. That's fine because she's more into wellness and preventative things than I am and that's just a reflection of our training. I'm becoming the procedure queen so anybody that wants a mole removed or this or that fixed, they go on my schedule.

Coordination also is characterized by the efficient organization of care efforts. This concept was demonstrated effectively by one dyad in their initiation of mutual chart reviews to ensure that each provider was utilizing similar, research-based treatment protocols.

DISCUSSION

A significant limitation of this study was the subjective nature of the definition of success in collaborative efforts. The yardstick for success was determined largely by the participants; thus, great variations were observed. Success as it relates to health care, and more specifically, to collaborative practice, has not been adequately defined in the literature. It was not the intention of this investigation to define success, but rather to isolate factors that enhance its existence. Future studies should look more critically at this elusive concept. Additionally, the respondents' comments could have been affected by their knowledge that their collaborative practice was viewed as a successful one by colleagues. Perhaps, a more intensive scrutiny of these collaborative practices, including field observation or use of available tools to measure various aspects of collaboration, would have revealed different results. Use of a larger, more diverse sample would have allowed for greater generalizability of the findings.

Despite these limitations, several conclusions can be drawn from the results. First, it is apparent that there is a great deal of congruency in the definition of collaboration, both in the literature and among the participants in this study. Common understanding of the concept establishes a more solid base on which to build a collaborative practice. There also appears to be consistency in the elements believed to be essential to fostering successful collaborations. Many of the respondents articulated that the same elements they described as essential to successful collaboration existed in their own partnerships. Because wide variations were observed in the interactional patterns, role perceptions, and logistical factors among the dyads, it may be hypothesized that success is a dynamic and varied phenomenon. A professionally satisfying finding in this investigation was the ease with which successful collaborations were identified.

Five themes appeared to be generalizable among the sample: 1) each of the professionals within the dyads expressed accurate perceptions of their environment, role, and relationship within the collaboration, as evidenced by the consistency in the comments between providers; 2) participants articulated, in varying degrees, the existence of the six critical attributes of collaboration identified by Norsen et al. (1995); 3) all of the dyads expressed similar philosophies in their approach to patient care and emphasized quality as their primary goal in providing care; 4) the APNs in this sample were both introspective and articulate, especially in describing their role and scope of practice, whereas the physicians were more matter of fact in their responses; and 5) many respondents emphasized the important role education plays in fostering successful collaborations through both teaching and role modeling of the skills necessary to collaborate effectively.

Studies of successful collaborative ventures provide many implications for education, practice, policy making, and research endeavors. Isolation of the elements that enhance collaboration provides the opportunity to expose professional students to this knowledge prior to their entrance into the "real world," thus increasing the probability of their success. Although not specifically asked during the interview process, some of the APNs discussed the impact mentors or "trailblazers" have had in shaping their practice. Additionally, two physicians in the study commented that effective collaboration was modeled during their training, thus underscoring the important role educators hold. Utilizing this information has the potential for positively impacting patient care. Understanding the dynamics of collaboration improves the ability of lawmakers to write more accurate and effective legislation, and greater interest in the concept ensures that constantly evolving questions of the concept will be investigated.

Several implications for future research remain. The concept of success needs to be investigated and defined more completely. An interesting approach would be to compare and contrast how success is defined by various groups, such as health care administrators, consumers, governing boards of health professions, as well as the professionals themselves. Additionally, because much of the literature examining the concept of successful collaborations is anecdotal, more detailed, investigational research should be pursued. Longitudinal research could investigate whether collaboration in stable relationships improves over time. Future research on this topic would be aided, as McLain (1988b) asserts by approaching the studies collaboratively, thus utilizing the unique perspectives of both the nursing and medical professions. Additional research on the relationship between the process of collaboration among health care providers and the outcomes of patient care is necessary. Last, continuing investigation of existing tools to measure collaboration and refinement of new tools that examine collaboration in specific practice sites such as in-patient hospitals, primary care clinics, and mental health care clinics should be pursued. Much of the literature on this subject has studied in-patient environments only. Continuing to research this concept will fuel increasing interest in its application to many health care environments.

Anderson, D. J. and Finn, M. C. (1983). Collaborative practice: Developing a structure that works. *Nurse Administration Quarterly, 8*(1), 19–25.

Avery, L. H. (1995). Nurses and physicians attempt to define collaboration and practice roles. *AORN Journal, (62)*, 1, 107–110.

Baggs, J. G. and Schmitt, M. H. (1988). Collaboration between nurses and physicians. *Image: Journal of Nursing Scholarship, 20*(3), 145–149.

Blickensderfer, L. (1996). Nurses and physicians: Creating a collaborative environment. *Journal of Intravenous Nursing, 19*(3), 127–131.

Briggs, N. A. (1990). The nurse practitioner: An expanded role within nursing. *NSNA/Imprint, 37*(1), 31–33.

Buchanan, L. (1996). The acute care nurse practitioner in collaborative practice. *Journal of the American Academy of Nurse Practitioners, 8*(1), 13–19.

Davidhizer, R. (1993). Self-confidence: A requirement for collaborative practice. *Dimensions of Critical Care Nursing, 12*(4), 218–222.

Dontje, K. J., Sparks, B. T., and Given, B. A. (1996). Establishing a collaborative practice in a comprehensive breast clinic. *Clinical Nurse Specialist, 10*(2), 95–101.

Gardner, H. H. and Fiske, M. S. (1981). Pluralism and competition: A possibility for primary care. *American Journal of Nursing, 81*, 2152–2157.

Hall, E. K. and McHugh, M. (1995). Family practice: Making collaborative practice a reality. *Nursing and Health Care: Perspectives on Community, 16*(5), 270–275.

Henneman, E. A. (1995). Nurse-physician collaboration: A poststructuralist view. *Journal of Advanced Nursing, 22*(2), 359–363.

Hilderley, L. J. (1995). Doctors and nurses-Are we still playing games? *Cancer Practice, 3*(2), 114–116.

Hughes, A. M. and Mackenzie, C. S. (1990). Components necessary in a successful nurse practitioner–physician collaborative practice. *Journal of the American Academy of Nurse Practitioners, 2*(2), 54–57.

Johnson, R. (1993). Nurse practitioner–patient discourse: Uncovering the voice of nursing in primary care practice. *Scholarly Inquiry for Nursing Practice: An International Journal, 7*(3), 143–157.

Jones, R. A. (1994). Nurse–physician collaboration: A descriptive study. *Holistic Nursing Practice, 8*(3), 38–53.

Koerner, B. L., Cohen, J. R., and Armstrong, D. M. (1986). Professional behavior in collaborative practice. *Journal of Nursing Administration, 16*(10), 39–43.

Lamb, G. S. and Napodano, R. J. (1984). Physician–nurse practitioner interaction patterns in primary care practices. *American Journal of Public Health, 74*(1), 26–29.

McLain, B. R. (1988a). Collaborative practice: The nurse practitioner's role in its success or failure. *Nurse Practitioner, 13*(5), 31–32, 34–35, 38.

McLain, B. R. (1988b). Collaborative practice: A critical theory perspective. *Research in Nursing and Health, 11*(6), 391–398.

National Joint Practice Commission. (1977). *Together: A Casebook of Joint Practices in Primary Care.* Chicago: Educational Publications and Innovative Communications.

Norsen, L., Opladen, J., and Quinn, J. (1995). Practice model: Collaborative practice. *Critical Care Nursing Clinics of North America, 7*(1), 43–52.

Polit, D. F. and Hungler, B. P. (1995). *Nursing Research: Principles and Methods.* Philadelphia: J. B. Lippincott.

Prescott, P. A. and Bowen, S. A. (1985). Physician–nurse relationships. *Annals of Internal Medicine, 103*(1), 127–133.

The Random House College Dictionary. (1982). New York: Random House.

Sebas, M. B. (1994). Developing a collaborative practice agreement for the primary care setting. *Nurse Practitioner: American Journal of Primary Health Care, 19*(3), 49–51.

Simborg, D. W., Starfield, B. H., and Horn, S. D. (1978). Physicians and non-physician health practitioners: The characteristics of their practices and their relationships. *American Journal of Public Health, 68*(1), 44–48.

Steel, J. E. (1981). Putting joint practice into practice. *American Journal of Nursing, 81*, 964–967.

Steel, J. E. (Ed.) (1986). *Issues in Collaborative Practice.* Orlando, FL: Grune & Stratton.

Stein, L. I. (1967). The doctor-nurse game. *Archives of General Psychiatry, 16*, 699–703, cited in Will, R. S. (1995). Nurse–physician collaboration: Dilemma or opportunity. *Canadian Journal of Nursing Administration, 8*(2), 30–42.

Weiss, S. J. and Davis, H. P. (1985). Validity and reliability of the collaborative practice scales. *Nursing Research, 34*(5), 299–305.

Interorganizational Collaboration

Coalition Building Among Diverse Organizations: Concept Analysis and Model or Theory Design

Toni J. Sullivan

INTRODUCTION

Understanding collaboration requires exploration of the topic of interorganizational collaboration, a topic of extraordinary complexity. There is an abundance of examples of collaboration in the form of coalitions, but there do not seem to be any clear parameters or principles governing their functioning.

Coalition formation and utilization is all about responding to change and complexity through connections. As discussed at length in Chapter 3, statewide, nationwide, and worldwide economic pressures, political forces, demographic shifts, changing family structures and gender roles, and fragmented family structures are combining to make our lives and our societies more hectic and disconnected than ever before. Narrow views of problems and concerns, and inadequate resources brought to bear on problems, are recognized as the old solutions and are rejected. In a White Paper entitled *Caring For People: Community Care In The Next Decade And Beyond*, the Department of Health of the United Kingdom stated, "It is essential that the caring services should work effectively together. . . . There is no room in community care for a narrow view of individuals' needs, nor of ways of meeting them" (Higgins et al. 1994, p. 269).

In the United States and elsewhere, it is tempting to attribute the movement to interorganizational collaboration in coalitions exclusively to cost-containment reimbursement, such as managed care or capitated care. Clearly, these models of reimbursement are influential. They are forcing competition in health care and are causing providers and provider organizations to behave differently than in the days of cost-plus prospective payment systems.

Wilford and Annison (1995) remind us that "[b]eginning in the '80s health care has had to learn to compete, and more recently providers have come face-to-face with the reality that they often have to [both] compete and collaborate with the same people and institutions simultaneously" (p. 28). Meservey (1995) opines that both managed care and a decline in health care resources have combined to create "the boundary-less organization," wherein hospitals are linked with myriad community-based organizations and other institutional services (p. 234). All the linking organizations are avoiding solo competition, which they cannot survive, and strengthening themselves and their competitive position through linkages. "In the days of cost plus reimbursement, independence meant strength. Now, institutional strength comes from collaboration, and the ability to work with a wide range of physicians, providers, hospitals, insurance companies, private businesses, and community groups" (Wilford and Annison 1995, p. 28). "Those who learn to manage both the competition and the collaboration will prosper; those who don't will be out of business" (p. 29). The goal of providers in linking together in a provider network or boundaryless organization is simply to provide the highest quality care (or at least adequate care) at the lowest possible cost. Tweed (1995) points out that it is only when providers work together over the full continuum of care that they can be successful in meeting that goal.

Yet, collaboration in interorganizational coalitions is not just about competition and saving money. It is about restoring our societies to good working order, and in the case of health care, it has to do with recognizing that no one discipline can effectively deal with all of health care. No longer can societies afford to squander their scarce economic resources on costly illness care while ignoring health promotion and prevention of illness care; rather, integrated, collaborative delivery systems are needed. Given how high the stakes are, those who are desirous of bettering society need to focus on the task at hand of learning how to formulate and conduct coalitions.

In the noisy milieus of coalitions, mixed signals abound. It is not always easy to make the right choices, given the sometimes conflicting demands of like-minded and diverse-minded members and of multipurpose goals versus those of advocacy, community empowerment, or community betterment. Making decisions, timing decision-making, and determining what works and what does not all are part of the complexity of coalitions.

The literature is filled with examples of local, state, national, and international formation and conduct of coalitions in response to health and health-related concerns and needs. Health promotion, policy advocacy, health care planning, intervention research, patient care delivery, and rural networks to increase access to care are but some of the reasons advanced for building coalitions. Clearly, coalitions are utilized pervasively in health care and health-related situations.

Collaboration was defined in Chapter 1 as "a dynamic, transforming process of creating a power-sharing partnership for pervasive application in health care practice, education, research, and organizational settings for purposeful attention to needs and problems in order to achieve likely successful outcomes." This definition also accurately defines a coalition and has stood the test of a comprehensive and exhaustive study of the literature in the database compiled for use in this book (see Literature Search later in this chapter). The term *coalition*, is, indeed, a surrogate term for *collaboration* and "seems to be widely used to describe two or more organizations joining forces to take joint action or resolve a mutually shared concern or reach a common goal" (Chapter 2).

In a coalition, the two or more organizations work toward meeting one or more common goals they would be unable to meet working alone. The goals are greater than the capacity of any one coalition member, and members often have to subjugate their own interests to the common goal. Sometimes, the coalition goal(s) responds to the self-interests of the members, such as in forming networks to compete successfully for patients and patient care revenue. Sometimes, the coalition goals are perceived to be incompatible with those of member organizations, such as in joint planning that requires some members to close or reduce enrollments in academic programs by which they have been known. Such a case example serves to show why widespread conflict sometimes occurs in coalitions. It also accounts for the blunt statement by the United Kingdom's Department of Health: "One reading of the most recent history of most . . . categories of joint activity would suggest it to be a chimera: a self-defeating illusion. In practice . . . , inter-agency and inter-professional relationships have been more marked by conflict and stand-off rather than productive cooperation" (cited in Higgins et al., p. 270).

The contextual discussion of what is going on in the larger environment, as well as the health care environment (for a review, see Chapter 3) gives meaning and even a sense of urgency to the topic of coalition. Not surprisingly, the rudimentary theory of collaboration put forward in Chapter 4 can serve to assist with organizing, designing, building, and evaluating coalitions. Nevertheless, there is a definite need to build on this firm foundation. The need is to focus specifically on the formation and conduct of coalitions. Virtually all the myriad factors that make up the concept are variable. This abundance of variable attributes bundled within the concept makes for both extraordinary detailed complexity and dynamic complexity (as defined in Chapter 4). Gray (1989), in her insightful book, states: "A theory of collaboration must account for how these processes organize a previously unconnected set of stakeholders to address common problems" (pp. 233–234).

METHODS

The methods used to develop and make specific the meanings of a coalition are 1) modified concept analysis using the evolutionary approach and 2) model and theory building as a continuation of the work in Chapter 4. Concepts, in the evolutionary method, are seen as dynamic and evolving—not fixed and static. They are context-dependent—not universally true. Certainly, this is the approach of choice for a concept that seems to be comprised of nothing but context-dependent variable attributes.

The analysis is modified in two ways. First, the categories of characteristics or attributes selected and defined for data extrapolation and organization have been varied from classic evolutionary concept analysis (see Chapter 1, p. 6) to assure capturing the richness of the topic. Second, the data are reported within the framework of a theoretical or conceptual model, as well as within the usual classic concept analysis reporting fashion of presenting a definition and then reporting on each of the definitional elements. Both of these modifications intend to build appropriately on, and advance the work discussed in Part I. In accordance

Processes: Described lists or sequences of actions used in forming, conducting, or evaluating a coalition (overlaps with characteristics)

Characteristics: Expressions of the concept as definitions or as descriptors or as processes (attributes*)

Conceptual frameworks, theories, or typologies: Either the use of a theory or framework to undergird the approach to understanding or the creation of a new framework or theory to organize understanding or influence meaning

Impetus for forming coalition: The catalyst or trigger that stimulates one or more actors to initiate a coalition (antecedents*)

Uses/applications/purposes: Closely related to impetus, the area of focus of the coalition; the actual situation to which it will be applied (references*)

Outcomes: Indicators, phenomena, or events that follow the formation of coalitions, and/or the conduct of coalitions by which the efficacy of coalitions may be judged (consequences*)

Surrogate terms: Means of expressing the concept other than the means selected by the researcher; they may be used interchangeably with the main term (Rodgers 1993, p. 83)

Related terms: Concepts that bear some relationship to the main concept but do not fully share the same set of attributes (Rodgers 1993, p. 83)

Philosophical/contextual background: The value-laden and/or larger, broader rationales for choosing coalitions to address human concerns

Benefits: Positive reasons stated for choosing to form coalitions, or the positive outcomes projected or achieved (overlaps with both uses and outcomes categories)

Barriers: The perceived or actual reasons given for inhibiting or preventing the formation of coalitions, and their successful conduct (overlaps with the categories of process, impetus, uses, and outcomes)

*Categories identified by Rodgers 1993, p. 83 that are similiar to the categories defined for use in this modified concept analysis.

Figure 9-1. *Definition of data categories.*

with the standard mode of evolutionary concept analysis, sample cases found in the literature are shared here. Figure 9-1 lists and defines the characteristics used for data gathering.

Literature Search

The entire database of 327 (mainly) articles and books on collaboration compiled for Part I of this book and selected later chapters was searched for the topic of *coalition*. As has been previously described (Chapter 1), all these works were entered into the computer database program, *Papyrus,* and the references were drawn from March 1982 to March 1996; *Medline* from 1992 to March 1996; and the *New England Journal of Medicine* from 1992 to July 1995. Although 310 of the articles were selected using the key words in each database that would yield the work on collaboration, purposive articles also were added, mainly on theory development, systems theory, and leadership and change. These 17 purposive works have been supplemented for this chapter by Gray's provocative book, *Collaborating: Finding Common Ground For Multiparty Problems* (1989), and by Williams' (1996) article concerning issues of coalition formation and conduct in the European Community. The database used for this chapter is thus comprised of 329 listings on collaboration or related topics.

In addition to entering key words named by the author into *Papyrus*, one of two research assistants read each article and also defined and listed key words they judged to best reflect the topics included in the articles. The author searched the directory of key words to initiate the process of selection of scholarly works focused on interorganizational collaboration. In total, 15 key words were searched, which accounted for 98 listings; a handful were duplicates. The key words *coalition, community coalition, interdisciplinary collaboration, interinstitutional collaboration*, and *service-education* yielded the great majority of the scholarly works.

The criterion for selection was that the article's primary focus be on interorganizational collaboration. Forty articles and one book fulfilled the criterion; 24 of the articles encompass widely varied purposes for interorganizational collaboration. The remaining 16 articles are all focused around service-education interorganizational collaboration; they are considered as a group in Chapter 10.

Data Collection and Data Analysis

Initially, the 25 scholarly works were read. Next, the data collection categories were defined. It was determined important that there be a separate data category relating to the impetus to establish a coalition because the later success of coalitions seems to be related directly to the circumstances of their initial formation. A category on conceptual framework or theory was deemed likely to help sort out the specifics of coalition from the generic topic of collaboration, and a category on process was created to help capture the myriad decision steps made in coalition formation and conduct. These categories proved useful in gathering data, although there was great overlap between the category of process and that of characteristics.

Armed with the data-collection categories, each article was reread for purposes of identifying and marking instances of data within the categories. Each datum was entered on a separate sheet of paper marked with the data category. Along with each entry was included the article code number from *Papyrus*, the author, and page number. This coding enables ease of citations in the text and ease of returning to the original source.

Following an extrapolation of data, intense study of the data sheets began. Themes, patterns, and issues were searched for. The data were reentered into a second round of data sheets, telescoping and combining initial entries. This procedure was repeated several times, as the author was searching for the variables that comprise a comprehensive research-based definition and the framework for a conceptual or theoretical model. The evolving definition and framework were tested for compatibility with the main definition of collaboration and the main theoretical framework.

One limitation of this process is that the author has acted alone. Reliability and validity of the data cannot, therefore, be addressed except as occurred by comparison with the main database on collaboration. Any errors of judgment are the author's alone.

FINDINGS

The first finding, already identified in the introduction, is the extraordinary detail and dynamic complexity of this topic. When, and why, and how should a coalition be formed? Who is and who is not the membership? How are the members brought together in coalition? How will the coalition approach problem-solving? What are the structures that best support coalition successes?

The second finding, closely related to the first, is that there are no clear answers to these questions because 1) a range of possibilities seems to exist in relation to each variable, 2) there is little or no evidence of systematic study of the subject using orderly research methods, and 3) the available literature includes only a few notable efforts to review the literature or organize a literature-based concept presentation (Butterfoss et al. 1993, Flower 1995, Gottlieb et al. 1993). Most of the literature is anecdotal, reporting on one or more coalition-formation projects.

The third finding is that the major focus of the literature is on coalition formation, rather than on coalition conduct or outcomes. The beginning work of deciding that a coalition is the way to approach resolving or addressing an identified need or problem and then going about the tasks of selecting and gaining members and building a structure that will support the members working in concert is extensive and extremely challenging. The strong implication gleaned is that the firm foundation constructed provides the bases for successes in conducting the coalition.

The fourth finding, not surprisingly, is that there is little or no evidence in the literature of successful outcomes of coalition activity. There are a few evaluation models, which will be shared, and there is thoughtful discussion of types of desired outcomes that extend beyond goal achievement. The notion of defining mission, vision, and goals and then setting about achieving them is, however, clearly articulated by many. The evidence of success in meeting goals is scanty. Part of the reason for this lack may be temporal; much of the literature reports on long-term, large-scale projects whose outcomes cannot be known until a later time.

Finding five, is that a crucial factor in successful coalition formation and conduct seems to be the degree of freedom or voluntariness members have in choosing to participate in the coalition and actively pursue its goals. This finding, perhaps more than any other, underscores the systems nature of coalition formation and conduct. Closely linked to voluntariness of participation is consideration of the impetus or trigger that caused people to come together at the particular moment in time to form a coalition. Those members who choose freely and voluntarily to join together with others in a coalition are more likely to participate actively in the coalition's work and to be actively committed to the coalition.

The sixth finding is that there is a wide diversity of reasons for forming coalitions, and there is great diversity of coalitions. Funding, or a lack of funding, is one major rationale for forming coalitions. Frustration with the lack of success in resolving problems and issues is a second major reason for coalitions. The increasing complexity of the health care and larger environments offers the third set of reasons for coalition formation and conduct. Problem-solving and even organizational survival for any one or a combination of these reasons bring organizations into coalition relationships. Coalitions may vary in size, be comprised of professional organizations only or of both lay persons and professional organizations, and may include any number of types of lay and professional groups. These are but a few of the variations of types of coalitions identified in the literature.

Finding seven, although not explicit in the literature but largely deduced by the author, suggests that the alternatives to coalition for myriad health care (service, education, research) enterprises seem to be less palatable to organizations and their members than are coalitions, particularly when voluntarily entered into. Acting alone, as an independently functioning entity, might be perceived as an ideal state. Most, however, recognize this perception to be a nostalgic wish to return to the past. The likely alternatives to coalition formation and conduct are 1) ownership by a corporate conglomerate such as Columbia HCA, 2) extinction of the organization and/or some of its programs, and 3) continuing neglect and likely worsening of difficult and complex socially related health and public health problems. This is a high-stakes topic of great importance to nurses, other health professionals, and society.

CONCEPT ANALYSIS AND THEORY BUILDING

The research definition of coalition, created as a result of this conceptual and theoretical analysis is the following: *Coalitions are complex dynamic human social systems strategically formed to respond purposively to identified needs and problems by the coming together of key representative members of two or more organizations within a formal organizational structure that supports a power-sharing partnership and facilitates designing and conducting interorganizational collaborative strategies and activities to pursue agreed-upon goals and outcomes that no one constituent could achieve acting alone.*

Also important to a basic understanding and defining of the concept is that coalitions are widely used in health care (practice or service, education, research) settings and health-related settings as an intervention strategy to achieve likely successful outcomes that are externally oriented to community welfare, such as risk reduction, or internally oriented to organizational welfare, such as scarce resource allocation. Undergirding the pervasiveness of coalition is the premise stated so well by Flower (1995): "If you bring together the appropriate people in constructive ways, with good information, they will create authentic visions and strategies for addressing the shared concern of the participating organizations and community constituents" (p. 22).

The model elements of coalition that represent the currently required necessary elements for configuring a coalition are purpose or reason,

Definition	Model Elements
Coalitions are complex dynamic human social systems....	
strategically formed to respond purposefully to identified needs and problems....	Purpose or reason, impetus for acting
by the coming together of key representative members of 2 or more organizations....	Membership, patterns of formation
within a formal organizational structure....	Structure of the coalition
that supports a power-sharing partnership....	Power-sharing partnership
that facilitates designing and conducting interorganizational collaborative strategies and activities....	Levels of collaboration, functions or tasks
to pursue agreed-upon goals and outcomes that no one constituent could achieve acting alone.	Outcomes sought and achieved

Figure 9-2. *Definition and model elements.*

impetus for acting at this time, approaches to problem solving, membership, patterns of formation of the membership, structure of the coalition, power-sharing partnership, levels of inter-organizational collaboration, functions or tasks performed, and outcomes achieved. A linear presentation of the definition and the model elements, placed in Figure 9-2, demonstrates their compatibility.

DISCUSSION

The model elements shown in Figure 9-2 interact in a dynamic systemic manner, as is depicted graphically later in the chapter. Description and discussion of each of the model elements can best increase understanding of their characteristics and characteristic complexity. As examples of coalitions, 15 sample coalitions were selected from the core 25 articles of the database. Although many more coalitions are named in these articles, these particular exemplars were selected to aid our understanding of the model elements because of the relative completeness of their descriptions. Tables 9-1 and 9-2 present aspects of coalition formation of the 15 coalitions. As the model elements are presented, these examples are cited, and the reader is referred directly to them for study.

(Text resumes on page 268)

Table 9-1. Coalition Formation: Purpose, Impetus, Approaches

Coalition—Author, Year, Description	Purpose	Impetus	Approach(es)/ Strategy(ies)
Cerne, 1993, Maine Health Care Forum—Consortium of Maine hospitals	Improve access to care achieving efficient resource utilization	Hospital Cooperation Act—directed hospitals to collaborate or state will decide collaboration	• Broad-based • Social planning • Strategic planning
Coluccio and Kelly, 1994, Partnership of rural hospitals and a university for a RN to BSN program	Fulfill nurse executives shared vision for accesible RN to BSN program and for BSN educated staff nurses	Shortage of RNs and agreement regarding vision (readiness to proceed)	• Broad-based • Social planning • Strategic planning
Flower, 1995, Community collaboration for determining Denver's future priorities and civic projects	Choose best ways to expend limited resources while achieving community consensus	Limited resources and citizen conflict led mayor to appoint citizens to a planning group	• Broad-based • Social planning & Locality-based • Strategic planning
Francisco et al, 1993, Project Freedom—Community Coalition to reduce substance abuse in Wichita, KS	Reduce substance abuse among 300,000 Wichita residents	Unsuccessful attempts to secure Robert Wood Johnson Foundation funding	• Broad-based • Social planning & Locality-based
Francisco et al, 1993, Project LEAN—community coalition to prevent cardiovascular disease	Educate citizens to improve diets and reduce cardiovascular risk behaviors	Began as partnership of Kansas, Dept. Of Health and 2 foundations to secure funding	• Broad-based • Social planning & Locality-based
Gottlieb, 1993, Smoke Free Class (SFC) of 2000-myriad coalitions of local, state, and national organizations and individuals to eliminate smoking by class of 2000	Increase community awareness of harmful effects of tobacco by focusing on students who entered 1st grade in 1988 and will graduate in 2000	American Cancer Society, American Heart Association, and American Lung Association seeking a way to increase national impact	• Broad-based • Social planning & Locality-based • Strategic planning

(continued)

263

Table 9-1. Coalition Formation: Purpose, Impetus, Approaches *(continued)*

Coalition—Author, Year, Description	Purpose	Impetus	Approach(es)/Strategy(ies)
Herman et al, 1993, MINNESOTA SAFPLAN—community-based family planning coalition	Achieve increased state funding for family planning	Loss of federal funding along with unchanged state funding	• Advocacy • Social planning • Lobbying/Political action
Humphries and Kochi, 1994, Coalition to improve access to consumer health information	Meet demand for consumer health information by library patrons	Patrons got attention of librarian after repeated requests	• Broad-based • Social planning & Locality developed • Strategic planning
Marosy, 1994, House Calls—coalition to provide services to frail elderly at home	Meet long-term care needs of frail elderly living at home	Visiting nurses noted that frail elderly didn't have physicians and couldn't travel to MD offices or clinics	• Broad-based • Social planning • Strategic planning
Meservey, 1995, CCHERS—Boston-based center for community health, education, research, services	Design and operate a seamless primary care education (research and service) system for nursing and medical students	Sought WK Kellogg funding in response to Kellogg Community Partnerships Project initiative	• Broad-based • Social planning & Locality developed • Boundryless organization • Shared governance
Oda et al, 1994, Coalition for research on public health nursing practice	Determine public health nursing profile for planning subsequent research studies	Readiness of researchers to commence work led to initiating relationships	• Broad-based • Social planning

(continued)

Table 9-1. Coalition Formation: Purpose, Impetus, Approaches *(continued)*

Coalition—Author, Year, Description	Purpose	Impetus	Approach(es)/ Strategy(ies)
Olden, 1995 NIEHS, National Institute of Environmental Health Sciences—affiliations with myriad other organizations	Fulfill agency priorities that mandate searching for ways to collaborate with other government and private sector organizations	New agency director committed to coalition building and planning	• Broad-based • Social planning • Strategic planning
Reed and Collins, 1994, Coalition of AIDS researchers, persons with AIDS (PWAs) and comunity-based AIDS service organizations	Facilitate conduct of AIDS research and research utilization	Years of frustration and conflict by AIDS researchers, PWAs, and community agencies	• Broad-based • Social planning & Locality based • Strategic planning
Ubbes and Pfohl, 1992, Partnership for evaluation research by researchers and clinicians	Conduct evaluation research of diabetes education program	Director of Diabetes Education programs requested that researchers and practitioners join forces	• Broad-based • Social planning • Strategic planning
Williams, 1996, PCN, Standing committee of nurses appointed by the governments of the nations of the European community and ACTN, an Advisory Committee on Training in Nursing, also comprised of appointed nurse leaders from the European nations	Enhance movement of RNs across European community nations through standards for education/certification; also participate in European Union health policy formation	Lobbying of European national governments by RNs led to realization of need (readiness to proceed)	• Broad-based • Social planning • Strategic planning • Political action

Table 9-2. Coalition Formation: Memberships Patterns of Formation

Coalition	Diversity/ Sameness	Type	Number	Voluntariness
Cerne 1993	Sameness	Professional	15 hospitals	(IV) Induced Collaboration
Coluccio & Kelley 1994	Sameness	Professional	8 hospitals and 1 university	(I) Freely and equally selected by all
Flower 1995	Diversity	Grass Roots	92 representatives of civic interests/organizations	(III) Last resort by all entities
Francisco, et al 1993 Project Freedom	Diversity	Combination	500 organizations	(II) Initiated by few organizations; others agreed to join
Francisco, et al 1993 Project LEAN	Diversity	Professional	70 organizations	(IV) Induced Collaboration
Gottlieb, et al 1993	Sameness	Combination	52 coalitions comprised of hundreds of organizations; thousands of individual members	(II) Initiated by few organizations; others agreed to join
Herman, et al 1993	Diversity	Professional	27 members, mainly clinics and professional associations	(II) Intiated by few organizations; others agreed to join
Humphries & Kochi 1994	Diversity	Combination	Several academic health sciences entities and some community organizations	(II) Initiated by library; others agreed to join

(continued)

Table 9-2. Coalition Formation: Memberships Patterns of Formation (*continued*)

Coalition	Diversity/ Sameness	Type	Number	Voluntariness
Marosy 1994	Sameness	Professional	2 organizations (2 disciplines)	(II) Initiated by one organization; other organizations agreed to join
Miservey 1995	Diversity	Combination	Several Boston-area hospitals, universities, communities, community health centers and Depts. of Health	(II) Initiated by few organizations; others agreed to join
Oda, et al 1994	Diversity	Professional	2 organizations	(II) Initiated by one organization; others agreed to join
Olden 1995	Sameness (in each affiliation)	Professional	9 federal agencies and several private sector agencies in separate affiliations	(II) Initiated by one organization, organizations agreed to join
Reed & Collins 1994	Diversity	Combination	1 university, several community service organizations, and persons with AIDS	(III) Last resort by all entities
Ubbes & Pfohl 1992	Diversity	Professional	1 university and 1 hospital	(II) Initiated by one organization, organizations agreed to join
Williams 1996	Sameness	Professional	11 European nations	(I) Selected freely and equally by all

Coalition Formation

Purpose and Impetus

Understanding the purpose for forming a coalition requires a response to the question, Why form a coalition? An opportunity or threat (or need, demand, problem) presents itself, and a judgment is made that forming a coalition is the way to respond. Opportunities or threats are abundant. Health promotion to reduce high-risk behaviors presents a common opportunity for community coalitions. Achieving increased government funding or changing public policy are common reasons for coalitions of professional organizations. Protection and maximization of scarce resources are frequent reasons for forming coalitions of health care providers. Frequently, increasing the support for research in community or service settings is cited by academicians as presenting an opportunity for coalition formation.

Specific examples cited in Table 9-1 include educating citizens to improve their diets and reduce cardiovascular risk behaviors (health promotion, Francisco et al. 1993), achieving increased state funding for family planning (government funding, Herman et al. 1993), improving access to care while achieving efficient resource utilization (maximize scarce resources, Cerne 1993), and facilitating conduct of acquired immunodeficiency syndrome (AIDS) research and research utilization (support for research, Reed and Collins 1994). Some presenting threats demand collaboration. For example, the agenda of increasing funding for family planning is not one that can be dealt with by any single organization (Herman et al. 1993). Other presenting demands, such as improved access to care for frail elderly, do not necessarily convince would-be-collaborators to unite in forming a coalition. Each potential participant needs to identify a rationale for joining.

The basis for coalition formation seems to be a belief that something to be gained by each participating member justifies the joining of the coalition and the participation in the coalition's activities. "A coalition effort can enable members to engage in activities and accomplish goals beyond the reach of any one organization or individual" (Herman et al. 1993, p. 334). Relationships that recognize a mutual need and are based on these mutual needs or concerns offer unique ways of combining efforts to bring to bear maximum resources (Fertman 1993). Conversely, when members do not perceive a mutual interest, coalitions are less likely to succeed in formation or conduct.

Merely having a purpose for establishing a coalition would seem to be insufficient rationale for actually doing so. In most instances described in the literature, an impetus or catalyst was also present that initiated the formation of a coalition. Impetus, as a model variable, responds to the question, Why form a coalition *now*? Frustration and conflict can be catalysts (Table 9-1, Reed and Collins 1994, Flower 1995); a common adversary can provide the impetus (Table 9-1, Herman et al. 1993); an opportunity for funding can mobilize potential collaborators (Table 9-1, Fransisco et al. 1993, Meservey 1995); a strategically placed actor may exercise leadership (Table 9-1, Olden 1995); and a group of leaders representing their organizations may share a common vision and feel ready to act on it by forming a coalition (Table 9-1, Coluccio and Kelley 1994, Oda et al. 1994, Williams 1996).

In the latter cases cited, the coalitions were internally initiated by the would-be coalition members. Coalitions also may be induced by an external source, such as happens with the enticement of external funding, or may be induced, and even forced, such as what happens with legislative mandates. As reported by Cerne (1993) (Table 9-2), legislation legally mandated that 15 Maine hospitals form a coalition to achieve increased access to care at cost-efficient rates or else the state would take over the decision-making regarding care delivery. In innumerable cases such as reported by Reed and Collins (1994), coalition formation often is perceived as a last resort. Flower (1995), in analyzing community coalitions around the United States, asks:

> Why were people beginning to collaborate? We searched for the visionary leaders who, like Moses, were bringing people to the promised land of collaboration, telling their followers the traditional way is too destructive . . . we have to do things in a different way. But we didn't find them. For the most part we found that people were collaborating because the other ways were not working. They moved into collaboration grudgingly, as a last resort. People backed into the collaborative movement. They felt they didn't have any other choice (p. 23).

It seems obvious that the impetus for forming the coalition will be a major influence on the success of the coalition. The degree of voluntariness exercised by coalition members, integrally related to the impetus for coalition formation, likewise is a major predictor of coalition success.

Approaches and Strategies

How the coalition will approach problem solving is the question addressed by this model. The variables have been organized into three clusters to aid understanding of approaches and strategies for coalition formation. The first cluster is focused on both the mission or goals of the coalition and the payoff to the members and nonmembers for achieving the mission and goals of the coalition. Advocacy, broad-based, and multipurpose are the variables comprising this cluster.

An advocacy approach to coalition formation and conduct has a preconceived agenda with a clearly defined mission and set of goals. There is little or no room for negotiation or compromise. Achieving a certain legislative victory, for example, is the preordained reason for coming together. Those who agree with the agenda are invited to join the coalition; those who do not agree are outsiders or even adversaries. There are winners and losers in advocacy approaches to coalition formation and conduct. The only advocacy example shown in Table 9-1 is Herman et al. (1993). Although the dearth of examples of advocacy approaches in the literature is surprising; on this basis alone, one should not conclude that advocacy is little used as an approach to coalition building.

Broad-based approaches to coalition formation and conduct also have one mission or focus and one related set of goals. They are, however, subject to shared planning and decision-making. Their missions may be shaped to appeal to a broader constituency. Their achievements lend themselves to a win–win perception both by members and nonmembers. Thirteen of the 15 examples in Tables 9-1 and 9-2 are of broad-based coalitions. Their purposes span almost all possibilities for establishing coalitions. Broad-based coalitions even allow for disparate membership. Thus, the beer company can collaborate with the department of health (Francisco et al. 1993) and the tobacco companies can cooperate with the public schools (Gottlieb et al. 1993).

Multipurpose approaches accommodate more than one mission and one set of goals. Butterfoss et al. (1993) note that multipurpose alliances are recent occurrences and that besides accommodating multiple missions and goals, they also direct their interventions at multiple levels, such as public policy, resource development and exchange, and ecological change (p. 316). Flower (1995) refers to multipurpose coalitions as civic will ventures. The Denver example (see Tables 9-1 and 9-2), wherein a task force of citizens seeks to achieve consensus on priorities for future development of the city and the acquisition and allocation of scarce resources, is a prime example of civic will at work. Gray (1989) presents another example of civic will, whereby disparate parties in a land use dispute work toward consensus on how best to develop the property in question (Chapter 1). It seems that an overriding vision or issue may bring parties together, such as the development of a city or the resolution of resource allocation issues, but the approach to problem-solving is an inclusive process of shared-visioning and shared decision-making. In these cases cited, bitter public acrimony was likely avoided and was replaced by self-governance of the highest order.

The second cluster of approaches may show the biases of the coalition formers regarding the authority for decision-making by the coalition members, as well as the logic inherent in membership selection. Approaches to decision-making may be recognized as *social planning, locality-developed,* or a *combination of both.* (See Francisco et al. 1993 and Goeppinger 1993 for further discussion of these concepts.) Planning and decision-making that is mainly top down and controlled by experts, such as social planners or health care providers, falls within the realm of social planning. Project LEAN (Francisco et al. 1993, Table 9-1), a community coalition of 70 organizations to improve diets and reduce cardiovascular disease is an example of a coalition that exclusively employs a social planning approach. Health care organizations banding together in provider networks seem to present another example of coalitions based wholly in the decisions of the providers—and perhaps the insurers. Cerne 1993 (Table 9-1) appears to represent a social planning approach by a hospital consortium.

Citizens who are affected by the decisions made may be negative toward such coalitions or at best weak in their support of them. Meservey 1995 (Table 9-1) speaks about the "town-gown" fears raised by the community when the experts from the university first approached the citizens about establishing the Center for Community Health, Education, Research, and Services (CCHERS).

A locality-developed approach to control over decision-making is the converse of the social planning approach. In this case, the citizens are empowered as decision makers from the start of coalition formation. The philosophical idea is that those most affected know best what is needed. Also, social planners and key persons in power recognize that active involvement in planning and decision-making is essential to later citizen support of the coalition and its mission. Such involvement not only gains citizen commitment, but it also develops in citizens the competence to achieve the coalition mission and helps to develop the social support network necessary to goal achievement (Goeppinger 1993). Community coalitions for health promotion (Francisco et al. 1993, Gottlieb et al. 1993, Reed and Collins 1994) are coalitions that are often wholly, or at least partially, locality developed.

A third possibility is for a combined approach of social planning and locality development. This approach seems to occur most commonly when experts want to establish a community coalition and turn to the citizens to invite their involvement. Examples of combined approaches outlined in Table 9-1 are Flower 1995, Francisco et al. 1993, Gottlieb et al. 1993, Humphries and Kochi 1994, and Meservey 1995. It is the author's experience that federal agencies or private national foundations lay out very directed guidelines (social planning) for conduct of projects but also require extensive local citizen involvement in all aspects of planning and conduct. Meservey (1995) writes about a W. K. Kellogg–funded community center that is a good example of national social planning and local control.

The third cluster, which has not been definitively formulated in this attempt to categorize variables, links a strategy for planning the conduct of the coalition to the purpose and impetus for formation, as well as to the approach to coalition formation. If this conceptualization has merit, others may identify and articulate additional strategies or rearrange these strategies. Those strategies identified here are *political action, lobbying, strategic planning/shared visioning, shared governance, and linkages in a boundaryless organization.* Thus when a coalition is formed for advocacy, the intent is that the coalition engage in political action in many ways (letter writing, media attention, citizen group formation, as examples) and in lobbying. A coalition that has a more general purpose, such as reducing substance abuse, and adopts a broad-based approach to problem solving is highly likely to engage in strategic planning. The term is used here to include shared development of mission, vision, goals, and actions.

A coalition engaged in strategic planning may carry out this strategy to its highest form and create a shared governance model. In shared governance, as described in Chapters 1 and 15, all participants are empowered as decision-makers and leaders in the coalition. Power is shared equally. Examples of coalitions utilizing strategic planning listed in Table 9-1 include Cerne 1993, Coluccio and Kelley 1994, Flower 1995, Gottlieb et al. 1993, Humphries and Kochi 1994, Marosy 1994, Meservey 1995—shared governance, Olden 1995, Reed and Collins 1994, Ubbes and Pfohl 1992, and Williams 1996. It is obvious that the purposes for coalition formation inviting strategic planning are numerous and highly varied. They range from international movement of nurses (Williams 1996) to conduct of research between one academy and one service center (Ubbes and Pfohl 1992) to national research and scientific priorities (Olden 1995) to a rural hospital consortium (Cerne 1993).

Linkages of organizations and individuals into seamless delivery systems is yet another strategy for coalition formation and conduct. This strategy is being used by providers to increase access to care while maximizing scarce resource utilization. This same strategy is often used as a survival strategy by organizations weakened in an economy of reduced resources and reduced resource utilization. The term *boundaryless* organization is used in the literature to describe a desired linkage state. Meservey 1995 describes the education and delivery system created by CCHERS as both a shared governance model and a boundaryless organization. Meservey discusses how negotiation of differences of opinion and mutually satisfactory resolution of those differences occur across the lines of the member organizations.

Tweed (1995) and Meservey (1995) both speak of seamless delivery systems in which integrated and networked providers overcome fragmentation of care by providing a continuum of care. Tweed notes that "providers are coming together to focus on delivering the highest quality health outcomes at the lowest possible cost. It is only when providers work together over the full continuum of care that they can be successful in meeting that goal" (p. 3).

Membership

Who will the members be? Who is and who is not us? What constituents will we represent? These are the major questions contained within the membership category. The literature speaks of three categories of members: *grass roots, professional, and a combination of both.* Not surprisingly, these categories parallel the approach to the problem solving category that defines social planning, locality-based, and combination of both. Locality-based approaches would include grass roots membership, social planning approaches would be conducted by professional members, and combined approaches to problem solving would be conducted by grass roots and professional members working in concert.

Ideally, the membership selected will depend largely on the purpose for coalition formation. Reed and Collins (1994) assert that would-be-members who recognize common cause and mutual benefit in coalition formation are the ones who can best develop the coalition into a lasting and successful organization. According to Butterfoss et al. (1993), those members who perceive the coalition as beneficial express satisfaction with their coalition membership and often collaborate more actively than those who are dissatisfied. A number of writers specifically encourage grass roots participation in community coalitions, as well as citizen participation in all coalitions that have an impact on citizens (Butterfoss et al. 1993, Francisco et al. 1993, Goeppinger 1993, Gottlieb et al. 1993, Meservey 1995, Reed and Collins 1994). The reader should note that many of the coalitions that use broad-based strategies have combination membership (see Tables 9-1 and 9-2).

Just what is meant by the term *grass roots*? Is it only consumers or are local organizations also defined as grass roots? The literature is not clear on this question. For the purposes of this chapter, the term is defined to include both consumers and local organizations. The term must be understood contextually.

A local, state, and national coalition such as Smoke Free Class (SFC) of 2000 (Gottlieb et al. 1993) logically will label the local school districts, along with the parent volunteers, as grass roots. The Three Communities Model to facilitate AIDS research and research utilization, which is a local coalition of academics, community-based organizations, and Persons With AIDS (PWAS), defines only the PWAS as the grass roots, whereas the community organizations are recognized as professional (Reed and Collins 1994). At the local level, community organizations such as county health departments or community clinics are recognized by citizens as professional and elite. It seems essential at that level that consumer participation in coalition formation conduct be sought and fully integrated in a combination approach.

In her discussion of coalitions or partnerships between professional organizations and lay people, Goeppinger (1993) describes these arrangements as pragmatic approaches whereby grass roots resources extend and complement professional resources (p. 4). She urges that lay membership not be equated with a victim-blaming mentality. The increasing usage of lay persons in health care is not a substitute for health professional services; "rather it does suggest they are necessary, complementary, additive—true partners" (p. 4).

Another variable used to describe the characteristics of the membership is their diversity, as compared with their degree of similarity, in mission, beliefs, goals, and values. Diversity also may refer to differences in skills, talents, and needs concerning a shared opportunity or threat. In both cases, great sensitivity is required to bring together organizations and individuals who can recognize a common vision and work toward common goals. Herman et al. (1993) notes that the work of the coalition must be defined so as not to infringe to any significant extent on the turf of any one member organization (p. 333). Butterfoss et al. (1993) note that the prior history of collaboration with each other among potential partners and their primary agendas will influence their ability to develop the necessary trust relationships (p. 325). The American Tobacco Growers Association and the U.S. Food and Drug Administration, for example, are likely to have a very difficult time joining forces and developing a coalition.

Clearly, the challenge of a diverse membership is to define and pursue a shared vision and goals in such a way that the philosophy, skills, talents, expertise, and resources of all members are respected and utilized (Herman et al. 1993, p. 332). When this challenge is met, the coalition is believed to be stronger and more effective (Butterfoss et al. 1993, Francisco et al. 1993, Gottlieb et al. 1993, Goeppinger 1993, Meservey 1995, Reed and Collins 1994).

Some writers recommend that coalition members be required to have similar beliefs and values as a prerequisite to joining a coalition. Tweed (1995) takes this position concerning building a boundaryless organization for seamless health care delivery. She stresses that partners should be sought who share the same vision and goals. They can then come together to define the mission and goals of the coalition and to agree upon coalition activities and resource sharing.

Of the 15 sample coalitions outlined in Tables 9-1 and 9-2, 9 have diverse memberships and 6 have similar memberships. Five of the similar members are professional-type memberships, counting the 11 European nations in the European Union and their nursing committees as professional (Williams 1996). There is disciplinary diversity among them, and there is the diversity between educators and researchers and educators and practitioners; however, they all share their professional talents and skills and their sense of mission and values for the coalition.

Interestingly, combination memberships of professionals and grass roots citizens and organizations can be classified as similar. This possibility seems to occur when both professionals and grass roots members agree strongly on a common cause, such as is present in SFC of 2000. In this case, hundreds of community-based organizations and thousands of individual members have come together with similar mission, goals, and values to create an SFC of 2000 (Gottlieb et al. 1993).

The memberships that are diverse offer endless combinations of members. The grass roots organizations that came together to advocate for family planning funding are surprisingly diverse. Herman et al.(1993) report that they represented many differing philosophical positions along the family planning spectrum. They represented local clinics, health departments, and professional associations. It was very difficult for them to present the united voice they set out to achieve; they had conflict determining who was their constituency. Francisco et al. (1993), on the other hand, report that the 500 organizations and individuals from Wichita, Kansas, who came together in Project Freedom to reduce substance abuse were able to develop a shared vision and agenda and to achieve many of their goals.

Meservey's (1995) report of success in bringing together several Boston-area hospitals, universities, communities, and community-based health services into CCHERS in a seamless organization functioning in a shared governance model is most impressive. Reed and Collins (1994) report that after many years of frustration and failure by all parties—especially the researchers—that PWAs, community-based service organizations, and university-based researchers were able to come together to create a coalition entitled The Three Communities Model. Since its creation, the three constituencies have planned and worked together to facilitate research design and conduct and research utilization. These and other examples of diverse membership coalitions are listed in Table 9-2.

The size of coalitions varies from two organizations in a local area to hundreds of organizations and perhaps thousands of individuals in national or combination local, state, and national organizations. There is very little consideration given in the literature to the size of the organization and its relationship to successful coalition formation and conduct. Butterfoss et al. (1993) point out that the coalition needs a sufficient number of members to have a "winning coalition" (p. 325). Also, the coalition needs a sufficient number of members to ensure that the defection of any one member will not make the coalition ineffective (p. 325).

Herman et al. (1993) caution that a large number of members [especially diverse members] may increase conflict over ideas, goals, and strategies; too few members, on the other hand, may make for a weak coalition with too few resources and talents, and minimal clout (p. 332). Membership size is perhaps a bit of a dilemma and spotlights the art of coalition building as opposed to its being a scientific endeavor. It does appear, however, that the size of a coalition is not nearly as important a consideration as is the diversity of the membership. Clearly, coalition members must be carefully selected. The success of the coalition depends on having the right members. The degree of voluntariness with which the would-be-members join the coalition is crucial to the success of the coalition. Consideration of this last identified variable concerning membership follows.

Patterns of Formation

Following study and data analysis a continuum typology of voluntariness of members joining a coalition was developed by the author. The reader has likely noted that Table 9-2 includes voluntariness rankings ranging from (I) to (IV). These rankings refer to a continuum of most voluntariness (I) to least voluntariness (V). Figure 9-3 presents the continuum.

Coluccio and Kelley (1994) offer an example of Level I voluntariness. The nurse executives in their rural hospitals already shared a vision for building a coalition to offer an RN to BSN accelerated educational program. When they agreed that they were ready to proceed, they sought an academic partner (Level II) and did so. Although they undoubtedly had to negotiate agreement on many particulars, there is no evidence of conflict presented in the literature. The story they tell is one of harmony and success. (See Chapter 2 for a case presentation of their coalition.)

(I) Selected freely and equally by all members; most voluntary; easiest configuration for forming coalition

(II) Initiated by one or more members; freely agreed to by other members; second most voluntary; second easiest configuration for coalition formation

(III) Collaboration after all other models fail; considered last resort by most or all members; third most voluntary; third easiest configuration for coalition formation

(IV) Induced collaboration by a force external to the members; fourth most voluntary; fourth easiest (second hardest) configuration for coalition formation

(V) Induced conflict by a force external to the members; fifth most voluntary (least voluntary); fifth easiest configuration (hardest) for coalition formation.

Figure 9-3. *Voluntariness.*

Williams (1996) also presents a Level I example of nurses from 11 European nations agreeing freely on the need for transnational standards for education and credentialing in order to facilitate international mobility. This example is complex because the nurse members of the two committees are appointed by their governments and the political authorities had to agree to the formation of the international committees. Nevertheless, the founding nurses seem to have been single-minded in their vision of a mobile international nursing profession and the importance of nursing leadership in making that happen. Level I voluntariness seems to represent the ideal pattern for coalition membership formation.

Nine of 15 coalitions outlined in Table 9-2 are of the Level II type; one or more members initiated the coalition, and others agreed to join. Project Freedom, for example, was begun by a few organizations who (unsuccessfully) sought funding. Others were then invited to join and did so until the coalition numbered 500 (Francisco et al. 1993). Smoke Free Class of 2000 was begun by three national organizations and then grew with their leadership and resources behind the growth to become a huge local, state, and national coalition (Gottlieb et al. 1993). In yet another example, Humphries and Kochi (1994) describe how the nursing service of a university hospital approached the university health sciences library head librarian to develop a consumer health information section. The librarian explored the topic, decided to proceed, and then invited several community groups and citizens to join the effort. A consumer health information center was then established.

Oda et al. (1994) describe a coalition formed to conduct research in public health nursing. There, the researchers initiated the relationship with the county health department. Similarly, the University of Missouri–Columbia Sinclair School of Nursing initiated the formation of a consortium of the school and three rural county health departments. The multipurpose consortium—Rural Health Consortium of Central Missouri—aims to advance rural public health and public health nursing practice in a managed care environment, and to advance community-based nursing education and nursing research. Also, the coalition aims to position itself to secure grant funding to meet its goals.

Who initiates the formation of the coalition is important. The initiators have the challenge and responsibility of motivating the members they attract to become fully committed and actively contributing members. Oda et al. (1994) point out that there is a significant difference in the collaborative process between whether a research program is requested of the researchers by the agency, or if it is conceived by researchers who are not a part of the agency. They urge involving the agency members in all phases of coalition building and conduct, including minute details of coalition functioning (p. 288).

Ubbes and Pfohl (1992), in developing a diabetes program evaluation research project, describe a similar process of joint planning. In this case, it was the program director from the hospital who invited the researchers to join forces—perhaps an easier process of initiation. Nevertheless, they urge "in-depth discussion;" development of philosophy, mission, and goals; establishing and maintaining excellent lines of communication; agreed-upon time lines; and anticipation of changes that may occur (pp. 362–363).

Fertman (1993), in a discussion of coalition formation between local community organizations and schools, observes that as long as a mutual need is recognized it does not matter which party (community or school) initiates the relationship. What is key is that the relationship addresses issues or concerns of import to both, and that efforts are combined to bring maximum resources to bear.

Meservey 1995, in describing the membership formation of CCHERS, which was initiated by one of the universities, opines that regardless of who initiates the coalition, the leader (initiator) must start out by sensitively recognizing the position that each potential member is in regarding the newly forming organization. The leader must understand the talents, resources, and needs of each organization. The leader must be "balanced, neutral, and open" (p. 235); roles, responsibilities, and accountabilities should be agreed upon at the start; and goals should be fostered that all members will desire to achieve. Level II seems to be the most common pattern of membership formation. The processes of initiating and joining are, therefore, very important components of coalition formation and conduct.

Two of the 15 coalitions described in Tables 9-1 and 9-2 are Level III types. These coalitions-of-last-resort offer challenges for membership formation. In the two examples provided in the tables, the membership is also wildly diverse. As well, if these examples are reflective of other, Level III types, the would-be-membership likely has a history of past conflict and animosity to overcome. The Flower (1995) example, already described briefly in the section on membership diversity, shows how severe conflict can be averted by bringing leading citizens in a community together to engage in community planning.

Reed and Collins (1994) describe several years of frustration on the part of researchers at the lack of community agency support for AIDS research and the lack of cooperation in research protocols by PWAS. Following several years of noncommunication with agencies and PWAS, the researchers decided to invite agencies and PWAS to attend a conference to discuss the issues. To the surprise of the researchers, they learned of equal frustration by the agencies and PWAS with the arrogant researchers. A lack of trust and perceived lack of respect by one group with the other was rampant. Following much relationship building and in-depth discussion of the issues and opportunities, all constituents came to realize that they would all benefit from collaboration. Research design and conduct, research utilization, and research funding benefiting all constituents could be achieved through the Three Communities Coalition.

Reed and Collins (1994) also describe the utility, in a case of collaboration-as-a-last-resort, of creating a social psychological model of interdependence. In order for each constituency to meet its individual goals, it must work in a linked model with the others. The parties need one another. They go on, however, to seek the additional inducement for collaboration of federal and/or state policy mandates or, better still, funding. This Level IV pattern of formation presents its own challenges, however.

Two Level IV cases are presented in the tables. In the first case listed, Cerne (1993) indicates that collaboration among 15 Maine hospitals was induced by the Maine legislature. Obviously, the legislature was dissatisfied with the level of collaboration that was—or was not—occurring or they would not have taken such directive action. The attention of the hospitals was clearly obtained. Cerne describes several collaborative ventures. He also describes how the hospital directors were initially afraid even to talk with each other. Their initial joint project was a cancer treatment center. That early success has led to other ventures and a growing sense of trust. Cerne also discusses the critically important leadership roles played by hospital trustees.

Cerne (1993) reports that the hospitals have not yet fully risen above their own self-interests and agendas; but they are trying. They have not yet met the challenge of convincing the various communities that the hospitals really care about the interests of the communities. He believes they must prove to the communities by their actions that they are more than a self-serving entity and that the needs of the communities are their top concerns (pp. 26–27). It also should be noted that the membership of this coalition is professional only, although Cerne reports that they are talking to various community members.

Project LEAN (Francisco et al. 1993) began as a partnership to secure funding by the Kansas Department of Health and two local foundations. Eventually, the coalition grew to about 5000 members. Community coalitions are widely used by foundations and government to induce collaboration by bringing together myriad community sectors that may or may not have worked together on community affairs previously. The idea is that the various key constituents will contribute to "locally defined problems and solutions" (Francisco et al. 1993, p. 403). (This is a social planning approach combined with a locality-based approach.) It can be extremely challenging to gain the commitment and active participation of the community membership in Level IV types of coalitions. Members need to see a benefit to themselves in participation that outweighs the time, effort, and resources expended.

The fifth type of membership formation, Level V, is induced conflict. This is similar to Level IV, induced collaboration, in that an external force has required the collaboration. What is different, however, is that 1) the would-be-collaborators definitely have a history of animosity toward each other, 2) the external force is usually legislative or legal pressure, and 3) one or more of the would-be-coalition-members perceive only negative consequences of cooperating in the formation and conduct of a coalition or some type of collaborative venture.

There are no examples of Level V coalitions in Tables 9-1 and 9-2. Chapter 11, "When Collaboration Is Legislatively Mandated," describes the Missouri experience of bringing a statewide task force of physicians, nurses, and pharmacists together in response to a legislative mandate and charging them with developing collaborative practice guidelines for collaborative practices statewide. This Level V case, illustrative of what is occurring throughout the United States, documents the tremendous conflict inherent when the criteria outlined are present, and it offers recommendations for management of such situations.

Clearly, formation of coalition memberships and coalitions are complex topics. These myriad and dynamic variables interact in causative ways. Making the right choices and processing the integration of these elements in a sensitive manner can spell success or failure in coalition formation and conduct. Fertman (1993) offers a set of questions to ask when contemplating a coalition: Who is involved? Should the membership be comprised of individuals and agencies? Should the membership be disparate or same? What is the (specific) purpose of the collaboration? What do people or organizations want to get out of the relationship? Who has the power? Is it shared? How will the relationship end? (pp. 32–33).

Butterfoss et al.(1993) assert that conflict and negotiation are inevitable in coalitions. They also assert that the type of membership formation provides a context for understanding conflicts [and for the severity of the conflicts and, perhaps, the potential for resolution]. It matters if the coalition is voluntary or forced, reactive versus proactive (crisis or planned), confrontation versus cooperation (an adversarial approach to power versus working within the power structure), consensus versus dissensus of the members [diversity versus similar], and single constituent versus multiple constituent [diversity versus similar] (pp. 319–325).

Coalition Conduct

Power-Sharing Partnership

The relationship that develops between the two or more organizations and individual members is one of partnership. During the formation phases, the newly developing partners hopefully have begun to develop a spirit of cooperation and a shared set of positive expectations for the coalition. Their perspectives on the coalition hopefully are positive and compatible. The work begun during the formation phase should continue, and the partnership hopefully will mature during the stage of coalition conduct. Lacking this maturity, the coalition will fall short of fulfilling its original purpose. The would-be-partners need to learn to share power, authority, and decision-making; to negotiate differences and resolve conflicts with mutual respect; to develop a relationship of trust; and to support the mission and goals of the coalition, which are bigger than, and perhaps dissimilar from, their own agendas.

Gray (1989) describes collaboration as an emergent process (p. 15). One can be more specific and substitute the term *partnership*, which is at the heart of a coalition or, indeed, any collaborative activity. Gray cautions not to underestimate the developmental character of the relationship and overlook the sensitive and delicate interactions that need to occur (p. 15). Goeppinger (1993) describes the partnership in coalition as "an active process; the informed, flexible, and negotiated distribution of power among all participants in the process of change (p. 2). By *informed*, Goeppinger means that each partner needs to know, to the extent possible, "their own and the others perceptions, rights, and responsibilities" (p. 2). Goeppinger urges putting one's self in the place of the other's and developing a "self-other-awareness" (p. 2). The final step of being informed is knowing the issues and the problems being addressed (p. 2).

Flexible partnership refers, says Goeppinger (1993), to the disparate members building on the uniquenesses of each participant and determining what unique contributions can be made by each and by each in configuration (p. 2). And finally, "because each situation demands different contributions at different times, the distribution of power must be negotiated at every stage of the change process. Negotiations, always deliberate and time-consuming and sometimes conflict-ridden, must occur during each stage . . ." (p. 3).

Negotiation, an important part of the process of decision-making in coalitions, may be defined in many ways and is a major conceptual topic in its own right. Although beyond the scope of this chapter or book to develop the topic fully as it relates to coalition, it will be helpful to define and briefly explore the meaning here. Gray (1989) defines the term *negotiation* in the broad sociological sense described by Strauss (1978, and cited in Gray 1989, p. 25), who observes stakeholders, through their talk, as trying to arrive at collective interpretations of how they see the world. Gray states: "Negotiation . . . refers to conversational interactions among collaborating parties as they try to define a problem, agree on recommendations, or design action steps. In this way they create a negotiated order" (p. 25). Not all negotiations in collaboration models lead to agreements for action, but when they do, they are arrived at by consensus. Consensus is achieved when "each of the stakeholders agrees they can live with a proposed solution, even though it may not be their most preferred solution" (p. 25).

Negotiated order refers to a context in which relationships and decisions made are negotiated and renegotiated on a continuing basis. Applying this conceptualization to coalitions recognizes the ongoing dynamic complexity of the organization and the behaviors required of the membership (Gray 1989, pp. 228–229). The partners in the coalition must take seriously the work involved in the partnership as informed, flexible, and negotiated distribution of power, as described by Goeppinger (1993).

Butterfoss et al. (1993) urge that regardless of the problem-solving approach used, the coalition milieu is enhanced when the processes for decision-making are defined clearly so that the resulting decisions made (solutions agreed to) do not conflict with the responsibilities of the individual participants (p. 325). These scholars go on to say that conflict is an inherent characteristic of coalitions because of four dynamic tensions: mixed loyalties of the partners to their own organization and to the coalition, the autonomy the coalition requires and the accountability it has to the member organizations, the diversity of interests of the members, and the lack of clarity about coalition purpose(s) as a means for specific change or as a model for sustaining the coalition (p. 325).

Wilford and Annison (1995) assert that the best indicator of whether a community coalition will have long-lasting benefits is the locus of decision-making and the degree of ownership. These authors specifically are urging that community members have full partnership powers of decision-making along with their professional colleagues. They describe a process called community betterment, which is analogous to the process of Level II membership formation, in which professional members initiate the coalition and then invite community members to participate. "This collaborative strategy can produce policy changes and improvements in program delivery and services, but it tends not to produce long-term ownership in communities or to significantly increase communities' control over their own destinies" (p. 31).

Collaborative empowerment, on the other hand, and again an example of Level II membership formation, has the community initiating the coalition formation. "Collaborative empowerment begins within the community and is brought to public, private, or nonprofit institutions. In this context, empowerment refers to the capacity to set priorities and control resources that are essential for increasing community self-determination. The empowerment approach can produce policy changes and improvements in program delivery and services. It is also likely to produce long-term ownership of the [coalition's] purpose, processes, and products in communities and to enhance communities' capacity for self-determination"(p. 31).

Trust is a critical element that enables power-sharing and mutual respect among the coalition partners. Trust, in fact, is the "indispensable ingredient" in the partnership (Wilford and Annison 1995, p. 29). (For an in-depth discussion of the communications and interpersonal relationships aspects of forming and sustaining a partnership, including the importance of taking time to develop a trusting relationship, and the ability to communicate clearly, honestly, and openly, see Chapter 1.)

There are numerous barriers to the development of trust. Within the coalition, the "institutional pride" (Wilford and Annison 1995, p. 30) one has in their own organization, which leads one to pursue their institution's interests at the expense of those of their partners or of the coalition, prevents trust from developing among the partners. Complexity is also a barrier to trust because it is hard to trust people or organizations that one does not understand (Butterfoss et al. 1993, Wilford and Annison 1993). Another major element of developing trust concerns being dependable and predictable in ways that invite trust. Although this sounds like a truism, it is an important notion. Having a clear vision and agreed-upon direction to which one adheres regardless of the pressures of the moment, definitely enhances trust.

During the establishment of a nurse-midwifery service at the University of Missouri hospital, a similar trust-building example occurred, wherein the medical school dean (the author's partner in the endeavor) reaffirmed his strong support for the service despite opposition from several medical faculty. Another important manifestation of dependability is seeing beyond one's own agenda to the larger agenda and supporting the larger agenda even when it may conflict with an individual organization agenda (Butterfoss et al. 1993, Fertman 1993, Flower 1995, Goeppinger 1993, Meservey 1995, Wilford and Annison 1995).

Fertman (1993) speaks eloquently about the importance of coalition members seeing beyond their own narrow interests. "Getting the big picture involves sensitivity to a variety of cultural, social, political, and economic factors. These factors provide the context for the collaboration. Often they influence, if not directly shape, the relationships and groups [coalitions]. Community agencies are particularly tied to such factors, as it is often their role to respond to needs identified in times of cultural, social, political, and economic changes" (p. 34).

Flower (1995) urges power-sharing partnerships in coalitions:

> How can you change something you can't control? What is the lever that can change complex dynamics in positive directions? If you want to make a difference in today's turbulent environment, you have to toss aside any ideas of hierarchical command-and-control-leadership as well as any ideas of building coalitions to advocate particular solutions. Your leadership must be rooted in true collaboration [—partnership] (p. 20).

Structure of the Coalition

Collaboration brings previously separate organizations into a new structure with a commitment to a common mission and shared goals

(Butterfoss et al. 1993, Gottlieb et al. 1993, Marosy 1994). Beyond this basic agreement, most authors diverge to discuss specific types of coalitions or specific elements of the structure. Some authors confine their descriptive statements of the structural aspects of coalitions to the physical and task-related aspects; others incorporate the human structural aspects, such as the relationship of the partners and the communication patterns. The approach to coalition structure chosen here is one that incorporates all aspects of the partnership with the impacting formation variables such as the degree of voluntariness or the approach to problem resolution. Although these topics are not discussed again, in the next major section of the chapter, the structural subsystem, comprised of the power-sharing partnership and the structure will be pictorially presented. As very human systems, this seems to be the approach of choice for conceptualizing the structure of coalitions. In a sense, this broad conceptualization invites a structural categorization of coalitions according to their approaches to problem-solving. The boundaryless organization and the shared governance model are two such examples.

Gottlieb et al. (1993) note that the complexity of purpose; degree of formality and degree of centralization of authority; and nature of leadership, decision-making, and communications "combine to produce a spectrum of structural types, ranging from loosely coupled coordinating networks to intense inter-organizational collaboration for problem-solving (p. 376)." In support of a common mission and goals, Sarason and Lorentz (1977) note that "[e]ach type of coalition, viewed within the context of exchange theory, must address the self-interest of each of the member organizations and provide for resource exchange" (cited in Gottlieb et al. 1993, p. 376). The purpose, degree of formality, type of authority, and leadership must be congruent or internally logical or the coalition will be structurally flawed.

Meservey (1995) describes the linking of hospitals with primary care, home care, and rehabilitation organizations "to better coordinate services and improve care with judicious allocation of financial resources" (p. 234) as the boundaryless organization. Meservey discusses the need for boundaryless organizations to have their own set of boundaries, however, and their own internally congruent structure. She opines that such an organization requires open, neutral, and mature leadership and management. The participating organizations must negotiate differences across traditional organizational boundaries. Meservey articulates four boundaries of the boundaryless organization: political, identity, authority, and task.

Within the political boundary, coalition members need to work at understanding how mutual gains will be realized and that without the consortium, these gains could not be achieved. A win–win or, at least, gain–gain situation is sought. Sometimes, one member needs to give more so that another member may gain. At a later time, the more giving member will make greater gains in this reciprocal relationship. The members of the boundaryless organization have a clear sense of identity. They are us. Those outside of the organization are just that—outsiders. They do not under any circumstances enjoy the privileges of being insiders (Meservey 1995) .

Authority within the boundaryless organization is a challenge. Meservey (1995) advises that one person must be responsible for each piece of work. Closely related to this idea of authority is the boundary of task. Who does what in the boundaryless organization? The combination of empowering transformational leadership that is open and neutral (see Chapter 15) with a strong system of coordination of the work and accountability for the tasks is a likely winning combination. It seems most congruent with the purpose, approaches, membership and partnership characteristics, and overall structure of the boundaryless organization. In contrast, Higgins et al. (1994) describe an effort to integrate nursing and social services organizations in Great Britain that failed badly. A joint management structure with strong central authority attempted to replace much of the extant management structure. Higgins et al. (1994) write that "The objective of a single operating base proved to be unattainable. It was suggested that the political and organizational obstacles were too great" (pp. 274–275).

The transformational leader approaches the work of coordination and task accomplishment from an empowerment perspective. Meservey (1995) states: "Bringing people together across the boundaries of each participating organization so there is a personal connection facilitates resolution at times of conflict. Effective leadership guides the new groups to define the work and divide responsibilities creating an ownership in the product. Further, anticipating the overlaps and gaps, and having the group attempt to resolve differences empowers each person. The outcome will be a positive group self-esteem and sense of collective accomplishment" (p. 236).

Butterfoss et al. (1993) cite several authors to document that early definitions of coalitions and collaboratives were of short-term, loosely structured intraorganizational and interorganizational alliances, and blurred distinctions with other types of relationships, such as networks and consortia (Levine and White 1961, Litwak and Hilton 1962, Gueztkow 1966, Aiken and Hage 1968, Schermerhorn 1975). They (Butterfoss et al. 1993) note that by more contemporary standards, coalitions are more formal working partnerships and are considered as more durable than short-term and ad hoc arrangements. Marosy (1994) uses the notion of a coalition as a durable interorganizational relationship to differentiate coalitions from other cooperative or coordinating relationships (p. 44). Use of ad hoc, and perhaps short-term arrangements, probably is increasing as organizations scramble to gain and assure a competitive edge in boundaryless organizations and other types of coalitions that ensure participating organizations market share or the maximum benefit from scarce resources.

Butterfoss et al. (1993) also reserve the definition of coalition to organizations that are primarily multipurpose as well as diverse in their membership. They define coalitions as "formal, multi-purpose long-term alliances that are issue-oriented, structured, focused to act on specific goals, and committed to recruit member organizations with diverse talents and resources" (p. 316). These authors go on to say that multipurpose organizations accommodate more than one mission or set of goals. Given this literature search and modified concept analysis, however, one cannot agree with such an assertion. The majority of coalitions reported on in these articles, which are drawn from a large sample of the mainstream health sciences literature, are broad-based coalitions approaching their broad but single mission from a strategic planning perspective. (The reader may wish to return to that discussion of approaches to problem solving earlier in the chapter, as well as reviewing Table 9-1.)

Regardless of the type of coalition, most authors stress the importance of carefully attending to the development and inclusion of several elements in the coalition structure. The specifics of coalition design ought to vary depending on the purpose, impetus for founding, approach to problem solving, and characteristics of the membership. The need for congruence between the formation and conduct features cannot be overemphasized. Marosy (1994) notes that coalitions require comprehensive planning; well-defined communication channels; determination of authority; and shared risks, resources, and products (p. 44). Gottlieb et al. (1993) list the following elements as structural: formal and informal agreements, rules, and sanctions; roles and responsibilities of members and staff; authority for decision-making; and a context for planning, communicating, managing, and evaluating (p. 376).

Once again, the importance of empowering leadership—organized as appropriate to the specific type of coalition—cannot be stressed too much. Regardless of the roles incorporated, the leader must be competent and effective. The leadership may spell the difference between effectively bringing a coalition to maturity and realizing its vision and mission or the coalition failing to meet its aims (Butterfoss et al. 1993, Gottlieb et al. 1993, Flower 1995, Higgins et al. 1994, Francisco et al. 1993, Olden 1995). In discussing leadership required in the boundaryless organization, Meservey (1995) notes that leadership must empower workers. The leader articulates vision, mission, and goals; has strong communications; evokes trust; and helps to create a positive organizational self-esteem (p. 236).

The empowering leader has much to do with the creation of an organizational climate conducive to effective functioning of the coalition. Butterfoss et al. (1993) define the organizational climate as "the group members' perceptions of . . . relationships, communication patterns, decision-making, problem solving, and conflict resolution processes" (p. 323). They assert that the "climate of the coalition is enhanced when leadership shares decision-making with the membership and when no one individual or organization has more authority or controls more resources than another" (p. 324).

Levels of Collaboration in Coalition, Functions, or Tasks

These elements focus on the work of coalitions. They will be discussed only briefly for two reasons. First, the internal logic required for coalition formation and conduct and the interconnections of all coalition elements within a systems framework mean that much of the conceptualization of the work of coalitions has already occurred. For example, the approaches to problem solving decision-making that occurs at the time of coalition formation encompasses the work-to-be-done in the conduct of the coalition. Second, the articles in this database focus, not surprisingly, on coalition formation far more than they focus on coalition conduct.

Three levels of activity in interagency coalitions are defined by Higgins et al. (1994): joint planning, joint management, and joint working on service delivery. Joint planning is most common. It occurs early in coalition formation. The stakes may not be too high, and individual organizations are participating without too much committed yet. Joint management implies a greater commitment with more at stake. Some integration of organizational structures is implicit. In a study of 12 coalitions with joint management, 5 factors were identified as necessary to ensure success: clarity of purpose, clarity of responsibility and assigned accountability, shared ownership and commitment to the coalition, strong joint management, and shared organizational learning (Hardy et al. 1992, as cited in Higgins et al. 1994, p. 270).

The third level of joint activity, working together or joint service delivery is relatively rare, according to Higgins et al. (1994), who cites various authors who speak of boundary or turf problems between professionals, services, and agencies; service overlap and duplication; and separatism giving rise to fragmentation and gaps in services (Renshaw et al. 1988, Brown and Wistow 1990, Hunter and Wistow 1990, Higgins and Young 1992, Meetham and Thompson 1992, Richardson and Higgins 1992, as cited in Higgins et al. 1994, p. 270). The multiple coalitions reported on in this chapter and as outlined in Tables 9-1 and 9-2 report myriad examples of working together to provide joint services in the forms of community education, health care delivery, research conduct and research utilization, collaborative health professionals education, and other activities. The author could also point to many coalitions personally known to her that offer joint services. These realities are in conflict with the assertion by Higgins et al. Yet, it is true, that the literature reports very little on successful outcomes of coalition joint activity.

Others define levels of activity more from a task perspective. Thus, Butterfoss et al. (1993, p. 318) speak of multiple levels of task accomplishment such as government funding and policy and ecological change. They also suggest that coalitions can even be categorized according to their differing functions, that is, information and resource sharing, technical assistance, self-regulation, planning and coordination services, service delivery, and advocacy. Herman et al. (1993) describe advocacy activities as lobbying in person, letter writing, phone calls to key decision-makers, and use of the media.

Herman et al. (1993) raise important concerns about gaining membership involvement in the work of the coalition. They seem to infer that only a small core group of coalition members will ever actively work to meet the goals of any coalition. Their report on their evaluation of SAF-PLAN, a coalition of family planning organizations to advocate for increased state funding (see Tables 9-1 and 9-2) presents several insights concerning member participation in the work of that coalition. Two thirds of the 70 members in that coalition never did anymore than pay their dues. The key predictor of level of involvement proved to be level of influence in formulating the coalition's mission and goals (p. 339). Other important variables were agency distance from activities occurring, time commitments and scheduling conflicts, discomfort and fear of lobbying, disagreement with goals or approaches of coalition by member organizations' boards, and feelings of inequality and inferiority by some members (pp. 349–342).

Outcomes Sought and Achieved

"Success in coalition work means first of all that the coalition actually gets off the ground, but beyond formation, coalition success can be measured in terms of its goals and longevity" (Staffenborg 1986, as cited in Herman et al. 1993, p. 342). This author has created a continuum of outcomes that can be used as both standards and criteria for analyzing and assessing the outcomes of coalitions. The continuum is presented in Figure 9-4.

The one-star level of outcomes represents success in the narrow or core sense of achievement of the mission and goals of the coalition. The two- and three-star levels are higher levels of achievement; they assume the accomplishment of the lower level(s). One may toy with whether level 2 should be level 3, or the reverse. In both cases, they represent high achievement that is beyond the narrow goals of the particular coalition. The partners have learned other perspectives and have grown beyond narrow self-interests.

As already discussed, the literature reports very little about successful coalition outcomes. This is in sharp contrast to the literature on collaboration among two or more persons for education, research, care delivery, and health care intraorganizational functioning. That literature reports an abundance of (mostly anecdotal) findings of successful collaboration (see Chapter 1). Two models for evaluation of coalitions are presented.

* Achieve goals of coalition; complete work

** Members see and commit to the needs and interests
of both the coalition and the larger society;
they have moved beyond self-interest

*** Members develop a true partnership that is lasting

Figure 9-4. *Levels of outcomes.*

Francisco et al. (1993), present an approach to evaluation of coalition conduct that mainly outlines both process and outcome measures. Their five process measures are: members recruited, planning products, financial resources generated, dollars obtained, and volunteers recruited. Each of these process measures is operationally defined; criteria for their assessment seems to relate only to the outcome measures. Outcome measures are: services provided, community action, and community changes. These measures are operationally defined; their criteria for achievement are the goals and objectives of the coalition. This model appears to be at the one-star level, that is, it will assess whether the coalition has met its objectives. It also will provide some clues as to issues within the coalition that inhibit or strengthen its functioning.

The second evaluation model attempts to relate the relationship of coalition structure and function to coalition performance. Gottlieb et al. (1993) designed this model to assess the performance of the 52 coalitions and their myriad members in the SFC of 2000 project. "Five composite variables were constructed for use in regression analyses. . . . Organizational barriers, personnel barriers, and formality of coalition structure are independent variables. Perceived effectiveness and perceived activity are the dependent variables" (p. 377). All the variables are operationally defined. The organizational barrier was defined to include 19 items, whereas the personnel barrier was defined to include nine items. Organizational barriers included items such as differences in agency fiscal years, local versus centralized control, and differences in agency philosophies. Personnel barriers included such items as expertise of staff and volunteers, volunteer turnover, and maintaining volunteer interest.

Formality of coalition structure included six items, such as written agreement, written mission statement, formal goals, and yearly objectives. Perceived effectiveness included effectiveness ratings on nine items such as fund-raising, teacher training, and product purchase decisions. Perceived activity was rated as a simple percentage of task accomplishment at the state or local or combined state and local levels on eight items, such as product purchase, fund-raising, and volunteer coordination.

The surveyors did indeed identify a multitude of barriers to successful coalition functioning. In that large and complex coalition, barriers were identified in all three barrier sets, and in a statistical analysis, all three clusters were significantly correlated with each other and personnel barriers and formality of structure were significantly correlated with perceived effectiveness of the coalition. On the basis of their study, Gottlieb et al. (1993) recommend that coalitions move to formalize interagency agreements, mission statements, and goals and objectives. They note this to be particularly important when there is high turnover of volunteers and other personnel and when the coalition is very large, as well as when there is potential for conflict between the member agencies and the coalition. Gottlieb et al. (1993) further recommend open dealing with issues spanning the agencies, and they recommend training coalition members to function effectively in "boundary spanning roles" (pp. 382–383).

This is also a one-star–level model. These useful models could be expanded by the addition of other evaluation methodologies, such as interviews with partners, long-range data gathering to determine continuing coalition functioning, and analyses of actions of member organizations in related spheres over time. These no doubt challenging activities also could be very enlightening as to whether coalition formation and conduct truly have changed organizational behaviors in ways that are foundational to the best interests of whole societies.

A SYSTEMS MODEL OF COALITION

The Model

The definition of coalition created as a result of this concept analysis begins with the statement that a coalition is a *complex dynamic human social system*. Conceptualizing coalition as such facilitates understanding of both the complexity of the system elements and their complex and integrally related connections. Coalition formation and conduct can benefit greatly from systems thinking and approaches. The work presented here represents only a modest beginning at articulating some of these concepts and relationships from a systems perspective. The propositions or relational statements put forward in the literature are incorporated in this presentation. Figure 9-5 presents an overall systems model of coalition. Figure 9-6 presents a more complex iteration that shows a coalition system as being comprised of four interacting subsystems: purpose subsystem, membership subsystem, structural subsystem, and outcomes subsystem. Finally presented are a few premises that undergird the coalition system and a few propositions relating to the subsystems.

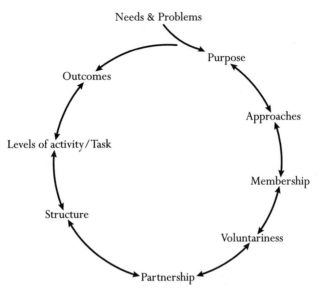

Figure 9-5.   *Coalition system.*

Premises

"If you bring the appropriate people together in constructive ways with good information, they will create authentic visions and strategies for addressing the shared concerns of the organization and the community" (Flower 1995, p. 22).

"The ability of varied discrete organizations with distinct but overlapping agendas to jointly pursue collective action is determinant of the degree of success movements for social change will have" (Herman et al. 1993).

"Partnerships [coalitions] between health care providers and rural residents are acceptable and effective strategies for health promotion in rural communities" (Goeppinger 1993, p. 1).

Coalitions approached as boundaryless organizations are effective for maximizing services while minimizing the use of scarce resources.

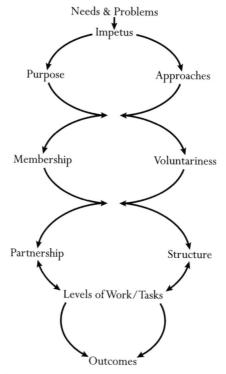

Figure 9-6.   *Coalition system and subsystems.*

Propositions: Approaches to Problem Solving

"Regardless of the problem solving approach used, the coalition milieu is enhanced when the [problem solving] process is defined clearly so that resulting solutions do not conflict with the responsibilities of the individual participants" (Butterfoss et al. 1993, p. 325).

Propositions: Approaches to Membership Formation

Potential coalition members who do not believe that the coalition will produce outcomes positive from their perspectives will refuse to collaborate, even if forced to join the coalition (Schermerhorn 1975, as cited in Butterfoss et al. 1993, p. 321).

The basis for coalition formation and for conduct that fosters positive coalition outcomes is a common goal or vision or mission that participants share and freely choose to pursue jointly.

A continuum of voluntariness of potential members joining a coalition can be articulated: the freer the choice to participate, the greater the likelihood of commitment to the goals of the coalition and the willingness to work for their achievement.

Propositions: Power-Sharing Partnership

"It is reasonable to hypothesize that positive relationships among members are likely to produce a productive milieu for the coalition" (Butterfoss et al. 1993, p. 324).

Partners who share fully and equally in all facets of coalition decision making are likely to have positive attitudes toward the coalition and actively work toward achievement of the goals of the coalition.

Propositions: Structure of the Coalition

The greater the degree of congruency between coalition purpose; degree of formality; degree of centralization of authority; and nature of leadership, decision-making, and communications, the more likely the coalition is to achieve its goals (Gottlieb et al. 1993, p. 376).

"The climate of the coalition may be enhanced when the leadership shares decision-making with the membership and when no one individual or organization has more authority or controls more resources than another" (Butterfoss et al. 1993, p. 325).

Proposition: Outcomes

Two or more organizations joined in coalition are able to achieve positive outcomes in relation to agreed upon goals and shared vision that organizations working alone are unable to achieve.

CONCLUSIONS AND RECOMMENDATIONS

Coalitions are indeed complex and varied. Within the health sciences, myriad coalition arrangements prevail. The most common type of coalitions seems to be those that are broad-based in their mission, diverse in their memberships, and engaged in strategic planning. These coalitions are usually initiated by one or more organizations but joined in by many others in Level II voluntariness. Their activities are very diverse. Despite these commonalities, many other combinations are also noted in health care delivery, education, and research. The boundaryless organization, usually an arrangement of integrated health care providers to increase access to services while economizing on scarce resources, is being widely used. This widespread usage is a recent phenomenon. Surprisingly, coalitions for advocacy purposes are not widely reported in this body of literature.

One of the major conclusions that may be drawn from this review is that one's involvement in the decision-making to join the coalition and one's influence over its purpose are critical predictors of the participant's future involvement. This in turn impacts on the likely success or failure of the coalition if the positive or negative members constitute a sufficient number to influence other members.

A systems approach to understanding coalition and systems thinking in designing and conducting coalitions seems to be most congruent with the attributes of coalition. One recommendation is for a systematic continuation by others of the systems model begun in this chapter. Second, research on coalitions is almost nonexistent. Research on coalition outcomes is greatly needed to document that the intense effort involved in coalition formation and conduct indeed results in positive outcomes. The case study method seems to be particularly in order to track the interrelation of the myriad complex variables, specifically the relationship of formation variables to conduct variables to outcome variables.

This modified concept analysis or a similar scholarly exercise could be conducted fruitfully again within 2 to 3 years. It will be important to see how lasting coalitions are in this era of turbulent change in society and in health care. Are coalitions durable or are they more ad hoc in nature, forming and breaking apart as soon as a new challenge or opportunity comes along? It will be important to focus on new and different kinds of coalitions. What will be the next new model?

References

Aiken, M. and Hage, J. (1968). Organizational interdependence and intra-organizational structure. *American Sociological Review.* 63, 912–930.

Brown, S. and Wistow, G. (eds.)(1990). *The Roles and Tasks of Community Mental Handicap Teams.* Avebury, Aldershot.

Butterfoss, F. D., Goodman, R. M., and Wandersman, A. (1993). Community coalitions for prevention and health promotion. *Health Education Research*, 8, 315–330.

Cagle, C. S. (1993). Commentary on health promotion for rural populations: Partnership intervention. *AWHONN'S Women's Health Nursing Scan*, 7, 6.

Cerne, F. (1993). Joining forces: Maine hospitals find that cooperation brings results. *Hospitals*, 67, 26–27.

Coluccio, M. and Kelley, L. K. (1994). Transformational partnership for delivery of RN baccalaureate education: A service/education leadership model. *Nursing Administration Quarterly*, 18, 65–71.

Department of Health (1989). *Caring for People: Community Care in the Next Decade and Beyond.* Cm 849. HMSO, London.

Fertman, C. (1993). Creating successful collaboration between schools and community agencies. *Children Today*, 22, 32–34.

Flower, J. (1995). Collaboration: The New Leadership. *Healthcare Forum Journal*, 38, 20–26.

Francisco, V. T., Paine, A. L., and, Fawcett, S. B. (1993). A methodology for monitoring and evaluating community health coalitions. *Health Education Research*, 403–416.

Goeppinger, J. (1993). Health promotion for rural populations: Partnerships interventions. *Family and Community Health*, 16, 1–10.

Gottlieb, N. H., Brink, S. G., and Gingiss, P. L. (1993). Correlates of coalition effectiveness: The Smoke Free Class of 2000 Program. *Health Education Research*, 8, 375–384.

Gray, B. (1989). *Collaborating: Finding Common Grounds for Multiparty Problems* (1st ed.). Josey-Bass, San Francisco, Calif.

Gueztkow, H. (1966). Relations among organizations. In Bowers, R. (ed.) *Studies on Behavior in Organizations.* University of Georgia Press, Athens, Georgia, pp 13–44.

Hardy, B., Turell, A., and Wistow, A. (1992). Innovations in community care management: minimizing vulnerability. Avebury, Aldershot.

Herman, K. A., Wolfson, M., and Forster, J. L. (1993). The evolution, operation and future of Minnesota SAFPLAN: A coalition for planning. *Health Education Research*, 8, 331–344.

Higgins, R. and Young, E. (1992). Evaluation of the Development Manager Role Within the Derby Elderly People's Integrated Care System (DPICS). Project Paper 1. Nuffield Institute for Health, Leeds.

Higgins, R., Oldman, C., and Hunter, D. J. (1994). Working together: Lessons for collaboration between health and social services. *Health and Social Care*, 2, 269–277.

Humphries, A. W., and Kochi, J. K. (1994). Providing consumer health information through institutional collaboration. *Bulletin of the Medical Library Association*, 82, 52–56.

Hunter, D. J. and Wistow, G. (1991). *Elderly People's Integrated Care System (EPICS): An Organizational Policy and Review.* Nuffield Institute for Health, Leeds.

Lenkman, S. and Gribbin, R. (1994). Multidisciplinary teams in the acute care setting. *Holistic Nursing Practice*, 8, 81–87.

Levine, S. and White, P. (1961). Exchange as a conceptual framework for the study of interorganizational relationships. *Administrative Science Quarterly* 5, 583–601.

Litwak, E. and Hylton, L. F. (1962). Interorganizational analysis: a hypothesis on coordinating agencies. *Administrative Science Quarterly*, 6, 395–420.

Marosy, J. P. (1994). Collaboration: A key to future success in long-term home care. *Journal of Home Health Care Practice*, 6, 42–48.

Meetham, K. and Thompson, C. (1992). Setting up the Scarcroft Project: the problems of joint working. *Caring for People.* 9, 6–7.

Meservey, P. M. (1995). Fostering collaboration in a boundaryless organization. *N and HC Perspectives on Community*, 16, 234–236.

Oda, D. S., O'Grady, R. S., and Strauss, J. A. (1994). Collaboration in investigator initiated public health nursing research: University and agency consideration. *Public Health Nursing*, 11, 282–290.

Olden, K. (1995). NIEHS perspective on collaboration among government, academia, and industry. *Toxicology Letters*, 79, 287–289.

Reed, G. M. and Collins, B. (1994). Mental health research and service delivery: A three communities model. *Psychosocial Rehabilitation Journal*, 17, 69–81.

Renshaw, J., Hamson, R., Thomason, C., Darton, R., Judge, K., and Knapp, M. (1988). *Care in the Community: the First Steps.* Gower, Aldershot.

Richadson, A. and Higgins, R. (1992). *The Limits of Case Management: Lessons from the Wakefield Case Management Project.* Working Paper 5. Nuffield Institute for Health, Leeds.

Sarason, S. B. and Lorentz, E. (1977). *The Challenge of the Research Network.* Josey-Bass, San Francisco, Calif.

Schernerhorn, J. Jr. (1975). Determinants of interorganizational cooperation. *Academy of Management Journal,* 18, 846–856.

Staggenborg, S. (1986). Coalition work in the pro-choice movement: organizational and environmental opportunities and obstacles. *Social Problems* 33, 374–390.

Tweed, S. C. (1995). Manager's corner: From competition to collaboration in home health care. *Home Care Nurse News*, 2, 3.

Ubbes, V. A. and Pfohl, S. Y. (1992). Collaborative health education research: Building university and hospital partnerships in diabetes program evaluation. *Journal of Health Education*, 23, 360–363.

Wilford, D. S. and Annison, M. H. (1995). The collaborative competitors—When the relationship is simultaneously collaborative and competitive. *Healthcare Forum Journal*, 38, 28–30.

Williams, S. (1996). Cross-country collaboration. *Nursing Standard,* 10, 17, 24–25.

Interorganizational 10
Partnerships: Mosaics
in a Changing Health
Care Environment

Rose Porter, Jill Scott, and Toni J. Sullivan

Contemporary health care requires proactive partnerships. Health care partnerships across organizations, across disciplines, and with communities are necessary to manage changing technology, increasing client acuity, an aging population, and diminishing fiscal resources (Nicholas et al. 1994). Health care professionals are integrating their and others' collective wisdom and responding creatively to increasingly complex health care delivery and education needs. By forging creative, committed partnerships, health care organizations are facing myriad challenges in the current environment.

Literally, *collaboration* is defined as "working together" (Styles 1984). In this cost-conscious era of health care redesign, collaboration between organizations is a rapidly growing phenomenon. Concomitantly, as a reflection of a larger movement toward collaborative partnerships, governmental agencies at all levels and the health care systems of the private sector are identifying new ways to optimize their collective resources.

Literature, once replete both with pleas for more cooperation and with laments regarding negative consequences of fragmentation and divisiveness (Styles 1984), is now filled with examples of organizations, big and small, coming together to face health care delivery challenges for the 21st century. Many organizations and providers are seizing the moment to seek new means of providing health care services expeditiously, emphasizing health promotion, disease prevention, and coordination of care delivery. This working together is leading to improved outcomes for populations served, and new wisdom and understanding of the health care delivery system is growing within organizations (Organek and Hegedus 1993).

Collaborative nursing service–education models traditionally have been between two organizations for quite specific purposes, usually skewed toward education or research goals. Table 10-1 presents a brief outline of 11 nursing education–service arrangements gleaned from the literature that demonstrate the traditional focus on education; only two are focused primarily on nursing services. Readily understood models such as unification and joint appointments seem to be giving way to more sophisticated and integrated partnerships across many disciplines and multiple organizational boundaries. These new mosaics are attending more to intradisciplinary and multidisciplinary collaborative practice and to service delivery. Distribution of shared resources within coalition partnerships is offering balance and stability within the chaos of changing environments (Coluccio and Kelley 1994).

Organizations are coming together. The need for interdependence in order to improve population health care outcomes and assure organizational survival is now recognized, and varied coalition models are encouraged. Similarities and differences among collaborating organizations are being acknowledged with common goals and consensus for activities overcoming past negative encounters. Organizational cultures are coming together for common cause in spite of their traditional potential for conflict (Baker et al. 1989).

Four foundational elements articulated by Styles (1984) still appear to be essential to the success of collaborative relationships: people, purposes, principles, and structure. Foundational to collaborative relationships are individuals who make things happen, those with vision. The purpose for coming together is critical to the ability to work collaboratively. The goal(s) must be clear, concise, and mutually valued. Principles are often the unspoken ground rules of the interaction. Those requiring patience and mutuality will foster success. Finally, structure involves the formal and informal roles and relationships of the organizations and of those with whom they serve.

Interorganizational partnerships are achieving success if their leaders and members work together in a true spirit of reciprocal respect and

Table 10-1. Education Service Partnerships

Reference	Collaborators	Coalition Activities	Coalition Results
Barrell and Hamric 1996	School of nursing, university hospital (different parent organizations)	Provide a structure in which education and service leaders jointly can address health care issues; increase nursing's voice in the university and faculty members' influence in hospital; and enhance education, practice, and research	Improved and increased communications, pilot units to test new delivery models, curriculum changes
Coluccio and Kelly 1994	Several rural community hospitals, small Christian university	Accessible, community-based RN and BSN program for place bound RNs employed by the hospitals	Increased professionalism of work force; improved RN recruitment and retention; more knowledgeable practitioners; improved employer—employee relations
Donnelly et al. 1994	School of nursing, university hospital (different parent organizations)	Joint appointment model to foster faculty practice so that faculty are grounded in practice and have opportunities for research and to increase exchanges between faculty and staff	Continual presence of faculty in clinical setting; improved communications, several funded research projects, new clinical programs; better placement of students; better blend of theory, practice, and research
Hills et al. 1994	School of nursing in university, four community colleges (Canadian)	Formalized commitment to develop new model of nursing education	Innovative curriculum based on health promotion in community and a humanistic (as opposed to Tylerian behaviorist) teaching or learning model
Karam and Niel 1994	School of nursing, nursing home	Collaborative research between students, faculty, and staff; and specifically, to implement a bowel management program that would decrease resident dependency on laxative and improve natural bowel function	Enhanced gerontological knowledge of students and staff, and improved bowel functioning of residents

(continued)

Table 10-1. Education Service Partnerships *(continued)*

Reference	Collaborators	Coalition Activities	Coalition Results
Keating 1994	Hospital nursing service, school of nursing	Implement a work study program to enhance recruitment of culturally diverse, well-prepared new BSN and MSN graduates	At end of 1st year, 65% of work study students hired by hospital; pass rate on NCLEX by work study students at 96%; students reported being well prepared for 1st position; hospital reported requiring less orientation
Organek and Hegedus 1993	School of nursing, university hospital	Collaborative project undertaken to design a model and prepare acute care nurse practitioners (ACNPs) for critical care and neonatal or perinatal nursing (impetus was the cutting back on medical residencies)	Collaboration between education and service; bridging of care–cure dichotomy; and preparation of ACNPs
Sherwood 1994	School of nursing in urban academic health center, school of nursing in rural area	Joining forces in a collaborative graduate nursing education model to educate advanced practice nurses for huge underserved, remote rural region	25 new multiethnic master's graduates, rural SON now has obtained approvals for MSN program, and faculty are available from new graduates

(continued)

Verderber and Urden 1994	School of nursing in university, eight community service agencies	Collaborative model whereby school and eight varied agencies —federal, state, and local—community based— and hospitals join forces to extend research into their service settings	Agreed upon listing of research priorities, achievement of funding by agency dues, and establishment of an Institute for Nursing Research
Verhey and Haw 1994	School of nursing, 80 clinical agencies	Partnership to design and offer a graduate-level course in quality management, students work in the setting to select actual QM problems and complete a major collaborative project	Students learn in real settings and resolve real problems; agencies benefit from projects conducted and by increasing their ability to recruit graduates
Wigginton et al. 1994	Four hospitals	Collaboration on continuing education by four hospitals in newly formed urban HMO; developed a critical care orientation course for new hires and a critical care consortium for teaching course	Several benefits such as cost effectiveness and better use of resources identified; have developed many other collaborative courses

ACNP, advanced nurse practitioner; BSN, bachelor of science in nursing; HMO, health maintenance organization; MSN, master's of science in nursing; NCLEX, National Council Licensure Examination; RN, registered nurse; SON, school of nursing.

peer influence. All involved organizations enter into equal partnership, regardless of size or resources available. Structures and systems formed by interorganizational collaboration of equal partners support collective inquiry and creative solution seeking. Sharing of knowledge and experience facilitates the development of innovative programs (Keating 1994).

Many leading national organizations are espousing the values of interorganizational collaboration. For example, the American Association of Colleges of Nursing (AACN) and the American Organization of Nurse Executives (AONE) have made national commitments to mentor and encourage collaboration across practice and education. "Collaborative relationships have been defined as substantive interchange of human and/or material resources for the purpose of advancing common goals in practice, education, and research" (Hegyvary 1991).

The "truth" of how to implement successful collaborative relationships is developing as each success story is shared. What is known is that achieving goals requires a commitment of time, energy, and resources. What has been shown are astounding positive effects for the recipients of health care and for health care providers (Hegyvary 1991).

Advantages appear to outweigh disadvantages in the forging of interorganizational relationships. The many advantages to collaborative partnerships include 1) cost-effectiveness, 2) improved utilization of scarce resources, 3) increased access to resources, 4) broader scopes of influence, 5) improved accessibility of services, and 6) increased networking and idea development (Wigginton et al. 1994). Disadvantages do exist but appear to be viewed as barriers to be overcome. Barriers include 1) conflicting organizational goals, 2) varied levels of commitment, 3) competition for decision-making authority, and 4) increased demands on participants (Wigginton et al. 1994).

A new set of factors facilitating organizational linkages identified by Hutchinson and Quartaro (1993) include the ethos of volunteerism; congruence of missions; maturity of organizations; structural similarities; regulatory requirements; homogeneity of clients, caregivers, and faculty; and ethical, social, and legal issues. A resurgence of volunteerism and community orientation is overtaking the health care system. Collaboration, as a means to share responsibility for all facets of planning, designing, and delivering health care, must be accomplished within a conceptual framework that recognizes the centrality of the recipient of care to these processes (Hutchinson and Quartaro 1993).

METHODS

A qualitative study with the goal of assessing the current state of interorganizational collaboration among service and educational institutions was completed. Key questions included, What is driving the efforts behind these new partnerships? What is facilitating success? What are stressors and barriers impeding success? It was anticipated that complex coalitions with many member organizations and multiple purposes would be described and that the organizations' leaders would describe many coalition arrangements occurring simultaneously. The study sought to describe what new collaborative arrangements and systems are evolving within the changing health care arena.

The study was set up as a two-phase process using semi-structured interviewing. Initially, key nurse leaders were interviewed; each key nurse leader identified three potential respondents who they thought to be exceptional partners (if they had three partners, and they all had at least three) for the second phase of interviews. The process resulted in five first-phase interviews and 10 second-phase interviews.

Samples and Procedure

Phase-one sampling

Initially, the executive directors of AACN and AONE were contacted for nominations of exemplary leaders in collaboration from both academia and service. The executive director of AACN provided a list of five nominees. The investigators chose three, giving consideration to achieving the broadest possible geographic distribution. The executive director of AONE directed investigators to the Robert Wood Johnson Strengthening Hospital Nursing Grant staff. A list of 10 nurse leaders from service were nominated by them, and again three were chosen. Of the six leaders chosen to represent academia and service, only one declined, as a result of unforeseeable circumstances.

The remaining five nursing leaders represented rural, urban, and suburban settings across the country. Each leader has been recognized at the national level as a role model in collaborative work between organizations. The resulting panel of respondents represented five regions: East–Central, Northeast, West, Southwest, and Midwest.

Phase-two sampling

In turn, each nurse leader who was interviewed identified three partnering organizations and representative outstanding partners. Semistructured interviews were sought with the representative partners of 15 organizations; 10 were completed. The nurse leader and the representatives of the partnering organizations identified by the leader became a set for the analysis phase.

The second phase of interviews provided many examples from across the country, thus providing an excellent opportunity to hear the stories of effective partnerships from diverse types of organizations as noted in Table 10-2. Of the 10 completed phase two interviews, six representatives were female and four were male; four were not providers of health care themselves, four were nurses in partnering institutions, and two were MDs.

Questionnaire development

Two interview tools were developed for the two-phase interview process, one for the nurse leaders and the other for the collaborative partners. Verification of content validity from experts within the field of collaboration was accomplished for each tool. Institutional Review Board approval was sought and obtained. Experts in both service and education reviewed the tools to verify that the choice of language used was appropriate to both settings.

Table 10-2. Partnering Organizations

An area agency on aging serving five counties (East-Central, rural)
Hispanic health center (Northeast, urban)
Metropolitan school system (Northeast, urban)
Five schools of nursing (Midwest, urban, suburban, and rural)
School of medicine (Midwest, urban)
National leader from medicine collaborating with national leaders from
    nursing (Midwest, urban)
A clinic caring for Native American women (West, rural)
A former nurse executive from a large teaching hospital (East-Central,
    suburban)
A principal in the public school system (West, suburban, rural)
A home health agency (Northeast, urban)

The first-phase tool, used with nurse leaders, sought to explore the context, process, and external forces influencing collaborative efforts within their organizations. The nurse leaders discussed how their organization had changed in the last 5 years, beliefs about collaborative efforts and how the efforts supported the organization in coping with change, and what were the trends in numbers and nature of collaborative relationships over time. Each of the collaborating partner sets, which include the nurse leader and the partnering organizations, was probed to learn their perspectives on structural issues related to collaboration. Structural issues explored were who were key players; what were their involvement, roles, and responsibilities; what incentives and rewards were offered, if any; what are the main activities, programs and services in the relationships; what are the missions and purposes of the arrangement; and what are the motivators or incentives, stressors, facilitators, and barriers of each partnership.

The second-phase interview tool focused the discussion at a more microlevel investigating collaborative interorganizational partnerships from the perspective of a partnering organization. Each respondent was asked to discuss how and why the arrangement had come into being. The respondents were also asked who are the key players, but with a new twist: When did they believe that the partnership truly became collaborative? Additionally, comparative information with the initial interview was sought within each set. Each organization's representative reported on their organization's main activities, programs, and services; implementation issues; expectations of the relationship; mission or purpose; and motivators or incentives, stressors, facilitators, and barriers. Finally, respondents were asked to discuss 1) what changes had occurred within their organization as a result of the collaborative arrangement, 2) what they projected as the future of the arrangement, and 3) whether they believed the arrangement was worthwhile in terms of time and effort expended in relation to outcomes.

Interviews ranged in length from 20 to 45 minutes. All respondents had received information before the telephone interview and were informed of the goals of the interview. They also received the tool in advance. At the beginning of each interview, and after they had reviewed the tool and understood what information was being sought, permission for participation was confirmed.

The principal investigator intermittently monitored the interviewing process to ensure the questionnaire was utilized as the study had intended. One of the investigators carried out all interviews and communication to respondents, ensuring consistent techniques and styles of probing across all interviews.

Interviews were taped, transcribed, and reviewed by two of the investigators. Review of the interviews and final notes were completed independently by two of the investigators and then compared and integrated for synthesis. Agreement on interpretation of each respondent's discussion related to the key questions as noted in key phrases for analysis was high, approximately 95%.

Data analysis

The goal of the study was to understand the lived experience of collaboration as perceived by nurse leaders and partner organizations; hence, a phenomenological approach was used. A naturalistic inductive analysis of the transcribed content was completed by the investigators, using constant comparative methods and analytic induction from the naturalistic paradigm described by Lincoln and Guba (1985) and Munhall and Boyd (1993). This analytic method began with the analysis of the transcript of each interview for information and categories to assist in answering the research questions. Phrases from the participants were analyzed and clustered in four rounds of progressive inductive analysis.

Phase One: Nurse Leaders

Placing interorganizational collaboration into context

In exploring the context of collaboration, a dichotomy existed within the initial nurse leader group. Change and responding to change was a constant theme. Four of the five nursing leaders spoke of change in terms of downsizing, consolidation, redistribution of work, managed care challenges, less hierarchy, and, most consistently, reduction of available resources. Current realities facing many nurse leaders interviewed mirrored the current state of health care. Collaboration was identified as a means to manage changes perceived as negative by pooling resources to achieve maximum benefit from scarce resources. Successful collaborative efforts were often supported by (or originated in a quest for) external funding, thus creating a mutually beneficial means of financial support.

The fifth nurse leader, from the Southwest, spoke of change in a different context. Change was perceived as the result of extreme growth.

Increasing the number of programs and faculty, procuring a new building, providing for an endowed chair, and creating a chance for seven disciplines to come together and produce truly multidisciplinary health sciences education were the opportunities envisioned. Collaboration within this setting was recognized as a means to develop and support an evolving system.

According to one nursing leader, the development of an intraorganizational culture is foundational for effective coalition formation and conduct:

> [I]t boiled down to a change in style and culture, a different way of communicating and managing, decreasing layers of hierarchy, and redistributing power throughout the new organization. Creating a culture of decision-making at all levels of operations, eliminating an intraorganizational competition related to decision-making. This initial intraorganizational preparation created the foundation for interorganizational collaboration to be successful. Improved communication, clear vision, trust, and a different sense of time were all critical in changing inside to work effectively outside the organization. The tools to collaborate and not compete facilitated effective partnering.

Regardless of the context of collaboration and organizational change, each nurse leader spoke of one overriding focus: the community and creating accountability that transcended organizational walls. Development of measurements to hold each other accountable were grounded in a framework of community betterment; for example, such areas as improvement of health care for adolescents, provision of perinatal care for Native American mothers, sharing nursing education resources, and making joint decisions about interdisciplinary support for community health improvement. Truly a new sense of organization within a context greater than their own organizations had been created. These organizations within communities were responding to larger issues by accepting obligations and responsibilities for population-based health care needs.

Collaboration was consistently discussed as a means to achieve stability and continued success when coping with organizational change. A dichotomy existed within the five nurse leaders. One nurse leader found that enormous change had threatened a long-standing effective collaborative arrangement. In this case, she and a partner were looking outward to establish other relationships; they were not turning to each other to meet their needs. "Enormous change had inadvertently led to deterioration of the long-standing relationship. Collaboration is like a beautiful garden needing to be fertilized and tended to. Nurture the garden or it will die of disuse."

One respondent suggested that coalition building and collaboration, on the one hand, and current changes within both service and academia, on the other hand, is a "chicken-and-egg" phenomenon. Is change creating the environment for successful collaboration or is successful collaboration bringing about successful change? "It is a circular relationship," according to this nurse leader from the Midwest.

Each nurse leader reported a significant increase in numbers of collaborative relationships. The number of ongoing active relationships across organization boundaries ranged from a modest four to the grand total of 30. To provide a foundation from which organizations could become successful collaborative partners, clear understandings and declarations of mission and vision began to develop across organizations. Consistently, comments of each nurse leader suggested common mission and vision as a critical antecedent to successful collaborative functioning. According to the nurse leader from the Northeast, clear declaration, understanding, and commitment to organizational mission creates a "dance card for other organizations to sign up on." Once the clear declaration of mission and vision is accomplished, an environment conducive to collaboration then becomes the framework for the effective conduct leading to successful collaboration.

These leaders described change as occurring within the environment as well as within the nature of their collaborative interorganizational relationships. Their current coalitions are clearly moving toward shared decision-making and shared accountability for services provided. The relationships described are truly equal partnerships. Specifically, one organization no longer acted in a paternalistic role as superior because of its size and fiscal resources. Equal partnerships are the norm. In addition, community or consumer participation is becoming commonplace, rather than having the provider organizations imposing their decisions upon the community. The nurse leader from the Northeast noted:

> [W]hen a marketing consultant told us that the community saw us as the organization where everyone worked together, we knew we had created an environment for collaboration to flourish not only within the walls, but within our community partnerships.

Moreover, coalitions are increasing movement from competition to collaboration, both across disciplines and across organizations. Combining their common missions and visions with a shared accountability to the community is facilitating the progress of individual organizations beyond traditional barriers to working together. The goal, according to the nurse leader from the Northeast, is:

> an integrated system, interdigitated and interdependent in nature with collaboration built into the system. . .providing a base or infrastructure for success to occur for both partners and the people which they serve.

Community, and a sense of serving larger societal needs, was a consistent theme noted and operationalized within the partnerships presented as exemplary.

The driving forces of successful collaboration

Not surprisingly, the forces driving the need to collaborate and those impeding effective collaboration were rampant. Within all organizations assessed, collaboration was a means to recreate the organization successfully and work with others in more desired ways. The driving forces motivating and focusing collaborative efforts were perceived to be critical by the nursing leaders. Analysis of such factors is fundamental to understanding successful movement into new collaborative partnerships. As noted in Table 10-3, many elements contributed to developing

Table 10-3. Driving Forces of Successful Collaborative Partnerships

Support of human resources
Visualization of the goal as greater than financial success
Restructuring and refocusing of the health care industry
Acknowledgment of community need
Seeing reward as community betterment more than financial gain
Top-down commitment, intensively felt by both parties
Long-term organizational commitment
Trust
Accountability

successful partnerships and changing how these organizations worked. Within the nurse leader sample, consistent themes that facilitated collaboration were noted.

Two driving forces internal to organizations or the communities they served were consistently described. Two circumstances—massive restructuring of the local health care system and refocusing of the larger health care system constituted the internal forces. A drive to obtain external funding was noted as a major driving force external to the organizations. The majority of efforts discussed by the nurse leaders involved interfacing with funding agencies, either to seek funds or to obtain grant monies. Once the coalitions were in the process of development, the two forces that seem to be most influential in the success of collaborative efforts are preparing and supporting human resources and seeing beyond the immediate financial ramifications of the partnership to the larger goals of meeting community needs.

Human resources: A key to success

Incentives, rewards, and motivators related to interorganizational collaboration focused upon mutual gain, a pooling of resources to obtain more personnel, a sharing of talent, and a new network of ideas. Qualified and committed human resources were described as both means and ends and were identified by nurse leaders as critical to collaboration at all organizational levels. Personnel educated and mentored in interdisciplinary and interorganizational communication skills provided one important means to ensure collaborative efforts could and would be operationalized. Staff, on the other hand, needed to see the benefit of working together for their organizations and their communities. Again, to create excitement for interorganizational partnerships, a clearly articulated mission and vision to which staff were committed was critical within the context of a goal of community betterment.

Supportive and effective human resources were not only indicated as a means to successful collaboration but also an end and motivating point. A "higher quality person" can be employed when resources are shared, that is, someone with higher credentials and greater expertise. It was further suggested by the East-Central nurse leader that in addition to the partnership's being able to afford a more skilled worker, there is the additional benefit of access to a network of ideas from both organizations that they serve. Moreover, enthusiastic and professional staff generate new successes and new opportunities for the coalition and its member organizations.

Visualizing the goal as greater than financial

All respondents indicated the existence of community needs that could be responded to by the services of an interorganizational partnership as a facilitator of enthusiasm, excitement, and commitment to working collaboratively across organizational boundaries. When both parties valued the goals and envisioned the gain as a mutual benefit, a shared understanding of need provided the milieu for development of an intense commitment. This sharing of goals, according to the nurse leader from the Southwest, must be primary to the relationship. "This is what we are about, are you?" appears to be a key question explored by would-be collaborators in establishing a successful starting point. The outcomes of collaborative efforts, or the vision of potential outcomes, also provided a driving force for these respondents. Clear articulation of the goals provided not only a means to hold each partner accountable but also served as a vehicle to pursue tangible, mutually satisfying outcomes.

The nurse leader from the Northeast discussed an "end-product" as more productive citizens. Often the gain, according to the East-Central nursing leader, was not directly financial to either partner but was a means to becoming more cost-effective and providing much needed interventions. In this way, financial consequences were minimized for each individual organization. Monetary incentives consistently were downplayed throughout the phase-one discussions. Rewards were listed as new resources, better services, or better access. Consistently, these nurse leaders saw the partnerships as vehicles to motivate the members to further their interorganizational collaborative work. The nursing leader from the West stated:

> [E]nthusiasm, excitement, opportunity to learn new things, and be involved in the change itself were the means of motivation. The partnerships provided renewal, reenergizing, and an opportunity to interact with new people.

The restraining forces to effective collaborative efforts

Just as some forces within organizations drive successful change, other forces slow down or prevent change. Restraining forces are real, according to the nurse leaders interviewed, and had to be balanced with positive forces or be neutralized in order to maintain the strength and momentum of the forces driving change. Restraining forces were perceived as having the potential to overcome organizations' abilities to manage change successfully. "Barriers provide the challenge," according to the nurse leader from the Southwest, "but they do not stop me, they are just a reality."

Restraining forces identified by nurse leaders are listed in Table 10-4. People themselves can be a barrier greater than any distance or physical obstacle, according to the nurse leader from the West. Lack of trust or of mutual understanding of the goal or of commitment all can result from improper planning and communication, as new interorganizational partnerships begin to form and develop. "Distance," according to the nurse leader from the West, "is not just measured in miles but in perspective." The distance perspective might be disparate goals or perhaps ignorance or fear of partnering.

The centrality of people to success

As discussed within the section on driving forces, people make the greatest difference. Because organizations are only enlivened by people, this is not surprising. Collaborative efforts require sharing of human resources, which without careful planning and monitoring may result in conflicting demands and too few people or organizations committed to the coalition. In the absence of clear understanding of purpose and goals and early involvement in the planning and decision-making process, both

Table 10-4. The Restraining Forces of Successful Collaborative Partnerships

Conflicting commitments, organizationally and interorganizationally
Partnering with those who are poorer than you
Logistics of consensus
Few tangible or traditional rewards
Multiple administrative structures
Territorialism
Thinking independently and not interdependently
Staying the same
Lack of time to grow and understand new relationships, cultures, and language
Lack of trust
Lack of money
Lack of understanding of the goal
Lack of energy, commitment, enthusiasm

leaders and staff members can become very threatened by these new relationships. Rapid changes require organizations and their people to be nimble and change quickly. The consistent message was there is no greater potential barrier or resource than people themselves.

The inability of people to communicate across organizational boundaries was identified as a significant barrier to success. New relationships, new language, and new cultures all present challenges, according to the nurse leader from the West. Time was an important related issue. Lack of time to invest in the new relationships only complicates the difficulties present in developing interorganizational skills in communication.

Organizations need to educate and develop their people and consider that not everyone will be an effective representative in an interorganizational partnership. Energy and motivation is essential; collaboration is not for those lacking enthusiasm and commitment. Commitment cannot be "half-way," according to the nurse leader from the West.

Another people-centered consideration is the threat to the status of individuals within their respective organizations. Some members of the partnerships traditionally have held more power and had more available resources, and perhaps control, than they will have in the new arrangements, according to the Midwest nurse leader. These are real barriers that require attention. Historical competitors coming together for a greater good, but with clashing financial interests, are very real, according to the nurse leader from the Southwest. The leader from the Northeast noted that territorialism is also an issue: people like to stay "inside their box." Territorialism can be seen not only among the staff but often in upper levels of both partnering organizations. Either the leadership or the membership or both may evidence territorialism. Leaders may come together with a vision; however, sometimes this vision may be viewed as threatening by employee groups. At other times, the friction might be within the leadership while the membership is ready to move ahead, according to the nurse leader from the Northeast. In both cases, the challenge to overcome the conflict requires organizational leadership.

Phase Two: Interorganizational Partners

Placing interorganizational collaboration into context

The analysis of phase-two interviews produced themes consistent with those discussed by nurse leaders interviewed in phase one. Unlike the phase-one sample, no dichotomy existed about the essence of interorganizational partnerships. The importance of community need and mutual vision and purpose again were noted as paramount rationale for these interorganizational partnerships to exist. "The overarching reason which triggered our coming together was a community assessment . . . which led to our conclusion that the community has needs and, with partnerships, we will have manpower and funds to meet them . . . ," stated a respondent from the East-Central area. All respondents indicated that community need was the reason partnerships formed. Each partner expected the other to enhance their ability to meet community need through sharing resources, both human and financial.

Despite the extensive diversity in the types of interorganizational partnerships, the power of working together to obtain mutually desirable outcomes was discussed as the engine creating momentum for engaging in partnering endeavors. Interorganizational partnerships were operationalized in many ways, as noted in Table 10-5.

Also, as noted by these leaders as well as the nurse leaders, top-down leadership and commitment were critical to the partnerships' success. A new twist for the phase-two interviews related to the question, What indicated to respondents that the partnerships had become or would be truly collaborative? A phase-two respondent from the East-Central area stated: "[D]on't exaggerate the depth of the partnership early on, they really fluctuate. . . . it becomes real when people in the partnership hear commitment and see action from someone other than me." Again, time was an important element, consistently noted as essential to ensuring a belief that the partnership was real and could be productive. "When you felt like you could really turn to each other then it felt real. . . . [T]his took about a year," according to a respondent from the Northeast.

Evidence of commitment was one critical indication of successful collaboration according to all phase-two respondents. Another critical indication of success was whether the participants from each organization took the time to know and understand their new partners at a personal level. Participants sought answers to questions such as those listed below.

- What are my new partners like?
- What are their priorities?
- Can I trust them?
- Will they take equal responsibility and accountability for the outcomes of the partnership?

Table 10-5. Main Purposes and Activities of Interorganizational Partnerships

Joint appointments between area agencies on aging and a school of nursing to stimulate age-sensitive research, education, service opportunities, and improved understanding of community-based services for the elderly. (Academic–community agency)

A Hispanic outreach clinic to facilitate outreach, education, and translation for adolescent mothers partnering with a local hospital for case management services and a means to meet the continuing unmet issues of a unique population. (Service–community agency)

Student volunteers working in the local hospital performing jobs that ultimately could lead to employable skills and future health care providers while supplying human resources to hard-to-fill employment areas within the hospital. (Service–community agency)

District educational model to support education of nurses, creating a pool of advanced practice nurses to fill primary care needs across a Midwestern state and enhancing research endeavors connecting nurse researchers across the state. (Academic–academic)

A consortium of care providers, payers, educators, and community business leaders as the vehicle providing cost-effective statewide primary care and providing all involved organizations education related to the new managed health care environment. (Academic–service–business)

A national interdisciplinary council role-modeling how disciplines can and should work together and providing joint recommendations related to primary care providers and labor issues in an era of health care reform. (Discipline–discipline)

A perinatal clinic for Native American women who lacked desirable alternatives to care recognizing long-standing issues of discomfort with traditional health care systems providing dignity and high-quality services for a vulnerable population. (Service–community agency)

An on-site children's health clinic next to the public school ensuring access for all in preventive and illness-related health care services. (Service–community agency)

Continuum-based care for high-risk patients from the acute care setting to the home care setting within a seamless plan of care for targeted populations such as patients with joint replacements. (Service–community-based service)

A joint partnership of academic and service leadership within a large teaching institution, ensuring one powerful voice for patient care by nursing. (Academic–service)

A public–academic partnership in psychiatry to provide a setting for developing clinical skills, upgrading educational level of current staff, and supporting the direct care staff of mental health facility. (Academic–service)

Another respondent, also from the Midwest, discussed how an outsider providing advice to the group solidified the interorganizational partnerships: Both organizations agreed that the outside consultant was incorrect and joined forces to dispute the consultant. Finally, a respondent from the West summed up how collaborative partnerships solidify; stating, "Initially, lots of talking without action . . . when the action finally started, I believed."

The driving and the restraining forces to effective collaborative efforts

As noted in the earlier discussion of data from phase-one respondents, successful change is driven by forces that ultimately are more powerful than those that restrain efforts to change. What was perceived to motivate and facilitate the success of the interorganizational partnerships from the perception of the phase-two respondents was consistent with those of their phase-one counterparts, as noted in Table 10-2. Also noted earlier, but stressed more emphatically by phase-two respondents, was an inability to meet community needs for reasons of inadequate resources, both human and financial. The perception was that this need drove their joining forces with often much "larger" partners. The fact that partnering organizations recognized and valued community needs provided a comfort-level in partnering with other organizations and taking the risk of coming together.

Forces noted to be potentially restraining were also consistent across both phases of the interviews, as noted in Table 10-3. Initially, one respondent from the East-Central area spoke of

a roller coaster of faculty commitment . . . [S]taff from the academic side change or semesters conclude leaving our staff turned off and wondering who will help tomorrow, what's going to happen next semester, or what will we do in the summer when the students and faculty are gone. . . . Where is the continuity?

Another respondent spoke of the stress of working with one hospital when there were two hospitals within the community serving—or underserving—in their area of concern. All but one spoke of the intimidation of high expectations and being the "tiny" organization working with a bigger partner. A respondent from the West actually discussed seeking out the larger organization and truly was in a position of guiding early formulation of the relationship. Noted earlier, and again stressed throughout phase-two interviews, was the challenge of navigating new systems and coming together from different cultures, perspectives, assumptions, and understandings. Organizational issues related to external regulation, internal financial systems, and adequacy of human resource were consistent across phases of interviews and sets.

What does the future hold for interorganizational partnerships?

All respondents have high hopes for the future of their interorganizational partnerships. Consistently, a future for the partnership was considered necessary and worthwhile. Most relationships are well beyond their first year in the partnership. Goals for the future are noted in Table 10-6.

Many of the respondents spoke of their collaborative partnerships as providing a means of rebirth for their own organization. New partnerships have expanded and redefined what many of the organizations in the sample can now do to support the health of their communities. "The coming together had created new systems," according to a respondent from the Midwest.

Table 10-6. Expectations and Outcomes of Interorganizational Partnerships

Improved and increased human resources to operationalize joint purpose

Consistent resources available to the communities they serve

Increased creative solutions with joint thinking and networking with the larger pool of colleagues

More power in contract negotiation within a managed care environment to ensure consistent high-quality care

More advanced prepared nurses to serve statewide needs

Collaborative training for all critical to the health of community

Expansion of services

A smoother flow of needed services and more local accessibility

A more productive community

Greater student achievement

Another 95 years to service our community in a high-quality, cost-effective manner

Systems that more clearly embrace and acknowledge the reality of the world will survive. Was the time, effort, and commitment worth it? The answer across both phases of respondents was a resounding yes!

"Risk-takers will be successful within the future of health care. Those who can leave their ego at the door and be open, listen, and facilitate a coming together of organizations for serving community health needs can be successful," according to a respondent from the Midwest. A respondent from the West summed up what interorganizational collaboration is all about.

> Forming partnerships is like gaining a new friend. You have to work together, solve problems together, associate with each other, strive to give each other something you both want. Then you do become friends, and once you are friends, you never want to give them up!

And, finally, from a respondent from the Northeast:

> People have been underexposed to one another. From a business perspective and a health care delivery perspective, a stronger product comes from collaboration. Choose your partners based on vision and like values and you both will be successful.

CONCLUSIONS

Interorganizational collaborative partnerships are thriving in the midst of changing technology, increasing client acuity, an aging population, and diminishing fiscal resources. Long-term coalitions are forming as a result of successful interorganizational partnerships collaborating to meet goals larger than themselves—goals of community betterment. The people within the partnering organizations, their mutual purposes and common principles, and the ability to overcome internal structural barriers with effective coalition building are all leading to successful coalitions.

The relationships described by our diverse sample all conveyed the essence of collaboration in their descriptions of dynamic, transforming, power-sharing partnerships. The resulting complex, dynamic relationships had all been strategically formed in response to community needs that each organization agreed were important. The coming together of key people from each partnering organization provided structure and support to accomplish that which each organization could not do on its own.

The lived experience of the nurse leaders and partnering organizations as told through this phenomenological inquiry exemplifies what successful health care communities are doing to overcome what appear to be overwhelming challenges to health care organization. Their purpose, their impetus, their problem solving approaches, their membership, their coalition structure, and their power-sharing all demonstrate model cases of effective coalition building.

Effective interorganizational partnerships have resulted in coalitions based upon a new paradigm of cooperation and collaboration, rather than competition and turfism with respect to the sharing of resources for care delivery and nursing education. This new ethos has created the necessary means for organizations to rise above their self-interests and see beyond themselves within a larger continuum of health care services necessary for each community. These partnerships of varied and creative mosaics are modeling community responsiveness to health care service needs and health care professional needs. They are demonstrating how to support the communities they serve effectively into the 21st century.

References

Baker, C. M., Boyd, N. J., Stasiowski, S. A., and Simons, B. J. (1989). Interinstitutional collaboration for nursing excellence. Part I, creating the partnership. *Journal of Nursing Administration, 19*(2), 8–12.

Barrell, L. M. and Hamric, A. B. (1996). Education and service: A collaborative model to improve patient care. *Nursing and Health Care, 7,* 497–503.

Coluccio, M. and Kelly, L. K. (1994). Transformational partnership for delivery of RN baccalaureate education: A service/education leadership model. *Nursing Administrative Quarterly, 18*(4), 65–70.

Donnelly, G. F., Warfel, W., and Wolf, Z. R. (1994). A faculty-practice program: Three perspectives. *Holistic Nursing Practice, 8,* 71–80.

Hegyvary, S. T. (1991). Collaborative relationships for education and practice. *Journal of Professional Nursing, 7*(3), 148.

Hills, M. D., Lindsey, E., Chisamore, M., Bassett-Smith, J., Abbott, K., and Fournier-Chalmers, J. (1994). University–college collaboration: Rethinking curriculum development in nursing education. *Journal of Nursing Education, 33,* 220–225.

Hutchinson, R. and Quartaro, E. (1993). Training imperative for volunteers caring for high risk, vulnerable populations. *Journal of Community Health Nursing, 10*(2), 87–96.

Karam, S. E. and Niel, D. M. (1994). Student–staff collaboration: A pilot bowel management program. *Journal of Gerontological Nursing, 20* (3).

Keating, S. B. (1994). Collaboration of practitioners and nurse educators in home care nursing. *Geriatric Nursing, 15*(2), 109–110.

Lincoln, Y. and Guba, E. (1985). *Naturalistic inquiry.* Sage, Newbury, CA.

Munhall, P. L. and Boyd, C. O. (1993). *Nursing research: A qualitative perspective.* (2nd Ed.). National League for Nursing Press, New York.

Nicholas, P. K., Leuner, J. D., Miller, D. F., Kellifer, D., Lynch, B., and Fitzmaurice, J. B. (1994). A collaborative program for international education. *The Journal of Continuing Education in Nursing, 25*(1), 41–45.

Organek, N. and Hegedus, K. (1993). Advanced practice: A model for neonatal/perinatal and women/child nursing. *Clinical Issues in Critical Care Nursing, 4*(4), 631–636.

Sherwood, G. (1994). Educational outreach in a rural underserved area. *Nursing Connections, 7,* 5–15.

Styles, M. M. (1984). Reflections on collaboration and unification. *Image: The Journal of Nursing Scholarship, 16*(1), 21–23.

Verderber, A. and Urden, L. D. (1994). A collaborative community model for nursing research. *Nursing Connections, 7,* 45–51.

Verhey, M. P. and Haw, M. A. (1994). Teaching quality management in a nursing graduate program: A collaborative university–agency quality team. *Journal of Nursing Care Quality, 8,* 48–54.

Wigginton, C. A., Miracle, V. A., Sims, J. M., and Mitchell, K. A. (1994). Partners in nursing education. *Journal of Nursing Staff Development, 10*(5), 245–247.

When Collaboration Is Legislatively Mandated

Toni J. Sullivan, Susan Morgan, Belinda Heimerichs, and Jill Scott

INTRODUCTION

When collaboration is legislatively mandated or externally induced in a forced manner, the process that follows is likely to be one of conflict and even rancor. The process can, perhaps, be described as a type of conflict-induced collaboration (Gray 1989), and the interactions that occur, at best, are a process of negotiation. These staged happenings, forcing key actors who would not otherwise interact to work together toward something defined by others external to the actors, are not rare. Powerful organizations and officials in government and in the private sector are increasingly forcing influential persons to the table, often as a last resort, to resolve seemingly intransigent problems. Such is the case with nursing and medicine agreeing upon rules for collaborative practice arrangements in Missouri.

Following a decade or more of conflict between organized nursing and organized medicine over collaborative practice by advanced practice nurses (APNs) and MDs (including doctors of osteopathy [DOs]) in primary care practice, and under the leadership of a reform-minded governor, the state legislature and administration faced the challenge of developing reform legislation. After a turbulent and often rancorous political process, House Bill 564, commonly but unofficially known as the Missouri Primary Care Access Package, passed the legislature and was signed into law in August of 1993. It allows that guidelines for collaborative practice *may* be promulgated for *geographic areas of practice, methods of treatment, and review of services.* The administration, the legislature, and the

325

organized medical community each (for their own reasons) were adamant that guidelines for collaborative practice arrangements be promulgated speedily. Organized nursing was less eager to come to the table to promulgate guidelines because they perceived they had little or nothing to gain by doing so.

The process of developing guidelines for collaborative practice arrangements for use in Missouri by registered nurses (RNs), APNs, and MDs to guide their conduct of collaborative practice in primary care practices and other community-based settings proved to be lengthy, arduous, and often acrimonious. The first meeting of representatives of the Boards of Healing Arts (Medicine), Pharmacy, and Nursing along with representatives of the state administration took place in a conference room in the governor's office on September 30, 1993. Subsequently, 48 meetings and events took place. Myriad documents were drafted and discarded, and thousands of support staff hours were expended. On September 30, 1996—3 years to the day from that first meeting in the governor's office—the collaborative practice guidelines went into effect as the *Collaborative Practice Rule.*

This chapter explores the approach of induced-conflict collaboration as occurring from a health care perspective. Both a theoretical perspective and a case study of the Missouri experience as exemplar are used to achieve in-depth exploration of what has become an important problem solving usage of collaboration. The Missouri experience is presented from three perspectives: 1) a historical context, 2) a temporal and documents overview of the events and materials that comprise the official record and serve to validate the experiences recalled by the key actors, and 3) a phenomenologically based research perspective that presents findings from loosely structured interviews and that discusses the data from conceptual and dramatic narrative perspectives.

The chapter concludes with recommendations for further study and research of this high-stakes topic and with recommendations for enabling successful collaborative outcomes when collaboration is legislatively mandated or otherwise forced.

HISTORICAL PERSPECTIVE

To understand the Missouri experience fully, the reader must have a sense of the political environment and events leading up to the decision for induced collaboration. This requires a brief review of events commencing in the mid-1970s. (This historical perspective is presented primarily from nursing's vantage point. Although every effort has been made to present a factual account only, it may be limited by the configuration of facts available to the authors.)

In 1975, the nursing community decided to revise the Missouri Nursing Practice Act (NPA), which had not been amended since the early 1950s. The nursing community believed that the statute reflected a very conservative and outdated viewpoint toward the nursing profession. The Missouri Nurses Association (MONA) lobbied for a model practice act developed by the American Nurses Association (ANA). The model act defined professional nursing as "the performance for compensation of any act which requires substantial specialized education, judgment, and skill based on knowledge and application of principles derived from the biological, physical, social and nursing sciences." The Missouri Nurses Association lobbied especially to remove the language requiring MD supervision over nursing practice.

The Missouri House and Senate passed the new practice act by a solid majority; however, then Governor, now U.S. Senator Christopher "Kit" Bond vetoed the bill. The nursing community, with MONA's leadership, undertook and was successful in overriding the governor's veto, an event that had not occurred previously in the 112-year history of Missouri government.

Approximately 4 years later, two nurse practitioners (NPs) employed by a Planned Parenthood agency in southeast Missouri were charged by the Missouri Board of Healing Arts (BHA) with engaging in the practice of medicine. Their collaborating MDs were charged with aiding and abetting them in the practice of medicine. Both NPs were educated for this role and practicing within their scope of practice. They primarily delivered well-woman care and provided medications to patients using standing orders and protocols.

The NPs brought suit against the state of Missouri. Their case went through the courts to the Missouri Supreme Court, which rendered a decision in 1983 in the matter of *Sermchief v. Gonzales* (Missouri Supreme Court Decision No. 646 92). This decision—the ultimate test of the NPA—ruled in favor of the nurses and nursing. In its decision, the court stated:

> The legislature substantially revised the law affecting the nursing profession with enactment of the Nursing Practice Act of 1975. Perhaps the most significant feature of the Act was the redefinition of the term "pro-

fessional nursing," which appears in RSMo 335.0168. Even a facile reading of that section reveals a manifest legislative desire to expand the scope of authorized nursing practices. Most apparent is the elimination of the requirement that a physician directly supervise nursing functions. Equally significant is the legislature's formulation of an open-ended definition of professional nursing. The 1975 Act not only describes a much broader spectrum of nursing functions, it qualifies this description with the phrase "including, but not limited to." We believe this phrase evidences an intent to avoid statutory constraints on the evolution of new functions for nurses delivering health services.

This decision was followed in 1987 by the passage of an amendment to the Healing Arts Practice Act (HAPA) stating that an MD would be disciplined for providing medication to a patient without first establishing a "physician–patient relationship." The purported intent of this amendment was to prevent MDs from prescribing medications for themselves, friends, and/or family members. The Missouri BHA, however, chose to implement this new law in a way that proved disastrous for collaborative practice between APNs and MDs. The BHA narrowly interpreted the new law as meaning MDs could not provide medications to patients without first "seeing" the patient and establishing a physician–patient relationship. In other words, RNs could not provide medications to any patients who had not first been examined by an MD.

The BHA then began investigating those physician practices in which the MDs were collaborating with NPs. It also began investigating MD practices that collaborated with county health departments by signing standing orders and protocols so that RNs could administer immunizations to well children. In myriad situations, the BHA charged the MDs with providing medications via standing orders and protocols to patients without the MDs' first establishing physician–patient relationships. Although few MD licenses were actually disciplined, the investigations and threat of disciplinary action by the Board had a very chilling effect on physician–nurse collaboration.

The Board of Pharmacy simultaneously conducted its own investigations to determine whether the prescriptions telephoned to pharmacists by RNs were legal. This also had a chilling effect on pharmacists' willingness to fill prescriptions telephoned to pharmacists by RNs.

By the late 1980s, concerned individuals such as physicians, nurses, attorneys, and agency representatives began meeting informally to consider strategies for countering the actions of the Boards of Healing Arts and Pharmacy. In 1990, MONA and the other participating organizations formalized this group into a strong coalition called the Health Care Access Coalition, which included representatives from approximately 15 agencies. This group decided to work toward a legislative amendment prohibiting MDs and pharmacists from being disciplined for practicing collaboratively with nurses who were functioning within the scope of their nursing license and education. This amendment successfully passed in 1990 but was vetoed by Senator John Ashcroft, then governor of the state, because of a high-cost fiscal note attached to the primary bill. The amendment passed again in 1991; this time, it was appended to a bill supported by the governor and became law. However, both the medical and pharmacy boards acted as though the law had not passed and continued their investigations and threats of disciplinary action.

It is important to note the coalition continued to attempt, without success, to collaborate with the Missouri State Medical Association (MSMA) in order to resolve these issues. Throughout 1992 and 1993, efforts to resolve these issues through legislative or regulatory action failed again and again. At the same time, the cries for health care reform in the state and nation were becoming louder and more demanding.

The election of Governor Mel Carnahan in November 1992 signaled a major shift in health policy because of his commitment to improving health care access in Missouri. He began his term in office by appointing a transition team who studied key issues facing the citizens of Missouri, including health care access. He appointed as director of his transition team an attorney who had actively participated in the Health Care Access Coalition and who had been directly involved in the *Sermchief v. Gonzales* Missouri Supreme Court case.

In late December 1992, the director of the transition team began convening meetings of the stakeholders in collaborative practice. The participating stakeholders included MONA, MSMA, the Missouri Hospital Association (MHA), and Missouri Planned Parenthood (MPP). (The Missouri Association of Osteopathic Physicians [MAOPS] was not invited because it was perceived as obstructionist to the process.) The purpose of the meetings, the director explained, was to reach consensus on the issue of collaborative practice. The governor planned to offer a legislative package that would codify collaborative practice in statute, as well as address other health care issues. Collaborative practice, with prescriptive privileges for APNs, was described as the linchpin of this omnibus legislation.

The Speaker of the House of Representatives agreed to serve as the sponsor of the bill. He contracted with a Missouri-based Health Policy Institute for development of legislative strategies for achieving passage of the bill. The bill was referred to by its bill number, HB 564, and also as the Missouri Primary Care Access Package. The strategy was to focus on the health professional shortage in Missouri; greater than 50% of Missouri counties were federally designated health professional shortage areas.

The stakeholder meetings in the governor's office continued, and HB 564 grew and addressed myriad topics in addition to collaborative practice. The collaborative practice section of HB 564 amended four statutes. Those statutes were the NPA, the HAPA, the pharmacy practice act, and the controlled substances act. The proposed amendments defined *Advanced Practice Nurse,* established a mechanism for collaborative practice, and removed barriers to collaborative practice including the problematic language of "physician–patient relationship." It also clarified the ability of pharmacists to accept and fill written prescriptions from APNs and telephone prescriptions from all RNs. Prescriptive privileges were indeed defined as a delegated medical act, but the proposed changes were meant to be strong building blocks in clarifying collaborative relationships among MDs and nurses.

The Missouri Nurses Association was guardedly optimistic about the collaborative practice portion of HB 564, as it had been lobbying for full prescriptive privileges legislation (HB 755), which had served to keep pressure on the legislators and, perhaps, kept them more balanced in their thinking. At this point, however, MONA was forced to make a critical decision whether to support HB 564 and abandon HB 755. Clearly, HB 755 would be difficult to pass, and because HB 564 was the governor's priority for 1993, it had a greater chance for success; organized nursing would be wise to support the administration. Therefore, the decision was made to sacrifice HB 755 and fully support the passage of HB 564.

Nursing's intent in lobbying for HB 564 was to clarify collaborative relationships among MDs and nurses. The administration's intent was to address the access to care issue from the perspective of the health professional shortage areas. Strongly opposing HB 564 was MAOPS, which took the position that codifying collaborative practice in statute would be devastating to the quality of health care in Missouri. The membership of MSMA was split on the issue; the MHA supported HB 564 because it was in the process of developing hospital-based rural health clinics that were federally mandated to be staffed by NPs.

On the evening of February 16, 1993, the governor's director convened another meeting of all of the stakeholders including MAOPS. At this meeting, the newly appointed director of the Department of Health was introduced and participated in the meeting as cochairperson. During this meeting, the issue of limiting the practice of APNs to the underserved counties within the state, including imposing mileage restrictions on collaborating professionals, was hotly debated. The MD groups would, not agree to support the legislation without such restrictions, whereas the other interests were strongly opposed to the restrictions. During the debate, it was restated by the administration's leaders that limiting the practice of APNs to geographic areas of the state or by placing a mileage radius limitation on their practice would not benefit the people nor would it ensure quality health care.

After debating this issue fervently for a considerable length of time, compromise language was proposed by the director of the Department of Health that would direct resolution of these and other problematic areas through joint rule making between the Boards of Nursing and Healing Arts. The joint rule specifically addressed three areas: geographic distance, review of services, and methods of treatment. The MONA representatives strongly objected to joint rule making, and pressure to accept this compromise language was brought to bear on them by several administrative and legislative key actors. In a private caucus, MONA representatives presented their perspectives on the dangers of joint rule making. They discussed the unequal balance of power the BHA had over the Board of Nursing and the lack of experienced Board of Nursing members who were knowledgeable about advanced practice nursing to debate these issues with members of the BHA. Despite these arguments, the strong message given to the nursing representatives by these appointed and elected officials was that "[n]ursing has power and nursing must use its power." It was clear from this discussion that the joint rule making would be included in HB 564 regardless of nursing's concerns.

HB 564 passed in the final hours of the legislative session ending mid-May of 1993. The bill was signed into law mid-August 1993, with the provision that collaborative practice could and would commence immediately. The signing of this historical bill closed one more chapter in the history of collaborative practice by physicians and nurses in Missouri and set the stage for the next act that would prove to be as formidable as the one that had come before.

METHODOLOGY

In order to best capture the essence of the Missouri experience, qualitative strategies were used to develop an understanding of conflict-induced collaboration. Official documents were vehicles for extrapolating a factual picture of events taking place over a 3-year period. The qualitative methodology of phenomenology was used to recreate the lived experience of conflict-induced collaboration, whereas emplotment was used to construct the stories of the three entities involved in drafting Missouri's Collaborative Practice Rule. Emplotment is a phenomenological strategy focusing on the beginning, middle, and end of a phenomenon presented as an ordered rendering of the sequence of events as a larger temporal whole governed by a plot (Mattingly 1994). The use of phenomenology enables the intensification and clarification of events as lived, whereas emplotment allows for the locating of self within an intelligible story to provide meaning to the experience.

Twelve individuals representative of the main constituent groups were invited to participate in the study; 8 agreed to participate, consisting of 5 nurses and 3 non-nurses. The 8 interviewees included representatives of the Missouri Department of Health, the Boards of Nursing and Pharmacy, and the Missouri Nurses Association. A loosely structured interview guide was used to prompt the participants to reveal their lived experience. The interview questions were designed to elicit a beginning, a middle, and an end to permit reconstruction of stories of the experience. The taped interviews were conducted by two graduate assistants with the 8 willing participants. Following verbatim transcription, the interviews were analyzed by the authors.

FINDINGS

Temporal Overview of the Rule-Making Process Using Official Documents

The rule-making process formally began on an unusually pleasant December day in 1993 and ended quietly in September of 1996, when the rule known as the Collaborative Practice Rule became effective. The rule, as legislatively mandated, was limited to "specifying geographic areas to be covered, the methods of treatment that may be covered by collaborative practice arrangements and the requirements for review of services provided pursuant to collaborative practice arrangements" (HB 564, p. 53).

The three entities (Board of Nursing, Board of Healing Arts [Medicine], and Board of Pharmacy) participating in the rule-making process each designated a singular task force to join with the others as one task force to draft a document for approval by all three full boards. The Board of Pharmacy was empowered by the original legislation to approve "any rules relating to dispensing or distribution of medicines or devices by prescription or prescription drug orders" (HB 564, p. 53). The Board of Nursing and the Board of Medicine held their first joint meeting on December 10, 1993. The histories of these two disciplines as they approached the conflict-induced collaboration table is most evident in the initial documents presented by each task force as their opening positions. These positions are presented in Appendix 11.1.

Twelve meetings occurred between December 10, 1993 and August 15, 1994, before the December 1, 1994 filing date of the initially proposed rule. A summary of the discussions that occurred during those meetings is presented in Appendix 11.2, within the three areas of rule making: geographic areas, methods of treatment, and review of services.

The Board of Nursing and the Board of Healing Arts basically reached agreement on the rule language on February 28, 1994. Language dealing with dispensing or distribution of medicines had been included in draft versions of the rule, and it was at this time in the process that the Board of Pharmacy took an active role in refining that language. A series of conference calls and meetings to negotiate acceptable language and to resolve conflicts finally resulted in agreement on August 15, 1994. Their proposed precepts may be reviewed in Appendix 11.3.

The draft rule then had to be approved by the boards involved. The monetary impact of the proposed rule had to be approximated by those entities that would be involved in the implementation process to be presented along with the rule. Following the required fiscal note impact and approval by the respective boards, the proposed rule was filed with the Secretary of State's office on December 15, 1994 and published in the *Missouri Register* in early January 1995.

In response to ongoing pressure by the medical, nursing, and pharmacy communities, the boards had agreed to hold public hearings regarding the proposed rule, which extended the comment period to March 23, 1995. Four public hearings were scheduled throughout the state, with 100 to 200 people attending each hearing. Testimony was accepted at all of the hearings; however, the respective task force members had agreed not to engage in discussion with those participating in the hearings.

A Final Order of Rule Making was submitted to the Joint Legislative Committee on Administrative Rules on May 19, 1995. The rule was immediately challenged by the MSMA, the Missouri Pharmacy Association (MPA), and MONA. A hearing before the Joint Committee on Administrative Rules took place on June 16, 1995. The Joint Committee was composed of three state senators and three state representatives. With the intent of keeping his fellow legislators within the bounds of their legislative mandate, one representative articulated the basis of statutory authority on which the committee could act:

> the absence of statutory authority for the proposed rule; an emergency relating to public health, safety or welfare; the proposed rule is in conflict with state law; or a substantial change in circumstance since enactment of the law on which the proposed rule is based. (Transcript of the Joint Committee on Administrative Rules, June 16, 1995).

Testimony revealed concerns that had not been openly addressed during the task force meetings and that extended beyond the bounds of statutory authority. Sample concerns were such as those expressed by Senator J. Schneider, who stated "but [as] a member of the public, I'm really concerned about the managed care corporations that are going to use all this" (transcript of the Joint Committee on Administrative Rules, June 16, 1995). A student from the Kirksville College of Osteopathic Medicine gave the following testimony: "I don't want to be told that in order to join an HMO or PPO that I must be held accountable for the work of several nurse health practitioners in order to become a member of that group" (transcript of the Joint Committee on Administrative Rules, June 16, 1995). Representatives from the Board of Medicine who had fully participated in the task force discussions gave testimony at the hearings against the proposed rule irrespective of the fact that their board had approved the proposed rule language.

The politicization of this legislated process became fully evident as testimony continued, and the Joint Committee ruled to suspend the proposed rule. Although it was frequently noted throughout the testimony by the Joint Committee members that they did not want to "write the rule," they elected to put forth four recommendations that called for more restrictive language. The recommendations were as follows: to "limit the number of 'extenders' a physician may 'supervise'," to "limit the geographic area to less than 100 miles or to geographic regions," to "consider recommendations from the testimony in regard to pharmacy," and to "make a requirement in the rules that a physician must see the patient at some time" (transcript of the Executive Session of the Joint Committee on Administrative Rules, June 17, 1995).

The rule was, therefore, withdrawn by the Boards of Nursing and Healing Arts on June 21, 1995. A meeting was then held in August in the governor's office. Participants included representatives of the Boards of Nursing, Healing Arts, and Pharmacy along with members of the professional associations and the Director of Policy Development for the Governor. Several additional meetings yielded a second proposed rule addressing the recommendations of the Joint Legislative Committee on Administrative Rules. The rule-filing process was repeated, with the boards giving approval to the proposed rule, filing the rule with the Secretary of State's Office, publishing the rule in the *Missouri Register,* and addressing the comments received during the official comment period. The Final Order of Rule Making was issued on May 6, 1996, with the Joint Committee on Administrative Rules receiving the rule on May 27, 1996. The rule was again challenged: however, no action was taken against the rule during the hearing held by the Joint Legislative Committee on June 12, 1996. This long, arduous process was reaching closure. Finally, three years after the date of the initiation of the process by the administration and following 48 meetings, conference calls, and hearings, the *Collaborative Practice Rule* became a reality.

The Lived Experience

Phenomenology is a methodology used to discover regularities within a phenomenon and for comprehension of the meaning of an experience (Miles and Huberman 1994). It is, thus, an acceptable method to discern commonalities and uniquenesses in the experience of induced collaboration. Following the transcription of the eight interviews, the researchers noted their initial reflections in the margins of the transcript. The unit of analysis was the sentence or a collection of like sentences. Major themes were then delineated and decision rules defined using the process as described by Miles and Huberman (1994). The researchers met twice to review the coding process and to reach consensus when coding discrepancies existed. Interrater reliability was determined to be 98% as evidenced by few disagreements on coding decisions. The data were considered self-evident, and after identifying patterns and differences, the researchers noted the presence of 12 themes.

The loosely structured interviews were designed to elicit aspects of the entire induced collaboration experience. Toward that end, questions were designed to address the beginning, the middle, and the end of the process. Perceptions of the experience were garnered from five nurses and three non-nurses who were involved in the collaborative practice dialogue. Positive and negative comments were included in each of the themes. Two hundred and seventy-six units were coded into the 12 themes. Table 11-1 presents the themes in rank order of number of nota-

Table 11-1. Themes of Conflict-Induced Collaboration

Variable	No. Beginning	No. Middle	No. End	No. Nurse	No. Non-nurse	Total
Role perception	10	9	18	26	11	37
Collaboration/ compromise	10	14	10	23	11	34
Negativism	9	7	14	17	13	30
Motive	4	4	21	21	8	29
Expectations/ optimism	15	2	12	21	7	28
Intention of Bill	6	9	9	12	12	24
Outside influence	5	8	8	14	7	21
Outcomes	1	3	17	15	6	21
Emotions	4	7	5	12	4	16
Turfism	3	4	9	8	8	16
Unprofessional behavior	1	4	8	5	7	13
Trust/mistrust	2	2	2	5	1	6

tions by the interviewees organized according to a sense of the beginning, middle, and end of the induced collaboration process.

Role Perception

Thirty-seven notations were made by the participants with regard to how they perceived their role, the role of others, or the role of a given board. Words used by participants to describe their individual perceptions of their role included "standard bearer for the profession," "peace maker," "mediator and negotiator," and "tracker of the process." Words used to describe how individuals believed they were perceived by others included "tough guy," "not being treated as professionals," "too soft," and "not a flag-waving liberal." Perceptions of others were noted in comments such as "I have yet to see physicians as a whole take a great amount of interest in prevention and care of the elderly and also care of the poor." "[T]he advanced practice nurses were identified as physician extenders." and "[W]e all heard about the money-hungry physicians and about the ignorant, uneducated and unqualified nurses who really were only fit to be physician's assistants." Two participants noted a sense of excitement about the role of their board with comments such as "Pharmacy in general was excited because this actually meant more cooperation by pharmacists in the rural areas and more work for pharmacists to participate in," "especially with the expanding roles in health care and the oncoming of health care [and] changes with HMOs and managed care, this was exciting to pharmacy itself and our organization was excited about it." The excitement, however, was not sustained as evidenced by a later comment to the effect of ". . . but when it got to the point where we were being degraded because of our education . . . there are some wounds that are going to take some time to heal."

Collaboration or Compromise

Comments regarding collaboration or compromise were noted 34 times in the participants' dialogue, clearly indicating that it was a key issue throughout the process. One participant expressed reservations about the process by stating, "nursing was not welcome at the table . . . the very beginning was not good," and another noted, "I figured that we would have to make some compromises but I thought that all of the actors were ultimately going to be very facilitating and would think in terms of what would really promote collaborative practice out in the remote areas." This thought was echoed by another participant, "I thought that it would be a collaborative process. I thought we were going to collaborate in order to come up with collaborative practice guidelines." Medicine was perceived as being an unwilling player at the table and obstructionist to the process by the participant who stated, "It was very clear to us that organized medicine was there against their will and had every intention of making it very difficult on us and had no intention of negotiating or compromising in any way, shape or form."

Another participant described the process as ". . . a very knock-down, drag-out negotiation process which had an entirely different set of rules and behaviors and operations in order to act it out." One participant's comments reflect the environment of the discussions in the statement, "[W]e're here to cooperate, we're here to work with everybody but you're not going to degrade our profession and tell us that you can practice just as well as we can without oversight." As the process reached conclusion, the interviewees expressed that actions had turned toward defending their positions rather than compromising and collaborating for the perceived intent of the bill. This is evident in comments such as, "I think one segment of the medical profession—the DOs—probably took it more personally than the MDs and they went out of their way more to make statements that just caused problems . . . when the nurses heard something against them and their educational ability and standards, then they got up and retaliated . . . that's how pharmacy got."

Negativism

Negativism about the process was pervasive and reflected changes in attitudes over time as manifested by statements such as "we were very open, but then as it progressed, it seemed people became very narrow in their viewpoints." "The process stunk." "I would advise them not to enter into joint collaboration of rules." "I was at a meeting where I heard a legislator get pretty nasty." and "[A]ll of us throughout were hampered in our ability to get together and strategize in secret." Several notations were directed toward the effect of Missouri's sunshine laws on the process. Comments reflecting the restraints of the law were made: "[S]trategizing, and in the back room plan[ning] your actions, plan[ning] your questions and agree[ing] ahead of time on what your actions were going to be or not be, what would be acceptable and what would not be acceptable. . . . [W]e were not able to do that in secret."

Motive

Terms used to describe the motivation of self included *highly motivated, committed, optimistic, discouraged, concerned,* and *deterministic persistence.* Descriptions of the perceived motivation of others are perhaps more revealing: "The pharmacists apparently were very afraid that APNs would be strategically placed all around the state in remote locations from physician colleagues who are by law allowed to dispense, and would become mini-dispensaries and put the pharmacists out of business." "Pharmacy wanted to review the collaborative practice agreement before they would fill any scripts written by an advanced practice nurse." "The motivation of the pharmacy board members was to extend health care to more Missourians. . . . [N]ursing just basically wanted a double standard." "[T]he physicians were very well motivated in trying to expand health care." and "The physicians don't care cause this didn't affect the physicians. . . . [T]his was a neutral bill for the physicians." Another view of the motive of the MDs offered by a participant was "I don't think the physicians and perhaps the pharmacists were ever motivated to achieve these collaborative practice guidelines . . . I don't think they ever were."

Expectations or Optimism

All participants spoke of being optimistic or positive about the process at the outset. Comments reflecting how expectations changed over time include "To see the opposition from the Pharmacy Association and the Osteopathic and Medical Associations and to have our own colleagues on the Board of Medicine testify against a bill that we had all agreed on was very devastating"; "[W]e had gone to that meeting with some very clear definitions of what we believed. Maybe they were a little idealistic, but they were defining definitions. They were never, ever addressed. The Board of Medicine just threw them across the table and wouldn't even look at them. That was a very big disappointment, because had we stuck to some definitions that we could have all agreed upon, it wouldn't have taken us three years." "Listening to how the Board of Nursing was starting out the process . . . it looked very good. Over time my expectations got less and less and my concerns got greater and greater as I watched the process develop." and "I went from thinking that we were going to be successful . . . to thinking that somehow we were never going to get this done. Thinking that any rules that were accomplished would be facilitating for collaborative practice."

Intention of the Bill

Lack of clarity on the intention of the bill is evident in seven transcripts. One participant repeatedly spoke of the fact that "[N]obody would take a stand and clarify the intent of that bill." Another participant commented, "the language in the statute was poorly crafted so we were half strung right from the beginning . . . because it was not clear how could we work collaboratively." Generally speaking, non-nurse participants spoke of the intent of the bill to be "to provide health care to the citizens of Missouri in deprived rural areas," whereas nurse participants viewed the intent more broadly, as evidenced by the statements, "It was to increase access to care." "[H]ealth care access is the ultimate goal. . . . [W]e're not out to replace the physicians."

Outside Influences

Outside influences included politicians, professional organizations, and practitioners of all three disciplines. A participant describes the impact of outside influences: "But when we started getting outside interference . . . the joint rules committee would throw out our rules and people that had no business getting involved got involved . . . ," and another describes the fear: ". . . that if we did not pass rules, some of the legislators would go back to the drawing board and do away with the legislation and replace it with far more onerous legislation." Nurse and non-nurse participants were aware of ". . . heavy political influence from outside the three boards. That had much more impact than we wanted or needed." One participant interpreted the outside political influence to be ". . . that if [we] wanted [our] budget process to go well, [we] needed to sit down and work out these rules and come to agreement." A second participant noted, "[W]e were getting a lot of pressure from the politicians and from the governor's office to get it done efficiently, quickly." The influence of the professional organizations is reflected in this participant's comment: "I think probably the biggest detour in reaching where we were going was the strong amount of lobbying that was done by the associations."

Outcomes

Lack of a positive outcome after 3 years of induced collaboration was evident in every transcript. Words used to describe the outcomes included *restrictive, barriers, negative, limiting, ridiculous, one group regulating another,* and *didn't meet objectives.* Descriptions of feelings about the outcomes included shame, disappointment, negativism, and displeasure. One participant did believe that the "rule and the statute have allowed improved access to occur," but balanced that comment with the statement that "we could have addressed more quality measures in the rule . . . more disciplinary actions in the rule than we did."

Emotions

Nurse participants spoke more about emotions than did the non-nurse participants. *Excited, frustration, anxious, anger, stressful, shock,* and *tense* were words used to describe emotions or an emotional state. Emotions expressed in the beginning of the process included more positive states such as "excited . . . with the whole thing" than those expressed as the process continued. One participant's comments of "[A]s time went on, the process became very wearing and it was very, very frustrating. . . . [A]fter a while . . . [it] was such a struggle that I think burn-out is a good way to describe where we were towards the very end of it," seems to capture the emotional scale of the experience.

Turfism

Sixteen references were made by participants regarding turfism. Although few in number overall, the comments were most pointed as demonstrated by comments such as "The physicians . . . were acting defensively and they were going to make sure that whatever they gave up, they were still going to protect their turf." and "[T]urf protection . . . total turf . . . the physicians thought that the nurses were asking for too much and the nurses felt that they were already doing it." Turfism seemed evident throughout the experience as described by one participant who noted "[T]hat's when all the turf protection started. Practically every meeting that we had, that particular issue was addressed and then we'd go on and try to resolve the problem but we'd always come back to that." Participants perceived the other entities to be engaged in turf protection as evidenced by one participant who reported, "[T]he pharmacists' position from beginning to end was very self-serving. . . . [T]hey were intent on maintaining the status quo." One participant noted "the matter of turf, to me, was the biggest thing. [P]hysicians were concerned about their pocketbooks and their territory." and another participant stated that the experience was "a debate around turf and money and control." This was echoed by another participant who "wondered how much influence the fact that managed care has become so prevalent and . . . that [it] has been eating away at the private practice of physicians . . . who feel they are losing control of their own practice because of some of the changes in the health care system that are coming down."

Unprofessional Behavior

Nurses and non-nurses both expressed feelings about their colleagues' unprofessional behavior as expressed in these statements: "As I watched the process I was amazed at how the Board of Nursing [representatives] were able to keep their professional demeanor and act in a professional manner the whole time. . . . [The other boards] said some very insulting things and the Board of Nursing took them very well, where on the other hand if anything was hinted from the Board of Nursing that they were interested in anything other than quality, or they had any other motive, their outrage was amazing."

Other comments verify the perceived unprofessional behavior. "To me, it was embarrassing. . . . [T]he Governor's office sent somebody to chair the meeting between us . . . because [we] couldn't work it out. That was embarrassing." Other comments: "I learned a lot about human behavior . . . but sometimes I was embarrassed to see it displayed so openly by my own colleagues. . . . " Finally: "I don't think the team, or nursing in general, was prepared for the tactics that organized medicine used. . . ."

Trust or Mistrust

Mistrust of the process was expressed more frequently by the nurse participants. All participants expressed a greater sense of trust in the beginning of the process, with trust changing to mistrust over time. This was evident in comments such as "I guess the bigger bump in the road . . . was that pharmacists were really leery of filling any prescriptions from someone [if] they didn't know whether or not they were a legitimate prescriber," and "[W]hen all of a sudden some of the conversations began to take place about what this NP could do, they (Medicine) began to dig in their heels and they weren't quite sure whether this was going to be competition, a threat to their practice, or could be used to enhance their practice."

DISCUSSION

The Story

Mattingly (1994) expands the notion of emplotment beyond the traditional archetypal plot structures of romance, tragedy, comedy, and satire and beyond Ricoeur's (1987) notion of life in time fundamentally related to the structure of narrative through the common bond of the plot to the arena of social action. Emplotted time is transformed by a plot into a meaningful whole with a beginning, middle, and end, with particular events gaining meaning by their place within the story and their contribution to the plot.

Nursing's story begins at the first noted official joint meeting of the three boards and is described by one of the nurse participants:

> We went to this meeting in St. Louis with our medical colleagues. We walked into the room. We were on time. We were not late, but they were already there, sitting together at one end of the table. They didn't say hello to us. They didn't welcome us. They didn't shake hands. Nothing. They thrust a document in front of our noses that was a regulatory document in which they had developed rules. It was stated in legalistic language, the way these documents ultimately come out, and it presented all of these rigid rules about the requirements for collaborative practice.

Nursing was reluctant to entertain the document offered by Medicine because of its perceived restrictive language; however, political realities and the clear message of power-control from Medicine created a negative situation in which nursing was unable to put forth the document successfully, which they firmly believed was an equitable beginning, and nursing's plot to begin the process with the least restrictive language was subverted. A participant noted:

> The Board of Nursing had an open meeting in which we strategized for this first meeting with the Board of Healing Arts representatives. We gave everybody an opportunity to share their best thinking about these areas of concern. At that meeting, we came up with a set of principles that served us well for the entire process.

To come forward with the most restrictive language possible set the stage for future discordant meetings, and Medicine's prospective story and power plot became evident. Pharmacy was initially an observer of the evolving plot, purporting to be a supportive player as revealed in the following dialogue:

> Once we were told that Pharmacy was to participate in this process, the Pharmacy Board made a commitment that we were going to cooperate in every way we could to help this to be achieved at the most cooperative

and fastest route. From day one, we entered into the fact that this was going to be a positive process and Pharmacy was going to play a positive role in it.

As additional meetings were held, the plot thickened and subplots emerged. The presence of outside influences, particularly in the form of legislators, enhanced the political plot, giving the appearance that all three boards were being equally "threatened" with budget cuts if progress was not made in a timely manner. The political plot was a diffi-cult plot to decipher for nursing. The reception of supportive messages from the governor's office was often incongruent with the messages put forth by various legislators, making political support for the least restric-tive language an uncertainty. This is evident in the following dialogue:

[T]he role of the politicians and the governor's administration in this process. They were warm and cold. They were in and out. Sometimes they were very facilitating, and sometimes they were absent. I learned in a way I had never learned before, how subject politicians are to the polit-ical whims of the day. They were not there for months, then they would come back in and say "you're not done yet? Let's get on with it or we're going to cut your budget, or the budget of the Boards." Then they'd be gone again.

The political plot was played out side by side with the "best position-ing" plot of the professional associations of each discipline. The Missouri Nurses Association, The Missouri Association of Pharmacy, the Missouri State Medical Society, and the Missouri Association of Osteopathic Physicians closely monitored the rule-making process and, at critical points in the dialogue, became intimately involved in the process by par-ticipating in hearings, speaking at task force meetings, or lobbying respective task force members or legislators or administration represen-tatives. Recognition of this plot is reflected in this nurse's comment:

Another thing is that we would reach agreement on something and then some medical group from out there somewhere would rise up and be totally in opposition and our physician colleagues would pull back and come up with what I can describe only as a new wrinkle and why things had to become more conservative or some tentatively agreed-upon lan-guage could not be used. The osteopathic physicians in Missouri were very nervous about all this. The DOs tend to practice more in rural areas and in primary care more so they perceived they had a great deal to lose. Another thing is that we had these public hearings. At one point where we did complete a draft set of guidelines, then we went through the process of filing them and we had agreed that we would have public hearings throughout the state. We had four public hearings and these were really three-ring circuses. We had hundreds of people there, all testifying and we had agreed that we would stay there as long as it took. We would make no comments, no discussion. We would just take someone's testimony. We had these people coming to the microphone and depending on their point of view, many of their comments were emotional.

Least restrictive language, power, politics, positioning—these plots were an integral part of the multiple discussions of the task forces and boards. It was inevitable that all could not prevail. One·plot would dominate and ultimately determine the final order of rule making and provide an ending to the story. That plot reached its climax in the hearing held by the Joint Committee on Administrative Rules (June 16, 1995) and is illustrated in excerpts of testimony:

SENATOR HOWARD: Dr. Bean.
DR. BEAN: You've seen the tip of the iceberg that we went through hearing all these opinions. Basically the legislature gave us the task of writing these rules but limited us to those three areas: geography [geographic distance], methods [of treatment], and requirements [review of services]. As a result we came up with rules that are rules based on intense compromise. You have compromise coming from groups with such diversion points. You have rules that really no one is happy with. I think that's probably a safe assumption
SENATOR SCHNEIDER: Mr. Chairman.
SENATOR HOWARD: Senator Schneider.
SENATOR SCHNEIDER: Why did you decide not to limit the geographic area where this would be applicable?
DR. BEAN: We tried. From day one we tried to initially limit them to federally designated underserved areas and we were fought tooth and nail. We tried. . . . The nurses wanted [a] basic plan as the geographic limit and we wanted at least something and we finally compromised. . . .
SENATOR SCHNEIDER: Your answer is the physicians wanted a limit but the nurses didn't. Is that your answer?

DR. BEAN: That is my answer.

SENATOR SCHNEIDER: So you couldn't get the nurses to agree.

DR. BEAN: We got them to agree on 100 miles.

SENATOR SCHNEIDER: And that was as far as—that's because the nurses wanted to do it even in St. Louis whether we need it or not. Correct?

DR. BEAN: Yes.

SENATOR SCHNEIDER: So the problem there is the nurses wanting to do something more than the physicians thought was appropriate.

DR. BEAN: Yes

SENATOR SCHNEIDER: And you felt compelled, in order to get a rule, to agree with the nurses because they had you over a barrel.

DR. BEAN: Yes

SENATOR SCHNEIDER: I gather that was used a great deal in order to convince you that you shouldn't limit the number of nurses. Did the nurses agree to limit the number or did they oppose you on that also?

DR. BEAN: They did not agree to limit the number.

SENATOR SCHNEIDER: Did you attempt to get an agreement to limit the number?

DR. BEAN: Yes

SENATOR SCHNEIDER: Was that another case in which the nurses just want everything they can get? And they don't want to be limited in supervision?

REPRESENTATIVE KLUMB: You believe that if this rule goes into effect, we will see an emergency relating to public health, safety and welfare?

DR. BEAN: My opinion is that will most likely happen. Yes.

REPRESENTATIVE KLUMB: I think it's not the role of this Committee to be critical; but it raises tremendous concern with me when you have voted for a rule, which now before the Committee you say if in fact goes into effect, will create an emergency for the citizens of this State.

A motion was made by Senator Schneider to suspend the proposed Collaborative Practice Rules. The boards were directed to incorporate four prescriptive recommendations into the rule. The power plot now dictated the roles of the actors in the succeeding events. It was clear that the rule would be very extensive and directive. The Board of Medicine, clearly aware of the dominance of their plot agreed to a facilitated meeting with a representative of the Governor's Office. Nursing's feelings of betrayal and dismay were typified by the following comments:

> I was very disappointed with my physician colleagues. I didn't feel that we could ever raise the level of debate to the issue of how do we all assure quality for the people we serve, our patients. So I was very disappointed about that. I was disappointed with the vehemence of the debate, and disappointed, frankly, at the whole health profession areas in Missouri. That we would have a debate that was so ugly and so negative about each other's skills that very little common ground could be found for the patient.

Nursing's plot was no longer a vital director of the story's ending. Following several additional meetings between the boards to incorporate the recommendations of the Joint Committee on Administrative Rules into the rule, a revised version containing highly restrictive language was submitted to the Joint Committee on Administrative Rules in February of 1996. This rule was accepted by the Joint Committee on Administrative Rules and duly filed with the Secretary of State's Office. The collaborative Practice Rule became effective September 1996. Another act or story has now ended and another is yet to unfold.

When we are little children, we fervently hope that wishing will make something so. That is not the case, as adults soon enough learn. Endings are uncertain. A story thus may be marked by suspense and by surprise. In efforts to shape events to achieve desired outcomes, particularly when the stakes are high and the other actors are dissimilar in their stories, "Enemies must be faced, risks taken. . . . Desire must be strong because danger is also present and one faces danger only when one wants something [or doesn't want something] very badly" (Mattingly 1994, p. 814).

In this case of viewing the series of events surrounding the establishment of collaborative practice guidelines in Missouri, it is difficult to conclude that any of the stories are even a partial success, although medicine's story demonstrates the successful assertion of power to achieve their agenda. Certainly from the perspective of developing a collaborative partnership to achieve mutually satisfying outcomes, these stories can be judged as outright failures.

It seems fair to ask, therefore, why tell these stories? What can be learned from the telling of failed stories? The answer seems to be that we *must* examine failed stories. As humans, it is our blessing and our curse to learn from our failures as well as our successes. From the philosopher Heidegger's (1962) perspective, we are always recreating ourselves. In our future-oriented humanness, we are in a position to shape a time ahead that is more to our liking. In short, we are more or less always trying to do better. As one of the interviewees stated:

> The idea of a professional endeavor . . . going through three years of intense work and coming out with nothing, I found very disconcerting. I don't know if some of that is even my own inclination for achieving results, and that I had a personal stake in that. . . . I really am counting on and looking forward to coming back to this within a year. . . . I'm really looking forward to this process over time improving. I would certainly do anything I could to facilitate that. I really hope that will be the case.

Relating the Findings to the Concept and Model of Coalition

Coalitions are defined in Chapter 10 as: *complex dynamic human social systems strategically formed to respond purposefully to identified needs and problems by the coming together of key representative members of two or more organizations within a formal organizational structure that supports a power-sharing partnership and facilitates designing and conducting interorganizational collaborative strategies and activities to pursue agreed-upon goals and outcomes that no one constituent could achieve acting alone.*

The model elements of coalition encompassed within the definition represent the necessary elements for configuring a functional coalition. These are *purpose or reason, impetus for acting at this time, approaches to problem-solving, membership, patterns of formation of the membership, structure of the coalition, power-sharing partnership, levels of interorganizational collaboration, functions or tasks performed,* and *outcomes achieved.* The first five elements are primarily concerned with formation of the coalition; their particular application or utilization will have an impact, negative or positive, on coalition formation and conduct. These elements will be briefly related to data from this case study, as the ways in which they are carried out in this case may be negative. Of the five elements primarily concerned with coalition conduct, power-sharing partnership is one of two focused in this case analysis. The expectation is that these group members had difficulty establishing a partnership. The second variable is outcomes achieved.

The variable purpose responds to the question: Why form a coalition? One or more would-be-members or influential persons or organizations perceive a value in bringing together two or more persons or groups or organizations to form a working interorganizational relationship. Impetus, as a model variable, responds to the question: Why form a coalition now? Catalysts for forming the coalition can range from a group of leaders representing their organizations who share a vision for joint action to an external mandate from a government agency. In conjunction with impetus for formation is the degree of voluntariness exercised by coalition members in joining in coalition. This pattern of formation—degree of voluntariness—is also a major predictor of coalition success. The freer the choice to participate, the greater the likelihood of commitment to the goals of the coalition and the willingness to work for their achievement. A continuum of voluntariness, described in Chapter 9, exists from most voluntary (level I) to least voluntary (level V). Level V is the level of conflict-induced collaboration.

Diversity or sameness of the membership refers to membership compatibility in mission, beliefs, goals, and values. Diverse members are not usually compatible in these core areas, whereas members who share sameness are compatible. This variable also can refer to differences in skills, talents, and needs. It is harder to bring diverse groups into coalition than it is to bring groups that are the same or similar in their makeup. In both cases, great sensitivity is required to bring together organizations and individuals who can recognize a common vision and work toward common goals.

The relationship that develops between two or more organizations and its representative members is one of partnership. During the formation phases, the would-be-partners have hopefully begun to develop a spirit of cooperation and a shared set of positive expectations for the coalition. The newly developing partners need to learn to share power, authority, and decision making; to negotiate differences and resolve conflicts with mutual respect; to develop a relationship of trust; and to support the mission and goals of the coalition, which are bigger than, and perhaps disparate from, their own agendas.

Gray (1989) describes coalition formation and the enabling partnership as an emergent process. She cautions not to underestimate the developmental character of the relationship and overlook the sensitive and delicate interactions that need to occur (p. 15). It is reasonable to hypothesize that partners who share fully and equally in all facets of coalition decision-making are likely to have positive attitudes toward the coalition and actively work toward achievement of the goals of the coalition. Partners who do not share decision-making in all areas of coalition conduct, conversely, will experience conflict and incompatibility.

Outcomes achieved are described on a continuum from agreed-upon goal achievement to a higher level of achievement that recognizes a new shared vision greater than the vision or mission of each participating organization or actor. The highest level outcome is defined as the development of a lasting power-sharing partnership that enables the participating organizations and their representatives to pursue their shared visions.

In this case of legislatively mandated collaboration, bringing together at least three disparate groups to accomplish externally imposed goals, it is not difficult to anticipate great difficulty in coalition formation and partnership development. It is also reasonable to suspect that this forced group may have much difficulty agreeing upon a course of action and achieving mutually beneficial outcomes.

In the Missouri case, there was no agreed-upon purpose by the Task Force members. The section of this chapter concerning the history that led to the passage of mandating legislation tells the reader that a joint rules committee to negotiate the terms of collaborative practice was a compromise measure to move the legislative process along. What that accomplished was a forced process of conflict-induced collaboration. The impetus that forced the coalition was the legislation that required that representative members of the nursing, medical, and pharmacy boards come together to work out an agreement. Because the participants did not share a common purpose or vision and were forced to meet, it is not surprising that they did not work well together or achieve a satisfactory result—by any standards.

Moreover, in terms of the voluntariness of the members coming together, the Missouri effort rates a level V on the degree of voluntariness continuum. In other words, this is the level of induced-conflict collaboration. Because these representatives of their respective boards were forced to come together, it is predictable in this case that there would be little or no commitment to the externally imposed coalition and that, to the contrary, all representatives would work to protect their disparate professional agendas.

Another very interesting aspect of this particular externally forced coalition, is that external interference *continued to be thrust upon the struggling members throughout the process, rendering it ever more arduous.* The comments of several interviewees testify to this assertion. One non-nurse interviewee stated, "[T]he interventions were very hard and rigid,being called into the governor's office with a number of folks and forcing resolution at that point. It is still . . . incredibly conflictual. . . . " A nurse interviewee who was not a board member stated,: "I think when it started . . . the nursing players were hearing from the Governor's office that often the best rule was no rule . . . [then] the political atmosphere changed, and some legislators decided there had to be rules . . . I'm aware that the boards, the regulatory boards, basically had their budgets held hostage to the process."

These coalition members were disparate. They had different agendas and purposes, and values and beliefs. With hindsight it is easy to question why anyone ever thought resolution to these issues could be achieved through a process of collaboration. Clearly, this forced coalition did not establish a power-sharing partnership. Rather, the group with the most power, MDs, refused to share power because they perceived no benefit in so doing. Again, with hindsight, we can realize that this venture had nothing going for it. There was no shared purpose. An external force mandated that the task force come together; their joining was involuntary; and there were great disparities in the agendas they brought to the table. Why would anyone think that given these conditions, a power-sharing partnership would be formed?

The answer to this rhetorical question is that perhaps no one thought they would form a partnership, but they did believe these representatives would finally settle down and develop a set of useful collaborative practice guidelines that would improve access to primary care for Missouri citizens. The emplotment theme suggests that the framers of the legislation may have intuitively tried to direct a plot leading to a desired outcome. Mattingly (1994) tells us that people as authors, directors, and actors may think:

> Even if our actions are taken up, reworked and redirected by the responses of other actors, we still have some success some of the time working toward endings we care about. And sometimes we are even able to negotiate with other actors so that we can move in directions cooperatively, cumulatively (p. 813).

As the presentation of data show, this was not quite the case. No member or representative group identifies a positive outcome. Some see mixed results; others are guardedly optimistic that the guidelines can be improved in the future. A pharmacy member states, ". . . [G]uidelines did not compare favorably to the boards initial expectations." A nurse representative of the health department states, "I guess [outcomes] are mixed. The law did give us prescriptive privileges." Another nurse non-board member asks, "Was it worth it?" and answers, "I don't know." Another nurse member was disappointed with the extent nursing had to compromise but seemed to believe the process had to occur. She states that "[i]t was a very worthwhile cause. If I had it to do over again, I would." Finally, another nurse member asserts, "This is a foundation."

Something was achieved, but it was not very satisfactory and it was achieved at a very high price. Gray (1989) points out that sometimes collaboration is not the desired approach. She identifies five questions that would be advisable for a would-be-collaborator to ask before committing to joining with others in a coalition. It would also be advisable for those with the power to force others into conflict-induced collaboration (level V) or induced collaboration (level IV) to ask this same set of questions concerning all the proposed players. These are the following:

1. Does the present situation fail to serve my interests?
2. Will collaboration produce positive outcomes?
3. Is it possible to reach a fair agreement?
4. Is there parity among the stakeholders?
5. Will the other side agree to collaborate?" (p. 59)

In the Missouri case, negative answers to these questions, predictive of negative outcomes of collaboration, would likely have been articulated even without benefit of hindsight. The authors have concluded that it is extremely difficult to answer these questions in a positive direction when one or several potential collaborators view the problem being addressed as economically driven and adopt protection of economic interests as their primary goal.

CONCLUSIONS AND RECOMMENDATIONS

The eight interviewed participants in the Missouri experience were very reflective about the experience and offered many thoughtful suggestions for those who might find themselves in a similar situation. They also reflected upon what they would do differently if they had it to do over again. Each comment that follows is made by a different interviewee. They said: "I would ask that all the parties have some tolerance of each other." "I'd spend more time with physicians having them experience collaborative practice settings that were positive and effective. I would spend that same amount of time with legislators, having them visit sites that are positive and effective." "I would [take] some steps for relationship setting, for openness of communication, for learning about each other's background, for developing some knowledge of each other and maybe some mutual respect. . . . For sharing up front without any kind of strings attached . . . what our goals and expectations for the process were . . . a lot more team-building up front could have helped considerably."

Additional comments were as follows: "I think that going in . . . some type of mediator or facilitator for the negotiation process. . . ." "How to negotiate without giving away the store. That's critical. . . . You have to be able to negotiate, but never lose sight of your ideals." "I learned . . . I need to be more flexible." Finally, one weary member placed the burden squarely with the inducers:

> The promoters of the process, and in this case it came out of a legislative mandate, it came out of a political agenda, so therefore I put this burden on the governor. The administration, I think should [have been] more informed about what we were moving into, and then of course, our professional people, have a responsibility to be better informed about what kind of a process we're moving into.

The first recommendation is a suggestion that would-be-collaborators ask the set of questions, previously listed, to elicit a judgment that collaboration is or is not a desired course of action. If the answers to Gray's questions are at all negative, serious consideration ought to be given to an alternative course of action. Although beyond the scope of this book, such actions might include a more clearly directed legislative mandate that would not require a collaborative act such as joint rule-making requires, or a dispute-resolution process. The latter, although taking on some of the trappings of collaboration, such as bringing people to the table, is more unabashedly a legalistic and formalized process of enforced negotiation.

Should a decision be made to induce a collaborative process, every effort must be made to depoliticize the process. All actors and external enforcers need to understand what they are setting in motion. Far greater sensitivity, such as that the actors involved in the Missouri experience were asking for, needs to be displayed. This increased understanding of and sensitivity to the process is the second recommendation. Third, in such difficult circumstances, it is recommended that conflict-induced collaboration only be used as a last resort and only after careful preparation.

Recommendation four is for team building. Those who force people to come together in coalition and those who are the would-be-collaborators need to respect the process and the time it takes to reach a common understanding and have mutual respect for each other's points of view. Collaborators have to be able to engage in open, honest, and guileless communication in order to develop a power-sharing partnership.

For those in other states and settings who find themselves in similar circumstances, we (the authors) offer the following summary set of guidelines:

1. Avoid a joint rule-making process, if at all possible; use only as a last resort.
2. Depoliticize the process.
3. Know what kind of a process you are getting into and prepare for it.
4. Use conflict-induced collaboration only as a last resort.
5. Be fully informed to the point of understanding the perspectives and positions of the other actors. (See Chapters 1 and 9 for discussions of power-sharing partnerships.)
6. Insist upon the presence of a negotiator or facilitator at all meetings.
7. Establish agreed-upon and clear ground rules for meeting conduct.
8. Focus and maintain focus on defining the problem in a way that is clear to all and, hopefully, mutually agreed to.

Finally, the authors offer a set of recommendations for research and scholarly development of induced collaboration and conflict-induced collaboration. First, additional case studies need to be completed using the coalition model as presented in Chapter 9. Gray's notions of conflict-induced collaboration need to be included and expanded in this conceptual framework. The emplotment notion is also judged by the researchers to be a dramatically vivid way to identify the human costs of this process when it is forced insensitively, as in this case. This methodology also can be profitably used, therefore, as a component of the additional case studies.

Second, we recommend that surveys be conducted to identify other instances of conflict-induced collaboration. Comparative analyses should then be conducted using qualitative methodologies and document reviews to determine which, if any, of those are reported as successful and make a determination as to why that is so.

The next recommendation logically follows. Interventions that promote coalition building in an induced-conflict model, based in empirical evidence, can then be articulated and tested in induced-conflict collaboration. Finally, evaluation research models for incorporation in induced-conflict models need to be designed and implemented as part of the intervention development and testing process.

Induced-conflict collaboration in health care is likely to continue to be widely used as governments at all levels and the corporate sector struggle with extraordinary changes in the organization, financing, and delivery of health care. We need to avoid it by substituting other actions to achieve our ends; modify it to take the negative elements out of the process, thereby making the process more truly collaborative, or use it as a last resort. But we must enter the process armed with understanding and skills and perhaps with interventions in hand that will facilitate reaching mandated agreements.

The analysis of the Missouri experience, using these research and theory building approaches represents the beginning of theory development in this complex, high-stakes area. The authors accept the challenge of continuing this work and hope the readers will also join in meeting this challenge.

References

Advanced Practice Nursing Task Force. (1993). *Official Draft document: Collaborative Practice.*

Davis, C. (January/February, 1983). On trial: Nursing judges rules, next step, The Supreme Court. *The Missouri Nurse,* 52, 1, 8.

Department of Economic Development. State Board of Nursing. (1995). Proposed rule making. *Missouri Register* (January 2, 1995; January 17, 1995; March 1, 1996).

Department of Economic Development. State Board of Nursing. (1995). Final Order. *Missouri Register* (August 1, 1996).

General Assembly of the State of Missouri. (1993). House Bill No. 564, p. 53.

Gray, B. (1989). *Collaborating: Finding Common Ground for Multiparty Problems.* Josey-Bass Publishers, San Francisco/London.

House Bill 564 (August 28, 1993). The Primary Care Access Package, Missouri Legislature, Jefferson City, Missouri: Signed into law by Governor Mel Carnahan.

Kellett, A. (June/July 1982). On trial: Nursing in Missouri. *The Missouri Nurse,* 51, 3, 2–3.

Kellett, A. Update: The case Missouri nurses make history. *The Missouri Nurse,* 53, 1, 8–9.

Legislative Nurse Power (February 1976). *The Missouri Nurse,* 45, 1, 3–8.

Mattingly, C. (1994). The concept of therapeutic emplotment. *Social Science Medicine, 38,* 6, 811–822.

Miles, M. and Huberman, M. (1994). *Qualitative Data Analysis,* 2nd Ed. Sage Publications, Thousand Oaks.

Missouri Association of Osteopathic Physicians and Surgeons. (1993). *Official Draft document: Collaborative Practice.*

Missouri Supreme Court Decision No. 64692. (November 1983). *Sermchief v. Gonzales.*

Official Minutes from the following:

Joint meeting of the Board of Nursing and the Board of Healing Arts (December 10, 1993).

Joint meeting of the Board of Nursing, Board of Healing Arts and Board of Pharmacy (January 4, 1996).

Joint meeting of the Board of Nursing, Board of Healing Arts and Board of Pharmacy (January 20, 1994).

Joint meeting of the Board of Nursing, Board of Healing Arts and Board of Pharmacy (February 7, 1994).

Conference Call of the Board of Nursing, Board of Healing Arts and Board of Pharmacy (February 17, 1994).

Joint meeting of the Board of Nursing, Board of Healing Arts and Board of Pharmacy (February 28, 1994).

Conference Call of the Board of Nursing and the Board of Pharmacy (March 16, 1994).

Conference Call of the Board of Nursing and the Board of Pharmacy (March 2, 1994).

Joint meeting of the Board of Nursing, Board of Healing Arts and Board of Pharmacy (June 6, 1994).

Conference Call of the Board of Nursing and the Board of Pharmacy (July 2, 1994).

Conference Call of the Board of Nursing and the Board of Pharmacy (August 15, 1994).

Joint meeting of the Board of Nursing and the Board of Healing Arts (April 26, 1995).

Joint meeting of the Board of Nursing and the Board of Pharmacy (May 15, 1995).

Advanced Practice Task Force (April 10, 1994).

Advanced Practice Task Force (August 18, 1994).

Official Transcript, Joint Committee on Administrative Rules (June 16, 1995).

Official Transcript, Executive Session, Joint Committee on Administrative Rules (June 17, 1995)

Official Transcript, Joint Committee on Administrative Rules (June 12, 1996).

On Trial: Nursing, The Supreme Court Hearing. *The Missouri Nurse*, 52, 5, 11.

Appendix 11-1. Opening Positions: Board of Nursing and Board of Healing Arts (Medicine)

Area	Board of Nursing Position (Concept Based)	Board of Healing Arts (Medicine) Position
Geographic areas to be covered	1. Availability of care in a crisis situation. 2. The use of all varieties of telecommunications. 3. Electronic device contact. 4. Recognition of the variations in rural communities. 5. Vary within the collaborating partners and the practice situation. 6. Development of a model that would interrelate the selected variables to include client population, health care problems, rural or urban, other resources available, transportation, and communication. 7. Development of mechanisms for referral and consultation. 8. Reasonable expectations within the context of realities.	1. APNS who perform delegated medical acts in remote practice sites shall be limited to medically underserved areas. 2. An APN shall not perform delegated medical acts during periods of time when a collaborating physician is unavailable. 3. The collaborating physician shall not, at any time, be more than 50 road miles by the most direct route from the remote site location. 4. The collaborating physician(s) shall be available for consultation as needed and shall be immediately available to the APN either personally or via telecommunications at all times, i.e. 24 hours a day, seven days a week. 5. The guidelines for an APN in remote sites will apply except in the Public Health Clinics functioning under federal guidelines, County Health Department clinics functioning under the Department of Health guidelines, and Family Planning Clinics. These clinics may provide services in areas not considered remote.
Review of services	1. Systematic and joint. 2. Development of a periodic mechanism of collaborative review such as CQI, Quality Assurance, Peer Review.	1. The collaborating physician bears the authority and the shared responsibility for the delegated medical acts.

3. Shall be written.
4. Collaborating partners will have plans for systematic review.
5. The plan for review shall be kept on file in the collaborating practice.
6. The collaborating partners shall decide the scope and detail of review based on the type of practice.
7. Jointly collect client care data and systematically analyze data for the evaluation of the practice and outcome of care.
8. Review process shall be documented and not a regulatory review.
9. Review shall be self review and peer review and not a regulatory review.
10. Patient care data should be kept on file in the practice for a designated period of time for legal and research purposes.

Accordingly, the tasks delegated to the APN shall be within the scope of those provided by the physician.
2. The collaborating physician must exercise oversight, direction and control of the services of the APN. It is the shared responsibility of the collaborating physician and APN to direct and review the work, records, and practice on a continuing basis to ensure that appropriate directions are given and understood and that appropriate treatment is rendered.
3. The collaborating physician and APN must annually review and renew protocols or practice guidelines to ensure they are current in regard to the collaborating partners' scope of practice, the range of medical acts delegated by the physician, and the evolving standards of practice.
4. Review of charts and records to determine the appropriate care of the patient and compliance with standing orders and protocols shall occur every two days by the collaborating physician. The collaborating physician shall cosign and date all patient's charts and records.

Methods of treatment

1. Professionals function within their specialized scope of practice.
2. Methods of treatment shall be the accepted current practice of nursing and medicine.
3. Scope of practice addresses both collaborating parties and is documented in the agreement.
4. Rule making in this area should not be dictated by reimbursement policies.

1. When off-site care is provided, transportation and backup procedures for immediate handling of patients needing emergency care and care beyond the APNs scope of practice must be established. The collaborating physician must have hospital privileges at a hospital in the

(continued)

Appendix 11-1. Opening Positions: Board of Nursing and Board of Healing Arts (Medicine) *(continued)*

Area	Board of Nursing Position (Concept Based)	Board of Healing Arts (Medicine) Position
	5. Practice guidelines to be used in the practice address methods of treatment, vary with the collaborating partners and the practice situation, and are on file in the practice setting.	state of Missouri.
	6. The number and specificity of the practice guidelines and materials is a decision of the practice partners.	2. No collaborating physician shall permit an APN to delegate medical acts to other APNs or PAs (Physician Assistants) in lieu of a collaborating physician.
	7. Consistent or standardized materials need to be present in the practice (such as history and physical forms).	3. The collaborating physician must provide direction to the APN to specify what delegated medical acts should be provided. These directions may take the form of written protocols, oral communication, in person, by telephone, or by other means of electronic communications.
	8. All shall practice within their specialization and within their scope of practice and in conformity with standards of practice within their profession.	
	9. Practice guidelines and/or protocols shall be kept on file in the practice and not monitored by regulatory agencies.	4. Protocols or practice guidelines must be developed by the collaborating physician and the APN to include guidelines describing and delineating the delegated medical acts. Protocols and practice guidelines should be specific in their guidance.
	10. Methods of treatment must be viewed at the highest level of abstraction.	5. Immediate physician consultation must be obtained for specified clinical situations and in situations falling outside those specified protocols or guidelines.
		6. Physician collaboration means that APNs only perform delegated medical acts and procedures that have been specifically authorized by practice guidelines or protocols and delegated by the collaborating physician.
		7. The collaborating physician shall see every patient at least annually or ever third visit, if

		the third visit is within a 12-month period or if there is a change in the patient's condition or symptoms.
Prescribing guidelines	None	1. The prescription shall include the name, address, and telephone number of the APN and that of the collaborating physician. 2. Prior to authority to prescribe, a standard medical pharmacology course shall be completed and successfully passed by the APN. 3. Protocols or guidelines for medications that can be used for patients by an APN shall be clearly written in the protocol or standing orders indicating follow-up care, dosage, quantity, and the number of refills, etc. 4. An APN shall not, under any circumstances, order controlled substances. An order for controlled substances must be initialed and written by the collaborating physician. The APN can dispense or administer controlled substances only after an order from the collaborating physician.
Additional dictates	1. Rule making must be consistent with access and cost containment and primary care. 2. Collaboration shall be defined in a preface and not in the rule. 3. The rule should be designed to improve access. 4. Delivery of care by multidisciplinary team. 5. Managed collaboration and care. 6. Focus of rule making must be consumer safety. 7. The rule must be stated simply and clearly.	1. The APN and collaborating physician shall have established a collaborating working agreement for a minimum of 6 months so defined by practice agreements prior to working in a remote location. 2. The APN shall wear a name badge at all times when working, identifying himself as an advanced practice nurse or registered physician assistant. The title of the individual shall not be abbreviated. Any

(continued)

Appendix 11-1. Opening Positions: Board of Nursing and Board of Healing Arts (Medicine) *(continued)*

Area	Board of Nursing Position (Concept Based)	Board of Healing Arts (Medicine) Position
	8. The following assumptions underpin the Bill: (a) care is safe, (b) joint liability for practice exists, (c) liability occurs through respective board sanctions and accepted practice guidelines (malpractice). 9. The rule sets the foundation for the future, not tomorrow. 10. The rule allows for the development of model practice situations. 11. Micro management language must be avoided. 12. May be multiple collaborative partners. 13. Modeling needs to occur to facilitate the intent of HB564.	marketing material of a service or site where an APN sees patients should post and clearly state the individual is not a physician, the individual's unabbreviated title and name, and the address and telephone number of the collaborating physician. 3. Notification of termination of supervision of an APN shall mean the primary collaborating physician shall notify the APN in writing, if he/she wishes to terminate the supervision of the APN or the collaborative practice agreement. 4. The Board of Healing Arts may cause a complaint to be filed against a physician in a collaborative practice arrangement with an APN for delegating professional responsibilities to a person who is not qualified by training, skill, competency, age, experience or license to perform them. 5. A physician shall not enter into a collaborative practice with more than two nurses.

APN, advanced practice nurse; CQI, continuing quality initiative.

Appendix 11-2. Summary of Meetings held December 10, 1993 to August 15, 1994

Date(s)	Geographic Areas to be Covered	Methods of Treatment	Review of Services	General Discussion
December 10, 1993	Advanced practice nurses (APNs) who perform delegated medical acts in remote practice sites shall be limited to medically underserved areas. An APN shall not perform delegated medical acts during periods of time when a collaborating physician is unavailable. The collaborating physician(s) shall be available for consultation as needed and shall be immediately available to the APN either personally or via telecommunication at all times, i.e., 24 hours a day, 7 days a week. A physician shall not enter into a collaborative practice with more then two nurses.	When off-site care is provided, transportation and backup procedures for immediate handling of patients needing emergency care and care beyond the APN's scope of practice must be established. The collaborating physician must have hospital privileges at a hospital in the state of Missouri. The collaborating physician shall not, at any time, be more than 50 road miles by the most direct route from the remote site location. No collaborating physician shall permit an APN to delegate medical acts to other APNs or PAs (Physician Assistants) in lieu of a collaborating physician. The collaborating physician must	The APN and collaborating physician shall have established a collaborating working agreement for a minimum of 6 months so defined by practice agreements prior to working in a remote location. The collaborating physician must exercise oversight, direction, and control of the advanced practice nurse. It is the shared responsibility of the collaborating physician and APN to direct and review the work, records, and practice on a continuing basis to ensure that appropriate directions are given and understood and that appropriate treatment is rendered. Protocols or practice guidelines must be developed by the	Operating from a document prepared by the Missouri Association of Osteopathic Physicians (MAOPS) presented by the Board of Healing Arts, discussion centered around definitions of *physician, advanced practice nurse, protocol or practice agreement, remote practice site, primary collaborating physician, secondary collaborating physician,* and *collaboration.* Although only three definitions would eventually be included in the rule (advanced practice nurse, collaborative practice arrangements, and registered professional nurse), this dialogue established terminology for use throughout the rule-making process. The introduction of the MAOPS document with its very restrictive language regarding the role of the

(continued)

Appendix 11-2. Summary of Meetings held December 10, 1993 to August 15, 1994 (*continued*)

Date(s)	Geographic Areas to be Covered	Methods of Treatment	Review of Services	General Discussion
	The collaborating physician shall see every patient at least annually or every third visit, if the third visit is within a 12-month period or if there is a change in the patient's condition or symptoms.	provide direction to the APN to specify what delegated medical acts should be provided. These directions may take the form of written protocols, oral communication, in person, by telephone or by other means of electronic communication.	collaborating physician and the APN to include guidelines describing and delineating the delegated medical acts. Protocols and practice guidelines should be specific in their guidance. The collaborating physician and APN must annually review and renew protocols or practice guidelines to ensure they are current in regard to the collaborating partner's scope of practice, the range of medical acts delegated by the physician, and the evolving standards of practice.	APN in a collaborative practice arrangement set the stage for a series of meetings in which extensive discussion occurred about the maintaining, rewording or deleting of pieces of the document.
January 4, 1994 January 20, 1994 February 7, 1994	The collaborating physician, or physician as designated in the collaborative practice arrangement shall be available for immediate consultation to the APN at all times, either personally or via	Methods of treatment selected and used by both parties shall be consistent with the scopes of practice of both collaborating professionals. Transportation and referral procedures for patients needing emergency care shall be	The collaborative practice arrangement shall specify a period of time during which the collaborating physician and APN shall practice together in one site prior to their practicing in geographically separate	Agreement had been reached on several contentious points; however, disagreement remained on several other points. Word was received from the governor's office to the various task forces that agreement in a timely manner

(continued)

telecommunication.

Sites where the physician is not present shall be within 50 road miles of the site where the collaborating physician is located unless the remote site where the nurse provides services is within a health profession shortage ara as defined by federal regulations under 42 U.S.C. section 254 or its successor.

established. The collaborating physician shall have hospital privileges (active, provisional, associate, courtesy) at a hospital in the state of Missouri or a border state.

The methods of treatment specified for registered professional nurses and APNs in a collaborative practice arrangement shall not be delegated to any other person except to a person qualified by Chapter 335 to accept such delegation if provided for in the collaborative practice arrangement and, except as provided in sections 338.095 and 338.198 RSMo, for the communication of prescription drug orders to a pharmacist.

locations.

The collaborating physician shall maintain accountability for authority granted in the collaborative practice arrangement. The collaborating professionals share responsibility for the collaborative practice.

It is the shared responsibility of the collaborating physician and APN whether engaged in single or multiple collaborative practice arrangements, to direct and review the work, records, and practice at least once every 2 weeks. At least once per month the physician shall conduct this review on site and shall be available for patient care during this review. This systematic review of services shall include but not necessarily be limited to: 1. the process of review which shall be on file and maintained in the collaborative practice setting, and 2. the collaborating professionals' determination

was expected. The Chief Counsel from the Governor's Office distributed a document containing proposed language to be considered addressing the concerns of the Department of Health regarding language in the draft document that could be interpreted to hinder its delivery of services. Members of the Missouri legislature addressed the board members, alluding to the fact that the budgets of the respective boards were controlled by the legislature and the legislature had a vested interest in a timely conclusion to the rule-making process.

Appendix 11–2. Summary of Meetings held December 10, 1993 to August 15, 1994 *(continued)*

Date(s)	Geographic Areas to be Covered	Methods of Treatment	Review of Services	General Discussion
			of the scope and detail of review based on the type of practice.	Concern by the Board of Healing Arts to "tighten" up the language regarding the registered nurse provided the opportunity to negotiate less restrictive language in the geographic area and review of services area.
February 17, 1994	The Board of Nursing expressed concern over the geographic area 50 mile restriction.	The Board of Healing Arts expressed concern over language dealing with the registered nurse.	The Board of Nursing expressed concern over the once a month review of services requirement language.	
February 28, 1994	The collaborating physician in a collaborative practice arrangement shall not be so geographically distanced from the APN or registered professional nurse as to create an impediment to effective collaboration in patient care or adequate review of services.	Prior to entering into a collaborative practice arrangement, the physician shall inform himself or herself as to the level of skill, training, and competence of the APN or registered professional nurse with whom the physician will be collaborating. The collaborative practice arrangement between a collaborating physician and an APN or registered professional nurse shall be within the scope of practice of the APN or registered professional nurse and consistent with the nurse's skill, training, and competence.	It is the responsibility of the collaborating professionals to determine a specified period of time during which the collaborating physician and APN shall practice together in one site prior to their practicing in geographically separate locations.	Although individual members of each task force were not entirely pleased with the agreed-upon language, each member was convinced that the language in the document on this date was the least restrictive language that could be agreed upon by all the boards. At this time, a series of meetings occurred with the Board of Pharmacy regarding finalization of the dispensing or distribution of medicines language.

Appendix 11-3. Summary of Meetings Between Nursing and Pharmacy

Date	Proposed Language	General Discussion
December 10, 1993	Nursing proposed that there be no language associated with prescribing. Medicine proposed: 1. The prescription shall include the name, address, and telephone number of the advanced practical nurse (APN) and that of the collaborating physician. 2. Prior to authority to prescribe, a standard medical pharmacology course shall be completed and successfully passed by the APN. 3. Protocols or guidelines for medications that can be used for patients by an APN shall be clearly written in the protocols or standing orders indicating follow-up care, dosage, quantity, and the number of refills, etc. 4. An APN shall not, under any circumstances, order controlled substances. An order for controlled substances must be initiated and written by the collaborating physician. The APN can dispense or administer controlled substances only after an order from the collaborating physician.	Prescribing and its associated acts were not considered in this initial discussion nor in subsequent meetings with the Board of Healing Arts (Medicine) who elected to defer to the Board of Pharmacy in this area. Discussions occurred peripherally between the Board of Nursing and the Board of Pharmacy over the course of meetings with the Board of Healing Arts (Medicine). Six meetings or conference calls took place between February 7, 1994 and August 15, 1994 between the Board of Nursing and the Board of Pharmacy specifically to determine language for the rule.
February 7, 1994	The prescription shall conform with present state laws and shall include the name, address, and telephone number of the APN and that of the collaborating physician. An APN shall not, under any circumstances, prescribe controlled substances. The dispensing or administration of a controlled substance by a collaborating nurse within the collaborative practice arrangement, shall be under the direction and supervision of the collaborating physician or physician designated within the collaborative practice arrangement and shall occur only on a case-by-case determination of patient needs and only after verbal consultation with the collaborating physician or physician designee. The required consultation and the physician's directions for the dispensing or administration of the controlled substance shall be recorded in the patient's chart and in the appropriate log by the collaborating nurse and shall be cosigned by the collabo-	Early language proposed by the Board of Pharmacy focused on controlled substances. The Board of Nursing contended that language in the original bill specifically stated that the APN shall not prescribe controlled substances, and additional language in the rule was unnecessary.

(continued)

367

Appendix 11-3. Summary of Meetings Between Nursing and Pharmacy *(continued)*

Date	Proposed Language	General Discussion
February 17, 1994	rating physician. Any dispensing or administration of controlled substances shall be in accordance with state and federal drug laws, rules, and regulations. A registered professional nurse may administer or dispense drugs and an APN may administer, dispense, or prescribe drugs, and the collaborative practice arrangement shall set forth the nature and scope of such activities. Where registered professional nurses or APNs are to dispense prescription medications pursuant to a collaborative practice arrangement, the following rules shall apply: 1. The amount of medication to be dispensed per prescription may not exceed one course for acute illnesses and "appropriate starter" supplies for maintenance of chronic illnesses. 2. Sites in which nurses receive drugs directly from drug distributors must be registered by the Board of Pharmacy and will be subject to periodic inspection. 3. A physician who is in a collaborative practice arrangement and supplies drugs to a nurse in the collaborative practice arrangement for the purposes of dispensing and whose inventory of transferred drugs exceeds lawful thresholds must be licensed as a drug distributor. In this event, no other registration by the Board of Pharmacy will be required of the nurse who is in the collaborative practice arrangement. 4. All state and federal laws concerning distribution and control shall be followed. 5. If a pharmacy is located within 15 miles of a practitioner, then no dispensing shall occur except for appropriate starter doses, emergency quantities, or samples. 6. All labeling requirements shall be followed.	Attention was now being directed to the role of the registered nurse as well as the role of the APN in dispensing. This is evident in the prescriptive language introduced by the Board of Pharmacy directed toward restricting the dispensing activities of both the registered nurse and the APN. Although this language was introduced and included in working documents of the draft rule, earnest discussions between the Board of Nursing task force members and the Board of Pharmacy task force members had not yet occurred. The Board of Nursing was fully aware of the activities authorized by the original bill regarding the registered nurse and was as reluctant to introduce language regulating the registered nurse's dispensing role as with the APN's dispensing role. Although the Board of Nursing was very much concerned about the limits imposed in this language, its

7. The types of medications to be dispensed by a nurse in a collaborative practice arrangement must be consistent with the scope of practice of the nurse.

8. Consumer product safety laws and Class B container standards shall be followed when packaging drugs for distribution.

9. Retrievable dispensing logs shall be maintained and a separate log kept for controlled substance dispensing. These logs shall include the following information:

   a. patient and drug identity
   b. sequential number
   c. date of dispensing
   d. manufacturer and lot number
   e. amounts dispensed
   f. directions for use
   g. daily signature of the dispensing nurse

10. All drugs shall be stored according to U.S.P. recommended conditions.

11. Outdated drugs shall be separated from the active inventory.

12. The name, address, and telephone number of the collaborating physician and advanced practice nurse shall be on a prescription.

The prescription shall conform with present state laws and shall include the name, address, and telephone number of the APN and that of the collaborating physician.

immediate attention was directed toward finalizing contentious language with the Board of Healing Arts (Medicine). The Board of Healing Arts (Medicine) had elected to remove itself from the one-on-one discussions about prescribing language and had gone on record stating it would approve language that had been approved by the Board of Pharmacy.

March 16, 1994

1. Medications may be provided without any restrictions on quantity to patients where the drugs are provided without charge or at or below wholesale cost.

2. An APN or registered professional nurse who engages in the retail sale of drugs at retail prices whose quantity exceeds 10% of the total dispensing log shall register their location with the Board of Pharmacy and shall be subject to inspection in accordance with Section 338.150 RSMo.

This language was proposed by the Board of Pharmacy to address the concerns expressed by the Board of Nursing on items #1 and #2.

(continued)

Appendix 11-3. Summary of Meetings Between Nursing and Pharmacy (continued)

Date	Proposed Language	General Discussion
March 30 1994	Items in which a change was proposed: 1. Medications may be provided without any restrictions on quantity to patients so long as appropriate in situations in which drugs are provided without charge or below prevailing market rate. The prevailing market rate shall mean the average retail price of the three nearest pharmacies. 2. An APN or registered professional nurse in a collaborative practice arrangement who engages in the retail sale of drugs at prevailing market rates whose quantity exceeds 20% of the total prescriptions entered in the dispensing logs shall register their location with the Missouri Board of Pharmacy and shall be subject to inspection in accordance with section 388.150 RSMo. Item #5 was deleted. The following item was added as #6: 6. The types of medications to be dispensed by a nurse in a collaborative practice arrangement must be consistent with the scope of practice of the nurse. An APN may delegate to a trained health care worker under his or her supervision authority to provide prepackaged prescription medications provided that such delegation is provided for in the collaborative practice arrangement and such medications are dispensed only to current patients with an existing prescription.	The Board of Nursing had concerns about the dispensing of "routine" medications such as prenatal vitamins or oral contraceptives and the effect earlier language would have on the ability of family practice and community sites to continue to allow clients to pick up their prescriptions on site for these types of medications. The Board of Pharmacy introduced language it believed would address this concern but was reluctant to change the focus of language already introduced.
June 6, 1994	Items in which a change was proposed: 1. Medications may be provided to patients so long as appropriate without registration in its	The first two items continued to be at the center of the dialogue between the two boards. The Board of Pharmacy was steadfast in its

with the Missouri Board of Pharmacy in situations in which the drugs are provided without charge or at or below cost.

2. An APN or registered professional nurse in a collaborative practice arrangement who receives funding from (titled monies) need not register their location with the Missouri Board of Pharmacy. Sites in which advanced practice nurses or registered professional nurses receive drugs directly from drug distributors must register their location with the Missouri Board of Pharmacy and shall be subject to inspection in with section 388.150 RSMo.

intent to retain highly regulatory language. The Board of Nursing continued to strive to have restrictions eased.

August 15, 1994

1. All sites where advanced practice nurses or registered professional nurses receive drugs directly from drug distributors must have their location registered with the Missouri Board of Pharmacy and shall be subject to periodic inspection in accordance with section 338.150 RSMo except as provided in paragraph (2)(G)2.

   A. Any and all information received by the Missouri Board of Pharmacy through inspections, including inspection reports, shall be forwarded to the Missouri State Board of Nursing for its review and disciplinary action if deemed appropriate by the Missouri State Board of Nursing.

   B. Missouri Board of Pharmacy and Missouri State Board of Nursing shall develop operational guidelines to form the basis of inspections by the Missouri Board of Pharmacy.

2. A physician who is in a collaborative practice arrangement and supplied drugs to a nurse in the collaborative practice arrangement for the purposes of dispensing, where the amount of transferred drugs exceeds lawful thresholds, must be licensed as a drug distributor. In this event, no other registration with the Missouri Board of Pharmacy will be required of the nurse who is in the collaborative practice arrangement.

This language, along with the consistent pieces from earlier discussions, was finally agreed upon, incorporated into the final draft rule and submitted to the appropriate body for processing through the rule making process. The rule was published in the *Missouri Register* on January 2, 1995 and on January 17, 1995. A 30-day comment period followed. Hearings were then held throughout the state. Comments and testimonial statements were reviewed in April of 1995. The final order of rule making was submitted to the Joint Committee on Administrative Rules on May 19, 1995. The rule was suspended on June 16, 1995 by the Joint Committee on Administrative Rules and withdrawn by the Boards of Nursing and Healing Arts (Medicine) on June 21, 1995.

(continued)

Appendix 11-3. Summary of Meetings Between Nursing and Pharmacy *(continued)*

Date	Proposed Language	General Discussion
October 30, 1995	1. The physician retains the responsibility for ensuring the appropriate administering, dispensing, prescribing, and control of drugs utilized pursuant to a collaborative practice arrangement in accordance with all state and federal statutes, rules, or regulations. 2. All labeling requirements shall be followed. 3. Consumer product safety laws and Class B container standards shall be followed when packaging drugs for distribution. 4. All drugs shall be stored according to the United States Pharmacopeia (USP) recommended conditions. 5. Outdated drugs shall be separated from the active inventory. 6. Retrievable dispensing logs shall be maintained for all prescription drugs dispensed and shall include all information required by state and federal statutes, rules, or regulations. 7. All prescriptions shall conform to all applicable state and federal statutes, rules, or regulations and shall include the name, address, and telephone number of the collaborating physician and collaborating APN. 8. An APN shall not, under any circumstances, prescribe controlled substances. The administering or dispensing of a controlled substance by a registered professional nurse or APN in a collaborative practice arrangement shall be accomplished only under the directions and supervision of the collaborating physician or other physician designated in the collaborative practice arrangement and shall only occur on a case-by-case determination of the patient's needs following verbal consultation between the collaborating physician and collaborating nurse. The required consultation and the physician's directions for the administering or dispensing of	New language was proposed to incorporate the recommendations of the Joint Committee on Administrative Rules and comments received after publication of the proposed rule in the *Missouri Register* on March 1, 1996. On April 26, 1996, the Boards of Nursing, Healing Arts (Medicine), and Pharmacy met to review and discuss comments received during the comment period. The final order of rule making was once again submitted to the Committee on Administrative Rules on May 27, 1996. The Joint Committee on Administrative Rules supported the final order of rule making and the rule was filed with the Secretary of State's Office.

controlled substances shall be recorded in the patient's chart and in the appropriate dispensing log. These recordings shall be made by the collaborating nurse and shall be cosigned by the collaborating physician following a review of the records.

9. An APN or registered professional nurse in a collaborative practice arrangement may only dispense starter doses of medication to cover a period of time for 72 hours or less. The dispensing of drug samples is permitted as appropriate to complete drug therapy.

10. The medications to be administered, dispensed, or prescribed by a collaborating nurse in a collaborative practice arrangement shall be consistent with the education, training, competence, and scopes of practice of both collaborating professionals.

Final Order Items added:

A registered professional nurse shall not, under any circumstances, prescribe drugs.

Item 9 was refined to read:

An APN or registered professional nurse in a collaborative practice arrangement may only dispense starter doses of medication to cover a period of time for 72 hours or less with the exception of Title X family planning providers or publicly funded clinics in community health settings that dispense medications free of charge. The dispensing of drug samples is permitted as appropriate to complete drug therapy.

Item 10 was refined to read:

The medications to be administered, dispensed, or prescribed by a collaborating registered professional nurse or APN in a collaborative practice arrangement shall be consistent with the education, training, competence, and scopes of practice of the collaborating physician and collaborating registered professional nurse or APN.

The final order carefully and precisely describes the roles of the registered nurse and the APN in the dispensing of medications.

International Collaboration

International Collaboration: Principles and Challenges $\boxed{12}$

Afaf Ibrahim Meleis
Genevieve Gray

INTRODUCTION

Achieving effective collaboration with one's peers in the international sphere is both a challenge and a rewarding experience. This chapter focuses upon international collaboration between nurses. Discussed are some of the key infrastructure supports that have facilitated effective international collaboration, the types or models of collaboration that are in place, and the strategies for fostering international collaboration. A great deal of the information provided emerges from the authors' personal experiences as international collaborators. Finally, principles for enhancing effective collaboration at the global level are proposed.

It is important to emphasize from the outset that there are many benefits to be accrued for the collaborators in any collaborative relationship. There is, however, a downside that must be recognized and planned for. It includes the burden of international travel, the investment of time necessary to maintain relationships, and of course the extensive resources required, including financial resources. In the authors' view, the rewards clearly outweigh the "costs" and include networking opportunities, opportunities for joint research and publication, and friendships that can prove both enduring and enriching.

WHY INTERNATIONAL COLLABORATION?

National events and even local events have ripple effects around the globe. Events in one corner of the world profoundly influence other regions of the world. Advanced modes of communication are instrumental in making local issues more universal and global. Universal issues require shared solutions, and shared solutions require collaborative approaches. Collaboration becomes ever more imperative as natural, economic, and human resources become scarce in one or another corner of the globe. Although access to computer networks, fax machines, and telephone conferencing is increasing, there are trends worldwide toward decreasing research budgets and downsizing health care systems. How to increase access to health care, how to provide culturally competent care, how to help marginalized populations become and remain healthy, how to support people while achieving organizational transitions, and how to support people's strategies for living with disease symptoms or disabling conditions are the type of important questions for which collaborative efforts may yield effective solutions and increase options. The solutions and the options are more likely to be productive and better reflective of population diversity if they evolve from different nations and different parts of the world and if they are shared and adapted in culturally sensitive ways. Internationalization of health care professions and disciplines is an issue of the 1990s and a major trend for the next decade.

Nurses have always been a significant force internationally. They comprise the highest numbers of workers in international health (Douglas and Meleis 1985). United States nurses are found in other countries in many settings. Examples include serving as members of health missions, as Peace Corps volunteers, and as health care providers in parishes. United States nurses may be sponsored by foundations, universities, church groups, or government, or they may be self-supporting. Countries that have limited human resources, such as Saudi Arabia, Kuwait, Brunei, and Hong Kong, import nurses from Egypt, India, Sri Lanka, and the Philippines. These same countries also export patients to institutions around the globe. Nurses are, therefore, often in a strategic position to initiate collaboration in answering shared clinical issues and in developing knowledge that reflects diversity in culture, ethnicity, religion, and language. Developing culturally sensitive knowledge requires collaboration between scholars from different nations. Utilizing such knowledge to enhance the quality of nursing care in different regions of the world calls for collaborative development, testing, and implementation of nursing therapeutics. Similarly, using models of education developed in different regions of the globe increases the educator's options. Collaborating in developing, evaluating or testing, and modifying models from different nations empowers educators to select and use the most advanced and culturally sensitive models.

COLLABORATIVE INTERNATIONAL NURSING CHALLENGES

The discipline of nursing and its mission and goals for enhancing health care of populations; for caring for people in their illnesses; and for supporting individuals, families, and communities during life and health transitions provide many opportunities for collaboration. Nurses may collaborate in developing models for patient care; models for education, strategic plans, and policies supportive of patient needs; and models for organizing systems of care. They may collaborate to test and evaluate these models. Collaborating nurses are challenged to develop and establish priorities for collaboration. International dialogue related to developing, deploying, and maintaining the valuable human nursing resource is needed. There is, however, a worldwide trend of encroachment on nurses' domain of knowledge and territory of practice. A united approach to developing guidelines for nurses' domain of practice may discourage the evolvement of other, less qualified clinicians to substitute for nurses and their expert practice. There is a universal and urgent need for answers about the most effective and productive models for the education of nurses, including for their advanced or graduate education.

Another universal nursing area of concern is the comparative socioeconomic status of nurses and patients and the impact of this socioeconomic status as well as cultural heritage on the type of care provided. Other concerns are that patients have access to health care and have quality of life. Models of care that are sensitive to diversity are needed worldwide and require the collaborative efforts of nurses.

Health care of vulnerable and marginalized populations represents another universal need for nursing knowledge development and practice. Issues related to women's health; to high morbidity and mortality of low income women; and to differences in the treatments of men and women, of the rich and the poor, and of central and the marginalized populations need to be discussed universally and require collaborative frameworks for solutions (Nelson et al. 1996).

Other models are needed for the development and testing of nursing therapeutics that are sensitive to alternative therapies and to local healers. Such models are more productive when options for health care are included that reflect the different regions and countries of the world.

INFRASTRUCTURE

Several organizations and activities are in place that support the development of collaborative efforts among nurses internationally. First, existing organizations provide opportunities for developing structures that allow the necessary dialogue. One example of such an organization is the World Health Organization (WHO), with headquarters in Geneva, Switzerland, whose role is to enhance the development of global solutions to shared issues. The WHO communicates with countries via a number of Chief Nurses in five world regions where a satellite WHO office exists; these are in the Middle East, Africa, the Americas, and Southeast Asia.

The International Council of Nurses (ICN), an organization that represents professional nursing organizations worldwide, offers another vital infrastructure reflecting the collaborative efforts of nurses. The International Congress of Nurses (the ICN's international meeting), which is organized every 4 years, provides many opportunities for international dialogue; for sharing educational, clinical, research, and organizational issues; and for identifying strategies for solutions. Collaborative efforts between nurses internationally, within the ICN, have resulted in the development of policy frameworks; for example, a universal ethical code for nurses; proposals for accrediting educational programs in nursing; guidelines for advancing nursing research internationally; a framework for transnational nurse regulation (Affara 1992) and, more recently, a proposal for a universal taxonomy for nursing diagnosis and intervention. Nurses use these frameworks to drive changes in policies in their respective countries or for the development or revision of policies within their continental or national organizations (Pratt 1995).

Sigma Theta Tau, nursing's International Honor Society, provides another important infrastructure for international collaboration. New chapters of Sigma Theta Tau are being established continually in different nations of the world. An international library, based at the headquarters of

Sigma Theta Tau in Indianapolis, Indiana, promises to be a catalyst for enhancing international collaboration. It is designed to facilitate access by nurses internationally to each other's research and publications. It is also designed to respond to the needs of nurses for international reviews of literature. Sigma Theta Tau's objectives for international scholarship reflect the increasing interest in American nursing toward internationalization.

Nurses in many corners of the world have recognized the significance of developing shared missions and shared approaches to actualizing these missions, and therefore, nurses are increasing their participation in international conferences. Although many U.S. conferences have always included international guests who sought opportunities to come in contact and dialogue with their U.S. colleagues, during the 1980s and 1990s there has been a phenomenal increase in the conferences that were intentionally labeled as "international." These conferences attracted more international guests, and in addition, the planning committees of these conferences deliberately invited international speakers to attract a more international conference audience. Countries other than the United States are also planning more regional and international conferences that attract presenters from different countries. The participants in these conferences better reflect the diversities within and between countries. Such events promote dialogue and sharing and make it easier for nurses representing different countries to network with each other. This, in turn, enhances collaboration.

Other forces also support and enhance international collaboration. While more accessible travel may have increased the gatherings of international colleagues, travel remains an expensive option for promoting collaboration. Travel can be tedious, requires funds, and necessitates taking time out of the already compacted lives of nurses. Recent increase in the use of electronic mail systems and of fax machines facilitates communication while decreasing the costs of time and money. Electronic mail facilitates and enhances dialogue, and as it becomes even more sophisticated and more accessible, exchanges between international colleagues will be even more possible, more rewarding, and less costly. For example, the planning of some international conferences has been accomplished through inviting nurses representing many countries to participate in brainstorming about the nature of the conference and the speakers to be invited. These international committees brainstorm, dialogue, identify goals, propose topics and speakers, and make decisions through consensus—all through electronic mail. In some instances, telephone conferences achieve similar goals; however, the time zone differences are a constraint for international telephone conferencing.

Recognition of the significance of collaboration in solving universal problems has prompted many institutions to develop supportive structures. Many such structures are evolving worldwide. The University of California Pacific Rim Research Program is one example. It was designed to increase the collaboration between the University of California (nine campuses) and colleagues from universities in the Pacific Rim region. Another similar structure is the Institute for Global Conflict and Collaboration housed at the University of California, San Diego, California. The goals of this institute are to bring together individuals from different disciplines, regions, and countries to identify problems and propose strategies to enhance peace and decrease political, economic, religious, and territorial conflicts. The premise upon which such programs are developed is that conflicts that are global can only be resolved through collaborative international dialogues, debates, and proposals and through international testing of the proposed solutions.

To stimulate intercountry collaboration, European countries have developed similar mechanisms. Among them are the European Research Group, which holds biannual meetings to identify common research areas and share research findings. It also provides opportunities to network and to develop collaborative alliances. Since both the collapse of the Soviet Union and the agreement between Western European countries to form the Economic Agreement, several initiatives have been instituted to enhance collaboration. Among these is the designation of funds to bring nurse educators, clinicians, and researchers together to discuss ways by which they can enhance the movement of nurses between the European countries to practice, teach, and do research. To achieve the goals of a common and collaborative Europe requires careful study of each other's systems, analysis of similarities and differences, and the fostering of common goals and strategies. Another major goal for the European Common Market Organization is to provide the necessary support for Eastern European professionals, including nurses, in their attempts to enhance their education and advance their practice.

These formal and informal structures are developed to provide frameworks pertinent to identifying universal issues and determining transnational solutions. Through them, international communication is fostered and collaboration is enhanced; however, barriers are present that have hampered international collaboration and threaten to continue to do so.

BARRIERS TO INTERNATIONAL COLLABORATION

Aside from the obvious barriers such as lack of knowledge of cultures or the limited proficiency in each other's languages, there are other more serious barriers. Research collaboration between members of a developed country and a developing country, for example, may be limited by the vast differences in the educational backgrounds of nurses and in the values surrounding research and science. Nurses' levels of preparation in research and of experience with data collection and data analysis may put some members of the collaborative team at a disadvantage. How research is viewed in one of the collaborating countries may also limit the type of designs proposed and used. Some researchers are trained in survey research or large sample research because this is the type of research that is valued in a particular country. When a research design is driven by the nature of the question and/or the power analysis for sample size calls for a qualitative design and/or for a small sample of research participants, the validity and significance of the research study may be viewed with suspicion in countries where science is defined very narrowly, meaning only using quantitative designs and large samples. The potential for collaboration may be severely limited or the integrity of the research project may be undermined to accommodate the scientific value system of the collaborating country.

The complexity of the institutional review board requirements and the demands for a consenting process that meets the expectations of the various boards (and their sponsoring organizations and nations) may also be another major deterrent to collaborative international research. Some review boards insist on written consent processes, whereas verbal consent may be the norm in some countries. When participants in research in a country are expected to participate for the first time in a consenting process imposed by an international review board or the review board of another nation, they may become suspicious of the intent and the refusal rate becomes disproportionately high. The collaborating member may become discouraged, and the whole effort is then aborted. Collaboration becomes more complicated when a U.S. board requires an approval letter from a collaborating international institution board when the latter such board does not exist. The collaborating team is left at a loss as to whom to seek approval from; ethical questions about the meaning of such approval may be too numerous to answer by the collaborating team and this may also abort the potential collaborative effort.

The development of collaborative educational models may also be impeded by the lack of knowledge of culture, of history, of education, of resources, and of the strategic plan of the country. Therefore, educational models may be dominated by the history and the resources of the United States or the United Kingdom, rather than being sensitive to the needs of a country at a particular historical moment.

Another major constraint to the development of international collaborative efforts is either the simple lack of availability of funds or the more complex lack of the knowledge of how to access designated funds. Many regions of the world are faced with decreasing budgets or downsizing of funds designated for enhancing collaboration; among them may be budgets for international travel or for support of international endeavors. Equally serious is nurses' lack of knowledge of available funds for initiating nurses' collaborative efforts. Many nurses in educational institutions around the globe are fairly new to the competitive processes for project funding. Unfortunately, as they are becoming more experienced in this competitive enterprise, the resources are becoming more limited. When new funding sources evolve, they are defined in ways that may appear on the surface to be less inviting to those interested in health care in general or to nursing's missions or goals in particular. The Pacific Rim grants at the University of California and the European Common Market funds in Western Europe are two such examples. The goals have now been redefined to include nurses' projects when nurses make application for resources for their proposed international collaborative projects.

Nurses who are interested in international collaborative efforts must realize that there are resources existing somewhere that are not well advertised. The challenge is to uncover them. Organized nursing must accept the challenge to make international resources more readily apparent to nurses, as well as to increase resources overall.

TYPES OR MODELS OF COLLABORATION

We propose three potential models for international collaboration. These are the formation of multipurpose partnerships among colleagues, limited-range collaborative projects, and sister institutions' alliances. Each is briefly discussed here.

Multipurpose Partnerships Among Colleagues

Multipurpose partnerships among colleagues offer multiple benefits to regions and nations and are becoming a common goal in institutional strategic plans. In western Sydney, Australia, for example, health care services and universities are cofunding positions of nurse academics. The aim of these positions is to bridge practice, research, and educational goals. These nurses have equal access to educational and service resources and are expected to enhance many strategic alliances between the institutions. When individuals in these prestigious positions (some are professors of nursing in clinical chairs) form collaborative relationships with international colleagues, other potential institutional alliances may be deliberately formed that could include a mix of practice, research, and education objectives. It is more likely that individuals in positions that seek to enhance connections between practice, education, and research will seek like-minded colleagues in similar positions internationally (Gray 1996).

The collaborative goals of these partners may be to develop or test culturally sensitive partnership models, to participate in the development of clinical knowledge, to enhance partnered educational strategies, or to provide complementary and supportive networks that could strengthen local partnerships (Greenwood 1996). An example is a project initiated by Professor Ingalil Hallburg from Kristianstadt, Sweden (personal communication, 1994). Supported by European Economic Market funds, the project included collaborators from Sweden, Northern Ireland, Spain, and the Republic of Ireland. The goals of the project included enhancing country-specific partners, as well as the potential formation of international partnerships. Educators, clinicians, researchers, and administrators from the four participating countries met in each participating country to discuss common topics of interest. They studied the situation of nursing in that particular country, they nurtured country-specific partnerships, and they supported the development of international collaborative projects.

Limited-Range Collaborations

Limited-range collaboration models are more project or issue specific. They are developed to meet the goals of, for example, a research project, an evaluation program, or a clinical program. These may be individually initiated and supported and bring together a team of international colleagues. Kathleen Dracup, for example, invited other colleagues from the United States, Australia, Taiwan, and Thailand to participate in a research project to study the delay in seeking treatment for diseases among women in the five participating countries (personal communication, 1996, 1997). Similarly, Meleis invited colleagues from Colombia, Brazil, Egypt, Mexico, and the United States to participate in a research project about women's abilities to integrate their roles and the strategies they use to maintain or promote their health. The collaborative efforts resulted in research studies conducted in each country and collaborative publications in international journals (Meleis and Bernal 1994, Meleis at Aly 1994, Meleis et al. 1994). The results have also been presented at a number of international conferences.

Other examples of collaborative projects from Australia include the conduct of specific education programs to facilitate nursing development in the host country (Gray and King 1993) and joint research into human caring between faculty at the Flinders University of South Australia and faculty at the Chulalangkom University of Bangkok, Thailand (A. Bartjes, Development in Western Samoa, personal communication, 1993).

Sister Institutions' Alliances

This third type of collaboration, of sister institutions' alliances, is broad in range and scope. It is, perhaps, modeled after the international sister city programs; it provides structures that facilitate collaboration. When institutions make commitments to an international institution to form an alliance, the speed by which decisions are made for joint collaborative effort is enhanced. Knowing about the sister institution is enhanced because of the long-term association that develops. Informal structures for decision-making are uncovered, together with traditional normative values, and this tends to facilitate future interactions and the joint recognition of the norms of reciprocity. Having the University of Alexandria as a sister university to the University of California, San Francisco, for example, increased the number of faculty who spent their sabbatical in each other's institution. The "sisterhood" facilitated the exchange of postdoctoral scholars, the collaborative supervision of dissertations, the initiation of collaborative research projects, the cosponsorship of conferences, and the further augmentation of sistership goals.

STRATEGIES FOR FOSTERING INTERNATIONAL COLLABORATION

Several strategies support the development of international collaborations; among them are establishing networks, nurturing established networks, and committing resources.

Establishing networks is a strategy to be considered and utilized deliberately or serendipitously. Colleagues for a particular collaborative effort or a project may be identified through the literature; during international conferences; or through selecting a special region, country, or institution and searching for the names of individuals within the particular area of interest. A deliberate process of finding a network of individuals with similar interest can then be systematically pursued. This process can be facilitated by computer searches, through Internet exploration, or through various modes of communication with other colleagues. For example, Professor Greenwood in western Sydney is seeking to establish an international network on "nurse thinking" through the Internet. Contacting interested individuals through the Internet and proposing collaborations could be a successful process in developing collaborative partnerships (Meleis 1994).

The potential for the serendipitous identification of individual colleagues to form collaborative partnerships and/or networks has not been fully explored. International conferences and exchanges and correspondences related to other goals and social activities may result in identifying potential colleagues, uncovering agreed-upon issues of concern, developing shared goals, outlining specific projects, or simply tabling the contact for future collaborations. Knowing and acknowledging that serendipitous contacts may result in future collaboration enhances awareness and support for seeking such contacts.

Establishing deliberate and serendipitous contacts and colleagues by itself does not lead to collaborative endeavors. Contacts and networks must be continually nurtured. Opportunities for collaboration with these newly formed contacts may not arise for a long while. In the meantime, supporting the relationship and its growth is important. This could be done by simply exchanging information, sharing new publications, identifying literature that is of mutual interest, or forwarding items of interest, or it may be more complex and take the form of having a prescribed plan for continual personal, collegial, or institutional contact. When an opportunity for collaboration arises, the nurtured contact then becomes an available resource for the collaboration. The preliminary work of knowing each other's values, interests, goals, resources, and context would have been already accomplished. Contacts that are not periodically nurtured are almost as unavailable for partnerships as nonestablished contacts.

Another essential strategy for fostering collaboration is the commitment of resources. Resources may be in the form of time, funds, literature, or opportunities for problem solving. To develop contacts or networks and/or to nurture them requires a commitment of energy and time, which are scarce commodities for women and for nurses. Such commitments may be particularly difficult for those individuals who may not be aware of the significance of contacts in fostering future collaborations, especially when that future is long-term rather than immediate. International collaborative efforts almost never yield short-term gains; nor is it immediately apparent which contact or network will be best suited for which collaborative goals. Therefore, a wider canvas of potential collaborators needs to be spread and colored, from which several small paintings may emerge.

Sister institutions need to have resources committed to encourage potential collaboration. Communication resources in the form of electronic mail, faxes, telephones, and regular mail expenses supported by both institutions are examples of commitment of resources. Resources for hosting international colleagues, for supporting travel, and/or exchanging reading material and publications are essential for fostering an international collaborative environment. Some of these may never materialize into collaboration—either short-term or long-term; however, they are imperative for the potential development of collaborative relationships that are more long-term.

PRINCIPLES OF EFFECTIVE COLLABORATION

A number of principles are essential for fostering effective international collaborations. Discussed here are the four most essential principles: mutuality, involvement, clarity, and reciprocity.

Mutuality

For collaboration to be effective, mutuality needs to be established and fostered. Mutuality is the principle of shared and agreed-upon assumptions and goals. It is ensuring that all the collaborative members have knowledge of the short-term and long-term goals for each participating member and their organization and that out of these diverse goals, there are some shared ones that drive the need for the collaboration. Mutuality supports the potential of more equivalence, which may then enhance a more effective and productive collaboration. Higher mutuality may also decrease the potential for developing dependent relationships in the collaborative team.

Involvement

The principle of involvement is to draw out and include all participants in the collaboration in all aspects of establishing, implementing, and/or finalizing the collaborative project. Effective and productive collaboration engages the energy, the time, and the resources of each collaborating partner in ways that reflect the abilities and the contractual agreements of each member (Sawyer et al. 1996). Involvement enhances equity in expenditure and in rewards. A collaborative research project may be proposed by one member; but to ensure cultural sensitivity and competence requires the active participation of all involved members in modifying all components of the research from the conceptualization of the question to the interpretation of the data. Lack of, or the limited involvement of, a collaborating member is likely to weaken the collaboration or render it less effective. For the collaborative effort to reflect the assumptions, the values, and/or the goals of each collaborating member requires the proactive participation of each member.

Clarity

We believe that clarity reflects a doctrine of precision in clarifying all components of the collaborative plan that we know may require a contracting and recontracting of expectations and goals. The less ambiguity there is in collaborative agreements, particularly in the early stages of collaboration, the more likely it is that collaboration will become more productive. Resentment will result from participating in international collaborative work that harvests neither acknowledgment nor rewards. Rewards may be more specific, such as coauthorship, or more general, such as invitations for other future collaborations, for visiting appointments, or for participation in conference planning, as well as other types of rewards. Discussion of collaboration must not shy away from dialogue about ownership of projects, periods of ownerships, collaborating in offshoot projects, authorship, and future and/or long term analyses and authorship.

Reciprocity

Reciprocity is the principle of give-and-take and of ensuring that the collaboration reflects a win–win situation for all collaborating members. The reciprocity is not exact in quantity or quality nor is it measured through short-term evaluations. An invitation to collaborate may be initiated by a person or an institution who is able to give more initially or for a while until the other collaborating member gets an opportunity to reciprocate. The nature and the amount of what is given may differ substantially from what is received at any one given moment, reflecting a different ability, resource, or approach. The extent to which the members in the collaborating team perceive give-and-take in the relationship will influence the level and the commitment of the members to the collaborative effort.

CONCLUSION

International collaboration is not an easy process, nor is it appropriate for everyone. It is time consuming and it requires patience, perseverance, and a vision for some tangible and intangible rewards. It allows for personal and institutional enrichment and growth that cannot be easily articulated or measured. Knowledge developed through collaborative efforts tends to reflect diversity of thoughts and of goals. As such, it is more congruent with the increasing population diversity that we experience in every corner of the world. Such knowledge becomes empowering to members of a discipline. Collaboration draws on the strengths of participating members, complements the weaknesses by the strengths of others, enhances knowledge of self and of one's own institution and country (Maglacas 1989a, 1989b; Meleis 1994). We tend to clarify goals, systems of operation, and values by comparing and contrasting ours with others' goals and values. Collaborative efforts between nations act as the catalyst to knowing and accepting our values and those of others. Complementarity in collaboration may also decrease the potential of repeating each other's mistakes.

Productive and credible international collaboration requires that special attention be paid to the principles of mutuality, involvement, clarity, and reciprocity. Actualizing these principles for each collaborative endeavor will enhance the potential for establishing coalitions and alliances that lead to effective collaborative projects and, indeed, may impact the quality of health professions education and of health care around the world.

References

Affara, F. (1992). Nursing regulation. Final Report Oja Worldwide project. *Bachelor of Nursing Program as a Contribution to Human Resources.* Geneva: International Council of Nurses.

Douglas, M. and Meleis, A. I. (1985). International Nursing: Challenges and consequences. *Mobius, 5*(3), 84–92.

Gray, G. (1996). Developing a research culture in Western Sydney. Conference abstracts. Second Academic Nursing International Conference, International Collaboration in Nursing: Working Together to Enhance Health Care, September 16–18, 1996, University of Kansas, Kansas City, Missouri.

Gray, G. and King, M. (1993). *The Planning and Implementation of an "In-Country" Bachelor of Nursing Program as a Contribution to Human Resources Development in Western Samoa.* Manila: World Health Organization.

Greenwood, J. (1996). Establishing an international network on nurse thinking. Conference abstracts. Second Academic Nursing International Conference, International Collaboration in Nursing: Working Together to Enhance Health Care, September 16–18, 1996, University of Kansas, Kansas City, Missouri.

Maglacas, A. M. (1989a). Health for all: Nursing's role. *Nursing Outlook, 36,* 66–71.

Maglacas, A. M. (1989b). Close encounters in international nursing: Impact on health policy and research. *Journal of Professional Nursing 5,* 304–314.

Meleis, A. I. (1994). Transcending national boundaries: Empowerment through international collaboration. In O. Strickland and D. Fishman. *Nursing Issues in the 1990's*. Delmar Publishing Inc., Albany, New York, pp. 544–555.

Meleis, A. I. and Aly, F. (1994). Women's health: A global perspective. In J. McCloskey and H. Grace (Eds.). *Current Issues in Nursing*, 4th ed. Mosby Year Book, St. Louis, 1992–1993, pp. 692–700.

Meleis, A. I. and Bernal, P. (1994). Domestic workers in Colombia as spouses: Security and servitude. *Holistic Nursing, 8*, 33–43.

Meleis, A. I., Arruda, E. N., Lane, S., and Bernal, P. (1994). Veiled, voluminous and devalued: Narrative stories about low income women from Brazil, Egypt and Colombia. *Advances in Nursing Science, 17*, 1–15.

Nelson, M., Proctor, S., Regev, H., Barnes, D., Sawyer, L., Messias, D., Yoder, L., and Meleis, A. I. (1996). The Cairo action plan. *Image: Journal of Nursing Scholarship, 28*:1:75–80.

Pratt, R. (1995). Controlling the profession's destiny. In: G. Gray and R. Pratt. *Issues in Australian Nursing*, vol. 4. Churchill Livingstone, Melbourne, pp. 3–5.

Sawyer, L., Regev, H., Proctor, S., Nelson, M., Messias, D., Barnes, D., and Meleis, A. I. (1996). Matching vs. cultural competence in research: A methodological note. *Research in Nursing and Health, 18*, 531–541.

International $\boxed{13}$
Collaboration:
The Strategic Key to
Building Healthy
Societies Throughout
the World

Patricia J. Blair

INTRODUCTION

Health care systems throughout the world are in transition. Health care providers struggle to redefine the essential components of health care required by the people within their systems in order to determine how these services can be provided in a manner that is cost-effective and has positive outcomes. Decreasing monetary support for human and material resources and increasingly complex problems in most nations and regions of the world provide the impetus for formation of new partnership coalitions.

In this time of international flux, it is necessary to create flexible, sustainable situations that balance three critical areas: access to care, quality of care, and cost-effectiveness of care. These three areas form the foundation that gives direction to the outcomes or results of health care programs. Each of the areas is dynamic and interactive with the other two.

393

To create workable health care systems, it is important to understand these variables, particularly as they occur in the context of regional and national cultures and social, economic, and political circumstances.

The literature indicates that one effective way of harnessing the dynamic interactions is to convene a coalition of stakeholders. Flower (1995) suggests that "if you bring the appropriate people together in constructive ways with good information, they will create an authentic vision and strategies for addressing the shared concerns of the organization and community" (p. 22).

For a health care system to be sustainable, it must achieve outcomes valued by all stakeholders. It must be rooted in the values, culture, and traditions of the community in which it is located. These principles are especially important when working with multiethnic groups, which may have extremely disparate community values and cultural norms. The coalition that seeks outcomes that address and balance the three critical health care areas of access, quality, and cost (as these are embedded in community values and culture) will likely achieve flexible, sustainable, and desired outcomes.

Definition of Coalition

For the purpose of this chapter, the author defines coalition as an alliance or union of stakeholders who share a vested interest in selected outcomes. Workable strategies to achieve the outcomes require a balance of access, quality, and cost. The outcomes as well as the strategies must be rooted in the values of the community, and the outcomes must serve the community interests, health, and welfare.

COALITION COMPONENTS NEEDED TO ASSURE SUCCESS

Stakeholder Inclusiveness

The coalition membership must include representatives of all organizations or groups who have a vested interest (stake) in the outcomes. The size or magnitude of the stake is not as important as the existence of the interest of the stakeholders and the good will generated by full participation. If some but not all of the stakeholders participate, those who do not participate will lack sufficient commitment to the coalition and may actually hinder the goals of the coalition. As time passes, the coalition likely will self-destruct.

Community Values

The community values ought to determine the meaning of health care access, quality, and cost as they are made operational by the community and its stakeholders. No matter how lofty the goals, the processes to achieve the goals must use the knowledge and skills of the people who will benefit from the outcomes. An unbalanced or unrealistic situation can be forced by an influx of money or by the imposition of high external standards (higher than are realistic for the community). In time, a project or coalition forced to accept such unrealistic conditions will burn itself out. Outcome goals relating to access, quality, and cost will only become tangible and achievable when embedded in community values and when the resources allocated to the coalition and its goals seem manageable to the stakeholders.

What are acceptable quality and access at a reasonable cost in rural Kentucky may not be acceptable quality and access in New York City. To a New Yorker, the Kentucky price might appear to be reasonable, but the quality and access purchased might not be acceptable. Paradoxically, and for example, the influx of large sums of money into a coalition in a poor community will likely lead to failure of the coalition in the long run, in part because participants have limited experience in handling big budgets. Also, they may not have resources available to them, even for a price. (A four-variable community values model is detailed later in this chapter.)

Partnership With Shared Decision-Making

In the 1950s, Deming introduced Japan to his management techniques of continuous quality improvement using the quality circle. In his manufacturing principles, the purpose of circular thinking and acting was to improve the quality of products continuously. His thesis is that the quality of a product or outcome is determined by the processes that are used to make the product or outcome and that all participants in the processes, even the most humble, impact the processes and, therefore, the quality of the product. To improve the product, therefore, all must participate (Deming 1982, Neaves 1990). His ideas revolutionized Japanese management and changed the world.

Coalition building in health care also must be composed of inclusive circles that are open to all participants who are already involved in, or have a stake in, services or outcomes. The process of coalition formation and conduct is time consuming, particularly that needed to involve all the stakeholders in any process. Once the stakeholders are all committed to the process, however, the results likely will be lasting.

Trust Development

Participants begin the process of coalition formation without trusting the others. As time passes, however, the development of trust is key to stakeholders' remaining involved and to the success of the coalition. The participants will earn each other's trust by being fair and open, and consistent and dependable. They also must demonstrate to each other their ability to transcend their own agenda and work toward the goals of the coalition. The investments of time and frequent interaction are prerequisite for building trust.

THREE AREAS OF FOCUS OF PROVED EFFECTIVE INTERNATIONAL COLLABORATION

International coalitions of organizations among nations have effectively addressed myriad policy, education, and research issues that transcend national borders. Effective coalitions may be regional, such as with the European common market community; hemispheric, such as with the Pan American Health Organization (PAHO); or worldwide, such as in the United Nations International Children's Emergency Fund (UNICEF) and the World Health Organization (WHO).

Three areas of focus can be used to categorize types of international coalitions. These are useful for increasing understanding of processes needed and strategies that may prove successful for coalition formation, conduct, and evaluation. Coalitions may be formed to 1) set standards,

2) address a problem identified by a community, and 3) implement a standard set externally by experts.

Examples of Standard-Setting Programs

In the European region, national nursing associations of member European Community nations have, for example, formed a coalition in the form of committees and task forces to address areas of mutual concern such as establishing educational and regulatory requirements for international movement. PAHO, in a hemispheric example of coalition conduct, holds annual meetings of surgeons practicing in nations within the hemisphere to exchange information on areas of mutual interest, such as the latest surgical techniques. WHO, in a worldwide example, has developed global pediatric immunization standards and has committed much of its resources and creative energy to their achievement.

Problem Identification by a Community-Based Coalition

In many parts of the world, community-wide and nationwide organizations (governmental and nongovernmental, private for-profit and not-for-profit) are forming coalitions within and across countries to address complex problems that individual organizations lack the expertise to resolve, the funding to implement, and the knowledge to evaluate credibly.

For example, the state of Oregon in the United States developed and implemented a community values health project using a community-based, multidisciplinary discussion and consensus-building process. This process was led by a coalition formed to establish priority rankings for health procedures and treatment to be covered by state Medicaid funding. More than 20,000 hours of discussion involved all stakeholders identified by the coalition members, as well as those who were self-identified. The diverse stakeholders included physicians, nurses, administrators, insurers, bioethicists, patients (consumers), educators, journalists, clergy, professional organizers, labor group representatives, and politicians (Fry 1994; J. Kitzhaber, personal communications from the former President of the Oregon Senate, and current Governor of Oregon, 1990, 1992, and 1995; Kitzhaber 1990; Thorne 1992).

The outcome of the process was a rank-order listing of medical procedures and treatment priorities. The estimated funds were then distributed theoretically along the list of priorities in accordance with the numbers estimated to be needing the procedures or treatments. The hypothetical funds ran out when the 486th procedure was reached. The first priority identified by the citizen coalition was child and maternal health. High-cost, high-risk procedures such as heart transplants were not included in the Oregon coalition's list of priority procedures. This model has subsequently been implemented amid much national publicity.

Standard Setting by External Experts

In another approach, national or international experts may set a standard for actions or services to be conducted locally, such as immunization of children. The standard is adopted with or without modification and then implemented by community-based coalitions formed for the purpose of meeting the standard. For example, a no-smoking policy was adopted at the San Jose airport in 1993 after a local coalition formed to mobilize support for the worldwide standard. The coalition included all the stakeholder governmental and nongovernmental and health professional groups.

The availability of a recognized international standard facilitated the introduction of the idea, the formation of a common vision, and the rapid implementation of the idea. Although helpful, the standard alone would not have resulted in a smoke-free airport. The implementation step required the local coalition to bring credibility and urgency to the standard. In addition, the local coalition had to adopt or internalize the standard as its own.

THREE CASE STUDIES OF INTERNATIONAL COALITION FORMATION AND CONDUCT

Three case studies are selected for presentation using the perspective of the three areas of focus—community-defined standard, community-identified problem, and externally imposed standard. In addition, each case is selected to represent one of three economic positions in the world as defined by international economists and policymakers. These are developed, developing, and in transition. These variables are interrelated in the description and analysis of each case. Finally, the variables outlined in Sullivan's model of coalition formation and conduct (see Chapter 9 for a comprehensive presentation and see Table 13-1 in this chapter for a listing and definition of variables) and a model of community values (see Figure 13-1), which is presented later in this chapter, are used as analytic tools to analyze each case and make judgments regarding the effectiveness of each of the coalitions.

Nations as Developed, Developing, or in Transition

There are 206 nations that report their economic status. Health care coalition design and conduct from an international perspective must take into account the membership characteristics of the stakeholders and the areas of focus as already outlined and described. In addition, the nation or nations forming the coalition must also be understood economically. The categorizations of developed, developing, and in transition help this understanding enormously. With respect to economic status, countries

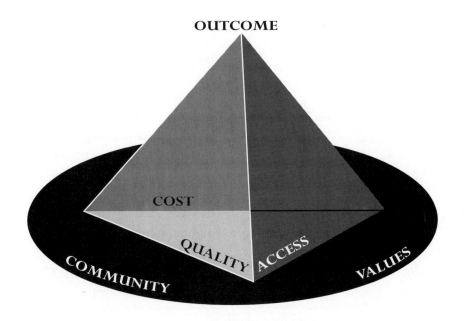

Figure 13-1. *A model of community values.*

Table 13-1. Sullivan's Coalition Model Components*

1. Purpose or reason	1. Opportunity or threat present, along with belief that joining together will be effective response
2. Impetus for action	2. Catalyst or trigger prompts immediate action
3. Membership	3. Those belonging to the coalition; may be diverse or same in their mission and goals; may be professional, grass roots, or a combination of both
4. Patterns of formation	4. The voluntariness of joining a coalition; ranges from freely and equally agreeing to join with others (level I) to induced conflict by an external authority mandating joining (level V)
5. Power-sharing partnership (trust)	5. Relationship that develops between members; preferably one of sharing, openness, honesty, familiarity, and trust
6. Structure of the coalition	6. Formation variables (1 to 5 above), organizational arrangements, and goals and outcomes sought
7. Level of collaboration	7. Focus on functions and tasks including joint planning, joint working, and joint management
8. Outcomes sought	8. Occur at three levels: one star (lowest), achieve goals of coalition; two stars (middle), members commit to needs and interests of the coalition and society; three stars (highest), members develop a true and lasting partnership

*For further discussion, please see Chapter 9.

may be considered on a continuum of high and growing economy (developed), a low or slowly increasing economy (developing), and a moderate, collapsing, or rebuilding (in transition) economy. Table 13-2 outlines selected variables of three exemplar nations in the three macroeconomic categories.

The developed countries are mainly in North America, Western Europe, and the Pacific Rim. The developing nations of the world are found in all regions of the world except North America and Western Europe. Three fourths of the world's nations are developing nations. The countries in transition are the nations of the former United Soviet Socialist Republic (Soviet Union). They are found in Eastern Europe. Because this third macroeconomic category is so new and the reader may not be familiar with the countries so categorized, and also because this author has done so much work with countries in transition, this category warrants some additional discussion. As well, the dichotomy of ancient cultures emerging in struggling new economic states (which describes the countries in transition) requires extraordinary skill, commitment, and sensitivity to establish effective coalitions.

Focus on Nations in Transition

Countries in transition were not recognized as such until 1991 and the collapse of the former Soviet Union, when 15 new nations emerged. The 15 newly independent states of the former Soviet Union are Armenia, Azerbaijan, Belarus, Estonia, Georgia, Latvia, Lithuania, Kazakhstan, Kyrghystan, Moldova, Tajikistan, Turkmenistan, Ukraine, Uzbekistan, and the Russian Federation. Each of these countries has a rich, ancient culture and proud heritage of language, the arts, and health care. Following the collapse in 1991, each of these nations found itself in a unique situation, with a worthless Soviet currency and an overbuilt system of Soviet-style health care. The Soviet health care system had emphasized the structure of medicine, with large numbers of physicians and large numbers of hospital beds, rather than access to care, health promotion and disease prevention, and a focus on positive outcomes of care.

During the 70 years of oppressive Soviet rule, one of the few positive social programs was the existence of a modest social safety net for the people of the Soviet Union. Lines were long and many hours each day were needed to acquire basic food supplies for a family. Both medications

Table 13-2. Socioeconomic Divisions of the Countries of the World*

	Developing (Sierra Leone)	In Transition (Republic of Georgia)	Developed (United States)
The Economy			
Gross national product (GNP), millions U.S. $	647	3071	6,387,686
GNP per capita, U.S. $	140	363	24,750
Inflation rate	72.3%	15%	3.5%
The People			
Population and Demography			
Area, km	71,740	69,700	9,363,563
Total population	4.7 million	5.4 million	266 million
Percent urban	32%	56%	75%
Population density, per km^2	62.9	149	75
Health Status			
Average Life Expentancy at Birth			
Overall years	43	72.6	77
Females	43	76.5	79.4
Males	44	68.9	72.7
Mortality			
Fertility rate (birth/woman)	6.5	2.2	2.1
Infant mortality per 1000 live births	135.6	17.8	8.3
Maternal mortality rate per 100,000 live births	Not available	39	7.8
Service Capacity			
Physicians per 10,000	.7	56.4	22.4
Nurses per 10,000	50[†]	103.9[†]	80[†]
Hospital beds per 10,000	30[‡]	98[‡]	33[‡]
Immunization Coverage	74%	36% in 1996 97% in 1991	84%
Literacy	21% 1 language	99% 2–4 languages	98% 1 language
Finance			
Health expenditure per capita, U.S. $	Not available	.81 (1994) 3.64 (1995)	3510 (1994)

*All statistical data is 1993 data unless noted otherwise.

[†]These nursing data do not capture the wide range of variability in who is labelled as nurse in these nations, or the wide range of education preparation.

[‡]These hospital bed data do not capture the degree of readiness of these hospitals to admit patients and manage their care to a reasonable quality standard.

Sources:
For Sierra Leone: *The Europa World Yearbook,* 1996, p. 2800; Rajewski, 1997; for Republic of Georgia: Johnson, 1997, p. 192; Tarkhan-Mouravi, 1996; for United States: Erhlich, 1996; Reddy, 1994, p. 974.

and health care were available without charge. Existence was possible: the price was constant vigilance and 24 hours a day of work to gain the basics for families.

This safety net vanished with the collapse of the Soviet Union. The 348 million citizens of the Soviet Union became citizens of 15 new nations. Although newly independent, many of these nations trace the history of their civilizations as far back as 3500 BC.

The rapid collapse of the Soviet economy and withdrawal of the Soviet Union from governance of these nations left the citizens of the new nations struggling to regain their footing (in most instances); these nations are experiencing unprecedented economic and social transitions. In many instances, the citizens have neither the material resources nor the skills needed to rebuild their countries. These nations represent a collapsed developed communist nation struggling to regain a measure of economic and political stability in a free-market environment. In addition to their characteristics common to developed countries (high literacy rate, low birth rate, high numbers of physicians per capita), they share many characteristics of undeveloped countries (high infant mortality, decreasing life expectancy). Moreover, the nations in transition share high rates of inflation and social chaos because of the absence of legal standards and absence of business acumen in a free-market environment.

Business is rudimentary at best. The systems of laws and business codes to govern business conduct are minimal or absent. Education curricula at all levels are in a state of change. In the communist world, the teachings of Lenin and Stalin were required at all levels. Although these nations now have the opportunity to develop new curricula, they lack the expertise and resources to do so.

Soviet-style health care, as previously described, dictated that big was good and bigger was best. Huge hospitals in a state of decay and unused beds are now frequently found attended by an oversupply of physicians and nurses. In the nation of Georgia, for example, there are more physicians and nurses per capita than in any other nation in the world. Although some of these health professionals are excellent, the educational process lacked rigorous clinical training or performance standards to guarantee well-educated health care professionals. Nursing education was particularly disadvantaged with the heavy focus on housekeeping-type tasks rather than clinical knowledge and skills. How to restructure education and training? How to introduce professional standards in a licensing and credentialing system? How to rebuild a health care system providing access, quality, and affordable health care to Georgians? These are the health care challenges Georgians are struggling to address.

Having reviewed the background of the countries in transition, we now can turn to the case studies. The developed countries are represented by the United States with its high and rapidly expanding economic growth pattern. The developing nations are represented by Sierra Leone, a West African nation with a low and only slowly increasing economy. The countries in transition are represented by the nation of Georgia with its collapsed and rebuilding economy.

Case Study No. 1

Summary: This is a case study set in a developed country, the United States, and concerns implementing an externally imposed standard. The immunization rate in Santa Clara County, California (Silicon Valley), in 1992 was less than 50% of children less than 2 years of age (author's knowledge). Standards set by WHO and the U.S. Standards for Pediatric Immunization Practice recommended by the National Vaccine Advisory Committee of the Centers for Disease Control and Prevention, approved by the U.S. Public Health Service, and endorsed by the American Academy of Pediatrics, call for 90% of all children less than 2 years of age in the United States to be immunized by the year 2000 (Peters 1997).

Reason for acting: The substandard rate for immunization of children less than 2 years of age was recognized by public health officials as an unacceptable rate.

Impetus for acting: The county health department identified the substandard situation with childhood immunization to myriad stakeholders in the community. The low level of immunization in one of the wealthiest and best educated counties in the nation was deemed unacceptable and demanded immediate action.

Membership: The coalition was formed by the county medical and hospital associations and by city and county public health officials and government officials by calling key stakeholders from government, public health, and the citizenry together to form a Steering Committee. This occurred as soon as immediate action was deemed necessary. The Steering Committee (of which the author was a member as Chair of the Board of Supervision of the Emergency Medical Care Commission) included health professionals who self-defined a large role and willingness to participate with pro bono (volunteer) investment of time and skills. These professionals included representatives of the Santa Clara County Health Department, Hospital Association, Medical Association, and Public Schools Association; several local nurses' associations; and the Santa Clara Emergency Physicians Association Medical Society. The Steering Committee also included key citizen stakeholders such as county-wide city managers and county supervisors, the mayor of San Jose, and the Emergency Medical Care Commission. In addition, political, religious, business, and media leaders in the many ethnic communities of Santa Clara County including Hispanic, Cambodian, Chinese, and Thai, and the mainstream media either joined or monitored the coalition closely. All were active participants in the ways in which they chose to be. Finally, Stanford University made available its mobile van for immunization in Hispanic communities with funding provided by a local television station.

Patterns of formation: As described in the membership section, the Hospital Association, the Medical Society, and the Emergency Medical Care Commission convened a broad-based group of stakeholders to address the problem. Initially, the Santa Clara County Health Department defined the problem. An Ad Hoc Task Force of the Steering Committee (appointed by the Steering Committee) developed a vision statement for the Steering Committee, which was approved by them at their fourth meeting. This level of voluntariness is level II. At this level, the coalition is initiated by one or more potential members, and other members freely agree to join. This is the second-most voluntary and presents the second easiest, and likely most common, way that members come together and join in coalition. It has a high likelihood of success in achieving coalition goals.

Power-sharing partnership (trust): This coalition was the second coalition this county had formed to address a community-wide problem. The first coalition comprised mainly 13 area hospitals with a traditionally competitive and often adversarial relationship. It achieved shared values and a common vision at the end of its work, but not at the start. Nevertheless, it did achieve its goals and facilitated the development of openness and trust from the start of this second coalition project. Also, this coalition began with a shared value for improving immunization rates and rapidly developed its shared vision.

Structure of the coalition: A Steering Committee structure using Ad Hoc Task Forces as deemed necessary provided a minimal, but functional, organizational arrangement. The Health Department provided much of the administrative and administrative support personnel and assistance. In addition, the patterns of formation of components already reported on, for example, membership, became part of the structure of the coalition. Various members of the coalition, such as the Hospital Association, accepted assignments and accountability for their accomplishment.

Level of collaboration: This coalition engaged in shared planning, work, and management. It was, therefore, a fully functioning coalition. The members of the Steering Committee and their respective organizations accepted their assignments and conducted the work accordingly. Steering Committee members assigned, and Health Department staff conducted, site visits on programs throughout the city and county to assess progress toward goal achievement and to seek and evaluate ideas for developing lasting model immunization programs. Reports and verbal presentations were provided by the Steering Committee at regular meetings of the committee in order to keep all members informed. In addition, the Steering Committee provided briefings to all community groups requesting them.

Outcome(s) sought: The short-term outcome was the design and funding of a program to bring Santa Clara County into compliance with the 2000 national standard of vaccinations for 90% of children less than 2 years of age. An intermediate goal was to develop model program sites to test coalition ideas. The long-term goal was to implement a sustainable countywide program to meet the 2000 goal and to sustain that level of immunizations thereafter.

The short and intermediate goals were met. Modest external funding was achieved to hire personnel for the health department to continue to monitor and evaluate model community programs. The members were able to act beyond their own agendas and address the common good. This coalition achieved a two stars outcome; time will permit an assessment to determine whether a lasting partnership has emerged (three stars).

Community values: This four-variable model considers the match between the goals or vision and the coalition members. The premise is that the closer the match, the higher the likelihood of commitment to the goals or vision and its accomplishment. The other three variables are the three critical elements to be balanced in any health care program—cost, access, and quality.

The Steering Committee formed rapidly because it perceived an unacceptable gap between the community value for high immunization rates and the surprising reality that over the years, inattention had allowed a situation unacceptable to the community to develop. The high national quality standard of 90% of all children less than 2 years of age to be immunized was matched by the community values for high-quality care.

One of the major contributions of the coalition was the establishment of conveniently located community access sites. Through the mainstream media and the smaller networks of ethnic media, the coalition was able to advertise locations, hours of services, charges, and transportation. It would have been cost-prohibitive and politically unfeasible for any one organization—even the Health Department—to do this single-handedly. The voluntary human resources and staff support of each of the coalition members significantly reduced the cost so that it was affordable. The influence of the many key stakeholders opened many community doors that would have otherwise remained closed.

The community-based model and coalition produced an unexpected bonus outcome. Infants newly born in Santa Clara County are now registered in a computer database, *Baby Calls*. The public health nurses use this information to call new mothers at 3-, 6-, and 9-month intervals to remind them of the upcoming need to have their babies immunized. The *Baby Calls* database was developed by the hospital and medical associations coalition members as their contribution to the immunization program's goals.

Conclusion: This example demonstrates that when the processes of forming and conducting a coalition are sensitively adhered to and when community values are in harmony with an issue, the marshaled resources of knowledge and skills, pro bono support, staff support, and media time can be mobilized. As long as it is embedded in community values and in accord with the stakeholders, an externally imposed standard can be implemented. Therefore, the Santa Clara County coalition had a very high likelihood of achieving its goals. The startup requires intensive commitment of time for planning, involving all stakeholders, responding to all members questions and needs to know, and developing the trusting power-sharing partnership. Once done, the potential for sustaining the project is built in and can be accomplished with minimal costs in time, money, and human resources.

Case Study No. 2

Summary: This case study is set in a developing country and concerns the imposition of an externally imposed standard. The immunization rate for children less than 2 years of age in the West African nation of Sierra Leone was 75% (The *Europa World Yearbook* 1996). This rate compared unfavorably with the international standard of 90% established by UNICEF. The Minister of Health of Sierra Leone, in collaboration with international private voluntary organizations (PVOs), decided to address the problem (The Europa World Yearbook 1996, Lisk 1996).

Reason for acting: The substandard rate of immunization for children under the age of 2 years was discovered and deemed unacceptable.

Impetus for acting: The Minister of Health of Sierra Leone identified the substandard situation. The UNICEF assisted the Minister and his department to gather and analyze data. The Minister was aware of the possibility of obtaining international assistance with improving the immunization rate and chose to seek that assistance.

Membership: The Minister of Health and his assigned staff and representatives of international PVOs formed the initial membership. Local PVOs were instructed to join the coalition, as were local village elders. The membership was composed, therefore, of government officials, international expert professionals, local expert professionals, and leading citizens. This configuration of members is broad-based and could form the basis of a successful coalition assuming the elements of *patterns of formation* and *power-sharing partnership* are managed sensitively.

Patterns of formation: The Minister of Health made the decision unilaterally to establish the coalition. He invited the international PVOs to join the coalition, and they agreed to do so. The local PVOs and the local elders were mandated to join the coalition. The goal of the coalition was already determined—90% immunization rates for children less than age 2 years—as was the membership. The level of voluntariness of joining the coalition for the local members was at level V.

Level V is the level of induced conflict. Some, or all, of the members are forced to join the coalition. They have had no say in the decision to establish the coalition; they might or might not agree with the coalition mission or goals. If the forced membership is in opposition to the goals, the likelihood of the coalition achieving its goals is minuscule. If the forced membership is merely indifferent to the goals, the coalition has a minimal chance to succeed.

Structure of the coalition: The variables already described are components of the coalition's structure. In addition, the organizational arrangements and the nature of the relationships among the members are major structural features, as are the goals and outcomes sought. The Minister of Health was in charge of this coalition. He set the goals, made the assignments, and determined the criteria for success. The international PVOs infused vaccines and cold-chain equipment into the nation. Initially, local PVOs could not identify or define a role for themselves in the coalition. Local community leaders began complaining that the citizens in their villages would not gain access to the immunizations. As local access and education of the citizens became a bigger and bigger issue, the local PVOs identified a role for themselves and they began to work in collaboration with the village elders. The Minister of Health, fortunately, began to realize the importance of involvement by all stakeholders. In the end, it was the credibility and support of the village leaders that saved the coalition and enabled it to meet its short-term goal.

Power-sharing partnership: The relationship began to develop into one of equality, sharing, and openness only when the top–down, authoritarian approach was threatening to destroy the project. Trust was earned very slowly by the village elders.

Level of collaboration: Joint planning did not occur until the project was well under way. Joint working was also retarded. Initially, the external experts were doing all the immunizations. The local villagers were not involved. Eventually, the international and local PVOs joined forces to educate the villagers to assist with immunizations. Joint management of the project did not begin until the project was threatened with failure. This project was an ambitious one, however, begun with excellent intentions and covering all components of project implementation.

Outcome(s) sought: The short-term goal of 90% immunizations has been met in the urban areas, but not in the rural areas thus far. The rural program was very decentralized by necessity and was cost-prohibitive until the resources of the local villagers were donated. Now that the village elders and villagers are involved in the planning and implementation, it is hoped that 90% of all children under the age of 2 years in the nation will be immunized by 2000.

Community values: Not all village elders understood the rationale for immunizing the preschool children. With time and education, the citizens came to value immunization. Only when the elders and the citizens valued immunization and their involvement was sought and respected, did they cooperate. The quality of care sought was high—a 90% immunization rate—but seemed reasonable given that the current rate in most places in the nation was a respectable 75%. Urban access was provided at local health department sites. Citizens were ordered to have their children vaccinated. In the rural settings, enforced participation proved to be cost-prohibitive and unwieldy. The education of the elders and their leadership in encouraging citizens to have their young children vaccinated at designated sites has begun to achieve the desired results. Despite the international PVOs supplying vaccinations, the project only became affordable when voluntary human resources and services by the coalition participants became available.

Conclusion: This case sharply demonstrates the importance of attention to coalition formation variables in order to develop a power-sharing partnership to engage in joint planning, implementation, and evaluation. This case also demonstrates the importance of community values being in harmony with externally imposed values. It was not until the elders and the local groups and citizens were included in the coalition's activities and they came to understand and value the goal of 90% immunization rates for their children that the coalition began to make acceptable progress toward its high goal.

Case Study No. 3

Summary: A nation in transition is selected for this case study. The coalition was built around the implementation of an externally imposed standard, again for immunizations. The nation is the Republic of Georgia of the former Soviet Union. Before 1991 and the collapse of the Soviet Union, the immunization rate in Georgia was a most impressive 97% (author's knowledge). After 1991 and the collapse of the public health system along with myriad other systems, immunizations became erratic, at best. Statistics are not kept in any reliable manner because of the difficult transformation from communism to democracy, so it is not possible to state a current immunization rate. In 1993, when this effort was under way, Georgia was very unstable politically and economically. As an example of this instability, there were four national Ministers of Health in 2 years.

Reason for acting: The rate of immunizations for children age 2 years was below the international standard of 90% (A. Jorbenadze, personal communications from the Minister of Health of Georgia, 1993 and 1994; T. Kerziladze, personal communications from the Regional Director of the World Health Organization, 1993 and 1994).

Impetus for acting: The international community was concerned, along with some Georgians, that in the near future, the rate of infectious diseases in the country would begin to rise rapidly. Following the collapse of the Soviet Union, the Georgians lost their social safety net, including free and accessible vaccinations for their infant children. These were most legitimate concerns, as the nation had experienced 3 years of erratic immunizations owing to lack of vaccine and cold-chain equipment, organized distribution sites, trained personnel and loss of all health records for persons displaced in their own country as refugees. In addition, the food, water, and sewage supplies were suspect at best.

Membership: The membership was composed almost exclusively of external experts and politicians. International PVOs and foreign embassies providing humanitarian aid decided that help was needed to prevent a public health crisis in Georgia, and they decided to intervene. This membership composition sets up the most challenging situation for establishing a power-sharing partnership. Grass root citizens and national and local experts are likely to resent being excluded and to lack trust in the coalition and its members.

Patterns of formation: The groups external to the country formed their own ad hoc group. They invited the Minister of Health of Georgia to participate, but the decisions made were controlled by the powerful international PVOs. Under the direction of a group of international donors, an expert children's immunization team from the United Kingdom came as consultants. The Minister of Health was invited to a planning meeting and faced with the choice of "do it our way or we won't pay." He agreed to their plans. The Georgian pediatricians, of which there are many, and the Georgian experts in infectious disease, were not partners in planning. They were told what to do by the international experts, who also possessed all of the funding and supplies for the project, but not the detailed knowledge that the local national experts did.

This level of voluntariness is level V, conflict-induced. It also contains aspects of level IV, induced collaboration. In both cases, a force external to the people experiencing the need mandated coalition formation and action. Often, level IV occurs because external funding is used as an inducement. People pursue the money, or they are reluctant to pass up the money. This level of voluntariness will lead to failure unless extraordinary efforts are made to gain the trust of those who have been induced into collaboration. At level V, collaboration is mandated or directed by an external authority. Persons forced to join have no choice in the matter. If the reason for having the coalition is one they value, there is a chance, as in the previous case study, that a real partnership can finally be developed. The more likely scenario is that the coalition will fail.

Power-sharing partnership: This did not exist in this coalition throughout it's brief life span.

Structure of the coalition: Structure includes all the formation variables already discussed, as well as the organizational arrangements and the outcomes sought. The international PVOs and the participating embassies provided the foreign aid and made all the decisions. Compliance with decision-making was expected by the Minister of Health and the Director of the Georgian Sanitation and Epidemiology Unit. No input was sought from Georgian pediatricians.

Level of collaboration: This variable concerns the extent to which shared planning, work, and management occurs. The greater the sharing, the greater the likelihood that the coalition will meet its goals. In December 1993, when the cold-chain refrigeration equipment and vaccine supply arrived in the country, the outside temperature was at freezing or below. There was only erratic heat in hospitals, homes, and schools. Electricity was on for only a few hours a day, at best. No international experts accompanied the supplies.

The Minister of Health had been told not to send the vaccines to any regional health care facilities or rural village hospitals until the cold-chain refrigeration units were in place and operating. The Minister of Health, however unfortunately, did not have the petrol or the trucks to distribute the refrigeration units and the vaccines. Thus, with only spotty refrigeration in the urban storage areas and no refrigeration (and no vaccines) in the outlying areas, the controlled temperatures required on the vaccines could not be ensured. The vaccines, therefore, could not be distributed or administered. A person with diphtheria entered the country from the outside in one of the port cities (the nation is on the Black Sea); without vaccination, 21 cases of diphtheria were reported with one known death.

Outcome(s) sought: This coalition failed to meet its goal because of the failure of coalition building. The international coalition neglected to include any Georgian stakeholders and developed a program that could not be implemented in Georgia.

Community values: The value of a 90% immunization rate by the year 2000 was shared by the international team and by the Georgians. The community value, however, of inclusion of local stakeholders on the coalition was not important to the international coalition members. The local stakeholders were not, therefore, able to contribute either their expertise or their political connections to the coalition plan. Consider the four-variable community values model. The quality of care ideal was high, and the funding was provided by international donations. The program failed, however, because the values of the Georgians were not respected and there was very poor access by those who needed the immunizations.

A new committee with Georgian stakeholders included with the international experts is now developing a modified program. This modification will address the prior weaknesses as discussed in relation to the coalition model and the community values model. It should prove to be a successful program.

ISSUES IN COALITION FORMATION WITHIN COUNTRIES

Within nations, the community values coupled with Sullivan's coalition model (see Chapter 9) provide a set of guidelines for success. Regardless of the socioeconomic status of the country, people know when their personal and community values have been disregarded. The concept of including all the stakeholders, large and small, and then letting them define their roles allows a voice to all. The time invested in allowing stakeholders to present their views is invaluable when they become vested in the work of the coalition.

Awareness and respect for the community values of the involved cultures is a reoccurring theme that is so obvious it seems impossible to miss; however, understanding another culture and observing its traditions out of respect takes time and involvement. Many cultures will not do business with strangers. You must first interact and become a friend. Small nuances, such as shaking hands or inquiring about family members' health, are vital to showing you know and respect the traditions.

When disaster strikes, international teams flow in to help. Not always is the help accepted, even when it is greatly needed.

In 1994, the Russian Federation requested that the United States stop all humanitarian aid to Russia because many of the leaders were deeply offended by the way in which the aid had been offered. Early in 1997, there were development and technical assistance programs in the Russian federation providing food, clothing, and medicines. These formed a life-sustaining chain for the Russian people. Many such programs, however, have now been halted by the Russian government. Well-known international PVOs have been asked to leave Russia or have had their licenses or visas blocked.

The desire to help is not sufficient in and of itself. This is a chilling lesson. We need to understand that in all nations of the globe, the laypeople and the professionals want the same things: to help peoples at risk. The lessons of coalition building, such as the higher degree of voluntariness that is more desirable and predictive of success in meeting goals, reinforce the need to understand and respect community values. Also of great import is the need to value and respect the internal structures and systems within nations. An immediate problem may be resolved, but if it is at the expense of the loss of respect for local leaders or the destruction of systems, the price paid is too high.

Sullivan's coalition model (Chapter 9) and the community values model are strong beginnings to building working partnerships with respect, dignity, and trust among members. When this occurs, the unleashed human resources that emerge can energize and complete any well-conceived project.

Members of coalitions achieve their goals, derive great satisfaction, and are willing to remain involved. Sometimes, as in the case of the Santa Clara County coalition, they are eager to use their newly found problem solving structure and relationship to address other problems within their community values perspective.

References

Deming, W. E. (1982). *Quality, Productivity, and Competitive Position.* MIT Center for Advanced Engineering Studies, Cambridge, MA.

Ehrlich, E. M. (1996). *U.S. Bureau of the Census: Statistical Abstract of the United States: 1996,* 116th edition. U.S. Government Printing Office, Washington, DC.

The Europa World Yearbook, vol. I (1996). Europa Publications Limited, London, UK.

Flower, J. (1995). Collaboration: the new leadership. *Health Forum Journal, 38*(6), 20–26.

Fry, S. (1994). Debate: do we have health care rationing? In McClosky, J., Grace, H. (Eds.). *Current Issues in Nursing.* Mosby Company, Saint Louis, MO.

Kitzhaber, J. (1990). Oregon act to allocate resources more efficiently. *Health Prog* June, 20–27.

Lisk, P. (1996). Popular participation in community health programmes. *World Health Forum, 17*(3), 294–295.

Neaves, H. R. (1990). *The Deming Dimension.* S.C. Press, Knoxville, TN.

Peter, G. (Ed.) (1997). *1997 Red Book: Report of the Committee on Infectious Disease Standards for Pediatric Immunization,* 24th edition. American Academy of Pediatrics, Elk Grove Village, IL.

Rajewski, B. (1997). *Countries of the World and Their Leaders Yearbook,* vol. 2. Eastword Publications Development Inc., Cleveland, OH.

Reddy, M. (1994). *Statistical Abstracts of the World.* Gale Research, Detroit, MI.

Tarkhan-Mouravi, G. (1996). *Human Development Report.* The United Nations Development Programme, Tbilisi, Georgia, USSR.

Thorne, J. I. (1992). The Oregon plan approach to comprehensive and rational health care. In Strosberg, M. A., Wiener, J. M., Baker, R. (Eds.). *Rationing America's Medical Care: The Oregon Plan and Beyond.* Brookings Institution, Washington, DC, pp. 24–34.

Facilitating
Collaboration

Collaborative Health Professional Education: An Interdisciplinary Mandate for the Third Millennium

14

Alice F. Kuehn

"All of us who have gone into space since the beginning of the space age were treated to a view of our planet that no photograph or television picture can convey. The scene floods your vision, as your entire view fills with the vivid colors of mountains, oceans, and land masses. At first you are inclined to seek out your home town, state or country. For the first day, as you see the sun rise and set 16 times, you go to a window whenever possible, to seek out the different countries and to match them against what you were taught in geography class. Then without warning, you are transformed . . . a special feeling evolves: you lose the urge to find boundaries between states and countries: the world becomes a globe . . . no longer do you think in terms of "my city" or "my country," rather you begin to sense that you are a part of something much larger . . . compelling us to live and work together toward making our planet a better place.

—*Sultan Al-Saud of Saudi Arabia*
Astronaut on Discovery, *June 1985*

The stories of astronauts and cosmonauts of their experiences reflect three consistent themes of collaborative learning:

- Development of a shared vision: "In space exploration we are united by our purpose" (Yuri Glazkov 1994, front cover).
- Shared insights into interdependence: "Just because borders are not visible from space doesn't mean they aren't real; however, solutions to problems must take the whole planet into account" (Collins 1994, p. 218).
- Shared experiences: "Space thinking" is the ability to think about the problems of humanity as a whole, about earth as a single inter-dependent world. Space thinking, a phenomenon described by Glazkov (1994), results from actual shared experiences in space. It has not only transformed those who have shared the experiences of space exploration but also has transformed the space programs of individual countries into an international, shared quest.

The purpose of this chapter is to explore the meaning, the challenge, and the potential of collaborative learning in health professional education. The development of "health care thinking," a shared vision of inter-

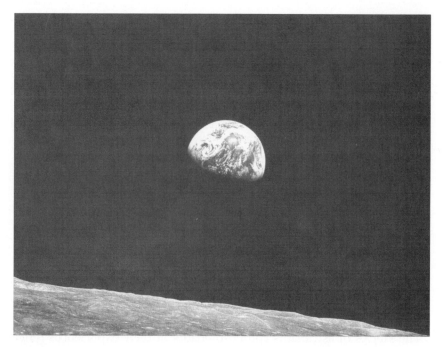

Figure 14-1.   *Earth, as seen from space, Christmas Day, 1968. (Photograph courtesy of NASA.)*

dependence inculcated in our health professional students, with human needs as the focal point, will transform not only our students but our health care world.

INTRODUCTION

The recent increasing emphasis on collaborative education is a product of expanding communication systems, global networking, diversity of providers and consumers, and the increasing complexity of health care. Toffler (1980) likens these changes to rivers flowing into a "third wave," an all-encompassing new paradigm of the world. This new world view, Toffler suggests, will require leadership that is more temporary, collegial, and consensual; decision division that is a shared decision-making that includes switching the locus of decision-making as the problems themselves require; and an environment that accommodates and legitimates diversity. Within this new wave is a *prosumer ethic* (a term used by Toffler to indicate the merging of consumer and producer as they share data and knowledge) in which "passive outsiders" become "active insiders" and the professional shifts from being the impersonal expert who is assumed to know best to being a listener, teacher, and guide who works with the patient (p. 269). Health care professionals cannot be prepared for this new world in the old world of disciplinary isolation; only collaborative, interdisciplinary experiences will adequately prepare tomorrow's practitioners for the complex, dynamic and ever-changing reality of their health care future.

HISTORICAL REVIEW OF COLLABORATIVE EDUCATION

Health professional education has a history of duplication, proliferation, fragmentation, and an increasing emphasis on specialization. Education for intraprofessional and interprofessional independence of practice has led to what has been described, for example, as the "Balkanization" of nursing, a scenario in which nursing is described as a discipline broken into smaller and often hostile groups, with practitioners educated within discrete programs and kept isolated until in practice or perhaps ad infinitum (Neuhauser and Norman 1996).

Little reference to collaboration is made in education during the first half of the 20th century. Medicine and nursing from early on emphasized the need to prepare an independent practitioner who could function within rigidly defined boundaries of professional practice (Neuhauser and Norman 1996). Mary Roberts (1954) , nursing editor and historian, described the period of the 1920s and 1930s as a time of increasing attention to nursing education and improved clinical practice status. Following the lead of the successful reforms of medical education and reforms flowing from the 1910 Carnegie Foundation's Flexner report on medical education, nursing leaders entered into a phase of "collaborative relationships" with MDs and hospitals as well as major health care foundations from which they sought funding to support reforms. Hospitals and MDs, however, were not particularly supportive because these reform proposals were perceived as taking nursing education away from service demands. In 1932, the president of the American Hospital Association commented that "hospitals had . . . 'sired' nursing," and that "nursing is the one and only legitimate daughter of hospitals" (Reverby 1987, p. 171). This was hardly the best way to develop a sense of collaborative partnership.

A more positive step toward collaborative education development was found in the recommendation of social work educator James Bartlett (as cited in Ducanis and Golin 1979). He urged participation of medical social workers in medical student education, noting that medical students needed to understand the need for and the complexities of teamwork before moving into practice settings. It should be remembered that it was also in the 1930s that the progressive educator John Dewey began to challenge the emphasis being placed on rote repetitive learning, stressing instead the capacity of the individual for identifying and solving problems. The educational reform movement Dewey stimulated proved foundational for later collaborative educational development (Dewey 1939).

In the 1960s, the launching of the Great Society, with Medicare and Medicaid and the surging development of the community mental health and primary health care movements led to a second wave of collaborative awareness and the beginnings of formalized approaches to collaborative education. The Surgeon General's report of 1963 emphasized, "[N]o health profession, health institution or community health service really functions alone. The education of nurses as well as of other health personnel must emphasize the interdependence of the professions in providing care" (United States Department of Health, Education & Welfare p. 35). The first nurse practitioner (NP) education program, begun in

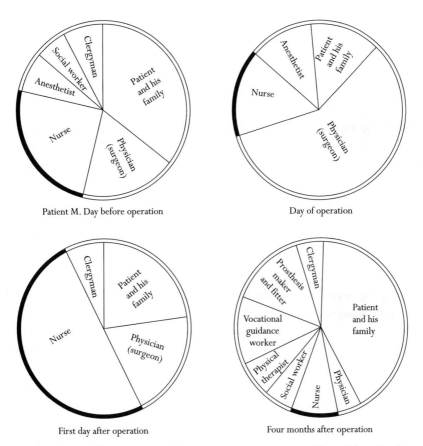

Figure 14-2. *Shifting roles in collaborative practice over time. Adapted from Henderson.* The Nature of Nursing. *Reprinted, by permission, from Macmillan Company.* © *1966 by Virginia Henderson.*

Colorado as a collaborative effort between medical and nurse educators, heralded an interdisciplinary approach to teaching primary health care. Although the learners were all nurses, the faculty were a mix of disciplines and their early writings reflected the cooperation and mutual respect each accorded the other profession (Ford and Silver 1967).

In Henderson's 1966 work, *The Nature of Nursing,* the interdisciplinary nature of patient care was clearly noted (see Figure 14-2). There appeared to be an inherent assumption in this text, however, that students would learn teamwork skills in practice, as there was no specific content for teamwork development provided.

The changes in social values flowing from the 1960s demanded professionals who were prepared as advocates for the improvement of society rather than only as providers of services. With the 1970s came the federally funded community health care centers and rural health clinics, both of which required a multidisciplinary approach to practice. The Area Health Education Centers (AHEC), founded in the 1970s and supported by federal and state funding, work toward alleviating the shortage and maldistribution of health care providers, providing needed resources and support for rural (and urban) clinical rotations of health care professionals. Since its inception, a major goal of AHEC has been to decentralize health professions education and clinical training by linking communities with academic health centers. Initially, it did not emphasize an interdisciplinary focus. Current objectives, however, require multidisciplinary and interdisciplinary clinical training responsive to community needs (AHEC 1995).

The 1960s and 1970s were a time of increasing interest in the new systems approach. It gained widespread popularity as a framework that could support the more interactive and changing environment of health care education and delivery that was evolving. These changes, coupled with a broad-based movement in higher education toward interdisciplinary interaction, prompted the examination of health professionals education from a broader, more interdisciplinary perspective. Piaget (1970) called for more of a collaborative approach in both teaching and research, harkening back to the problem-solving active learning approach stressed by Dewey.

In 1971, the Rockefeller Foundation Task Force on Higher Education added its voice by calling for changes in professional training, emphasizing the stifling effects of rigid curricula that inhibited any movement toward interactive and/or creative educational endeavors (Newman 1971). In a 1972 Carnegie Commission profile of the nature of higher education, Schien proposed a lessening emphasis on professional boundaries, a holistic approach, and a call for "curricular bridges" across disciplines to combat what he described as the inherent parochialism of professional education.

In 1972, the National Academy of Sciences of the Institute of Medicine, in examining interdisciplinary education in the health professions, proposed the following recommendations:

- every academic health center has an obligation to engage in interdisciplinary education;

- faculty members have a responsibility to develop new skills in interdisciplinary teaching and to demonstrate in their practice new role models for a variety of health care delivery systems; and
- public and private funding agencies should be encouraged to support interdisciplinary programs (Institute of Medicine 1972, p. 22).

With matched emphasis came a 1973 National League for Nursing position statement on nursing education proposing that nursing education programs

> institute interdisciplinary and intraprofessional planning . . . establish ways for nursing faculty to collaborate with faculties preparing practitioners for other health professions and occupations, and for nursing students to share learning experiences with students in other health disciplines (cited in Pennington 1981, p. 8).

Two studies in the 1970s, while exploring the current status of interdisciplinary education, also noted some inherent problems associated with such a complex model of education. One study, sampling 175 schools of allied health, dentistry, nursing, medicine, and social work, reported overwhelming support for the idea, but found only 34% of respondents reporting any such curricula or courses in their institution. Nursing programs, for example, while reporting that the idea of interdisciplinary work was "integrated throughout present courses," offered no explanation or examples as to what this really meant (Ducanis and Golin 1979).

A second 1970s study reported on perceived MD and nurse faculty risks and benefits if involved in interdisciplinary efforts. The 118 educators reported "risks" including workload stress, intense activity demands (planning sessions, time with students), lack of academic acknowledgment and/or institutional support, and sometimes overwhelming complications with clinical arrangements. Acknowledged benefits to faculty included personal growth, learning to teach in a collaborative setting, and learning about other professions (Pennington 1979).

Throughout this period, one major area of interdisciplinary educational development was in the field of gerontology. David Satin, MD, of Harvard Medical School wrote extensively, served as editor of the newsletter of the American Association for Gerontology in Higher Education (AGHE) and, in conjunction with AGHE, provided numerous faculty development conferences and seminars. The major emphasis he and his colleagues stressed in interdisciplinary education was the need to understand and work with other disciplines while preserving the identity of each discipline (Satin 1986).

During this period, this author had the opportunity to develop and teach an interdisciplinary course for associate degree nursing students and practitioners of each of three participating disciplines. During their fourth and final semester, the nursing students had an emphasis area on care of the elderly. A nutrition specialist, a speech therapist, and a nurse educator (the author) designed an elective evening course that would present an in-depth look at eldercare from our three perspectives. Students from the three disciplines participated. The course thus was interdisciplinary from both a student and faculty perspective. As faculty, we learned a tremendous amount about each other's disciplines as we developed the course. Because the course was elective, we could more freely allow the course to flow from our shared perspectives. This sharing then extended to the class sessions and involved both faculty and students. In this way, we were able to role-model collaboration to the students, and they were able to engage in collaborative activity. Major impediments to course survival included the small size of the class (due to its elective nature) and the overload status of the course on each of the participating faculty. For these reasons, the class survived only two semesters.

During this same period, the author also had the opportunity to meet with interdisciplinary colleagues in the Association for Gerontology in Higher Education, including David Satin, and dialogue with him and other interdisciplinary colleagues during a seminar session. One of the overriding concerns discussed that day was the dilemma of the lack of academic recognition for interdisciplinary courses and acknowledgment of the workload of shared courses. The bottom line was the economic concerns regarding academic credits generated and credited to the faculty of each participating discipline. The question remaining was, "Who gets credit for teaching a course taught by faculty and attended by students from more than one discipline?"

As the 1980s progressed, educators from many disciplines noted an increasing isolation of professional schools related to the continuing explosion of specialization within each profession and resulting in an increasing number of departmental and disciplinary boundaries. Health care professionals in many disciplines tended more and more to treat a very specific type of patient, creating more subspecialties and levels of professionals to address patient needs falling outside their usual parameters of expertise. For example, the pediatrician possibly moved into pediatric gastroenterology; the pediatric NP may have shifted into a specialized emphasis on acute care pediatric otolaryngology. Changes in academic curricula, certifying requirements, and professional practice acts reflected this pendulum swing back to specialized isolation in the name of professional autonomy, making interdisciplinary efforts almost heroic. The major question became how to preserve disciplinary identities while striving for a collaborative approach (Mechanic and Aiken 1982, Satin 1986, Schien 1972, Siegler and Whitney 1994).

During this same period, the University of Missouri–Columbia health sciences faculty (the institution with which this author is affiliated) worked at collaborative educational efforts in both the NP program and in the field of gerontology. Guest lecturers from medicine, sociology, pharmacy, and physical therapy (PT) provided students with a multi-disciplinary, broader perspective of health care, and clinical precepting by MDs in addition to NPs also provided opportunities for collaborative learning in the field. In gerontology, faculty from allied health, medicine, nursing, and sociology joined together in the creation of an adult day care center on campus (which still operates). Possible curricular innovations that could provide a collaborative foundation for students from each of the participating disciplines were designed in joint grant-writing initia-tives. When grants were approved without funding, however, and there was no broad-based administrative umbrella of support, the efforts became those of dedicated faculty from disparate disciplines who continued on their own time to dialogue and plan possible collaborative strategies.

The third and current wave of collaborative education awareness and perhaps the most powerful has come with the 1990s' rush to control the economics of both health care and health professionals education. Managed care, case management approaches, and primary health care echo the systems approach of the 1970s with a call for continual im-provement through collaboration, reflection, and change (Moore et al. 1996). Although interdisciplinary education has been in place since the 1970s, it was not until the 1990s that innovative models began to be seri-ously designed. During this decade, foundation support has aggressively addressed the development of collaborative education approaches. Inter-disciplinary training grants supporting development of training materials, dissemination of educational materials, preceptor training, and develop-ment of interdisciplinary, rural practice projects have recently received federal support through the Public Health Service (Health Resources and

Services Administration [HRSA]) and AHEC. Two additional major foundation initiatives are the Pew Health Professions Commission report (O'Neil 1993) and the Robert Wood Johnson program, *Partnerships for Training*, which proposed the development of interdisciplinary education and training models for NPs, nurse-midwives, and physicians assistants (PAs).

The Pew Foundation, in a 1995 report on progress toward interdisciplinary education, noting how difficult it was to change established patterns of professional education, stressed the absolute need for collaborative approaches. The *Journal on Quality Improvement* of the Joint Commission on Accreditation of Health Care Organization (JCAHO) devoted an entire issue to "Collaborating for Change in Health Professions Education" (Institute for Healthcare Improvements, Interdisciplinary Professional Education Collaborative 1996). This issue reports on collaborative education initiatives supported by the Institute, the Bureau of Health Professions of the HRSA of the Department of Health and Human Services, and the Pew Health Professions Commission of the Pew Charitable Trust. This rapidly expanding broad base of support for interdisciplinary education continuing into the third millennium undergirds the necessity for our full understanding and our acknowledgment of the significance and credibility of collaborative education and health care delivery.

A CONCEPTUAL FRAMEWORK FOR COLLABORATIVE EDUCATION

Health professional education aims to prepare knowledgeable and skilled practitioners able to deliver health care services that are satisfactory, appropriate, and cost-effective. Education traditionally has been grounded within each discipline based on a consistent belief in the need for personal mastery of a discrete body of knowledge and skills. Individual professions emphasize unique identities, specialized knowledge base, and autonomy of decision-making. Focus is upon socializing their future colleagues within a distinct culture and disciplinary-oriented educational format. This traditional approach has produced a model described as "chimneys of excellence" (see Figure 14-3), a health care scenario in which practitioners from each discipline are educated in isolation from each other and, although well prepared to make singular contributions, find their educational preparation a total mismatch for the complex, interactive world into which they graduate and practice (Headrick et al. 1996).

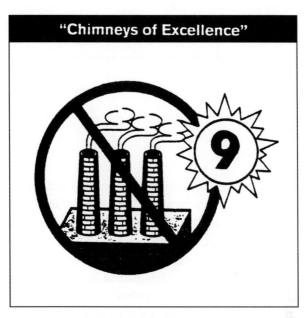

Figure 14-3. *In this logo, designed by Duncan Neuhauser, Ph.D., the chimneys represent the disciplines of health administration, medicine and nursing. The number 9 stands for the ninth of Edward Deming's 14 points, "break down barriers." Reprinted, by permission, from Neuhauser and Norman in* The Joint Commission Journal on Quality Improvement. *© 1966 by the Joint Commission on Accreditation of Healthcare Organizations.*

A Collaborative Educational Continuum

Collaborative education can be visualized as an interactive teaching or learning experience occurring along a continuum of unidisciplinary or intradisciplinary, multidisciplinary, interdisciplinary, and transdisciplinary interactive models of increasing interactive complexity (Piaget 1970) (see Figure 14-4). For example, collaborative educational models of PT programs frequently have been described within a unidisciplinary context of PT students collaborating with other PT students on different educational levels (Reynolds 1996). In nursing literature, the emphasis on educational collaboration frequently focuses on unidisciplinary partnerships of faculty with students, students with students, students and faculty with staff, and students with patients; however, multidisciplinary and interdisciplinary efforts at both undergraduate and graduate levels have also been reported (Pennington 1981, Siegler and Whitney 1994). Until recently, medical education literature has focused more on a need

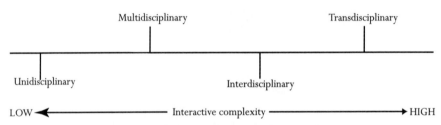

Figure 14-4.   *Collaborative educational continuum.*

for collaboration among its many specialties and between the basic and applied sciences, rather than on interdisciplinary educational approaches, although they, too, have had a consistent albeit lean offering of literature on collaborative educational models, particularly in shared content areas such as gerontology, ethics, medical informatics, health care systems, public health, and primary care (Adams and Miller 1995, Pew 1995a and b, Satin 1987, Siegler and Whitney 1994).

At the *unidisciplinary* end of the spectrum lies each health profession. Within this discipline-specific model may be found a number of collaborative combinations designed to prepare students for the interactive world of practice with the security of working with students, faculty, and practitioners of their discipline. Support is strong for the continuation and expansion of collaboration at this level for beginning students. The collaborative approach within a single discipline can assist neophyte students to develop a shared vision of their discipline with their professional colleagues, to share common goals for patient care delivery, and to assist in learning team skills and developing understanding of group dynamics. At the same time, students will be developing personal mastery of professional knowledge and skills, an essential prerequisite for effective functioning at more complex interactive levels. Peer support, confirming and validating ideas and information, provides students with a sense of mastery and comfort with basic discipline-specific knowledge essential for personal mastery. Core values and abilities ideally developed at this stage include

- sensitivity to diversity,
- openness to learning and change,
- trust throughout conflict resolution,
- shared goals and focus,
- time management and planning,

- cooperation versus competitiveness,
- sense of connection, cohesiveness, and
- responsibility to others.

Clinical experiences at this level assist in achieving the core values and abilities. Parallel practice opportunities also can foster an awareness of and respect for the contributions of other disciplines in practice.

At the next level, multidisciplinary, interaction begins to occur between or among professionals of different disciplines. Information may be exchanged; however, there is no presumption of change or enrichment to any of the participants. Learning goals are met by many health care professionals working toward the same goal through each fulfilling a discipline-specific role. This level exemplifies the "chimneys of excellence" approach in which all three chimneys work toward producing the desired effects but in "isolated splendor" (Headrick et al. 1996). Work is accomplished not by a team but by a collective of professionals, a scenario often referred to in the literature as "parallel play." Although learning at this level is very discipline specific, the parallel practice and educational encounters can increase awareness of, and toleration for, professionals of different disciplines. These increasing opportunities for interface with providers of a number of health care disciplines can mark the beginnings of dialogue leading to the interdisciplinary level of collaborative learning (Adams and Miller 1995, Pennington 1981, Piaget 1970).

Interdisciplinary education is created within an integrated teaching or learning environment in which health professionals are working together toward a shared vision transcending each discipline's boundaries. Each participant is expected to share discipline-specific expertise within a broader perspective in order to facilitate the cross-fertilization of ideas and group ownership of the results. Learning at this level requires a noncompetitive stance and is highly dependent on a supportive environment; personal readiness of each participant whether faculty, staff, or student; a conducive mix of participants; and the timing, pace, and direction of the educational effort. A proposed framework of collaborative education at the interdisciplinary level (Figure 14-5) portrays the movement of core personal values through a filter of professional knowledge and skills toward a focal point that coalesces the many inputs into a shared goal of quality patient care. Shared core values carry along through the funnel of discipline-specific perspectives on care. These core values coalesce as interdisciplinary learners focus on a shared goal.

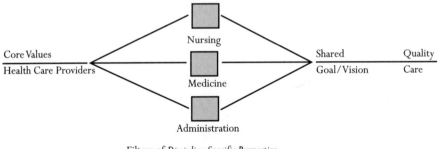

Figure 14-5. *Proposed framework of collaborative education at the interdisciplinary and transdisciplinary levels.*

The most complex level of collaborative education, *transdisciplinary,* is a system without professional boundaries (Adams and Miller 1995, Ivey et al. 1988, Pennington 1981, Piaget 1970). At this level, each participant—health care provider or patient—possesses and shares certain knowledge not bound within disciplinary or traditional walls. Going beyond an interaction of disciplines, practice becomes a synthesis of knowledge and practice. At this level, health care educators, students, and practitioners must rise above their fears of being subsumed as disciplinary boundaries disappear and individual visions join to become a new shared vision. Collaborative education at this level might be visualized as a hologram, a three-dimensional picture produced by a split coherent beam of light. Each piece of the picture contributes to the whole; however, because each piece also reflects the whole, when pieces are added together the image does not change but becomes more intense (Senge 1990). For example, as each professional, patient, and family member shares in the learning process of chronic illness management of arthritis, each becomes as a holographic piece, reflecting the totality of the learning but in a unique way. Each contributor maintains integrity of self, but the resulting learning and plan of care is owned at once by all. There is no turf because the goal of quality patient care transcends it.

The historical tendency for "professional posturing" has socialized faculty into a fear of losing autonomy and the possibility of one discipline emerging as "leader" when curricula merge. As the number of participating disciplines increases, the resulting increased diversity may dissipate the focus if members feel their own vision doesn't matter or the "vision" has already been predetermined by another discipline. The resulting polarization could lead right back to the unidisciplinary level. Faculty as well as students must be well-grounded in core values for any level of collaborative education to succeed.

Collaborative Education Defined

Collaborative education is an active learning experience crossing institutional, professional, and historical boundaries. The collaborative mix of participants lies on a continuum from a simple set of two to an infinite set of interdisciplinary complex combinations. It requires an interactive group of at least two people who come together as equals, participate in meaningful dialogue, and take ownership of a shared, external goal. As an active learning community, a collaborative accelerates the shared learning process into a synergistic experience during which participants discover a totally new interdependent perspective of both the problems and the solutions, sharing successes, failures, and resources in their search (Covey 1989, Headrick et al. 1996, Senge 1990).

Attributes of Collaborative Education

The attributes of collaborative education, emphasized in the literature and personally experienced in our collaborative education developments at MU include action, context, parity, dialogue, shared vision, and ownership. These attributes have been identified as critical elements by faculty and students alike for the success of any collaborative endeavor. In this section, each attribute is described, with illustrative cases demonstrating the essential role each plays in the success of any collaborative educational endeavor (see Figure 14-6).

Action is the essence of collaborative education. This attribute, hearkening back to Dewey's "learning by doing," is consistently recognized in the literature as essential by faculty and students alike. Faculty, it is suggested, become experts in the collaborative process only by immersion in it through actively working with each other in its design (Headrick et al. 1996). Faculty need to participate actively in the joint development of programs as well as with the students in shared activities. For example, in a collaborative course developed by the Oregon Health Sciences University, medical and nursing faculty initially served as course facilitators;

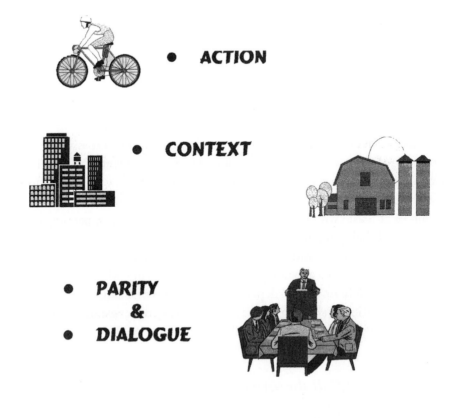

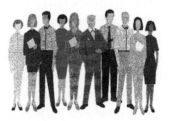

Figure 14-6. *Attributes of collaborative education.*

however, they increased their level of interaction within the course following midcourse evaluations indicating that students wanted more active faculty participation (Siegler and Whitney 1994).

Collaborative learning occurs only through interaction among and between participants. A "lived experience" is essential for collaborative interaction to become more than an exercise in rhetoric; it is foundational to the development of ownership of a shared vision. The dialogue essential to collaboration will develop only as participants gain experience dialoguing. Competence in teamwork requires active practice in the skills of teamwork. Students learn from role models; actual collaborative role modeling in team building and shared visioning must be available for their observation and critique; students must actively participate in team-building exercises and role-playing scenarios such as conflict resolution. To begin to develop the ownership of a shared vision, they must actively participate in its creation.

Only through experience in developing and teaching interdisciplinary courses can faculty gain the expertise in collaborative teaching; only through actual experience in classroom and shared clinical practice and community projects will students gain expertise in collaborative practice. As one student noted, "[T]hough the difference is difficult to define in words, the experience gained from working on the project is much richer than working on a textbook case" (Moore et al. 1996).

Collaborative learning is situation specific, *context-bound*. Within the classroom, the environment created by faculty is key to creating a collaborative success. Readiness of faculty, learners, and the environment will determine the degree of collaborative interaction that will occur. Lessons, clinical cases, and role-playing scenarios, placed in the context in which they will be used, afford students the opportunity to test approaches and apply lessons learned. The goal is to prepare students to work in an environment into which they will move after graduation.

The clinical learning context is a result of the dynamic interplay of the educational institutions and the health care setting. In one example, nursing students noted competition among team members, as well as institutional policies on workload and release time that failed to support interdisciplinary treatment plan development as resulting in little enthusiasm for the collaborative approach (Snyder, 1981, as cited in Siegler and Whitney 1994). In contrast, students participating in another venture, the Institute for Healthcare Improvements (IHI) Interdisciplinary Professional Education Collaborative (Collaborative), completed a force-field analysis of the driving and opposing forces impacting on interdisciplinary efforts. Armed with this new awareness, they focused their energies on their clinical settings, reporting "considerable success working together in an interdisciplinary environment . . . in settings [which] were incredibly diverse. . . . We had instructors from disciplines as diverse as our own, and their ability to cooperate and their sense of shared vision was important for us to observe" (Alexander et al. 1996,

p. 204). The context of the total learning experience overrode whatever differences existed among settings and practitioners.

Parity of participants reflects an absence of boundaries or a noncompetitive stance in which there is respect for varying types of expertise. Parity is dependent upon readiness of the participants. Each must have a well-developed sense of personal mastery to create a balance of contributory efforts. Parity requires active learning partners, each assuming equally active learning roles. The group membership, although diverse, requires a balanced mix of disciplines. For example, a group with medical students and graduate nursing students, or another with medical students and undergraduate nursing students, may have difficulty in establishing an interdisciplinary approach because there may be an imbalance in the educational and/or clinical background and experience of the participants. Imbalances in *numbers* of students from each discipline may also exist. Beatty's (1989) study (as cited in Siegler and Whitney 1994) found undergraduate nursing students, feeling inadequate and as lesser-valued members of the health care team, attributed these felt deficiencies to a lack of teamwork skills, poor self-image, self-doubt, shyness and unassertiveness. Students and faculty alike from the IHI Collaborative educational project re-emphasized the need for parity.

> Shared core values became important to the faculty and we realized that a commitment to role parity was essential. All voices were important, and we recognized the importance of our individual autonomy in the presence of our interdependence on each other. We valued "shared leadership" (Harman et al. 1996, p. 191).

Parity of content is relevant as well. Whether in the classroom or clinical setting, participants must avoid implications that certain content areas are considered less important, especially if they are predominantly emphasized by only one discipline. Parity requires an environment of mutual learning supporting a pluralistic approach to problem-solving in which each participant has personal mastery of a focused knowledge or skill area and contributes to a shared vision and in which the contributions are equally valued as essential for the success of the whole.

When faculty come together to design a collaborative educational experience, or students come to share in one, they find meaning in the interaction only when it becomes a shared vision of all participants. The emphasis in the literature is for each participant to share in a vision, a goal, which is outside and beyond any singular discipline's mission or goal. If this were not so, there would be no need for the team in the first place. The Institute for Latin American Concern (ILAC), an interdisciplinary health care experience for students and practitioners, requires a preliminary weekend retreat to provide for team development. "The success of the team's early cohesion is based upon a belief in a common mission, a shared commitment to the program's objectives, and planned team interaction" (Vinal 1987, p. 258).

In designing a model of collaborative education between a school of nursing graduate program and an anesthesia certificate program, in another example, distinctly different initial proposals were submitted by each of the participant groups. A consultant was called in, and over a period of 2 years, work focused on developing a cohesive faculty work group whose members could value and appreciate each other's knowledge and expertise. One solidifying factor was the shared belief by all participants in the value and critical need for this collaborative curriculum (Chamings et al. 1989).

For interdisciplinary students to create a sense of shared mission with each other is critical, and opportunity for this to occur must be included in the curricular design. In the W. K. Kellogg Community Partnerships Program in Boston, students make a commitment to a singular community for 4 years. During the first 2 years of the experience, all disciplinary students are taught together and share the same clinical experiences resulting in a "cohesive team spirit" that carries them together through the 4 years (Curley et al. 1994). Shared vision, shared mission, cohesiveness, collegiality, and teamwork; each of these terms illustrates the same sense of joint effort within which each participant becomes partner to the other and boundaries disappear.

Dialogue is described by Senge (1990) as a "free and creative exploration of complex and subtle, issues, a deep 'listening' to one another and suspending of one's own views" (p. 237). Nowhere is this attribute more necessary than in collaborative education. Anywhere along the continuum, whether between student and student of one discipline or among faculty of many disciplines, team learning is collective and all players must simultaneously be open to each other's perspectives and ideas. Dialogue cannot coexist in a hierarchical environment. At New York University, the Division of Nursing and the Medical School described their collaborative efforts as "mutual explorations . . . in identifying the professional intersects and those areas where the disciplines are distinct"

(Barnum 1990, p. 89). In another collaborative project, third-year medical students and nursing student externs participated in weekly humanistic discussion groups in which views presented were defended through dialogue or in-depth conversation regarding the issues (Forbes and Fitzsimmons 1993). Learning to work collaboratively as colleagues demands experiential learning in the art of dialogue.

Any project imposed by another will become a task or duty, with lack of participant ownership limiting its effectiveness. (See Chapters 9 and 11 for exploration of forced collaboration and induced-conflict collaboration.) Not one report of successful collaborative education has failed to stress the significance of each participant's "buy-in" to the project. Each faculty member and student must believe in the project and have a sense of personal contribution. David Satin (1987) described four gerontological interdisciplinary programs as "three failures and one success." In his one reported success, the "curriculum was developed and faculty and student participants selected by the participants themselves, without strictures from institutions or faculties unsophisticated in and unmotivated by interdisciplinary ideas" (p. 61). Development of a common curriculum by faculty participants has been reported time and again as a sine qua non of success; likewise, ownership of the educational experience by the students is a critical factor in building a commitment to participation.

Impact of a Successful Collaborative Education Process

As learners experience a simultaneous shared reception of knowledge, ideas, or problems, each processes the information within his or her professional knowledge base. Discipline-specific knowledge is described as convergent, that is, moving toward one viewpoint with narrowly focused technical jargon, style of thinking, and approach to problem solving. Because the collaborative educational scenario reflects the reality of practice—a divergent, open-ended world, the resulting sharing and interaction between and among participants may be likened to a collection of individualized streams flowing into a pool of common meaning of great vigor (Schien 1972, Senge 1990). Each practitioner, faculty, and student is professionally socialized to "go with the flow." As they interact within the collaborative educational environment, they move toward the more divergent, interdisciplinary pool of shared learnings within which they are more able to address the nuances of unique and complex health

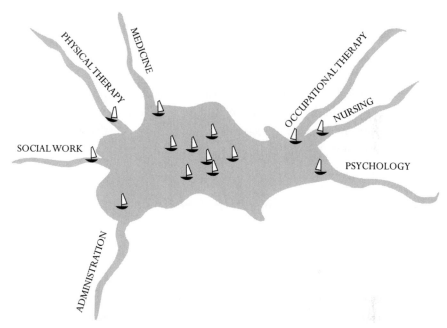

Figure 14-7. *Interdependent disciplinary flotilla on the pool of shared learnings. As participants emerge from a sampling of discipline-specific "streams," they do not dissolve into a single pool as streams into the pool, but join together as a "flotilla." Preserving their individual identities, they join to become an interdependent reality focused on a shared goal.*

care issues and problems. They do not lose their personal identity, but together create a new interdependent identity (see Figure 14-7). This new creation represents educational movement from an independent state to the interdependent, interdisciplinary paradigm described by Covey (1990). The new reality becomes a boundaryless, transdisciplinary mode of collaborative education focused on a shared goal of quality patient care (Pennington 1981).

EXEMPLARS OF COLLABORATIVE EDUCATION

Through the 1980s and into the 1990s, publications, presentations, and national and international conferences have reflected an increasingly enriched storehouse of stories and case examples of collaborative and interdisciplinary educational programs and projects. Three cases, two from the literature and one from personal experience, have been selected as exemplars of the collaborative education process. Case 1 describes interdisciplinary education as experienced in an outreach project to Latin America, case 2 illustrates the attributes of collaborative education as they unfold within a shared project between two universities, and case 3 presents the development of a collaborative educational process within a complex educational environment that has slowly expanded to now include schools of nursing, social work, psychology, health-related professions of PT and OT, and both allopathic and osteopathic medicine.

Case 1: The Institute for Latin American Concern Experience

The ILAC, described by Vinal (1987), began with an interdisciplinary educational focus. Designed as an annual summer experience, the project trains teams of undergraduate students, graduate students, and educators and practitioners from medicine, nursing, pharmacy, and dentistry to provide health care and health promotion activities to families in the Dominican Republic. In addition to the 80 participants in the summer sessions, additional teams are created and sent to the same remote clinics in November, January, and March to maintain some degree of continuity of care. Selection of participants is highly competitive, and the selection process is designed to maintain an interdisciplinary team balance carefully. Nursing students selected receive five semester credits for the experience (listed as an interdisciplinary course) specifically for having completed the clinical practicum, daily log, and program evaluation; they must also have completed a Spanish language course before the program. (No mention is made of similar requirements for participants from other disciplines.)

The experience begins with a mandatory "retreat week-end" during which teams are formed and opportunities for team interaction begin. "The success of the team's early cohesion is based upon a belief in a common mission, a shared commitment to the program's objectives and planned team interaction" (Vinal 1987, p. 258). For the students, the summer program of 8 weeks begins with 2 weeks of orientation to the country, language, customs and culture, and current issues and concerns of the people of the Dominican Republic. Additional team development activities are also scheduled for the students during this period. The professional practitioners arrive toward the end of this period for their orientation and team assignments. The students, after 2 weeks of living with native families "in-country," are given leadership roles in orientation activities for the health professionals because by this time they have had considerably more orientation and experience in living with the local people of the rural villages. This inequality is deliberately designed to create an environment of parity between the student and professional participants; the students have an edge in the cultural or experiential scene and the professionals have the edge in professional knowledge and work experiences. Additional student leadership is also established in the clinics in which one student assumes responsibility for the safety of the team and the logistics of the project for that setting. These student leaders are chosen very early in the year so that they may be in a position to receive additional instruction in group process and dynamics.

As cases and projects unfold throughout the experience, leadership of health care service delivery or health promotion activities shifts according to the expertise needed. The value of each profession as equally important and complementary to the success of the whole is emphasized throughout the experience. "Continuous consultation among the student/professional participants allows for a truly integrated interdisciplinary approach to health care" (Vinal 1987, p. 259). The cooperation needed for the team to function promotes a sense of interdependence and trust among students and professionals. Weekly conferences called "reflection meetings" allow team members to discuss daily activities, review the daily journal (recorded daily by team members taking turns), refresh and restore their sense of mission and commitment to the program goals, and validate their achievements to date.

The lived experience that forms the core of this case clearly reflects the *action* attribute of a collaborative educational experience. Both the challenge of the setting and the planned timing of student or professional interactions *(situational context)* work toward creating *parity* among participants. The commitment that each brings to the project evolves into a sense of personal and joint *ownership* as team members design the number and nature of clinic visits, home health visits, and health education projects that they believe will achieve the goals of the program. Through "reflection meetings" and shared clinical and village life experiences, the *dialogue* and sharing with each other leads them to discover their inevitable interdependence as team members. The faculty designers of this program believe the cultural dissonance experienced by the participants in working to deliver health care in a Third World country provides a unique framework for development of a positive interdisciplinary experience. Sharing of common problems of living and working within a new cultural context result in a "cohesiveness that is uncharacteristic of most health care teams" (Vinal 1987, p. 258).

Team comradery strengthens with the realization that their work has been more effective because of the pooling of their competencies and a shared accountability for decisions and outcomes. Although they come with a *shared vision,* a commitment to providing holistic health care, they also come with narrowly focused disciplinary and cultural viewpoints. Through the immersive, experiential nature of this experience, however, they are transformed. "Through its transcultural experience . . . [ILAC] . . . enables participants to realize an ethnocentric model of health care different from their own" (p. 259).

Case 2: The George Team

George Washington University (Washington, D.C.) and George Mason University (Fairfax, Virginia), described by Harman et al. (1996), have collaborated in shared curricula for medical, PA, and NP students since 1974. However, when invited in 1994 to participate in the Collaborative sponsored by the IHI, they received a special opportunity to deepen and enrich their interdisciplinary efforts. This educational model uses an adult education approach based on learning as a change of behavior, attitude, knowledge or belief (Knowles 1990); Deming's (1991) principles of data-driven decision making; and Senge's (1990) five disciplines of learning: personal mastery, team learning, shared vision, mental models, and systems thinking. Settings selected for the shared experiences are those with an already established relationship with one or both of the academic institutions. The two sites, George Washington University Health Plan and La Clinica del Pueblo, were chosen because faculty and medical residents already had practices there and both were involved in a diabetic care project, one with which students could relate.

The focus for the teams, care of the diabetic communities served by these clinics, became a shared vision of excellence for the students. Student teams of primary care residents, graduate students in Health Services Management and Policy (HSMP), PA and NP students joined with the clinic staff of physicians, nurses, diabetic educators, nutritionists, and administrative staff to work together on the project.

The collaborative educational experience is one of *action*. Only through active experience in the classes and at the clinical sites were students able to develop a sense of teamwork. They learned to acknowledge shared core values, noting in their diaries such values as a "whole system approach," sensitivity to diversity, trust, hope for accomplishing the project goal of improving patient lives, and the need to keep patient outcomes as the *shared focus* of group activities. They developed team skills as well as clinical expertise as a result of experiencing the classroom and clinical realities of a cooperative, rather than a competitive environment. Students noted, "I have no experience or training in team building and meeting skills. . . . [T]his meeting further solidified the group members into a functional team. . . . I feel that I am really a part of a team. . . . I feel connected and responsible to the other team members" (Harman et al., p. 195).

As students assumed personal ownership of the project, teams for each setting created their own "opportunity statement" relating to the clinical goal of meeting health care and preventive needs of diabetic patients. An example is the statement of the team of La Clinica del Pueblo, serving a culturally specific, indigent population: "An opportunity exists to develop a strategy that will bring diabetic care to an indigent population diagnosed with non-insulin-dependent diabetes mellitus (NIDDM) into line with the American Diabetes Association guidelines" (Harman et al., p. 190). One major issue in interdisciplinary education is the competing or nonarticulating programmatic requirements of each academic program.

To support student development of *shared ownership* and a sense of *parity* in the project workload, faculty worked to minimize any negative effect of discipline-specific programmatic requirements. They assigned to specific disciplines the primary responsibility for components of the project that required their particular expertise and could meet at least part of their particular academic requirement. For example, the HSMP students served as facilitators of the project, sharing their knowledge of continual improvement and teamwork facilitation. The PA students used the project as satisfaction for their Masters of Public Health project requirement and the NP students were allowed to have the project serve as part of their requirement for community service and research. Unfortunately, the medical residents were given no shift in job responsibilities. With project responsibilities perceived as an addition to their current clinical load, they had neither a sense of equal parity nor of administrative acknowledgment of their potential contribution and work release needed for equal participation in the project. As a result, project work became low priority and they failed to develop any sense of project ownership.

In addition to developing a sense of ownership for the *clinical project,* the faculty also needed to develop a sense of ownership of the *collaborative educational goal,* namely, to teach students to function in their professional roles as an interdisciplinary team. The first step involved faculty commitment to professional parity by acknowledging the contributions each makes, the core values that they all share, the interdependence on each other for project success, and the recognition that faculty were learners with the students. "We taught and clarified concepts, and the students learned. The students applied the tools and work with the community sites, and we learned" (Harman et al. 1996, p. 191). The first challenge in their development as an interdisciplinary faculty team, finding time when all faculty could meet on a consistent basis, was solved by scheduling luncheon meetings:

> Once the faculty development process was formed, maintaining our focus depended on our ability to share our vision, and on why it was different and important. . . . As with the students, *shared vision* was essential to faculty interdisciplinary team building. We had to stay committed to the task and not get squelched by bureaucratic logistics" (p. 190). (emphasis author's)

The role of faculty was to model interdisciplinary teaching and collaboration. They were able to do this only after extensive, open discussions and *dialogue* regarding the vision and the logistics of realizing it, conversing about priorities, agendas, scheduling, and support from the administration for student time allotments and faculty time. No faculty release time was given; only their commitment to model development for interdisciplinary education kept the program alive.

Students also developed the art of conversation, of *dialogue* about the meaning and direction of the project. They realized quickly the faculty did not have all the answers, and within this context of an open learning environment, the "students immediately became more active learners. . . . This project was energized by the students. . . . They would look at the faculty somewhat quizzically and say, 'Why is this so innovative? Why haven't we been doing this all along?'" (Harman et al., p. 191).

The report of the "George Team," as they called themselves, mirrors well the essential attributes of collaborative education. Their accomplishments include strengthening of their collaborative commitment, successful changes within their educational institutions to accommodate interdisciplinary education requirements better, and subsequent receipt of a 3-year collaborative grant from the Pew Health Professionals Schools in Service to the Nation project. Their goal is to have all first- and second-year medical students, NP, and PA students—a total of 500 students—working on interdisciplinary projects by the completion of the 3-year grant-funding period. Their report highlights the need for and benefits of a positive and pleasant environment. They valued the time taken to "lighten up" and enjoy each other's company. "We shared our knowledge, our experiences, our questions, and our answers. (We also consumed large quantities of chocolate and made sure that the last session of each semester was a celebratory one, with chocolate *and* pizza)" (p. 191; emphasis in original). Their student-generated motto says it all: "Blessed are the Flexible—and the Perseverant!" (p. 197).

Case 3: Developing a Rural Collaborative Experience in Missouri

The current rural collaborative educational programs of the University of Missouri–Columbia flow from a number of previous interdisciplinary experiences, such as joint grant-writing initiatives and educational projects. Medical family practice faculty and NP faculty began to *dialogue* seriously in the late 1970s and early 1980s during development and early expansion of the NP program. They served as guest lecturers for each other's programs, although nursing's contributions to medical courses were more limited than medical contributions to nursing courses. These same faculty also worked together at a volunteer evening clinic for the working poor, serving as preceptors for students and providing direct care. During the middle and late 1980s, medical, nursing, social work, PT, and OT faculty met regularly to discuss possible development of additional collaborative educational opportunities in gerontology. Although grants written at this time were not funded, the continuing dialogue among the faculty laid the foundation for future successful collaborative endeavors.

As state legislative initiatives in the early 1990s addressed the need for collaborative professional education, workforce planning, and removal of barriers to collaborative practice, these same medical and nursing faculty found themselves working together on statewide task forces to address primary care health professional education needs. Together, they developed policy papers on workforce and educational issues, testifying before Missouri Senate and House committees regarding collaborative practice legislation. Building on this work, a rural collaborative education pilot project was successfully launched in 1993.

Funded by the Public Health Service, this pilot placed students in medicine, nursing, occupational therapy, and PT in two rural sites, namely, Ironton, Missouri, in the summer of 1994 and Bolivar, Missouri, in the winter of 1995 (Kuehn 1995). Faculty of each participating discipline *shared a vision* of an interdisciplinary practice model that would better serve residents of rural Missouri. Their goal was to provide reality-based classroom and clinical interactions that would assist students to develop this interdisciplinary approach to practice. Interdisciplinary interactions at Ironton included morning rounds at the local hospital, collaborative work on patient cases, weekly team meetings, socializing, and a community project. In Bolivar, the interactions were similar; however, the discussion of clinical cases moved from a case-study format to problem-based learning (PBL), the format that the medical school had just adopted for their curriculum. The NP faculty already used a case-study approach and readily supported the PBL format. Orientation sessions were expanded to include practice sessions for the PBL format of interdisciplinary case discussion.

The *context* of the learning, classroom or clinical, has been a critical consideration in planning and operationalizing the experiences. The rural context of the learning experiences was designed specifically to enhance collaborative learning in the reality of a rural setting, with clinical experiences scheduled together as much as possible. The PBL cases were designed by faculty from all participating disciplines, and weekly case discussions were moderated by an NP in Ironton and a nurse educator at the hospital in Bolivar. Students began developing a *shared vision* of health care planning and delivery as they focused on the cases together. They also shared clinical vignettes with each other from personal experiences at their respective clinical sites.

Students began to claim *ownership* of the projects as they reported to the faculty their decisions regarding the cases, particularly when their decisions involved cases they chose from the current clinical patients they were seeing. In addition, students identified and then completed a community project of their choice at each site, leading to an even greater sense of personal ownership of the project. Five of the eight students in the Ironton experience stated they had not worked in an interdisciplinary health care team before and all cited the case-study conferences as a very positive experience. Student comments included, "Learned more about family medicine, rural medicine, NPs, and PTs" and "different perspectives increased understanding of a given situation." Students in the Bolivar experience noted, "This experience was positive because of learning from other professions" and "working with this group did take extra time commitment and several clinical experiences had to be missed for team meetings, projects, etc. . . . but I think this time was also beneficial and not necessarily detrimental to my clinical experience." One student of the five at Bolivar reported the experience as not positive, stating that "[t]he team did not work together well due to widely divergent goals"; apparently from this student's perspective, the shared vision never materialized.

This developing model of collaborative action has focused on *active* reality-based experiences from the start. Collaborative accomplishments of these two pilot experiences included interdisciplinary interactions in classroom and clinical settings; academic, clinical, and community collaborative initiatives; measures of student attitudes regarding rural practice; and a computerized database of actual clinical encounters of each type student practitioner (Kuehn 1996). Provision of community housing allowed students to socialize together, and computer, phone lines, and Internet linkages with faculty and health sciences center and national and international resources facilitated student learning at the remote rural sites.

Following successful completion of these two pilots, faculty moved to incorporate their model into the newly funded AHEC at Rolla, Missouri. This site was chosen by the group as a region fairly new to the University, one which might be open to development of clinical sites and preceptors willing to work with the faculty and students within their interdisciplinary framework of practice. The participant group expanded at this point to include both allopathic (MD) and osteopathic (DO) physicians as well as graduate psychology students. Previous attempts to facilitate undergraduate students in social work had not been successful owing to scheduling, preceptor difficulties, and faculty shortages that precluded earlier social work involvement in the interdisciplinary experiences. Social work student rotations at the graduate level are now being planned.

One challenge has been the shortage of clinical sites. Few NPs currently practice in some of the rural AHEC areas, and medical preceptors are kept busy with medical student rotations. Because of this dilemma, the three participating NP students have traveled daily to distant sites for their clinical experiences; however, faculty are working to cultivate new sites and students are willing to travel in exchange for the interactive experiences they are experiencing in the PBL sessions. Faculty continue to work to develop sites at which students can see and participate in interdisciplinary practice. The number of participants in the winter of 1997 increased to 20, creating a need for two groups evenly representative of the disciplines. Although there were three NPs, one PT, one OT, and one psychology student, there were 14 medical students. Thus *parity* of discipline representation was not possible.

Although parity of disciplinary impact has been a consistent goal of the faculty group, it has been challenging to operationalize it for these reasons: 1) funding for the PHS grant was managed through the medical school and 2) funding for the AHEC grant is funneled through the AHEC offices at the two cooperating medical schools, with the funding emphasis on medical student education. The AHEC project managers and participating faculty at the MU Health Sciences Center, committed to the interdisciplinary concept, however, work diligently to facilitate broad-based interdisciplinary participation. Parity among faculty and students is developing steadily. One medical faculty who served as a PBL session moderator noted that he had not been a strong believer in the whole collaborative process. After his session with the students he changed his mind, however. He found that the medical students whom he had expected to do well did so, but so did all participating students who were right on "top of the case." In fact, the cases often seemed too elementary for the NP students. "I applaud their abilities and achievements in this collaborative project" (personal communication, February 1997).

What has been most dominant as a parity issue outside of the parity of discipline representation has been parity of the educational and experience level of the participants. One PT student commented during a PBL session that there "was not a level playing field," referring to the fact that NP and medical students are all postbaccalaureate status. Nurse practitioner student comments focused on the lack of clinical experience of the medical students and the simple intellectual level of the PBL cases; however, as one noted, "I keep telling myself it's not the content that's important, but the process," referring to the teamwork process developing among the students. Another student observed that PBL cases were nothing new but were reflections of the way nurses think all the time, similar to care plans. What he found most rewarding in the experience was the camaraderie, the behind-the-scenes working together, and the gathering of everyone at the student residence after clinical rotations to eat, enjoy TV, and socialize together (personal communications, February 1997).

Although age has been mentioned as another possible source of imbalance in groups, the University of Missouri collaborators have not found it to be an issue. Faculty continue to work at achieving greater *parity* among the students through a balanced mix of participating disciplines, appropriate matches of educational level and clinical experience, and increasing opportunities for faculty, students, and preceptors to share in the interdisciplinary activities. Rural settings and interdisciplinary group participation for student experiences provide an environment that will foster a transformation of these students into practitioners well-grounded in the realities of rural practice and the potential of an interdependent practice model.

THEORETICAL FRAMEWORK FOR ACTION

In collaborative education endeavors, successful programs and academic institutions have followed a rather similar and consistent blueprint for success consisting of three basic components: preparation for change, design and implementation, and evaluation of impact (Moore et al. 1996, Batalden 1996).

Preparation for Change

The collaborative learning environment is created from a complex mix of academic, clinical, political and professional forces. Using the force-field analysis approach of Lewin (1952), Schien (1972) proposed a model for examining the strength and relevance of driving and restraining forces impacting educational systems of professional disciplines. Driving forces have been portrayed as overt, positive, logical, and economically driven in contrast to a view of restraining forces as covert, emotional, negative forces arising from more of a psychosocial base (Covey 1989). Driving forces, however, can also be emotionally charged and restraining forces can be economically driven. What is critical for the design of a realistic plan is that each be identified, discussed, and rated within the context of the given situation. The primary focus of change, the point of entry into the system at which you will begin the change process, should be on those restraining forces that are significant, relevant, and changeable. Do not waste energy on forces most difficult or nearly impossible to change. Neither should you spend time on reinforcing positive strategies; they will come along on their own as the key negative forces are defused. Points of intervention into the system to begin change should be based on the following five criteria:

- Access to the target entry person;
- Power linkages of the target entry person (not necessarily the hierarchical leader) to the system;
- Suitability of the initial change project or target for your specific intervention (for example, is the academic course chosen as the inaugural target for change, such as pharmacology, conducive to the interdisciplinary approach?);
- Leverage upon the entry point person, based upon personal influence, previous positive history of working together, or disciplinary connections such as family practice medicine with family nurse practitioners; and,
- Openness of the system to change at this time (Schien 1972).

Planned change in health professional education requires a serious examination of the forces supporting and opposing such change. Driving forces moving collaborative educational efforts forward come from a multitude of forces both external and internal to the educational system (AHEC 1995, Moore et al. 1996, Schien 1972). Satin (1987) described a successful interdisciplinary project based upon the positive driving forces of faculty commitment, trust, collegial respect, and integrity to the program design despite competing loyalties or goals. Planning, administration, and teaching were accomplished by the core faculty group without institutional interference; their pilot course did not interfere with or compete with other disciplinary requirements. Restraining forces working to prevent or inhibit collaborative educational change are legion as well (Moore et al. 1996, Culmon 1996, Siegler and Whitney 1994). In his frank discussion of the difficulties of interdisciplinary education, Satin (1987) described the highly competitive, traditionally conservative world of academia as one teeming with vested interests, scarce resources, and even scarcer examples of honesty, trust, and respect.

Because of administrative lack of support and competing interests for academic resources, "interdisciplinary education is not allowed to disrupt the status quo" (p. 66). Faculty, although dedicated to the concept, will let it go when it competes with survival or advancement. In describing three failures of interdisciplinary education, Satin (1987) emphasized the lack of support or overt hostility demonstrated by both faculty and administration toward the interdisciplinary efforts. Trust among members frequently was undermined, often because of conflicts relating to student rotations, research areas, patient, populations, or turf issues causing colleagues to return to a posture of disciplinary loyalties. An illustrative force-field analysis of driving and resisting forces impacting upon collaborative education can be seen in Figure 14-8.

Many of these resisting forces continue to plague current efforts in collaborative education projects, including our own. Despite faculty workload and recognition concerns, however, many driving forces are moving us toward even more successful levels of collaborative education. Administrative support at MU health sciences school and college levels, including crossover support for tenure of participating faculty from different disciplines, has assisted us in developing stronger interdisciplinary ties. In addition, there is an increasing awareness and support of these issues by institutional administration due largely to the Health Sciences Leadership Group. This committee of deans, chairs, and faculty leaders from health-related professions, health services management, medicine, nursing, social work, and veterinary medicine joined to network and support initiatives in interdisciplinary education, research and practice. Faculty interest and support also continues to be high as reflected by the recent development of a World Wide Web page, "The Virtual Health Team" created by the Health Related Professions faculty to carry the concept of our interdisciplinary PBL case approach to the world. Although the political climate in Missouri is in flux regarding advanced practice nursing, as preceptors of different disciplines move toward a more cooperative educational and practice stance, historical turf issues may begin to defuse.

Design and Implementation

The design of a collaborative, interdependent "learning community" mirroring the "learning organization" of Senge (1990) and the inter-

Driving Forces	Present Level of Collaboration in Education	Restraining Forces
Past history of interdisciplinary work →	←	Turf Issues Academia/clinical autonomy gate-keeping roles
Institutional support →	←	Professional posturing regarding provider functions
Foundational funding initiatives →	←	Scheduling conflicts
Mandates from foundation reports →	←	Competitive stance of educational institutions
Federal funding initiatives →	←	Academic credit concerns
Increasing pool of collaborative education models →	←	Discipline-specific accreditation concerns
Increasing interest/support in academia →	←	Faculty workload/tenure concerns
Commonalities in educational concerns across disciplines →	←	Traditional emphasis on individualistic approach and recognition
Increased clinical emphasis on teamwork →	←	Insecurity in assuming a parity role
Increasing complexity of health care delivery →	←	Fear of own discipline being subsumed and another emerging as sole leader
Knowledge explosion →	←	Emotional resistance to a team approach
High level of interest and motivation among faculty →	←	Faculty bias toward own profession's superiority
High level of interest and support among students →	←	Lack of administrative commitment
General public and media push for health care system and economic reform →	←	Lack of faculty skill in team approach
Managed care →	←	Lack of experience and/or insecurity in shared and equal recognition between disciplines and/or faculty and students
Demand for graduates with interdisciplinary skills →	←	Lack of motivation, interest, and/or resources at program level
		Lack of faculty interest

Source: Adapted from Schien 1972. Schien, E. H. (1972) *Professional Education: Some New Directions.*

Figure 14-8. *A force-field analysis of collaborative education.*

dependent synergy of Covey (1989) flows directly from cognitive or organizational theories of learning. In considering collaborative, professional
education, the cognitive approach grounded within clinical experience,
interrelated situations, and interactive dialogue is essential for achieving
the more complex syntactical, contextual, and inquiry levels of learning
(Bevis 1988). Dewey's (1939) premise of the need for learners to understand the nature of the problem; German Gestalt psychologists' emphasis on the role of perception, the problem-solving process, and the
context-driven nature of problems (Bower and Hilgard 1981); and
Piaget's (1970) subsequent description of cognitive development, further
developed by Perry (as cited in Valiga 1988), all are foundational to the
current emphasis on inquiry and diversity in management and education.
Core concepts of this cognitive theory base to be attended to in your
design and implementation model include the following:

- readiness of the learner
- stimulating environment
- acknowledged sequential, predictable, and progressive stages of
  development, and
- the interactive nature of learning at the more complex levels of
  learning (Covey 1990, Senge 1990, Valiga 1988)

Readiness of the learner

Readiness for collaborative learning is the sine qua non at any level of
complexity. Regardless of the type of educational format, whether formal, informal, or even spontaneous, the outcome will depend on the
readiness of each participant for the unique shared learning experience
in which he or she participates.

In the history of American space flight, the astronauts first moved
from solo flights to pilot pairs and then to groups of three to four male
pilots from different services (Navy, Air Force, Marines) working as
teams. Later developments took a quantum leap when nonpilot scientists
began to be invited, and an even more significant move forward was seen
with the presence of women and scientists from other allied nations and
ethnic backgrounds on the space exploration teams. But all of these paled
in significance when compared with the tremendous forward leap that
collaborative space travel took when the Russians and Americans began
flying shared missions. None of these changes occurred, however, with-

out a close examination of the supportive forces and definite action taken to defuse the resisting forces. Even more importantly, each stage of increasing complexity of collaboration was preceded by a planned educational agenda to prepare the voyagers for that "new" level of team effort or "new" composition of the team. Particularly important for the joint Russian and American flight was the education needed on both sides to understand the differences in language, in mission approach, in tools, and in skills. To succeed as a singular endeavor, each needed to be masters in their own right while clearly understanding and valuing the expertise of the others in order to merge their collective efforts into a shared mission. Preparation was key, and their successes attest to its thoroughness. The transformational level of shared understanding achieved by astronauts and cosmonauts could not have occurred without each having a sense of personal mastery, being well-prepared for the team effort, and possessing an openness to growth.

The level of readiness needed for each level of collaborative education is not universally agreed upon. At the undergraduate level, however, where role socialization begins, collaborative experiences designed within a single discipline (unidisciplinary) allow for development of core collaborative values and skills while providing students a more limited interactive environment within which to develop personal mastery. Core values and skills possibly developed at this level are listed earlier in the chapter. Students of different disciplines could also readily share courses focusing on common areas of clinical practice, patient issues, or team building. Clinical experiences might be single discipline activities between different levels of students and/or between clinical staff and students or multidisciplinary, providing parallel practice opportunities that foster an awareness of and respect for the contributions of other disciplines.

In moving to the design of educational experiences with other disciplines, consider the listing of curricular content to be team taught. Content on group dynamics, role theory, organizational change theory, conflict resolution, and assertiveness skills along with role playing and storytelling have been recommended as prelude for shared clinical learning experiences. Additionally, seminars to debrief with peers following interactive clinical rotations are suggested to assist learners to analyze the personal, social, and organizational variables operating in such a collaborative environment (Joel 1988, Hamric et al. 1996). At the graduate level, readiness preparation includes validating student skill levels in collaboration, communication, and joint problem solving. Building on that, faculty can move to more intense group process and team-building activities and shared clinical experiences at higher levels of disciplinary interaction, such as transdisciplinary. The level of readiness required of participants for this level of interaction is highly debated in the literature; however, this author would suggest parity of participants, whether faculty, students, or preceptors, in relation to their personal mastery strengths and developed set of core values as a fundamental criterion.

A stimulating environment

Covey (1990) stresses the responsibility of each stakeholder for providing an environment that fosters trust, empowers the learner, and supports cooperative creativity rather than competitiveness. The mix of participants and the timing, pace, and direction of the educational effort are highly dependent on the educational goals within the context of the academic and clinical learning environment. Developmental steps toward creation of a supportive environment for interdisciplinary education include institutional initiatives to provide faculty support and reflect administrative buy-in; establishment of a continuing mechanism for dialogue among all participants such as a permanent committee with designated goal, mission, meeting schedule, and administrative support; curriculum changes within each discipline that support interdisciplinary approaches; creation of new interdisciplinary collaborative practice models between preceptors of the disciplines; and continuing exploration of cross-disciplinary curriculum innovations (Bevis 1988, Ducanis and Golin 1979). In preparing a supportive environment for collaborative education:

1. Consider the impact of external and internal forces on the development of a program.
2. Conduct a force-field analysis to identify driving and restraining forces relating to the interdisciplinary plans.
3. Carefully appraise the readiness of the faculty, administration, and program for the change.
4. Consider well how you will orchestrate the initiation of students and clinical preceptors into the project.

Cognitive theories of learning help us to understand why and how collaborative education will work. Creation of a facilitative environment will allow it to flourish.

Sequential, predictable, progressive stages of development

Perry (1970) described cognitive development as a movement through dualism, relativism, and commitment. Dualism reflects a learner's view in which there is only black and white, right or wrong. Within relativism comes an awareness that much of knowledge is uncertain; however, overwhelming experiences at this stage could lead to retreat from this level of awareness to a safer, less flexible set of beliefs or, at best, a temporary holding pattern. In commitment, the most advanced level of development, the learner carefully considers options of others, evaluates alternatives, and then makes choices with an awareness and acceptance of the consequences of those choices. Experiences with diversity, exposure to uncertainty, and discomfort in dialogue are essential at this advanced level, reflecting Schien's (1972) suggestion that "an important part of the training of a professional is what some sociologists have called 'training for uncertainty,'"(p. 44). In a similar vein, Covey (1989) admonishes us to put first things first, moving the learner from a stimulus-response paradigm to a proactive model, progressing from self-awareness and a personal mission statement, through an affirming state of personal independence, to an interdependent, interpersonal level of synergistic success. As he describes it, "It is the crowning achievement of all the previous habits . . . effectiveness in an interdependent reality" (p. 283). Likewise, mastery of Senge's (1990) core disciplines—personal mastery, mental models emphasizing reflection and inquiry, shared vision, team learning, and systems thinking—results from a progressive development of cognitive and linguistic capacities, and new values and operating assumptions grounded in the practices, principles and essence of the five disciplines (p. 377).

Interactive nature of learning

From a Gestalt framework, we are told that the "solution occurs more quickly if all the parts which need to be brought into relationship are simultaneously present in perception" (Bower and Hilgard 1981, p. 319). Senge (1990), building on this concept, has emphasized the need to explore complex issues from many points of view, describing the synergistic nature of dialogue among participants as a flow of simultaneous perceptions of learners into a pool of common meaning (see Figure 14-7). We are asked to "go with the flow" without losing our sense of personal integrity and identity. Within this framework, the focus is on learning outcomes rather than on instructional delivery. Health care becomes the context for health professional learning. Participants become part of a "learning organization" with synchrony (simultaneous coexistence) between education and health care institutions through a singular focus on health care. A clinical learning context is created as a result of the dynamic interplay of both entities. Newer models of collaborative learning, focusing on a continual learning (systems) approach, emphasize neither the specific discipline of the participants nor outstanding individual performances. Rather, they focus on the capacity of the faculty team to change and improve the educational process and the capacity of the students to acquire the knowledge and skills needed for continuous improvement of health care (Moore et al. 1996).

At the University of Missouri–Columbia, the evolution of interdisciplinary activities has been supported and advanced by the continuing interaction of health professional leaders, dedicated to the improvement of health care access, quality, and cost-effectiveness. Because the faculty and staff continued to work with each other on state and university task forces, advisory panels, and grant proposal efforts, they began to know each other in a personal way different from the professional formality of previous encounters. They developed a sense of comfort, confidence, and trust to the point where they could truly dialogue without feeling threatened or appearing defensive; however, this did not happen overnight. It was a result of 4 years of working at learning to dialogue, to trust, and to establish a comfort level that would allow each to speak openly and honestly regarding our concerns or issues. It was a humbling, and at the same time exhilarating, experience as letters, drafts of documents, and dialogue across the table became more open and honest; sometimes painful but never hostile.

EVALUATING THE IMPACT

Evaluation of the impact of collaborative education (assuming a clinical component) involves two major considerations: impact of the program upon the students and impact upon the outcomes of care delivered by the collaborative team. Although evaluation literature has been sparse, there has been a recent and noticeable increase in attention to development of evaluation tools.

The impact on students has been the most frequent type of evaluation reported. Using a team-effectiveness scale, Slack and McEwen (1993) measured the extent to which the interdisciplinary program affected nine dimensions of team development. Analysis of reports of two separate 10-week experiences found all students showing a gain in all nine dimensions (including utilization of resources, trust and conflict, leadership, interpersonal communication), but none were statistically significant at $P < .05$. Student descriptions of the experience included, "One of the most satisfying experiences of my life" and "[We w]ill take a piece of each other's disciplines with us" (p. 256). The time at which students noted their sense of "coming together as a team" differed with each student. Facilitating factors for team development identified by the students included having a team goal, openness to others' opinions, and informal time shared.

A study of the Idaho Rural Interdisciplinary Training project (RITP), started in 1991, analyzed changes in student perceptions of interdisciplinary practice relative to both their own discipline and other health-related disciplines. The Idaho program places students from 10 academic institutions over a five-state region. Students from nursing, pharmacy, PT, medicine, social work, and counseling complete clinical rotations at one of these sites for periods ranging from five to 16 weeks. Prior to the clinical rotations, students completed a pretest of perceptions of interdisciplinary rural practice, viewed an orientation video, and received computer training for using a bulletin board system. Collaborative interaction included weekly seminars, presentation by each student of one case study to the team, and networking through the computer system on rural issues and clinical experiences. Upon completion of their rotation, students completed a post-test using the Interdisciplinary Education Perception Scale (IEPS) of Luecht et al. (1990). Reliability and validity were established in the original study; reliability was established for this study as well. Male and female students showed a significant change in perceptions of both professional competence and autonomy of their own and of other disciplines and of actual cooperation and resource sharing within and across disciplines following their interdisciplinary experience (Hayward et al. 1996).

The evaluation component of the George Washington University and George Mason University George Project addressed impact both on students and on patient outcomes. Faculty team dialogue, project reports and student diaries were tools of formative evaluation used to assess the effectiveness of team community projects as health care interventions. Summative evaluation was conducted using outcome data from the projects: medical records, glycosylated hemoglobin levels, and health assessment tools. Limitations noted included a lack of feedback on certain of the curriculum components and methods. They recommended use of pretest and post-test learning tools and assessment of team effectiveness and group dynamics to study the impact of team experience on student learning (Harman et al. 1996).

The evaluation process at the University of Missouri–Columbia has focused on student outcomes. Pretest and post-testing of the groups at Ironton and Bolivar assessed changes of perceptions of health professional students related to their three areas: rural life, rural health care practices, and interdisciplinary health care practice. Results from both groups ($N < 13$) indicated very slight changes in perceptions regarding rural life. A slight increase in post-test scores reflected a greater perception of the clinical site as rural, offering location and population as their criterion. In addition, their perceived level of health care knowledge of rural people decreased at both settings, suggesting a growth in awareness of some unique health care needs of rural Missourians. Perceptions regarding interdisciplinary health care practice included three students' concerns that the interdisciplinary commitment took valuable time from learning. There was an increased level of importance and value attached to the interdisciplinary experience from the first to the second group, due probably to the faculty's improved planning of the second experience.

Student diaries offered insights into comfort levels and viewpoints regarding the interdisciplinary process. Comments were generally positive, although some did express concern that the "team activities" took too much time away from their "real learning needs." Following the Bolivar experience, the five students submitted a joint overview of the project in which they stated:

> [O]pen communication between all members of a team is a prerequisite for that team to reach its stated goals. . . . Physicians, nurse practitioners, occupational and physical therapists and other allied health professionals vary greatly in their training, philosophies of patient care and abilities. Unfortunately, these professionals often work in a vacuum as they care for patients within the context of their specialty. . . . Our time spent in Bolivar has allowed the participating students an opportunity . . . to not only learn more about the specific methods of treatment offered by students of other specialties, but . . . the opportunity to follow the thought processes that went into implementation of treatment (Johnson 1995, p. 11).

Variables associated with collaborative learning include time involved, effort involved, faculty cost, learning experiences required, value of resultant learning, decisions made from shared learnings, lessons from failures, unexpected learnings, and cost per student . Each component should be evaluated, testing its contribution to the achievement of goals set (Cleghorn and Headrick 1996). Questions to be asked relate to changes occurring in their effectiveness as an intervention team, team-building skills, understanding of the issues related to interdisciplinary collaboration, difference in outcomes from nonparticipants, and numbers of students staying on as rural providers upon graduation.

Methodological problems of studying the effects of teams relate to problems of internal and construct validity of study designs. Studies frequently attribute the impact or outcome noted to the team effect without controlling for the numerous variables within the team setting. Suggestions for improving internal validity include random assignment to teams and control teams; time series design; pretesting and post-testing; and use of equivalent groups. Construct validity requires controlling for confounding variables, including knowledge and skills of different team members, communication patterns, target populations served by the teams, organizational context, team effect versus usual care, family effect, or having only a single team as the study group. When a "team" is the independent variable, it is a very complex, multidimensional variable. It is necessary to study a full range of potential outcomes that can be directly related back to the educational strategies chosen (Schmitt et al. 1988).

CONCLUSION

As learning more and more becomes a shared process, the diverse participants discover much about themselves, each other, and the world beyond. Because of the interactive nature of the experiences, each learning situation is a unique process, a creation of new learnings from the participants themselves. This shared learning is most effective when focused on a common purpose, much like the coherent light of a laser beam. Unlike the scattered light rays of the ordinary light bulb, the laser captures the oscillations of atoms, shaping their energy into a singular, transformed, powerful beam.

Collaborative education can be our "laser of opportunity," transforming the diffused educational efforts of our diverse health care professions into a powerful unified force. In the rapidly evolving world of health care, the discipline-specific health care approach will merge into a global one as we lose the urge to find boundaries. No longer need we stress "my professional autonomy" because of the reality that we are each an integral part of a larger "health care world."

Adams, L. J. and Miller, M. E. (1995). *Interdisciplinary Teams Training Project Resource Manual.* Denver, CO: University of Colorado Health Sciences Center, Colorado AHEC System.

AHEC (1995, April). *Area Health Education Centers: A National Resource,* 2nd edition [Brochure]. Rockville, MD: AHEC and Special Programs, Department of Health and Human Services.

Al-Saud, Sultan. (1994). United nations. In Association of Space Explorers. *The Greatest Adventure.* Sidney, Australia: C. Pierson Publishers, p. 140.

Alexander, G., Fera, B., and Ellis, R. (1996, March). From the students: Learning continuous improvement by doing it. *Joint Commission Journal of Quality Improvement, 22*(3), 198–205.

Barnum, B. (1990, Feb.). At New York University the Division of Nursing Develops a Model for Nursing and Medical School Collaboration. *Nursing and Health Care ,11* (2), 89–90.

Batalden, P. (1996). Stakeholders and reflections on improving health professions education: What's next? *Joint Commission Journal of Quality Improvement, 22* (3), 229–232.

Beatty, P. R. (1989). Attitudes and perceptions of nursing students toward preparation for interdisciplinary health care teams. *Journal of Advanced Nursing, 12,* 21–27.

Bevis, E. (1988). New directions for a new age. In *National League for Nursing Curriculum Revolution: Mandate for Change,* Pub. 15-2224. New York: National League for Nursing, pp. 27–52.

Bower, G. and Hilgard, E. (1981). *Theories of Learning,* 5th edition. Englewood Cliffs, NJ: Prentice-Hall, Inc.

Chamings, P., Maree, S., Hodges, L., and Marce, N. (1989, May). Anesthesia nursing: A collaborative model for graduate education. *Nursing and Health Care, 10* (5), 270–275.

Cleghorn, G. and Headrick, L. (1996, March). The PDSA cycle at the core of learning in health professions education. *Joint Commission Journal of Quality Improvement, 22* (3), 206–212.

Collins, M. (1994). "100,000 out." In Association of Space Explorers. *The Greatest Adventure.* Sidney, Australia: C. Pierson Publishers, pp. 217–218.

Covey, S. P. (1989). *Seven Habits of Highly Effective People.* New York: Simon and Schuster.

Covey, S. P. (1990). *Principle-Centered Leadership.* New York: Simon and Schuster.

Curley, T., Orloff, T. M,. and Tymann, B. (1994). *Health Professions Education Linkages: Community-Based Primary Care Training.* Washington, D.C.: National Governor's Association.

Deming, W. E. (1991). *Out of the Crisis.* Cambridge, MA: Massachusetts Institute of Technology, Center for Advanced Engineering Study.

Dewey, J. (1939). Experience and education. In S. B. Merriam (1984) (Ed.), *Selected Readings on Philosophy and Adult Education.* Malabar, FL: Robert E. Krieger Publishing Company.

Ducanis, A. J. and Golin, A. K. (1979). *The Interdisciplinary Health Care Team.* Germantown, MD: Aspen Systems Corporation.

Forbes, E. J. and Fitzsimmons, V. (1993, July). Education: The key for holistic interdisciplinary collaboration. *Holistic Nursing Practice, 7* (4), 1–10.

Ford, L. C. and Silver, H. K. (1967). The expanded role of the nurse in child care. *Nursing Outlook, 15* (8), 43–45.

Gelmon, S. (1996). Can educational accreditation drive interdisciplinary learning in the health professions? *Joint Commission Journal of Quality Improvement, 22* (3), 213–222.

Glazkov, Y. (1994). Space Thinking. In Association of Space Explorers. *The Greatest Adventure.* Sidney, Australia: C. Pierson Publishers, p. 138.

Hamric, A. B., Spross, J., and Hanson, C. (1996). *Advanced Nursing Practice: An Integrative Approach.* Philadelphia: W. Saunders.

Harman, L., Carlson, L., Darr, K., Harper, D., Horak, B. and Cawley, J. (1996). Blessed are the flexible: The George Team. *Joint Commission Journal of Quality Improvement, 22* (3), 188–197.

Hayward, K.S., Powell, L. T., and McRoberts, J. (1996, Fall). Changes in student perception of interdisciplinary practice in the rural setting. *Journal of Allied Health, 25* (3), 315–327.

Headrick, L. A., Knapp, M., Neuhauser, D., Gelmon, S., Norman, L., Quinn, D., and Baker, R. (1996, March). Working from upstream to improve health care: The IHI Interdisciplinary Education Collaborative. *Joint Commission Journal of Quality Improvement, 22* (3), 149–164.

Henderson, V. (1966). *The Nature of Nursing.* New York: The Macmillan Company.

Institute for Healthcare Improvements, Interdisciplinary Professional Education Collaborative (1996, March). *Joint Commission Journal of Quality Improvement, 22* (3), 149–232.

Institute of Medicine. (1972). Educating for the health team. *Report of the Conference on the Interrelationships of Educational Programs for Health Professions.* Washington, D.C.: National Academy of Sciences.

Ivey, S., Brown, K., Teski, Y., and Silverman, D. (1988, August). A model for teaching about interdisciplinary practice in health care settings. *Journal of Allied Health, 17* (3), 189–195.

Johnson, T., Belanger, M., Hartman, C., Glover, K., Nall, W., and Shoemaker, D. (1995). *MU/CMH Interdisciplinary Program, January 23–March 17, 1995.* Unpublished manuscript.

Joel, L. (1988). Impact of DRGs on basic nursing education and curriculum implications. In *National League for Nursing Curriculum Revolution: Mandate for Change,* Pub. 15-224. New York: National League for Nursing, pp. 9–26.

Knowles, M. (1990). *The Adult Learner: A Neglected Species.* Houston: Gulf Publishing Company.

Kuehn, A. F. (1995, July). An interdisciplinary education and collaborative practice pilot in rural Missouri. A paper presented at the 21st Annual Conference of the National Organization of Nurse Practitioner Faculty (NONPF). Keystone, CO.

Kuehn, A. F. (1996, June). *Documentation of Patient Encounter Using a Database Program.* Paper presented at the 1st International Nursing Education Conference. Hamilton, Ontario, Canada.

Lewin, K. (1952). Group decisions and social change. In Swanson, G. E., Newcomb, T. M., and Hartley, E. L. *Readings in Social Psychology.* New York: Henry Holt and Company, pp. 459–473.

Luecht, R. M., Madsen, M. K., Taugler, M. P., and Peterson, J. (1990, Spring). Assessing professional perception: design and validation of an interdisciplinary education perception scale. *Journal of Allied Health, 19* (2), 181–191.

Mechanic, D., and Aiken, L. (1982, Sept. 16). A cooperative agenda for medicine and nursing. *New England Journal of Medicine* 307 (12), 747–750.

Merriam, S. B. (1984) (Ed.). *Selected Writings on Philosophy and Adult Education.* Malabar, FL: Robert E. Krieger Publishing Company.

Moore, S., Alemi, F., Headrick, L., Hekelman, F., Neuhauser, D., Novotny, J., and Flowers, A. (1996, March). Using learning cycles to build an interdisciplinary curriculum in CI for health professions students in Cleveland. *Joint Commission Journal of Quality Improvement, 22* (3), 165–171.

National League for Nursing (1973, May). *Nursing Education in the Seventies* [a statement approved by the membership]. New York: National League for Nursing.

Neuhauser, D. and Norman, L. (1996). Accepting the Galvin challenge: Increasing efficiency and productivity in health professions education. *Joint Commission Journal of Quality Improvement, 22* (3), 223–227.

Newman, F. (1971) (Ed.). *Report on Higher Education.* Washington, D.C.: U.S. Government Printing Office.

O'Neil, E. (1993). Health professions education for the future: Schools in service to the nation. San Francisco: Pew Health Professions Commission, Pew Charitable Trust Foundation.

Pennington, E. (1979). Interprofessional education for physicians and nurses [Doctoral Dissertation, Columbia University 1979]. *Dissertation Abstract International 40* (09), 4218B.

Pennington, E. (1981). *Interdisciplinary Education in Nursing.* New York: National League for Nursing.

Perry, W. G. (1970). *Forms of Intellectual and Ethical Development in the College Years: A Scheme.* New York: Holt, Rinehart and Winston.

Pew Health Professions Commission (1995a). *Critical Challenges: Revitalizing the Health Professions for the 21st Century.* San Francisco: Center for the Health Professions UCSF.

Pew Health Professions Commission (1995b, January). *Interdisciplinary Collaborative Teams in Primary Care.* San Francisco: WCSF Center for the Health Professions.

Piaget, J. (1970). The epistemology of interdisciplinary relationships. In L. Apostel (Ed.). *Interdisciplinarity: Problems of Teaching and Research in Universities.* Nice, France: Organization of Economic Cooperation and Development, pp. 127–139.

Reverby, S. (1987). *Ordered to Care: The Dilemma of American Nursing 1850–1945.* Cambridge: Cambridge University Press.

Reynolds, J. (1996, Feb.). Collaborative Learning. *PT Magazine, 4* (2), 47–53.

Roberts, M. (1954). *American Nursing.* New York: Macmillan.

Satin, D. (1986). *Association of Gerontology in Higher Education Faculty Development Conference Report, June 2–6.* Kennebunkport, ME.

Satin, D. (1987). The difficulties of interdisciplinary education: Lessons from three failures and a success. *Educational Gerontology 13,* 53–69.

Schien, E. H. (1972). *Professional Education: Some New Directions.* Profile sponsored by Carnegie Commission on Higher Education. St. Louis: McGraw-Hill.

Schmitt, M. H., Farrell, M.P., and Heinemann, G. D. (1988). Conceptual and methodological problems in studying the effects of interdisciplinary geriatric teams. *The Gerontologist, 28* (6), 753–764.

Senge, P. M. (1990). *The Fifth Discipline.* New York: Currency Doubleday.

Siegler, E. and Whitney, F. (1994). *Nurse-Physician Collaboration.* New York: Springer Publishing Company.

Slack, M. and McEwen, M. (1993). Pharmacy student participation in interdisciplinary community-based training. *American Journal of Pharmaceutical Education 57,* 251–257.

Snyder, M. (1981). Preparation of nursing students for health care teams. *International Journal of Nursing Studies, 18* (2), 115–122.

Toffler, A. (1980). *The Third Wave.* New York: Bantam Books.

United States Department of Health, Education and Welfare. (1963) *Toward Quality in Nursing: Needs and Goals. Report of the Surgeon General's Consultant Group on Nursing.* Public Health Service Publication 992, Washington, D.C.: U.S. Government Printing Office.

Valiga, T. (1988). Curriculum Outcomes and Cognitive Development: New Perspectives for Nursing Education. *National League for Nursing Curriculum Revolution: Mandate for Change,* Pub. 15–2224. New York: National League for Nursing, pp. 177–200.

Vinal, D. (1987, June). Interdisciplinary Health Team Care: Nursing Education in Rural Health Settings. *Journal of Nursing Education, 26* (6), 258–259.

Transformational 15
Leadership

Toni J. Sullivan

INTRODUCTION

In the first part of this book, especially Chapters 1 and 2, and again in Chapter 9, a compelling case is made for the importance of transformational leadership to the strength and viability of collaborative practice systems in health care settings. Planned systems of collaboration, encompassed within supportive, albeit complex, environments were recognized as the structural and functional collaborative models that would thrive and would achieve likely successful outcomes. Leadership—especially transformational leadership—was recognized as central to the type of supportive environment required to facilitate collaboration.

This chapter, because of the centrality of transformational leadership to collaboration, is devoted to transformational leadership. The intent is to inform and educate collaborators and leaders and would-be-collaborators and would-be-leaders about this exciting and important leadership model. Specifically, transformational leadership is described and defined from a structural perspective. The characteristics of transformational leaders, group members, and environment are explored. Considered are some ways that transformational leadership and an environment structured by transformational leadership can facilitate collaboration. Also considered is the important topic of how to go about developing or becoming transformational leaders. Finally, presented in this chapter is a brief case study of the author's experience in participating in the creation of an environment enriched by transformational leadership in the university school of nursing at which she serves as dean.

This chapter merely presents a sampling of this rich topic; it is not meant to be exhaustive. The reader's attention is called to the expert references listed at the end of the chapter. Those who wish to pursue this topic more extensively would be advised to turn to these carefully selected references.

WHY TRANSFORMATIONAL LEADERSHIP?

In a global era of instant and massive communications, rapidly expanding and exploding sociotechnical acumen, international and boundaryless markets, and increasing awareness that tried and true paradigms of human systems of functioning do not work any longer; change—rapid, complex, dynamic—is the new reality. Change is the constant; all else is motion.

Coping with change in any complex organization, not surprisingly, requires the best effort initiatives of a multitude of workers—all the workers in an organization (Koetter 1990, Porter-O'Grady 1993, Porter-O'Grady and Wilson 1995.) A diversity of skills and people are needed in organizations to make necessary changes. The more disparate the talents and skills of the players in the organization, the more effective the participants can be in addressing the challenges of change and the more successful the organization can be in responding to its service needs and adjusting to, coping with, and managing change.

A central feature of modern organizations, according to Koetter (1990), is interdependence, whereby no one has complete autonomy of functioning and most employees are tied to many others by the work, technology, management systems, and hierarchy. In patient care delivery, health care providers are increasingly tied together by the complexity of care needs and the integration of care delivery and payment systems (see Chapter 3). The organization cannot change or evolve unless the wonderfully disparate members become unified in their diversity or align to achieve common goals in their quest of their vision. Working together in an interdependent system requires effective interpersonal and professional relationships. Connections between working professionals and their knowledge, skills, and talents must be made and sustained.

The function of leadership, increasingly in the decade of the 1990s and as we approach the millennium, is to make change happen, set the direction for change, and position an organization to prosper in a challenging and extraordinarily competitive marketplace (Koetter 1995). The way to lead change in this changing world is to empower the workers, to develop them as co-leaders in the enterprise. Transformational leadership is the empowerment model of leadership (Evans 1994). Its central feature is to develop the members as self-directing, actively participating, practicing experts on behalf of the organization and the mutually agreed upon vision and goals.

As the transformational leader succeeds in empowering the workers as described, the leader's behaviors must undergo substantial transformation from a superordinate style of functioning to a peer style of functioning. "In today's socio-technical organizations, the culture is collective (team), the expectation is involvement and investment, and the style of implementation is facilitative and integrative" (Porter-O'Grady 1993). No one person has the only best strategy, vision, or methodology. All participants are recognized as full partners in the organizational venture.

PROFILE OF TRANSFORMATIONAL LEADERSHIP AND THE TRANSFORMED ORGANIZATION

Transformational leadership is helping a group create their vision in alignment with each individual group member's sense of purpose and values, thus assuring the motivation to achieve the vision and to meet the goals of the organization (Koerner and Bunkers 1992). That is all, but that is a lot. What are the qualities needed to be a transformational leader? How does a transformational leader accomplish the task at hand?

Various scholars have listed the desired qualities of transformational leaders: that they possess high self-esteem and are self-confident, self-directed, honest and straightforward, highly energetic and persistent in pursuit of goals, loyal and committed to the welfare of those in their sphere of influence, and committed to the people and the welfare of the organization with which they are associated (Flarey 1993, Koetter 1990, Porter-O'Grady 1993). These qualities are needed because, more than any other member of the group, the leader must cope with lack of control over direction and outcomes and with constant change over which he or she presides precariously. The analogy that comes to mind is riding a tiger or having a tiger by the tail. Such dynamic ambiguity, moreover, usually is very public and universally experienced.

Nevertheless, the leader's job is to get the people in the organization to follow the leader into a new collective place where they are not sure they want to be. The personal qualities—*strengths*—of the leader, along with professional qualities ought to add up to *credibility*. The group needs to believe the messages of the leader, even though the transformational leader does not begin to have all of the answers.

Porter-O'Grady (1993, p. 54) offers a thoughtful set of professional/personal behaviors transformational leaders evidence:

1.   The ability to call the players together to construct a common vision which reflects the values and participation of those affected by it.
2.   The insight to obtain a high level of participation from a broad cross section of players with the skills necessary to achieve successful outcomes.
3.   A well developed service focus that reflects the core values of the health care enterprise in ways that can be expressed and validated. [Although written for a patient care setting, this precept applies to all categories of health care.]
4.   Low control needs, e.g., the ability to allow expression of accountability from a variety of places in the organization depending on the issue and on the place where decisions can most effectively be made.
5.   A high level of trust in all members of the organization is evidenced by encouraging opportunity-finding, solution-seeking and risk-taking to occur.
6.   Openness to exploration of different ways to do day-to-day work, achieve outcomes and serve the community more creatively.
7.   Willingness to model vulnerability and openness to what she or he doesn't know and to practice equity in both role and relationship.

Vision, participation, value-laden, freedom to act responsibly and creatively, trust, openness, and learning are the attributes of the transformational leader and the transformed organization. The organization is comprised as a community of varied people with various positions but with common cause. They engage in teamwork to do their work, recognizing working together as the only way to accomplish their mutually agreed upon goals. Decision-making in the transformational organization is by consensus, with the group working through issues and reaching a decision. Even though it may not be everyone's first choice, all members abide by the consensus decision.

The organization with transformational leadership in place may be referred to as a shared-governance model. A surrogate term for collaboration, *shared governance* is defined in Chapter 2 as an organizational arrangement with a highly participatory staff empowered to function cooperatively with both management and colleagues, and leadership that empowers staff. The organization could be referred to as a learning organization. The learning organization, according to Senge (1990), is an organizational system requiring systems thinking to function within it. It is a system of people who undergo a profound shift from seeing themselves as individual and separate from other workers to seeing themselves as connected to the others in the organization (and world). Whereas problems were seen as caused by someone or something beyond the self, they are now seen as connected to themselves. "We" are part of the problems and "we" are part of the solutions. This is a paradigm shift in organizational behavior and requires a paradigm shift in organizational leadership.

Learning organizations are flexible organizations. They are able to respond speedily to opportunities or threats. Organizational structures that do exist aim to facilitate both rapid response and team decision-making. Organizational hierarchy is, therefore, minimal to nonexistent, as are standing staff committees. Most of the work is accomplished by formally or informally organized teams and ad hoc committees. The organization as a whole can usually best be described as an adhocracy, rather than a bureaucracy.

In a beautifully simple presentation of the characteristics of successful leaders of the late 20th century, Bennis (1984), after exhaustive study, identifies four traits. Although not labeling these 90 leaders studied as transformational leaders, the traits of these leaders would appear to apply to that paradigm. Successful leaders evidence management of attention, management of meaning, management of trust, and management of self (p. 146). Management of attention refers to the ability to get the attention of the group through a compelling vision that brings others to a place they have not been before. Bennis (1984) and Koetter (1990, 1995) both stress in their own styles that the vision need not be elegant or complete; it is better, in fact, when it is not detailed fully and when it is not mystical. But it must get the attention of the group and motivate them to want to pursue the direction of the vision and want to participate in both further creating the vision and in fulfilling the vision.

Koetter (1995) tells of one organization's vision statement that was excruciatingly complete with detailed objectives, procedures, and strategies outlined. The organization was never enthused about it and quickly became buried in the trivia of the details. Bennis (1984), on the other hand, relates a story of a great cellist and his protégés. The pupils told Bennis why the cellist was so great: "He doesn't waste our time" (p. 147). The idea is that the cellist knew what he wanted. His expectations for the pupils were clear. They had a shared vision with him of their potential and went about the business of working to achieve it. The vision may be an idea, a goal or goals, a sense of outcomes, or a direction.

Management of meaning refers to the ability to use a metaphor to make your vision clear to others; the ability to communicate ideas; to create meaning. If the leader lacks the ability to convey the vision, the leader will not successfully lead the group. Although at first glance, this may seem a silly and trivial idea, rather, it is exactly on target. Whatever linguistic device is used, the vision must be made clear.

Management of trust is an essential element of leadership in all organizations. Bennis (1984) likens trust to reliability and constancy. People in the organization need to be able to depend on the leader. Regardless of the dynamic change that is swirling around them, the leader is reassuringly there for them. People count on the leader. Comments, such as, "Whether you like it or not, you know where she is coming from," are reflective of the ability of the leader to inspire trust.

Management of self, the fourth trait identified by Bennis (1984) as characteristic of the 90 successful leaders he studied, refers to knowing one's skills and deploying them effectively. Bennis also discusses the importance of keeping one's own counsel concerning doubts and misgivings. The leader is a sower of seeds and needs to be careful concerning which seeds she or he sows.

Leaders know themselves; they have a realistic perspective on their strengths and weaknesses. They are secure in their abilities to succeed in leading others. Leaders do not have a concept of failure. They may make mistakes, early and often, but these are not failures. They are learning experiences and are growth opportunities. They focus on achieving success, not on avoiding failure. They do not necessarily play it safe; they take risks. Leaders are mature, talented people.

Before turning to a discussion of the attributes of group members, a brief discussion of how leaders motivate participants will serve to complete the profile of transformational leaders. Clearly, the leader's ability to articulate and communicate vision is a major motivational act. The whole set of behaviors that leaders engage in with their colleagues in the organization also should serve as motivational tools.

Koetter (1990) tells us that leaders motivate by 1) articulating vision in a manner that stresses the values of the audience; 2) involving people in deciding how to achieve the vision, which gives them a sense of control over their work; 3) supporting employees' efforts to achieve the vision by coaching, feedback, and role modeling, which enables professional growth and higher self-esteem of workers; and 4) rewarding success, which increases the sense of belonging and accomplishment of the members. What is most exciting about this conceptualization of motivational leadership is the assertion by Koetter that when all of these elements are in place, work itself becomes intrinsically motivating.

A major feature of this paradigm of transformational leadership and the learning organization, in fact, is that work itself takes on new meaning. Work is no longer merely viewed as instrumental—something one does to earn wages; work is viewed as sacred—something one does because it has intrinsic benefits (Senge 1990, p. 5). This is not a new idea. Plato viewed work as sacred over 2000 years ago. Work is seen as the highest expression of human being. It is a good, and it leads to good. Work, in this paradigm, can be fun. It is always worthwhile. It energizes us. Leaders and group members will evidence bursts of energy propelling them toward grand accomplishments. The resulting accomplishments are extraordinarily satisfying and empowering!

EMPOWERED ORGANIZATIONAL MEMBERS

People in an empowered organization know that people are the significant components of the organization; they are important members of an organizational community: their work is exciting and important; and learning and competence matter greatly to the organization (Bennis 1984). The staff of an empowered organization become well-integrated adults. They trust others and they themselves are trustworthy. They treat others with respect and consideration and expect the same treatment in return. They are not fixated on equity but expect fair treatment by leadership and peers.

The members of the organization need information and data about the organization, just as does the leadership. Lacking the big picture, members are unable to participate in consensual decision making or assume leadership and accountability in a particular sphere of the organization's work. Members are not able to support the vision unless they have all the information necessary to make informed and intelligent decisions.

The members of the organization, as has already been mentioned, are a varied and diverse group by design. In health care organizations, the norm has been, and will largely continue to be, that workers are also an intellectually talented and highly educated group. A group such as this must have good and timely data available to them. The group also must learn to be a team or teams, and to think and act as a team. In learning organizations, individuals do not make decisions; teams do. Individuals do not achieve organizational goals; teams do. Leaders are not solely responsible for the successes of the organization; all members earn and receive an appropriate share of the credit.

Bill Russell, the great basketball center for the Boston Celtics in the 1960s, is eloquent on the subject of teams: "By design and by talent," he wrote about the champion Celtics team, "we were a team of specialists, and like a team of specialists in any field, our performance depended both on individual excellence and on how well we worked together. None of us had to strain to understand that we had to complement each other's specialties; it was simply a fact, and we all tried to figure out ways to make our combination more effective. . . ."

"Every so often," Russell further stated:

> [A] Celtic game would heat up so that it became more than a physical or even mental game, and would be magical. The feeling is difficult to describe and I certainly never talked about it when I was playing. When it happened I could feel my play rise to a new level. . . . It would surround not only me and the other Celtics but also the players on the other team, and even the referees. . . . At that special level, all sorts of odd things happened. The game would be in the white heat of competition, and yet I wouldn't feel competitive, which is a miracle in itself. . . . The game would move so fast that every fake, cut, and pass would be surprising and yet nothing would surprise me. It was almost as if we were playing in slow motion. During those spells, I could almost sense how the next play would develop and where the next shot would be taken. To me, the key was that both teams had to be playing at their peaks, and they had to be competitive (Russell and Branch 1979, quoted in Senge 1990, pp. 233–234).

In this marvelous anecdote, Bill Russell describes professional relationships and communications, teamwork and team alignment toward mutually agreed upon goals. The result is an exquisite focus on team excellence in playing the game. Although there are enormous bursts of energy in rising to new heights, there is no wasted energy on individual agendas or on group members whose goals are out of alignment with those of the rest of the team. This team clearly loves its work and is just as clearly having a good time.

The September 15, 1996, edition of the *St. Louis Post-Dispatch*, in reporting on the settlement of the 99-day strike between the union and management of the McDonnell Douglas Corp. had a headline and sub-headline stating: "McDonnell's new teams mean challenges for machinists: Old work rules will disappear" (p.1, Section E). The article describes that when the workers return to work on the coming Monday, they will find that their jobs have changed. Many of the rules that governed their work in the past are going to disappear. Teams called High Performance Work Organizations will manage the daily work activities.

The article reports that a lot of the machinists are angry. They have a history of believing they have been treated unfairly by management and do not trust them. Middle management is very fearful of the new teams. They see the teams as threatening their power in the organization. The article continues in the same vein. There is no discussion of preparation or education or consultation or test runs or shared planning. It is terribly difficult to believe a major corporation could be so naive. Time will tell. Although beyond the scope of this chapter to present fully, developing staff as a team is a time-consuming and challenging task. One brief model will have to serve as an overview of the venture that is team development.

Heim (1993), cited in Mason (1994), discusses a four-phase process model of team building. Occurring over a substantial period of months or years, the phases overlap and disappear and reappear depending on several factors. New members, new tasks, and new opportunities as well as group accomplishments and group disappointments may bring into focus a phase that the group was done with for a while. The phases are forming, storming, norming, and performing. The group and the leadership would like to be and remain at the performing level, and works to that end, but it is not always feasible or realistic to plateau at that high performance level.

In stage, or phase, 1: *forming*, team members-to-be feel all the behaviors of newness—excitement, enthusiasm, anticipation, and perhaps anxiety. (Leaders at this stage need to provide clear direction and perhaps structure to the group work.) In stage, or phase, 2: *storming*, feelings of the group may include discomfort with newness; members may be resistant to change and feel frustrated about the work required or the chances of success. Group members may be annoyed or bored with each other. Communications may be distorted by ego-driven behaviors and personal agendas. (Leaders may also become discouraged, but cannot give up. It may be time for an external consultant. In any event, the lines of communication must be kept open by any means available, whether using a time-out, humor, or even food.)

Phase 3: *norming*, includes the new ability to communicate openly and constructively with each other. Criticisms of past practices or current approaches can be made with mutual well-being in view. There is a sense of relief that the team has progressed to this point. A new perception of team cohesiveness characterized by team spirit and harmony pervades group meetings and activities. This is the time when the group should seriously plan its future endeavors. Group members' activities and responsibilities need to be clarified. The team members' goals need to be developed as team goals, hopefully coming into alignment. (The leader is a full participant in this stage, either from the sidelines or as a team member. Clearly, the leader approves or delegates approval of all the major decisions made by the team. The main roles of the leader, however, are more as coach, mentor, and cheerleader.)

The last phase (stage 4) of team building is *performing*, a phase of implementation and accomplishment of goal-directed activities. Members have insight gained from actual experience of teamwork. They have a better understanding of each other's strengths and weaknesses. The team may evidence a strong sense of team pride and satisfaction with team progress. At the same time, the team may be tackling constructive change in their structure and functioning. (The leader's job is to allow the team maximum freedom and flexibility in performing, hold out high expectations, reward success, and see to it that the team has necessary supports to continue performing at a high level.)

Although this model is useful for conceptualizing team building, it is frightening to contemplate movement back over the early phases once the team has moved ahead to the performing phase. Movement is not likely to go from performing to norming and stay there until it progresses ahead again to performing. It certainly is not going to move backward from performing to forming while skipping norming and storming. It is a risk that movement backward from performing is more likely to degenerate into storming.

It is this author's experience that in terms of leadership behaviors, much of the time is spent supporting progress made and avoiding storming behavior. Integration of new staff into an organization and its team(s) through a carefully planned orientation program can avoid the storming phase. Also, individuals who have matured to become self-assured team members and productive contributors to the team's and organization's goals will not regress in their behaviors—not for long in any event. These people would be more likely to resign from the team than to behave in ways that would not meet their high standards.

Culture of Leadership

Every team and every team effort in the organization requires leadership at the level at which the decision-making has occurred and the work has been planned. Leadership, in fact, must be evidenced in all places within and outside the organization where the work of the organization intends to have an impact. Leadership, then, is the prerogative of many people in many different places throughout the organization. The organization is essentially a community of many leaders and many followers, frequently changing places depending on the particular activity that is occurring. Many staff who are leaders in one or more activities are also followers in one or more activities. Both positions are of great importance and valued by the organization.

Transformational leadership in a transformed organization ultimately matures into a leadership-centered culture in which myriad mature professionals, skilled in teamwork and team learning, committed to the organization's vision, and proficient in the work of the organization exercise energetic leadership throughout the organization. In a leadership-centered culture, leadership and leaders are valued and leaders support and encourage each other. Although open and vulnerable regarding their strengths and limitations, and their accomplishments and mistakes, they are not alone. Their leader peers rally to their side in difficult times and let them know how they, too, experienced similar challenges and how they learned from them.

Institutionalizing a leadership-centered culture is the ultimate act of leadership (Koetter 1990). The transformational leader not only focuses on the work output itself but also on the context in which the work occurs and the relationship of each team member to the work (Porter-

O'Grady 1994). The leader has to analyze and critique the performance of tasks and the accomplishment of work objectives from both a team perspective and a developmental perspective. The traditional focus on task alone as achieved by the individual worker—who is held accountable—is inappropriate in a leadership-centered culture. (The exception to this precept is, of course, the transformational leader, who is held accountable for the organization's overall performance in achieving the vision.) Individual and team commitment to a project, quality of team interrelationships and interactions, extent to which team members worked together to complement each other's strengths and limitations, and the leadership provided by the team or project leader are all elements to be considered in an evaluation process. An ongoing feature of transformational leadership is professional and team development. The organization—a learning organization—is, in fact, one big learning laboratory.

Both the leader and the staff in a learning organization have to learn the "fine art" (Peterson 1994) of problem solving together. The leader has to learn to solicit information, ideas, and assessments (input) from the staff and must learn to listen carefully and respectfully. The staff have to learn how to provide input that focuses on finding solutions, not just on articulating problems. Staff input that places blame or is ego driven is simply not allowed within the communication guidelines (unwritten, but universally understood).

If the organization, in fact, values and encourages risk taking and the leader welcomes the empowerment of staff, then the leader and the organization must accept mistakes and occasional subpar performance as lessons to be learned by others and by the self (leader). How the leader behaves when criticism must be tendered is probably the greatest test of the leader and of the strength of the organization. The leader allows herself or himself to be open and vulnerable when assessing and critiquing her or his part in an organizational mistake or disappointment. The leader faces up to the difficult task of evaluation, as described. At the same time, clear expectations for future performance by both team and individuals are laid out, and team and individual progress is monitored as specified.

Although beyond the scope of this chapter to lay out a framework for performance assessment in a learning organization, it can be said that the leader can be very patient and developmental with both teams and individuals with respect to the work to be accomplished as long as they show that they are open to growth and change and to being fully participating teams and members of the team. To return to the framework proposed by Heim (1993) for team building, a staff member who does not progress beyond the storming phase when the rest of the team has moved beyond that phase should probably be removed from the team and, perhaps, should leave the organization.

Environment

The environment—organizational, instrumental, physical, and cultural—should be obstacle free. Systems and structures in place and supported should facilitate the leaders' and members' achieving the vision and goals of the organization. Too often, Koetter (1995) tells us, an elephant seems to be blocking the pathway to achievement. Sometimes the elephants are actual; sometimes they are perceived. In either case, they are real. Various job categories may be outdated, performance appraisals may assess inappropriate behaviors while the leader gives lip service to team behaviors, bosses may refuse to change their behaviors; the list could be very lengthy. Much of the work of the transformational leader is to keep the environment as free of roadblocks as possible.

As described already, both a decentralized organizational structure and transformational leadership as a major component of the environment support decision making at the team level and enable the members to develop their leadership and membership skills. Obviously, a culture that is committed to change, to leadership, to shared decision making, and to staff development must prevail at all levels of the organization. A culture that learns from mistakes rather than punishing failures facilitates achieving desired outcomes. Flarey (1993) quotes Kanter (1991), who speaks of a culture of pride: "Positive views of people's abilities can cause improved performance as well as result from it. A culture of pride, based on success, increases confidence and motivation. It's a virtuous cycle [note the systems thinking]: performance stimulating pride stimulating performance" (p. 158).

The instrumental structures, procedures, tools and technology, and allocation of resources need to be designed and used in support of the learning organization. In a sense, the leaders and members of the organization need to be vigilant sleuths in ferreting out ways to support the work of the organization. Shared decision making by the transformational leader and the staff is important for reaching consensus about the best use of scarce resources. One of the noticeable features of a mature learning organization is the commitment of the staff to, and their success in, stretching or increasing scarce resources, rather than merely complaining about the scarcity. If an element of the environment is dysfunctional, fix it. If resources are inadequate; earn more. Much of the environment, in an empowered organization, is within the control of the members of the organization.

COLLABORATION IN AN ENVIRONMENT OF TRANSFORMATIONAL LEADERSHIP

Transformational leadership, as already noted, facilitates the creation of a shared governance model of organization, which is, as we have also noted, an organizational form of collaboration. In shared governance, the members of an organization work together as partners and peers in meeting the mutually agreed upon goals of the organization. Such an organization is a fertile field for collaborating partnerships (of two or several members) to develop and implement practices to advance patient care, education, service, research, and interorganizational endeavors, from intradisciplinary, interdisciplinary, and multidisciplinary perspectives.

The reader will recall that this organizational model celebrates diversity and valuing of each member's unique or special expertise. This means that collaborators have information and/or skills that the other(s) lacks. It means that each adds their special contribution to the whole, making collaboration an imperative for this holistic, systems view of reality (Koetter 1995). People who hold this perspective and want to achieve success in their endeavors are, thus, motivated toward collaborative functioning.

The organization, which of course, exemplifies this world view, is organized to support collaboration over time with both understanding and guidance as well as resources. It is okay for new collaborators to experience growing pains, to make mistakes, to become discouraged. We know because we have experienced all of these feelings and places, too. Many of the issues that individuals experience in working alone, such as the need to prove one's self as worthy or even superior to others and the need to "know it all," can and should disappear in a transformational environment. This point of view is extremely supportive to would-be-collaborators. In a patient care environment and, in fact, in every health care environment, the focus can instead turn to the patients and their care, or to the research design or the education of students, instead of focusing on the very real concerns that others will find one wanting or that our turf will be supplanted by others.

DEVELOPING TRANSFORMATIONAL LEADERS

An organization steeped in transformational leadership is, as stated before, a great big learning laboratory. It is a marvelous setting in which to learn to become a leader. The decentralized structure affords "junior" employees the opportunity to participate fully in project development and in shared decision-making. Much sooner than would be likely in traditional organizations, workers have an opportunity to try on leadership skills by assuming team leadership on occasion.

In addition, the transformational leader focuses far more attention on the way in which the work is performed (as well as on the product) than does the traditional leader. The staff person, in this way, is given ongoing leadership seminars by the leader.

A scenario for leadership development starts with staff recruitment. People with self-confidence, enthusiasm, and energy for the work and goals of the organization, apparent communication skills, and knowledge and skills in areas of expertise required to achieve the vision of the organization—at a level appropriate to their professional growth and development—are people sought as new recruits to the organization. Once new staff enter the organization, a comprehensive orientation needs to occur. Many members of the organization ought to participate. One senior member of the organization, however, ought to be a mentor and act as a mentor over the first year or more of service to the organization.

Generally, challenging opportunities should be provided to junior staff, first through team membership and increasingly through team leadership. Internal seminars and individual guidance sessions, as well as ongoing opportunities to attend external professional meetings and programs, are a deliberate part of the leadership development plan. Organizational resources are, of course, allocated to professional and leadership development as a priority activity.

THE TRANSFORMATION OF A SCHOOL OF NURSING: A CASE STUDY

The last section of this chapter is a brief case study of one school's approach to transforming from a very traditional model of leadership and faculty organization to a model of transformational leadership and an empowered faculty intending to provide national and international leadership in university education in nursing well into the 21st century. This case study is adapted from a presentation entitled "Transforming a School of Nursing" that was offered by the author in conjunction with two colleagues at the American Nurses Association (ANA) convention, June 16, 1996. This case study is not intended to offer a formula for success. It is but one school's approach, and it is provided so that the reader can choose from it whatever portion(s) he or she would like to use. It also demonstrates that members of one organization were able to learn and grow together. In the process, they did many things wrong and experienced many growing pains. They, nevertheless, persevered and have achieved many successes including an organizational transformation of which all are excited and proud. The case study offers a framework and process for change; it is an overview of outcomes of this ongoing change process.

In one school-wide evaluative exercise, faculty were asked to describe transformational changes that had occurred in the school (over a 7-year period). The five transformational changes they identified are outlined in Figure 15-1. Additionally, faculty were asked to use phrases that archetypified the way they see themselves now. The five top phrases are shown in Figure 15-2. At present, this faculty and this school have no shortage of energy, enthusiasm, brainpower, and opportunities. Making wise choices in pursuit of our shared vision is our greatest challenge.

It was not always so. Seven short years ago, all faculty and staff were discontented with the school's direction (or perceived lack of direction) and were dissatisfied with their work assignments and the lack of challenges coupled with the abundance of frustrations they experienced in their day-to-day functioning. While the school had strong and well-established baccalaureate and master's programs in nursing, the faculty had sought fruitlessly over a 14-year period to establish a doctoral program in nursing. In addition, although a Carnegie Research 1 university, the school had little or no funded faculty research. Despite the presence of a long-standing and well-regarded nurse practitioner program, faculty practice was not a priority, and it was not recognized by the faculty as such. Like many state universities, the budget was being cut, rather than expanded. Over a 3-year period beginning some 7 years ago, the budget of the school was cut by 12%. Salaries that were already too low could not be raised as they should have been. A mentality of retrenchment, rather than growth, frequently poisoned the atmosphere despite the best efforts to remain upbeat.

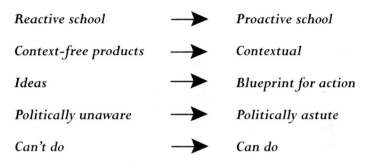

Reactive school	⟶	*Proactive school*
Context-free products	⟶	*Contextual*
Ideas	⟶	*Blueprint for action*
Politically unaware	⟶	*Politically astute*
Can't do	⟶	*Can do*

Figure 15-1. *Transformational changes (as defined by faculty).*

"Transformed, but becoming"

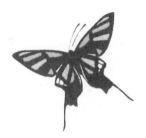

"Create our own future and don't wait for it to happen"

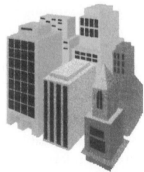

"Opportunities chase us"

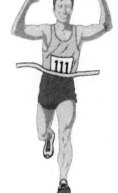

"Bricks build structure instead of walls"

"We are Mighty Morphins that metamorphose"

Figure 15-2. *Phrases describing faculty (as defined by faculty).*

Planning
Strategic
Niche
Environment
Physical
Organizational
Instrumental
Cultural
Leadership
Transformational
Faculty
Community
Shared meanings
Shared vision
Shared goals

Figure 15-3.   *Transformational change processes.*

Some of the actions taken on the author's part as dean may be attributed to experience; others, to philosophical conviction, dumb luck, openness to learning from others, and the persistence that comes from a growing attachment and commitment to the organization and its people. The University of Missouri–Columbia Sinclair School of Nursing was and is a fine school of nursing. This case study is about growth and change of direction; not about rescue. In doing a retrospective analysis for the ANA presentation, four major elements were identified as comprising the transformational change process. They are outlined in Figure 15-3. In interaction, they complemented and facilitated the efficacy of each in a synergistic way. The terms used in the school, rather than the terms more commonly used in the literature, on transformational leadership, are used here. *Developing a shared vision* is thus referred to as *strategic planning* (an older term, but one that works well), and *shared governance* is referred to as *community* (a term that accurately presents the members of this case study).

Planning

Beginning with the interview process and continuing through the myriad individual meetings, a consistent theme heard was a yearning for change and growth. Although there was great disagreement, of course, on the what, how, and who of change, there was, however, universal agreement on the need for movement from the status quo. The author had shared with faculty, staff, alumnae, and university administration the conviction that the school could be a fully established and leading university school of nursing—with a doctoral program in nursing, a strong profile of funded faculty research, exemplary faculty practice in advanced roles— and be a force in the academic health center. Too many of the faculty did not see themselves or the school as existing on that high plane. They simply did not believe in themselves or these possibilities. Why not? The analogy that comes to mind is of the major league pitcher, Tug McGraw, who pitched the New York Mets to the pennant. His mantra for himself and his team was: "Ya Gotta Believe!"

In May of 1990, the entire faculty, professional staff, and school administration went away together for a 2.5-day retreat, the purpose of which was to begin to develop a strategic plan for the school. The intended agenda was to begin to bring everyone's ideas for the school into focus and begin to develop a common agenda. Many faculty were shocked by this event. Never having participated in such an activity before, they could not see how it would help; they saw it as a waste of the school's scarce resources. Other faculty thought it was okay but that the time could be better spent grading papers or completing other tasks. A minority were enthusiastic about the potential for the event.

The retreat was extremely successful; almost everyone participated with some enthusiasm. One of the guidelines that was implemented consistently—and still is—is to give everyone an opportunity to be heard. Everyone contributed something to the thinking and planning and, therefore, began to feel some sense of ownership and pride. The planning model and documents that emerged from that retreat were modeled essentially the same as those used to this day. They consist of a mission statement, priority goals, ongoing 5-year objectives, and a resource assessment (repeated annually). In a later year, we began to outline strategies for pursuing the goals and achieving the objectives.

The strategic planning definition printed in our school's handbook is the classic definition by Drucker (1973):

> Strategic planning is a continuous systematic process of making risk-taking decisions today with the greatest possible knowledge of their effects on the future: organizing efforts necessary to carry out these decisions:

and evaluating results of these decisions against expected outcomes through reliable feedback mechanisms. (p. 125)

It lives and works for us. New faculty are oriented to our concept of planning and to our plan. Continuing faculty are very conversant with both planning and our plan.

Dating from that first landmark retreat, the entire faculty, professional staff, and administration meet together in workshops and planning sessions three times annually, 3 days in May, 1–2 days in January, and 2–3 days in August. The purposes of the meetings are simply to learn together, to grow together, and to plan together. The sessions, which are jointly planned by faculty and the dean, include educational activities conducted by the faculty and/or by external experts; lively group discussions on current topics of importance; group processes to foster consensual decision-making; and review, updating, and approval of the school's plan (mission, goals, objectives, strategies). At the August workshop, an annual resource assessment of the school's fiscal performance from the prior year is reviewed by all. A major component of this assessment is an analysis and critique of the allocation of our precious resources during the prior year. (A Faculty Budget Advisory Committee also meets with the dean quarterly to advise on budget matters.) Finally, the workshops are a marvelous time to recognize individual and group accomplishments. We do this with a spirit of celebration and do it without fail.

Sometimes, because they are really very busy, certain faculty complain about having to use their time for the workshops. The ad hoc committee that plans the workshops, in turn, schedules them to be "chock full" and doesn't schedule unnecessary sessions. Mostly, however, we are all good-natured about the workshops, recognizing that the time together is essential to our continued successful functioning as a community of like-minded professionals pursuing our vision of becoming a top-ranked school of nursing. We jokingly admit that while we might complain about the time spent, we would miss the workshops if they were not held.

Faculty and staff, through this planning process, have developed a shared vision and a set of priority goals. They are in alignment about the direction the school is moving in and even the strategies to use to achieve the goals and vision. The continued existence of our undergraduate program and the numbers and qualifications of the students is one example. Clearly, some faculty are more committed to the undergraduate nursing education program than others. Every May, a straw vote is taken by the faculty to test the commitment to the bachelor of science in nursing program. Every year, an overwhelming majority vote to keep the program. By consensus, then all agree to support the program and the program continues to thrive. The numbers of admitted students are, however, controlled at a moderate level both to protect the scarce resources of the school and assure an outstanding undergraduate population. Similar exercises are engaged in with other academic programs. The clinical nurse specialist student enrollments were capped at lower numbers, while the nurse practitioner student enrollments were increased, for example.

Figure 15-4 presents the 10 priority goals of the school. Although arranged by the faculty in logical order, all goals are of equal priority to the school. The goals collectively present our shared vision. The achieve-

Priority Goal No. 1.   Offer a full range of academic nursing programs: baccalaureate, master's, doctoral, postdoctoral, and continuing education offerings responsive to changing health and health care delivery needs.

Priority Goal No. 2.   Increase significantly the fiscal, human, and material resources to accomplish the mission of the School of Nursing.

Priority Goal No. 3.   Foster collegiality and scholarship.

Priority Goal No. 4.   Develop and implement a strategic plan for information management, technology, and nursing informatics to enhance teaching, scholarship, service, and administration.

Priority Goal No. 5.   Strengthen and build cooperation among School of Nursing, the MU Health Sciences Center, and the other MU academic units.

Priority Goal No. 6.   Strengthen existing state and national ties and form additional international linkages with external constituencies.

Priority Goal No. 7.   Increase the ethnic and cultural diversity of academic, research, and service activities of the School.

Priority Goal No. 8.   Increase the visibility and enhance the reputation of the School of Nursing for excellence in academic nursing.

Priority Goal No. 9.   Strengthen the position of the School of Nursing within the University.

Priority Goal No. 10.   Increase state, national, and international leadership of the School of Nursing to improve nursing and health care delivery.

Figure 15-4.   *Priority goals.*

ment of all 10 priority goals spells excellence and recognition as a leading school of nursing in the nation and the international community. Each of the priority goals is accompanied by a set of (usually) measurable objectives. Also included for every priority goal is a set of strategies that everyone agrees to for meeting the objectives.

Figure 15-5 presents priority goal 3 and its objectives and strategies as an example. One cannot stress strongly enough how real to us these are and how much direction they provide. As an example, historically, the faculty and the ARPT (Appointment, Retention, Promotion, and Tenure) Committee had not played an aggressive role in recruitment of faculty. Because the School of Nursing did not have a Ph.D. program or an active research faculty, the school had only limited success in recruitment of outstanding faculty. The objective, "Recruit and appoint faculty to com-

Foster collegiality and scholarship

Objectives

1.   Recruite and appoint faculty to complement existing faculty with respect to priority goals.
2.   Provide an environment that fosters the development and retention of faculty.
3.   Provide an environment that fosters socialization of students as nurse scholars.
4.   Strengthen the research support infrastructure.
5.   Enhance intellectual partnerships between and among students, faculty in the school, statewide, nationally, and internationally.

Strategies

Involve faculty in active, vigorous recruitment with leadership from ARPT Committee.

Recruit and appoint faculty experienced in doctoral nursing education; further develop the extant faculty's skills in doctoral education.

Support undergraduate nurse scholars program and full development of mentoring programs for undergraduate and graduate students.

Foster faculty development with undergraduate students in the campus summer research program of minority students.

Refurbish School of Nursing beginning 1998.

Promote visibility of graduate student accomplishments through the Graduate Nurses Association.

Attend to ongoing excellent communications as a day-to-day imperative.

Continue to develop and support research consulting services.

Figure 15-5.   *Priority goal No. 3.*

plement existing faculty with respect to priority goals," is very aggressively pursued as the strategy to "involve faculty in active, vigorous recruitment with leadership from ARPT Committee" is enacted. Consequently, the school now is enjoying great success in recruiting outstanding faculty who are complementary to our strengths.

The objectives and strategies are not as perfect in form as they could be, nor are the strategies always plotted out with an explicit blueprint for action. We like our goals and strategies as they are. They work for us. Every member of the community can make a contribution to them, and they also enable us to maintain a great deal of flexibility in pursuing opportunities as they occur, if we so choose. The school has not made one decision about new ventures over the past several years that did not appear first in our objectives and/or strategies. Consequently, support and commitment have been staunch and virtually universal for all new ventures—despite the extensive shift of human and material resources that some of our new ventures have required.

When the university experienced several budget cuts by the state government from 1990–1992, they were implemented at the university level by central administration and the Board of Curators (governing board of the four-campus university system), requiring each campus to cut programs and each school to show how they would cut their programs. It was necessary to engage in a lengthy retrenchment planning exercise three times. Although these were unpleasant and difficult exercises, our strategic planning process enabled us to be well prepared to present ourselves in the most favorable and politically astute manner. The dean [the author] and faculty endeavored to keep us in control of our fate, rather than be taken over by an externally imposed plan that would destroy our vision. It was—and is—crucial to keep the vision before us regardless of external obstacles as long as we can assert with objectivity and conviction that our vision is in the best interests of the university, the profession, and society. It is not in anyone's best interests for the school to be forced to mediocrity. We capitalized on that awareness. We escaped that era with a 12% budget cut and a conviction that we would increasingly have to generate our own revenues.

A new chancellor was appointed to our campus and began his tenure late in 1993. He, too, understood that universities would increasingly have to generate their own revenues, and he made his expectations for increased revenues known—early and often. He was not in favor of program cuts per se; rather, he was in favor of the university and its schools and divisions identifying their unique niches and channeling both school and university revenues to supporting the unique niches. The next externally imposed challenge the faculty, staff, and administration then faced was identifying our unique niche. The chancellor defined niche planning in this way:

> Our approach to strategic planning—the development and funding of unique niches—is a modification of practices used in the modern corporate world. The metaphor involves considering each unit—department, school, or program—as if it were a separate business in a major corporation. Its customers can be several: the scientific and scholarly world; the world of employers; or the educated public.
>
> The approach is to build upon strengths to position ourselves in unique niches that address issues or problems commonly perceived to be very important ones. In doing so, we raise our aspirations, develop feasible pathways to success, and get people working at common purposes. The fact that the process leads to addressing important problems helps to capture national and state attention and attracts the attention and cooperation of both private donors and granting agencies.
>
> Our niches become our priorities and our resources become focused on them, not only between units but within departments and within schools. Because very high aspirations are required, several iterations of a proposed plan are typical. (Charles Kiesler, Chancellor 1994 unpublished)

Once again, we were required to respond to externally imposed authority to decide our destiny. We twice developed extensive niche plans and are now working on the third such round. Niche planning has been very helpful to us. We reflected long and hard on the what, where, how, and why of many of our programs and ventures. We identified that much of our work in education, research, and practice was occurring in rural areas with rural dwelling persons. Through niche planning we have sharpened our focus on rural nursing and health care. In a brief iteration, the school's niche is stated as "Excellence and leadership, statewide and nationally, on advancing nursing: education, research, and practice . . . for rural America and rural areas internationally." We are now considering identifying the school as a Center for Rural Nursing within Community.

It has been a challenge for us, in a niche-planning environment, to hold fast to our vision of a school of nursing that offers a full range of professional nursing education programs responsive to changing health and health care delivery needs. It is, perhaps, unfortunate that this school has been coming into its full maturity as a university school of nursing while two different retrenchment strategies were enacted. (Niche planning is a very sophisticated retrenchment strategy that is also a growth strategy.) We never wavered, however, and the school's ongoing planning process and our vision is still entrenched in our school. As we have achieved some major successes, central administration is increasingly attentive to our plan.

Environment

A major component of transforming the school has been to attend to environmental factors. Many elephants were blocking the pathways toward transformation, to use Koetter's graphic image. Early on it was discovered that faculty dreaded coming to the dean's office, and because it was needed anyway, the office was completely redecorated. The dean's office is a very comfortable place; many faculty and staff visit frequently, by appointment or during open office hours and, for the most part, they are quite at ease. A dreary lounge, decorated in 1970s' brown and orange plastic furniture that lined the walls, was redecorated with alumnae support and renamed in their honor. Colored in blues and mauves (probably now outdated) and furnished with movable tables and chairs, bright lights, and many live and silk plants, the room is heavily used. It is the main setting for most of our school-wide planning.

In keeping with our commitment to our students, a Student Affairs Office was established and made attractive and welcoming. Several classrooms have been completely refurbished to create pleasant and conducive learning environments for both faculty and students. Faculty and staff now have complete kitchen facilities; coffee and tea is always available free of charge. Attention to the physical environment is a visible and relatively simple way to create an environment conducive to collaboration and communications. Faculty offices are being renovated one by one. A plan is being developed for continued refurbishment of the entire building, although scarce resources prohibit moving ahead more quickly with these renovations. We want our building to be more reflective of our excitement and enthusiasm for academic nursing.

The structure of the organization, as has already been discussed, can contain a whole herd of elephants. Without repeating obstacles already named, allow me to share who a few of our elephants were and how we removed them. One complaint we found to be universal to the faculty was the complexity and perceived inequities of the faculty workload model. A new model was speedily designed in collaboration with faculty. With periodic review and reaffirmation, along with minor changes, it has served very well since 1990. It is a model that is appropriate to faculty in a research university. It allows for a reasonable allocation of faculty time to teaching, research, and service. It also specifies a different allocation of work for faculty on a tenure track and faculty on a clinical track.

The creation of a clinical track (with subsequent approval through the ranks all the way to the system president) represents sending another huge elephant to the zoo—where it belongs. Prior to creation of the clinical track, those instructors on the faculty who were not on the tenure track perceived themselves as inadequate and inferior to their tenure-track colleagues. Those on the tenure track, unfortunately, often treated their non–tenure track colleagues as if their knowledge, skills, and authority in the organization were, indeed, inferior. Moreover, although a few of these faculty had been employed as instructors in the school for 10 or more years, they were all convinced that their positions were insecure. The clinical track is a parallel track to the tenure track. It includes rank, the opportunity for promotion, and a requirement for scholarship. Multiple-year contracts can be awarded. The clinical track is another model for excellence in academia.

A third example, which is mentioned only briefly (although it could be a chapter in itself), is the recreation of our research infrastructure. Using a "bottoms up" total quality management type approach, the faculty completely redesigned, and the author (dean) subsequently approved, a faculty-led team approach to meeting our goal and objectives for research and research funding. The school no longer has an associate dean for research. Two faculty, who complement each other's strengths in research expertise, serve as codirectors of the Office of Research. They are complemented by an external consultant for research. This seasoned research scientist spends about 2 days per month at the school in planned activities with individuals or teams of faculty or with doctoral students.

Over the years, an ongoing objective was to develop the faculty to join together in a team approach to research. Progress was being made and the implementation of the new infrastructure brought the team approach to research into focus. Two research interest groups were formed: Women's Health and Gerontology, both with a strong focus in rural nursing and health care. In addition, several research teams focused in specific projects are flourishing. Faculty had perceived many obstacles to research productivity; increasingly they came to recognize that the obstacles were within, as well as external to, themselves. The new infrastructure not only removed elephants from the pathways that were blocking productivity, but also removed all small animals. This particular change, perhaps more than any other in the school, signifies the growth and development of the faculty, as well as their commitment to the vision.

Equipment and supplies are another important element of the supportive environment. Keeping the elephants at bay in this case means making a major commitment to the latest state-of-the-art computer equipment. With the guidance of a school-designated Chief Information Officer, a half-time technology specialist, and a faculty-staff Task Force on Technology we have made the technology-enriched environment a priority for allocation of scarce resources. Every staff member and every faculty member has a computer on their desk. They range from 2-year-old models to today's latest Pentium models. A set of guidelines helps to determine the logical placement of the computers. We also have student offices with one or several computers, a state-of-the-art telecommunications classroom, and two very sophisticated technology learning laboratories for students.

In a few short years, the approach to environmental supports in our school has changed radically. One new faculty member, for example, requested a piece of equipment to support her physiological research costing several thousand dollars. We agreed that she had to have it—and purchased it. We wouldn't think of bringing in a new faculty member without outfitting them up front with a computer, probably a printer, and a handful of requested software packages.

This commitment has been very demanding of our resources. Some other activities, such as additional refurbishment of the school, take second priority to equipment and supplies. Fortunately the school became an endowed school in 1994. An annual fund (relatively modest), as one component of the endowment, is available for use for the physical plant, including the purchase of equipment. Also, central administration is helping the schools with annual competitive grants to earn either revenues to purchase equipment or equipment itself.

When we set out to begin to achieve our shared vision, we had no idea how we would be changed in the process. We knew, not exactly to what extent (and still do not), we would change the school. Changing ourselves was not contemplated early on. As the dean, of course a more enthusiastic and cooperative faculty was desired and one that was informed about their school. The author thinks leaders starting out with a deliberate plan to implement transformational leadership and a learning organization would be far more aware of empowerment processes and probably more efficient in achieving success.

Involving faculty in planning early on, developing a shared vision, sharing data about the school openly and comprehensively, encouraging teamwork in education and research, fostering a consensus decision-making process, and embarking on a vigorous faculty development pathway along with removing many organizational obstacles are most of the actions that undergirded the empowerment of our faculty and staff and the development of teamwork or shared governance or a learning organization, whatever it is called. In any event the faculty, staff, and administration of the school have developed a culture of pride, of continual learning, of empowerment, and of community.

We are a culture of leadership. About two-thirds of the faculty hold important leadership positions in the school. This reality evolved over time as the teams became more effective and as the work of the school became increasingly comprehensive and diverse. Faculty serve as course, level, and program coordinators; as committee and task force chairs; as Principal Investigators on research or special projects; as mentors to new faculty; as representatives to professional organizations; as directors or codirectors of activities or programs the school offers; and the list continues almost endlessly. Lacking faculty leadership, the school could not be functioning as it is nor having the successes it is enjoying.

We have used Weisbord's (1992) model of environment or adaptation to explain why we must behave as we do. Weisbord describes the environment as turbulent and projects that it will remain so well into the next century. Turbulent environments are fraught with unexpected changes, uncertainty, unintended consequences, and complexity. The active adaptation principles called for by the organization and its people in a turbulent environment are flexibility, innovation/creativity, social responsibility, and participation or collaboration. A flat organizational structure, a preponderance of ad hoc committees, a team approach to our work, a shared plan, and shared vision are the products of our growth and development. So, too, are great energy and enthusiasm for our work and the achievement of many innovations and successes (see Figure 15-6 for a listing of some of our innovations and outcomes).

We define our school community as "A group of professionals committed to utilizing their individual and collective expertise to conduct

Academic Programs

Established a Ph.D. in Nursing; enrolled first students in January, 1994; had first graduate, December 1996. (This program is collaborative with the other schools of nursing in the university system.)

At the masters level: established a nurse-midwifery area of study; a public health nursing area of study; a chronic illness case management model curriculum; a telecommunications outreach masters option, and doubled enrollments in our Family Nurse Practitioner area of study while either suspending or reducing enrollments in several clinical specialty areas of study. Curriculum reform has occurred in all areas of masters study.

At the postmasters level, established a one year "fast track" Family Nurse Practitioner area of study; have graduated 2 classes and are working with the third class. At the baccalaureate level, implemented a Scholars Program. At present 22 BSN students are scholars. We are aiming for increasing those numbers very substantially.

Selected Funded Faculty Research and Special Projects
(Current funding exceeds 4.5 million dollars, and is about 1.5 million per annum.)

Gerontology Team
- Well-being and Health Promotion in Three Rural Populatons
- High-Risk Residents In Nursing Homes
- Family Involvement In Care

Women's Health
- Breast Feeding Intentions of Low-Income Women
- Older Rural Widows' Experience of Home Care

Health Policy
- Missouri Pew Health Professions Partnership
- RWJ Colleagues In-Caring Work Force Design in Northeast Missouri
- Advanced Practice Nursing Statewide Database

Nursing and Medicine Joint Funding
- Missouri Rural Area Health Education Centers (MRAHEC).
- Primary Care Rural Initiatives of Missouri (PRIMO)
- Missouri Integrated Advanced Information Management Systems (MIAIMS)

Program Support
- MU School of Nursing Nursing Center at MACC (a local community college) (a primary health care school owned and operated service setting)
- Rural Telecommunications Outreach
- Public Health Nursing Specialist Program
- Family Nurse Practitioner Expansion to Rural Areas
- Nurse-Midwifery Education and Service

(Continued)

Figure 15-6. *Innovations and outcomes.*

Faculty Practice

MU Nurse-Midwives Service
MU School of Nursing Nursing Center
Seniors Team at University Hospital
Myriad faculty practices in hospital outpatient and community-based settings. (All practices are revenue-generating.)

Other Innovations
Collaborative affiliation with Alcorn State University in rural Mississippi for faculty and student education and research programs.

A Central Missouri Rural Health Consortium with Three Rural Health Departments.

An Expeditions in Rural Practice undergraduate residential rural clinical practicum.

Figure 15-6.   *Innovations and outcomes. (Continued)*

the work of the organization to advance their agreed upon goals and enact their shared vision; a group of professionals who care about the welfare of the others and assume a full share of responsibility for group welfare and organizational achievement" (Faculty and Administration 1996, unpublished work).

Acknowledgment

I would like to acknowledge the input and participation of Dr. Rose Porter, Associate Dean, and Dr. Alice Kuehn, Associate Professor in developing this case study.

References

Bennis, W. (1984). The 4 competencies of leadership. *Training and Development Journal,* August, pp. 144–149.

Drucker, P. (1973). *Management of Tasks, Responsibilities, Practices.* New York: Harper and Row.

Evans, J. A.(1994). The role of the nurse manager in creating an environment for collaborative practice. *Holistic Nursing Practice, 8*(3), 22–31.

Flarey, D. L. (September 1993). The changing role of the nurse manager: redesign for the 1990s and beyond. *Seminars for Nurse Managers, 1*(1), 41–48.

Heim, P. (April 1993). The empowered team. Presented at the 26th Annual Meeting of the American Organization of Nurse Executives, Orlando, FL.

Kanter, A. A. (1991). Transcending business boundaries: 12,000 world managers view change. *Harvard Business Review,* May–June, pp. 151–164.

Koerner, J. G. and Bunkers, S. S. (1992). Transformational leadership: The power symbol. *Nursing Administration Quarterly, 17*(1), 1–9.

Koetter, J. P. (May–June 1990). What leaders really do. *Harvard Business Review,* 103–111.

Koetter, J. P. (March–April 1995). Leading change: Why transformation efforts fail. *Harvard Business Review,* 59–67.

Mason, J. M. (1994). Building the team during consolidation. *Seminars for Nurse Managers, 2*(4), 203–208.

Porter-O'Grady, T. (April 1993). Of mythspinners and mapmakers: 21st century managers. *Nursing Management, 24*(4), 52–55.

Porter-O'Grady, T. (January 1994). Building partnerships in health care: Creating whole systems change. *Nursing and Health Care, 15*(1), pp. 34–38.

Porter-O'Grady, T. and Wilson, C. K. (1995). *The Leadership Revolution in Health Care.* Gaithersburg, MD: Aspen Publishers Inc.

Russell, W. and Branch, T. (1979). *Second Wind: Memoirs of an Opinionated Man.* New York: Random House.

Salsbury, G. (1994). *Transformational Leadership: The Fine Art of Making a Difference.* Salsbury Enterprises.

Senge, P. M. (1990). *The Fifth Discipline.* New York: Doubleday.

Weisbord, M. R. (1992). *Discovering Common Ground.* San Francisco, CA: Berrett-Koehler Publishers.

Articulating Nursing 16 for Advanced Practice Nursing

Victoria T. Grando

The reorganization of the health care delivery system of the 1990s is resulting in an explosion of managed care companies orchestrating health care in the United States. Although this change developed as an American response to the ongoing problems with quality of care, access to care, and cost of care, the predominant thrust of managed care companies has been cost containment. This focus is shaping changes in the delivery of health care that include a reduction in overall services provided, the increased utilization of primary care providers as gatekeepers to health care services, a decrease in hospital care with a simultaneous increase in outpatient services and home health care, and an increased utilization of unlicensed assistive personnel.

As the nation struggles to adjust to the managed care environment, advanced practice nurses (APNs) have the opportunity and challenge to take the lead in providing quality, cost-effective health care for all Americans. Nonetheless, as nurses strive to fulfill their social mandate, there remains an uncertainty about the purpose of advanced practice nursing and its boundaries with other health care providers. Indeed, nurses themselves are often not in agreement about the role of APNs and have difficulty articulating what advanced practice nursing encompasses. This

499

chapter addresses these issues and attempts to delineate benchmarks for advanced nursing practice by analyzing the views and perceptions of leading nursing scholars, educators, and clinicians.

METHOD

This descriptive study sought to identify the meaning that "advanced practice nursing" held for nurses intimately involved with expanded practice, either directly as APNs or indirectly as nurse educators and administrators. It aimed to elicit their unique points of view and personal perceptions of advanced practice nursing based on their individual lived experiences. Special attention was given to identifying how these nursing leaders and experts articulate APN roles. Their accounts present a rich portrait of advanced practice nursing in the late 1990s.

The sample consisted of 16 APNs and nurse educators, many of whom played a prominent role in the development of advanced practice nursing over the past 30 years. Included in the sample were family, gerontologic, and pediatric nurse practitioners; certified nurse-midwives; and mental health, adult health, and child health clinical nurse specialists. The subjects' views were gathered through in-depth interviews conducted in 1996. Nine open-ended questions were mailed in advance to the subjects. The researcher conducted the interviews by phone. The interviews were recorded and transcribed for analysis. The data were than analyzed and synthesized to explicate the parameters of advanced nursing, its boundaries with other health care providers, and the forces that have influenced its development. For the purposes of this study, advanced practice nurses were defined as certified nurse-midwives, clinical nurse specialists, nurse practitioners, and nurse anesthetists. In addition to the interviews, selected articles were reviewed to provide a historical background on advanced practice nursing.

HISTORY OF ADVANCED NURSING PRACTICE

Advanced nursing practice has a long tradition. It began in the late 1880s with the development of nurse anesthetists. Since that time, roles in other clinical specialty areas have emerged, including nurse-midwives in the early 1930s, clinical nurse specialists in the 1940s, and nurse practitioners beginning in the mid-1960s (Bullough 1992, Menard 1987). Each of these developed uniquely and with differing emphases. Nonetheless, one thing united them, namely: advanced *clinical* practice. But it also set them apart from other nurses. Neither nurse generalists nor nurses with advanced expertise in education, research, and administration are considered APNs because advanced practice nursing refers to advanced clinical practice. This distinction has been stressed by both the American Association of Colleges of Nursing (AACN; 1996) in *Essentials of Master's Education For Advanced Practice Nursing* and the American Nurses Association (1995) in *Nursing's Social Policy Statement.*

According to Bullough (1992), advanced practice nursing emerged from two models. The first, a nursing model, is the foundation of the clinical nurse specialist. It has a strong basis in nursing science and research, the psychosocial sciences, and education. Clinical nurse specialists focus on helping people achieve optimum health by improving nursing care and often by working at the system level to improve organizational responsiveness to care needs. Their scope of practice is broad, encompassing an array of activities including direct and indirect practice, patient and staff education, management, consultation, and research (Page and Arena 1994). The second model, the collaborative model, is the basis of the nurse practitioner, nurse anesthetist, certified nurse-midwife, and the mental health clinical nurse specialist. This model has a strong emphasis on nursing science, medical science, research, psychosocial sciences, and education. The nurse practitioner, certified nurse-midwife, nurse anesthetist, and mental health clinical nurse specialist roles are more circumscribed, focusing predominately on improving health by providing direct care to patients (Page and Arena 1994). They engage in primary health care, management of chronic health problems, patient education, and research (Page and Arena 1994, Elder and Bullough 1990).

Since the inception of the roles of clinical nurse specialist and the nurse practitioner, there has been continued controversy over which model is most appropriate for nursing (Ford 1982, Mauksch 1975, Rogers 1975, Elder and Bullough 1990). Some nursing leaders believed that the nurse practitioner role was an extension of medicine and was not nursing, whereas others saw it as nursing's future (Mauksch 1975, Rogers 1975). Recently, these arguments have diminished, and there is growing discussion about the possibility of merging the two practice areas. An increasing number of nurses argue that the similarities in the education and practice between the two areas of advanced practice outweigh their differences (Elder and Bullough 1990, Forbes et al. 1990). Still, others propose one title to encompass all advanced practice nurses.

In spite of the recent embracing of all advanced practice roles by nurses, the debate over advanced practice nursing continues. The question no longer concerns whether the nurse practitioner movement takes nurses away from nursing into the realm of medicine, but it now centers on exactly what constitutes advanced nursing practice. In 1988, while arguing for the need to redefine expanded nursing roles, Mechanic did not differentiate between the clinical nurse specialist and the nurse practitioner. She proposed, however, a distinction between the *extended* role of the nurse and the *expanded* role of the nurse. Mechanic stated that the extended role involved performing activities that were once solely in the realm of medicine. These included such tasks as defibrillating patients or prescribing medications. Mechanic believed that the expanded role of nursing had grown from an early focus on advanced health assessment to one that now included health promotion and protection, disease prevention, and episodic care of uncomplicated illnesses. These areas of practice are encompassed within a model of nursing autonomy and authority and in collaboration with other health care workers. She made the point that advanced nursing practice was a way of thinking and that it went beyond the disease model; it focused on health.

Watson (1995), in a similar vein, has argued ardently to "[c]larify advanced practice of nurses [that is designed to meet medical care and cure services] and differentiate such from *nursing* practice within a *nursing qua nursing* [caring–healing–health] paradigm" (p. 82). She calls for nursing to move away from the predominant illness model of cure by redefining nursing and health care. Watson also advocates that nurses adopt a caring–healing–health paradigm in order to meet society's health needs.

THE DOMAIN OF ADVANCED PRACTICE NURSING

The meaning of advanced practice nursing is rapidly evolving in the current health care environment. This study provides a snapshot of the state of advanced practice nursing as it is being lived, practiced, and articulated. This analysis begins by examining the question: What is the domain of advanced practice nursing? The informants were asked to identify what they believed made up the domain of advanced practice nurses.

A domain is the area of responsibility and concern of a discipline. It derives from the ideas, values, goals, technology, and knowledge of the field (Hahn 1995). The domain of the APN is extensive, encompassing a large arena of activities and knowledge. Moreover, it varies according to the APN's scope of practice, knowledge, and expertise. For example, the certified nurse midwife is concerned with the health of the childbearing family, whereas the mental health practitioner is concerned with the mental health of individuals, families, and groups. Likewise, having prescriptive authority is vital to nurse practitioners, but it is not as important to the practice of clinical nurse specialists. At the same time, there are many aspects of the APN domain that are shared by APNs in differing specialty areas and with differing scopes of practice. For instance, whether the APN works in primary care or acute care or chronic care all are involved in health education and referral.

Consequently, the APN's domain is multifaceted and diverse. Even so, there emerge core aspects of the APN's domain: the APN's concern for promoting the client's health and wellness; the APN's responsibility for providing direct care to individuals, families, and groups; and the APN's management of a patient's self-care systems and illnesses. These echo Jean Watson's *caring–healing–health* paradigm for nursing (Watson 1995). As APNs treat a failed self-care system or assist a woman giving birth or teach the importance of physical fitness or manage a diabetic's insulin, they are involved with providing care, promoting healing, and achieving health.

From these core concerns of nursing—health, caring, and healing—flow other important subcomponents of the APN domain. Those interviewed identified the following phenomena and functions as being within the APN domains of practice:

> Clinical Domain
> Primary, secondary, and tertiary prevention
> > Self-care
> > Primary care, acute care, and chronic care
> > Case management
> > Outcome management
> > Program design
> Specialized practice arenas such as well-women or child care, mental health, oncology, or public health
> Health assessment, diagnosis, treatment (nursing or medical) and evaluation or revision

Caring or healing interventions including conventional (pain control, self-care management) and nonconventional care (therapeutic touch, imagery)
Frequently mentioned specific interventions
    Prescribing drugs
    Ordering or interpreting of diagnostic tests
    Offering guidance with socioeconomic issues
    Promoting healthy lifestyles
    Providing nutrition counseling
    Providing health teaching and coaching
    Providing counseling and psychotherapy
Professional Domain
    Consultation and referral
    Research
    Clinical leadership in nursing
    Staff development

Besides these phenomena, the domain of advanced practice nursing also encompasses actions and behaviors that are part of each specific APN's scope of practice. At present, these are rapidly changing as health care delivery is being reshaped. They include traditional nursing behaviors as well as behaviors historically a part of medicine's domain. Alice Kuehn, Ph.D. (taped interview on advanced practice nursing; unpublished raw data, October 1996), a gerontologic nurse practitioner, described the diversity of APN's activities as follows:

> The list of tasks and activities that APNs engage in could be endless depending on the type of APN and where they are located. If you're in a busy practice that has all kinds of specialists, what you do in your practice is going to be totally different than if you have a rural practice.

Indeed, many of those interviewed believe APNs could do anything they were educated to do and believe this is an exciting time to be an APN.

Advanced practice nurses were seen as being well-positioned to move into new territories and take on new tasks competently because of their broad nursing background and past history of delivering quality, cost-effective care in new arenas. A sampling of current APN activities include, but are not limited to, conducting social skills training for the persistently mentally ill; performing medical procedures such as Papanicolaou smears, colposcopes, and minor surgery; guiding people as they develop their self-care systems; teaching teenagers about sexually transmitted diseases; and managing asthmatics' drug regimens.

THE INTERSECT OF ADVANCED NURSING PRACTICE AND MEDICAL PRACTICE

In addition to delineating the concerns of a field, domains are also social constructs that provide boundaries between professions and disciplines. Typically, boundaries may be thought of as distinct and rigid, but they are not. They overlap and continually change and evolve with time (Mechanic 1988). As a consequence, different professions frequently share similar interests, and what may be part of one field or profession can also be part of another. Moreover, a phenomenon once viewed as solely the domain of one discipline can become part of another with time. One family nurse practitioner interviewed, Beth Geden, Ph.D. (taped interview on advanced practice nursing; unpublished raw data, October 1996), stated that she struggled to differentiate between her practice and that of an MD. What she came to realize was that she was trying to make a differentiation where none existed; that there were many elements of primary care and health problems to which both attended. Whereas both treated common illness similarly, she as an APN had a different emphasis such as patient self-care management and patient integration of new activities into those of daily living.

The subjects identified aspects of the APN domain that they believed overlapped with MDs and other health care providers. They held that many, if not most, aspects of their domain overlapped with MDs'. Advanced practice nurses and physicians shared primary care, the management of acute and chronic illness, assessment and diagnosis, psychotherapy, well-woman and well-baby care, medical treatment (cure model), and prescriptive authority, to name a few. Nonetheless, one area is not shared at present: major surgery.

Some of those interviewed accounted for the overlap between the two professions as a sharing of tasks but not of philosophies. Moreover, they insisted that although both had a commitment to helping people and performed many of the same behaviors, they had distinctly differing approaches and emphases. For example, when caring for persons with diabetes, the subjects viewed the APN's concern as going beyond the disease management to include the individual's complicated self-care problems. On the other hand, the subjects believed that the MD caring for a diabetic would focus on unstable or complicated medical problems. In another example, both certified nurse-midwives and gynecologists treat menopausal women with estrogen, but certified nurse midwives often report better results because of their close contact with their pregnant women and their families. They explore in more depth how their well women manage their hormonal replacement therapy and thus are able to improve care outcomes. Loretta Ford, Ed.D. (taped interview on advanced practice nursing; unpublished raw data, December 1996), co-founder of the first Pediatric Nurse Practitioner program at the University of Colorado, summed up these beliefs as follows:

> APNs and MDs do so much in common, they collect and use data similarly, share the same tools, and perform the same procedures. However, they process the data differently and set different goals, which influences patient outcomes. And this relates to their differing philosophical orientation.

ADVANCED PRACTICE NURSES' UNIQUE PHILOSOPHY

As discussed previously, many areas of nursing's domain overlap with the domain of other health care providers such as MDs, psychologists, and social workers. Therefore, what sets nursing apart? What specific values, beliefs, philosophies, orientations to practice do APNs hold that are uniquely nursing's?

The responses to these questions revealed four distinct orientations that the subjects perceived as specific to nursing philosophy. The first is the APN's relationship with the patients. Many remarked that this was different from that of the MDs with whom they worked and observed. As Loretta Ford, Ed.D. (1996) put it: "APNs bring values of consumer partnership, of listening to consumers, and considering consumer goals that I don't see medicine doing." Others interviewed also saw themselves as being in a partnership with their patients and went on to relate that a bond developed between nurse and patient as they worked together toward the same goals. They used terms such as *person-centered* and *family-centered* to describe the nurse–patient relationship. In many situations and practice arenas, they had the time to listen to what their patients say and believe and to learn their patient's views about their life situations. They held that the APN puts greater emphasis on the patient's story, how the patient sees it, and what is the client's context. Moreover, those interviewed believed that APNs honor and respect their clients' points of view, values, and rights to participate in decision making. Beth Geden (1996) emphasizes this by the following statement:

> Honoring the person is the overriding philosophical position [of advanced practice nursing]. It includes the belief that individuals make the best judgments they can make about caring for themselves and the appreciation that they are trying to do the best they can for themselves. With this kind of a belief you are not in a position to be a critic, but you're in the position of a helping relationship.

The subjects also believed APNs value their patients' autonomy, putting the emphasis on working *with* people rather than doing *to* them. As was poignantly explained, the certified nurse-midwife participates with the patient as *the woman* gives birth to the baby, rather than delivering the baby. Also articulated was that the family nurse practitioner is first willing to meet the patient's overriding need to be recognized as a person before engaging the person in treatment issues. It can be concluded that the APN and the person receiving care share a collaborative relationship, not a paternalistic one.

The next characteristic setting APNs apart from other health care providers is their health perspective. Over and over those interviewed stressed that APNs focus on their patients' health states. Indeed, they took the position that APNs put the emphasis on their patients' health even though they treat their illnesses. For example, one pointed out that APNs routinely go beyond illness care and actively promote health and self-care strengths. They then build on these, rather than solely looking for and treating disease.

Viewing their patients holistically was another attribute of the APN philosophy. It was pointed out that APNs operate from the integration of multiple sciences and multiple ways of knowing, which affords them a holistic perspective (Geden 1996). It also was stressed that APNs see those who are the recipients of their care within the context of their total environment and culture, including their families, neighborhoods, and larger communities. Donna Scheideberg, Ph.D. (taped interview on advanced practice nursing; unpublished raw data, October 1996), a certified nurse-midwife, described that her holistic view of her clients differed from her MD colleagues as follows:

> When I see my patient, I don't just see my 18 year old patient that comes in for birth control. I see her but also take into consideration that she may be a senior in high school, her family might not know she uses birth control, she may not have money for pills, she may have a child at home, and her boyfriend may be battering her. I consider all of these as I work with her.

She thus goes beyond the typical medical focus of birth control and the possibility of sexually transmitted diseases. She also notes the young woman's lifestyle, family situation, relations with others, social issues, or whatever else might seem appropriate. To emphasize: APNs are interested in their patients' health and illness, self-care competency and self-management behaviors, healing and coping strategies, stress management, lifestyle and patterns of daily living, and socioeconomic issues.

Another aspect of APNs' holistic care is knowing the communities where their patients live. This knowledge assists APNs to glean a good notion of their patients' other health issues. They are more likely to identify mental health problems that may hinder their patients' abilities to manage their health and may exacerbate their illnesses. They also work at empowering their patients. They help them negotiate the health care system, access resources for assisting them to improve job skills and education, and assist them in learning and accessing health information. All of these are part of the holistic orientation of APNs.

Last, the APNs' commitment to collaboration with other health care providers sets them apart. The interviewees were in agreement that APNs practiced within collaborative relationships. They believe their collaborative orientation sets them apart from other health care providers. Some of the subjects questioned the notion that any health care provider practiced independently of others. Many believe that collaboration between APNs and MDs is necessary for quality health care and is mutually beneficial for APNs and MDs. They saw APNs referring patients to MDs when the MDs' greater depth of knowledge in pathology was needed, but they also saw that MDs often referred patients to APNs when patients had problems managing their self-care systems or their health states or had difficulty coping with emotional, personal or family issues. One pediatric nurse practitioner interviewed, Debra Gayer (taped interview on advanced practice nursing; unpublished raw data,

November 1996), explained how this played out in her practice. She saw the wellness focus as her strong point. But she also treats illness effectively and refers patients to her MD partner when the disease problems become too complicated for her level of expertise.

ADVANCED PRACTICE NURSE/ MD RELATIONSHIP

Given that APNs and MDs share a similar domain but have differing orientations to practice, how has their relationship developed? This is an important issue because APNs do not practice in a vacuum. The APNs' relationship with their MD colleagues will certainly influence the APNs' own practice. This is especially true in light of the historic control that MDs have exerted over all other health care providers, including nurses (Freidson 1970).

Those interviewed believe changes are occurring in how APNs and MDs interact. They stated that the past 20 years have been marked by competition between the two groups of professionals. This competition increased as APNs became more involved in primary care and were increasingly seen by MDs as competitors for patients. Four of those interviewed developed this theme in this way: Nurses had been performing expanded roles within hospitals for a long time and MDs were not concerned; they became concerned when APNs moved into primary care. Physicians saw this as a challenge to their exclusive control over gatekeeping for access to health care. Furthermore, MDs had initially assumed a supervisory position over APNs. Some believed that APNs were, and had to be, dependent on MDs. This occurred in part when APNs referred patients outside their scope of practice to specialty MDs (a practice commonly existing within the medical community). This, however, was interpreted as a reflection of their inability to provide primary care rather than as instances of appropriate referral.

In spite of continuing differences between APNs and MDs, there was agreement that changes were occurring, especially at the individual level, between nurse and doctor. Many of those interviewed believed that APNs are currently enjoying true collaborative relationships with MDs and that care is becoming increasingly interdisciplinary. As a result, nurses are experiencing greater appreciation from their MD colleagues within collaborative relationships. This is exemplified by the fact that

MDs are beginning to model the practice of APNs and find that they can learn from them. Dr. Donna Scheideberg (1996) has experienced this in her midwifery practice. She related how MDs she knows are learning from nurse midwives to "labor sit" and appreciate the benefits of allowing laboring women to remain in their rooms rather than taking them into the delivery room hours before they were ready to deliver.

Advanced practice nurses are also beginning to experience a new spirit of collaboration and respect with their physician colleagues. One interviewee remarked that it is a new era, especially in regards to changes in the types of patients with whom APNs are working. Initially, most of their patients were from underserved groups—the poor, vulnerable, elderly, and rural. But more and more APNs are caring for persons of all backgrounds. MDs are asking APNs to join them as partners in collaborative practices because they are finding consumers are interested in the kinds of care APNs provide.

WHAT HAS PROMOTED AND HINDERED ADVANCED PRACTICE NURSING GROWTH AND ACCEPTANCE?

Besides investigating how nursing leaders and clinicians view advanced practice and the relationship APNs have with MDs, the subjects were asked to identify what factors have promoted advanced practice nursing and what factors have hindered it over the past 20 years. This knowledge will aid understanding of the present position of advanced practice nursing in society and can help guide the nursing profession as it changes to meet society's caring–healing–health needs of the future.

Those interviewed identified numerous professional and societal forces that played a role in the development of advanced practice nursing. Surprisingly, in many instances, the same factors that were seen as promoting advanced nursing practice by some were seen as barriers by others. This occurred in part because some tended to focus on achievements made, whereas others looked to the challenges ahead. Moreover, some forces that were barriers early in the development of advanced practice nursing later promoted the development of these roles.

Professional forces identified included both intraprofessional (within nursing) and interprofessional (between nurses and physicians). The subjects named several intraprofessional forces that have shaped the growth of advanced practice nursing. One important driving force was the efforts of nurses themselves, especially the efforts of the visionary leaders who spearheaded advanced practice nursing in spite of early opposition from other nurse educators and leaders. Over time, the development of graduate-level education with a focus on clinical nursing helped promote the role. Dr. Alice Kuehn (1996) emphasized that in the last 10 years, nursing academia, including organizations such as the AACN, have done much to promote the role of APNs. Second, many nurses tenaciously pursued advanced practice even though barriers existed initially. And last, nurses have effectively networked across the country to achieve legislation that has supported and expanded advanced practice nursing, such as the right to prescriptive authority.

Another driving force within nursing that furthered expanded practice has been the maturing of nursing's paradigm through theory and knowledge development and research. This has provided APNs with a clearer nursing perspective, a knowledge-based rationale for care, and a rapidly developing nursing science. Furthermore, a substantial body of research has promoted APN roles by documenting the quality care that APNs bring to health care delivery.

Interprofessional driving forces include the many MDs who believed that advanced practice nursing could improve health care and who supported the early development of the role. The interviewees related that early endeavors at providing advanced practice often hinged on finding MDs who would practice with APNs. Fortunately, many MDs were willing to do so. And today, the many MDs willing to share joint practices with APNs make possible myriad collaborative partnerships. Organized medicine was also seen as promoting APNs at times. One example given of this was the efforts of the MDs in the American College of Obstetrics and Gynecology to gain public recognition and support of certified nurse-midwives and their contributions to women's maternal health.

In addition to these compelling professional influences, many societal issues also helped expand the role. Three major driving forces have been the ongoing problems with health care: costs, quality, and access. Advanced practice nurses have proved that they provide effective solutions to these concerns. At present, they are increasingly being utilized to help keep health costs down while increasing access to care and improving the quality of care. These interviewees stressed that APNs have influenced access to care in several ways: by increasing the number of primary care providers; by consistently providing care to the undeserved, poor, elderly, and rural; and by their commitment to health promotion. Legislation and regulation have also played an important part in expanding the utilization of APNs in two major ways. First by increasing sources of reimbursement for APNs through Medicare and Medicaid regulations and second, by changing nurse practice acts to allow APNs to increase their scope of practice. Two other major societal trends that have fueled the growth of advanced practice nursing have been consumer demand, which is increasing as more and more people have contact with APNs, and managed care, which has created new opportunities for APNs.

Barriers to advanced practice nursing were also identified as both professional and societal. Intraprofessional obstacles were identified as numerous. Disagreement among nurses concerning the appropriateness of advanced practice nursing was seen as a major barrier. Early in the development of the advanced practice nursing roles, some nurses, nurse educators, and leaders were ambivalent and not supportive of initial efforts for advanced clinical expertise, especially those for nurse practitioners. This led to the development of continuing education programs outside of nursing that began preparing "advanced practice nurses." Unfortunately, these fueled yet another barrier, the continuing confusion over differentiation of practice, credentialing, and what exactly is it that APNs do. Finally, the large numbers of nurses without advanced nursing education, who lack nursing knowledge or a nursing paradigm, were viewed as hindering the development of advanced nursing practice. A current concern to these interviewees is the proliferation of nurse practitioner programs, many of which, they say, lack qualified faculty and adequate clinical teaching sites.

Organized medicine was identified as another major deterrent. Although individual MDs and some specialty medical organizations have promoted APNs, organized medicine, especially through the American Medical Association, has continued its efforts to control advanced nursing practice. A few of those interviewed believed that APN students and medical students should share some of their educational experiences, didactic as well as clinical, as a way to break down this long-standing obstacle. They believe collaborative learning represents a long-term solution to MD opposition to APNs.

Societal barriers were also seen as numerous. Many believed that a large number of consumers still remained uninformed about advanced practice nursing and the types of care APNs provide. In addition, stereotypes still remain about what is nursing. Others described how reimbursement issues have hindered the growth of APNs. Advanced practice nurses (and their MD colleagues) have had difficulty receiving reimbursement for health promotion and disease prevention activities. Also, APNs have had great difficulty being recognized by insurers as preferred providers, which would enable them to bill directly for their services. Lack of funding sources for reimbursement of APNs, in turn, limits consumer choice of providers.

Many states have laws that continue to limit the practice of APNs, especially limiting prescriptive privileges. For example, APNs in some states may not be legally authorized to prescribe even low-level narcotics or may be required to prescribe from a limiting drug formulary. Institutional bureaucracies with their paternalistic mindset were also identified as a barrier limiting the potential of expanded nursing roles. They often do not develop incentives for advanced nursing practice, nor do they provide positions that allow APNs to practice to the full potential of their expertise.

CONCLUSIONS

The nursing profession is now, as it has been many times before in its history, at a pivotal place. As new models of practice emerge, the direction that advanced nursing practice takes is vital. It shapes nursing's place within the health care delivery system and its relevance for meeting Americans' health care requirements. Of great importance is nurses' ability to articulate their role, for nurses have an important opportunity to clarify their domain and philosophical orientation to others. This will help make their unique contribution better understood by both colleagues and consumers alike. Based on the insights of those nursing leaders and clinicians interviewed for this study, it is evident that advanced practice nursing is meeting these challenges.

Although controversy still lingers over the roles APNs play, these nurses were able to articulate clearly their domain and scope of practice. The subjects related how they played important roles in helping their patients heal. They were firm in their belief that they promoted their patients' health. Furthermore, they had no difficulty articulating their mission to provide advanced nursing care bridging nursing and medical practices. Indeed, they held a distinct nursing philosophy even while performing traditionally medical tasks. And last, they clearly identified their philosophical underpinnings—collaboration with their patients and other professionals within a holistic health perspective. Most important, these APNs see their APN practices as a vital and valuable addition to America's health care.

References

American Nurses Association (1995). *Nursing's Social Policy Statement*. Washington, DC: American Nurses' Association.

American Association of Colleges of Nursing (1996). *Essential of Master's Education for Advanced Practice Nursing*. Washington, DC: American Association of Colleges of Nursing.

Bullough, B. (1992). Alternative models for specialty nursing practice. *Nursing and Health Care, 13,* 254–259.

Elder, R. G. and Bullough, B. (1990). Nurse practitioners and clinical nurse specialists: Are the roles merging? *Clinical Nurse Specialist, 4,* 78–84.

Forbes, K. E., Rafson, J., Spross, J. A., and Kozlowski, D. (1990). Clinical nurse specialist and nurse practitioner core curricula survey results. *Nurse Practitioner, 15*(4), 43, 46–48.

Ford, L. C. (1982). Nurse practitioners: History of a new idea and predictions for the future. In L. H. Aiken (Ed.). *Nursing in the 1980s: Crises, Opportunities, Challenges*. Philadelphia: Lippincott, pp. 231–247.

Freidson, E. (1970). *Profession of Medicine*. New York: Dodd, Mead and Co.

Hahn, R. H. (1995). *Sickness and Healing: An Anthropological Perspective*. New Haven, CT: Yale University Press.

Hockenberry-Eaton, M. and Powell, M. L. (1991). Merging advanced practice roles: The NP and CNS. *Journal of Pediatric Health Care, 5,* 158–159.

Mauksch, I. G. (1975). Nursing is coming of age . . . through the practitioner movement: *American Journal of Nursing, 75,* 1834–1843.

Mechanic, H. F. (1988). Redefining the expanded role. *Nursing Outlook, 36,* 280–284.

Menard, S. W. (1987). The CNS: Historical perspectives. In S. W. Menard (Ed.). *The Clinical Nurse Specialist: Perspectives on practice*. New York: John Wiley and Sons, pp. 1–7.

Page, N. E. and Arena, D. M. (1994). Rethinking the merger of the clinical nurse specialist and the nurse practitioner roles. *Image, 26,* 315–318.

Rogers, M. E. (1975). Nursing is coming of age . . . through the practitioner movement: *American Journal of Nursing, 75,* 1834–1843.

Watson, J. (1995). Advanced nursing practice . . . and what might be. *Nursing and Health Care: Perspectives on Community, 16,* 78–83.

Consumers as Allies or Partners in Care

Jane M. Armer

The crescendoing health care costs in the United States combined with the epidemic of inadequate access to health care have created an urgent demand for health care reforms in this country. An essential step in designing much-needed widespread health care reforms is the research-based assessment of perceptions about health care and receptivity to change among consumers of health care. Only through better understanding of the consumer's perceptions of the current system and their expectations for future health care delivery can policymakers and health care providers develop responsive health care programs that will meet local and national health care needs and be acceptable to consumers in the decades ahead. This is an especially urgent consideration in view of the current expanding and aging population and growing health care needs at a time of diminishing economic resources (Mitchell et al. 1990). With government poised on the brink of monumental changes and reductions in support of health care, the timeliness and urgency of such research are evident.

RELEVANT BACKGROUND: CONSUMER INVOLVEMENT IN HEALTH CARE

In the decade of the 1970s, as consumers of health care became more informed, organized, and assertive of the right to be active participants in the health care delivery system (Stoller 1977), much research focused on consumer satisfaction with, and utilization of, the health care system (Flexner et al. 1977, Linn 1975, Olsen et al. 1976, Stewart and Wanklin 1978). The Aday et al. (1977) and Andersen et al. (1976) national surveys in 1963, 1970, and 1976 of individuals' utilization of, and attitudes toward, health care were three of the few studies to focus on future rather than past utilization of health care services and programs. Focusing on health care expectations of the public, these surveys were used to analyze the public attitude toward health policy proposals of national health insurance. Satisfaction with health care and responses to expanded nursing practice were also examined. Andersen et al. (1971) found that three-fourths of the families sampled agreed that there was a crisis in health care in the United States, although only 10% indicated they were dissatisfied with the quality of care they had recently received.

In the decade of the 1980s, there was continuing concern among consumers and providers about spiraling health care costs; diminished access to health care among the rural, the poor, the elderly, and minorities; and questionable quality and quantity of care (Boston 1990, Preziosi 1989, Sovie 1990, Wakefield 1990). The National Governors' Association declared escalating health care costs and access to care to be top priorities for the 1990s (Bocchini 1990).

Missouri, where the research reported on here was conducted, is a state ranked 48th out of 50 in terms of the health of its citizens based on 22 health factors such as percent of population covered by health insurance and per capita health care payments (Morgan et al. 1993). The state of Missouri continues to grapple with the politically sensitive issue of health care reform in an era of cost constraints. A prominent debate by regulatory boards and professional associations centers on state regulation of the advanced practice nurse role, a role shown to provide cost-effective, high-quality primary care (Aiken and Salmon 1994, Office of Technology Assessment 1986, Ramsey et al. 1982, Spitzer 1984). Indeed, it is estimated that 50% to 90% of care provided by primary care MDs could be provided by nurse practitioners (NPs) at a fraction of the cost. Clear validation of consumer acceptance of care by NPs is key to designing a restructured health care delivery system that meets the expectations and needs of the consumer.

One widespread and reportedly successful approach to resolving the current access and cost crises has been the development and implementation of a collaborative model of practice with NPs providing primary care in partnership with MDs in medically underserved areas and health professional shortage areas. Following intense lobbying and legislative jockeying, prescriptive privileges within written collaborative practice arrangements for advanced practice nurses (APNs) were recently approved by the Missouri legislature and passed into law by the governor. (A research-based report on the Missouri experience in advancing APN–MD collaborative practice through the legislature and regulatory process may be found in Chapter 11).

Consumer satisfaction with care provided by nurse practitioners has been found to be high (Banahan and Sharpe 1982, Kweskin 1979, Moraine 1992, Stone 1994, Thompson et al. 1982). Little research has focused on the perceptions and responses of consumers to collaboration and the collaborative model currently in place. In order to design and implement a model of health care delivery responsive to the needs of consumers in general, and underserved populations in particular, prospective investigation of consumer perceptions, satisfaction, and receptivity to the proposed model is essential. Social surveys of health care consumers have the potential to influence the health care policy decision-making process by clarifying and informing (Aday et al. 1977). Inclusion of the consumer as a partner in planning, developing, and participating in the collaborative health care model of the future is integral to the success of the new model.

SELECTED LITERATURE REVIEW ON THE CONSUMER ROLE IN COLLABORATIVE PRACTICE: AN OVERVIEW

Because the definition of collaboration is dealt with thoroughly in earlier chapters, it is here but briefly summarized to provide a platform for the discussion of consumer involvement in the collaborative partnership. Collaboration, according to the American Nurses Association (1980), is a "true partnership, in which the power on both sides is valued by both, with recognition and acceptance of separate and combined spheres of activity and responsibility, mutual safeguarding of the legitimate interests of each party, and a commonality of goals that is recognized by both parties." Note in this historical definition the implicit assumption of the existence of a collaborative dyad (NP and MD), rather than a triad inclusive of the consumer.

Patzel and Smith (1994) point out that neither physicians nor nurses are prepared by traditional education to operate as partners in collaborative practice. Perhaps because of tradition as well, the models and examples of collaborative practice almost uniformly fail to focus on a vital partner in the endeavor of care: the consumer. Johnson's (1993) qualitative study of nurse practitioner–patient conversations serves as an important exception to this tendency to exclude patients by describing collaboration between provider and patient: "The relationship between the NP [nurse practitioner] and patient was viewed as a partnership. . . . An element of camaraderie was viewed as positive and *not* in opposition to maintaining a professional stance" (p. 155).

Patzel and Smith (1994) view collaborative practice as a way to promote egalitarian practice, expand knowledge, and enhance skills, while promoting patient-centered care and improving outcomes. Reifsteck and D'Angelo (1990) document the relationship between communication and collaboration. Communication requires collaboration that is vital to patient care and education. Ideally, in collaboration, each member of the team, including the patient, participates in setting goals and priorities and in joint decision-making.

Existing literature claims impressive results from sound collaborative care, including better outcomes for patients, increased job satisfaction and improved communication among providers, and enhanced efficiency and coordination of care (Evans 1994, Norsen et al. 1995, Saur and Ford 1995, Velianoff et al. 1993). Miccolo and Spanier (1993) argue that collaborative practice is mandated by 1) articulate, knowledgeable consumers who question the quality and cost of health care; 2) professionals worried over fragmented, inaccessible care; 3) accrediting bodies emphasizing interdisciplinary care; and 4) the constraints of changing reimbursement patterns that call for increased efficiency.

Cahill (1996) identifies collaboration as a necessary precursor to patient participation in health care; in turn necessary for effective, ethical illness care and/or health promotion. Among the defining attributes, without which patient participation cannot occur, is "a narrowing of the appropriate information, knowledge and/or competence gap between the [provider] and patient using suitable modalities in different contexts" (p. 565). Educating consumers about collaboration and the roles or credentials of providers, as well as about health promotion and illness prevention or treatment, is seen as an important activity for nurses (Patzel and Smith 1994).

Research Findings: Patient Responses to the Advanced Practice Nurse Role

Despite the absence of studies that deal directly with consumers' perceptions of collaborative practice, research on consumers' perceptions of APNs (especially NPs) has been under way for some time (Armer 1993, Banahan and Sharpe 1982, Kviz et al. 1983, Hogan and Hogan 1982, Zikmund and Miller 1979). In a survey of users and nonusers of rural health clinics in Mississippi, Banahan and Sharpe (1982) found that only 56% of the nonusers were acquainted with the term *nurse practitioner*. After defining the term with an emphasis on NP–MD collaboration, 83% of the consumers expressed a willingness to receive services from an NP. The findings are consistent with the observation that familiarity with collaborative nurse–physician practice results in acceptance and appreciation (Mauksch and Campbell 1987); similarly, familiarity with the NP role has been crucial for gaining public approval.

Zikmund and Miller (1979) contend that acceptance of NP care in a given population would depend, in part, on what options in health care are available and how the consumer compares the options. In a factor analysis of the attitudes of 205 rural Oklahoma adults about the possibility of NP care in communities that currently had only one or no doctors, three dimensions of care were identified: 1) competency in role, 2) interpersonal relations, and 3) relative performance (or trust, when NP care was compared with MD care). Respondents generally believed that NPs would be competent but were uncertain about their diagnostic skills. Respondents viewed interpersonal skills of NPs as moderately favorable and held the expectation that NPs would educate and counsel. More uncertainty was exhibited regarding matters of relative performance of NPs when compared with those of MDs.

Two surveys of public opinion (Hogan and Hogan 1982, Kviz et al. 1983) in two differing populations, employees of a Midwestern university and rural residents of six Midwestern states, focused on specifying which primary care services were more or less acceptable to consumers when offered by an NP. Both studies supported overall acceptance of NP functions, with over 90% of respondents agreeing that they would allow the NPs to take a health history, give injections, and teach about health care (or explain the doctor's diagnosis, as one study stated). The two least acceptable NP functions (prescribing medication, performing complete routine physical examinations) were identical for the two groups. A significant portion of respondents in each study, however, would allow NP to prescribe medications and perform routine well care. Kviz and associates found 45% of their population would allow an NP to prescribe medication for a minor illness or injury, and Hogan and Hogan (1982) found that 37% of consumers would allow the NP to prescribe medicine for them. Similarly, 43% (Kviz et al. 1983) and 50% (Hogan and Hogan 1982) would allow the NP to perform a complete physical examination.

In the 1980s, Kviz et al. (1983) determined that rural consumers expressed a strong acceptance of a broadly defined NP role. Both Kviz et al. and Hogan and Hogan (1982), however, found that acceptance of the NP was greater for functions that were part of the traditional nurse's role than it was for less traditional functions such as complete routine physical examination. For example, respondents were much less willing to permit the NP to order routine tests, to suture lacerations, or to prescribe medicine and especially to perform a complete physical examination (Hogan and Hogan 1982). Hogan and Hogan (1982) also found that respondents felt that NP services were synonymous with providing support to underserved areas, spending time with the patient, and NP availability for home visits, all of which are care aspects that appeal to the patient as a consumer.

Public understanding of the APN role has evolved with the 1990s (Evans et al. 1995, Garrard et al. 1990, Hueston and Rudy 1993, Nugent 1992, Oakley et al. 1995, Olade 1989, Reed and Selleck 1996, Shaffer and Wexler 1995, Sebas 1994). Betancourt et al. (1996) compared MDs and patients in their knowledge of the roles and functions of NPs. Although the study is hampered by a small nonrandomized patient sample and a low return rate among MDs (25%), a comparison of 52 MDs and 55 patients offered an update to earlier studies regarding which primary care functions the public finds appropriate to NP practice. While performing physical examinations was viewed as an appropriate part of the NP role in 1996, prescribing medication, suturing minor wounds, and ordering and interpreting laboratory tests and X-rays were still viewed by both groups as outside the NP role. Only one significant difference between the two groups was found: NPs' ability to perform obstetric and gynecologic exams was recognized by MDs but not patients.

Similarly, Armer (1993) found that the majority of respondents from a Midwestern community supported the expanded nursing role, as evidenced by positive responses to selected advanced practice nursing activities, such as management of follow-up treatment and chronic illness and performance of physical exams. Armer further determined that without exception, farm-dwelling respondents showed the greatest percentage of support for all categories of advanced practice nursing.

Consumer Satisfaction With Advanced Practice Nursing Care

Notwithstanding some degree of reluctance among some potential users of services, reports from the era of the early 1980s support consumer acceptance and patient satisfaction with services rendered by family NPs (Kweskin 1979, Thompson et al. 1982). In a journal interview with a MD leader from the Oakland Kaiser-Permanente Medical Center, an innovator in utilizing NP to provide primary care, patient satisfaction was emphasized: "Patients are not obliged to participate in the NP program, but most have chosen to do so" (p. 19). Results of patient satisfaction surveys at Kaiser-Permanente were in concordance with a report from western Washington state (Thompson et al. 1982), where members of a consumer-owned health maintenance organization (HMO) recorded higher satisfaction with care in an outpatient clinic when the provider was an NP than when the provider was a MD. Likewise, Banahan and Sharpe (1982) and Thompson et al. (1982) found that patients were just as satisfied with treatment by NP as with that by MDs. The patients were more satisfied with waiting times for and the cost of care by NPs than with MDs.

In the decade of the 1990s, patient satisfaction has been a continuous thread in the APN literature. Morain (1992) reports a patient who is followed by a NP rates her NP an 11 on a scale of one to 10. In a review of the literature, Stone (1994) summarized, "Patients appear to be more satisfied with the care they receive from NPs than the care received from MDs in regard to several factors: personal interest exhibited, reduction in the professional mystique of health care delivery, amount of information conveyed, and cost of care (p. 21)."

Several factors are identified in the literature as influencing consumer satisfaction with advanced practice nursing care. Chang et al. (1984) found that patient participation in planning care had the most significant effect on patient satisfaction. When the patient was encouraged to participate in decision making, the visit was more satisfactory than when NPs made all of the decisions. This research supports the active involvement of patients in care-related decision-making in order to bring about greater satisfaction.

Studies conducted by D'Angelo et al. (1984) showed an 86.7% satisfaction and acceptance to care provided by NPs. Some of the identified reasons for satisfaction were that the NPs spent more time with them and that there was less waiting time for appointments, continuity of care, professional skills, education and teaching, and interpersonal support. Of these respondents, 97.5% would recommend an NP to others.

Kviz et al. (1983) demonstrated that a patient's age is the best predictor of NP acceptance. They go on to report that young males with low incomes are more willing to use NP services. Nurse practitioners are accepted in performance of traditional nursing duties and diagnosis of minor illness and injuries, but young adult males are less accepting of NPs performing minor surgery or physical examinations and prescribing medications or treatment.

Consumers tend to exhibit more positive acceptance and satisfaction once they have knowledge and understanding of the APN role. Kviz et al. (1983) concluded that lack of acceptance is related to lack of knowledge and public awareness by the consumer. Other studies (Hogan and Hogan 1982, Mackay et al. 1973, and Diers 1985, Ohliger 1985, Shively 1975) reported similar findings, in that there was less acceptance by those unfamiliar with the APN. Conversely, a high majority of patients felt confident in and satisfied with an NP as their primary care provider after they had experience seeing one. More than 10 years later, Armer (1993) found a substantial proportion of respondents who were "uncertain" about the appropriateness of selected advanced practice nursing tasks, leading us to conclude that the need for consumer education about the expanded nursing role continues.

This literature review demonstrates what little research has been done on consumer perception of actual collaborative practice. As with the role of NPs, the consumer must first be educated on collaboration before an accurate portrayal of satisfaction can be obtained.

Clients as Allies: Research on Consumer Perceptions of the Nurse Practitioner Role

Among the few prospective studies of consumers' views of the health care system is a series of studies conducted and reported by the author

(Armer 1993, 1997). The overall aim of the most recent study was to describe Midwestern residents' expectations and perceptions of health care. The specific research purpose was to describe and examine local and statewide public opinion about current satisfaction with health care, acceptance of the APN role, and prospective utilization of the APN for care for oneself and one's family. The project represented an extension of earlier research (Armer, unpublished data 1993) examining expectations and perceptions of health care in two Midwestern communities.

The majority of Midwestern respondents queried in 1991(Armer 1993) supported the expanded nursing role, as evidenced by positive responses to selected advanced practice nursing activities, such as management of follow-up treatment and chronic illness. Highly favorable responses (70%–94% agreement/strong agreement) to three of the selected examples of advanced practice nursing activities were found. The least favorable response (45% agreement/strong agreement) was found with the function often associated with the office nurse (licensed practical nurse or registered nurse), medical assistant, or receptionist who triages phone calls and, in effect, limits access to MD appointments. Urban and rural, male and female, young and old respondents favored the advanced practice nursing role, with a statistically nonsignificant trend toward increased agreement by rural (farm dweller), older, and male respondents. Without exception, farm-dwelling respondents showed the greatest percentage of support for all categories of advanced practice nursing, and this group was the only one that had a majority in agreement with the function of deciding whether the patient needed to see a doctor (56% agreement).

Two years later, the study was extended through use of a statewide randomized telephone survey. As in the 1991 county-wide study, support for the advanced practice nurse roles was high throughout the state (Figure 17-1). Overall, 85% supported the concept of an NP ("a nurse with special advanced training and certification") performing "well care" such as a health assessment and physical examination; 55% agreed the NP was qualified to decide if a doctor needed to be seen; 78% supported the NP in providing follow-up care and treatment; and 77% supported the NP in providing routine prenatal and infant care.

In a follow-up question, respondents were asked if they themselves or family members would personally use the services of an NP for each of the four activities. Percentages of prospective utilization were consistently within 2%–4% of the corresponding percentage of support in the preceding question (81%, 53%, 76%, and 74%, respectively). Findings

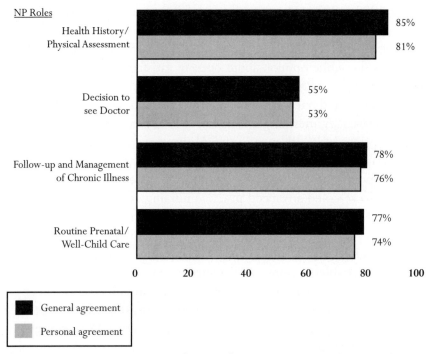

Figure 17-1.   *Overall percentage of support for nurse practitioner roles (N = 891).*

of NP support were generally consistent (statistically similar) across the variables of interest (age, gender, education, residence, income, insurance, and medical debt) (Table 17-1). Exceptions follow.

A significant association between the independent variables of age, education, gender, and income and the NP role of health history and physical examination was found. Education alone was shown to be related to positive response, with higher education related to a more positive response (74% approval for educational level of eighth grade or less; 85% approval for those with some high school and high school degree; and 89% approval for those with some post-secondary education, $P = .005$). When these four variables were looked at together via logistic regression, however, education did not help predict response in the presence of the other variables. Males (89% versus 82% for females, $P = .002$), those above poverty level (87% versus 77%, $P = .003$), and the younger two age groups (87% and 87% versus 76%, $P = .001$) were more likely to be positive.

For the NP role of delivering routine prenatal and well-baby care, age was associated with acceptance. A higher proportion of positive

Table 17-1. Variables Found to Significantly Predict Nurse Practitioner Support (N = 891)

NP Roles		Age	Gender	Education	Residence	Income	Insurance	Medical Debt
					Independent Variables			
Health History/ Physical Assessment	Relationship	+/-	+	+		+		
	Chi-Square	15.0/13.75	9.24	12.81	1.39	9.05	0.50	0.85
	Probability	P = .001*	P = .002*	P = .005*	P = .50	P = .003*	P = .82	P = .36
Decision to See Doctor	Relationship						−	
	Chi-Square	6.24	0.37	1.13	0.08	0.16	7.08	1.99
	Probability	P = .04	P = .54	P = .77	P = .96	P = .69	P = .008*	P = .16
Follow-up and Management of Chronic Illness	Relationship		+					
	Chi-Square	0.95	9.09	3.87	1.96	0.01	0.43	0.23
	Probability	P = .62	P = .003*	P = .28	P = .38	P = .92	P = .51	P = .64
Routine Prenatal and Well Child Care	Relationship	+/-	+					
	Chi-Square	9.6/9.7	5.42	5.69	1.22	0.05	0.08	0.51
	Probability	P = .008*	P = .02	P = .13	P = .54	P = .824	P = .78	P = .48

* $P < .01$.

525

responses was found among the middle age group (82%) than for the younger (74%) or the older (71%) ($P = .008$). The difference between the older and younger groups was not significant. Gender had borderline significance ($P = .020$), with males (at 81% approval) slightly more positive than females (74%).

The NP follow-up role was found to have a significant relationship with gender (positive responses by 83% of males versus 74% of females, $P = .003$). For the decision of whether patients needed to see a doctor, there was a relationship with insuredness. Among those without health insurance, 64% supported NPs making this decision, as compared with 53% of those who were insured ($P = .008$).

Findings of this statewide survey are consistent with the literature, which supports the generally high level of acceptance of community-based nurses and NPs by the consumer of health care (see, for example, Aiken and Salmon 1994). Overall support for the APN role was extremely high, with greater than 75% approval across three of four activities by gender, age, education, and rural/urban residence. The finding of overall high support and relatively few differences among groups when variables such as age, gender, residence, education, insurance, income, and medical debt were considered is a most positive finding in terms of its implications for both practice and policy. Residents of rural and urban communities; young, middle-aged and older adults; males and females (especially males); the insured and the uninsured; those above and below poverty level; households with and without medical debt; and persons at all educational levels are receptive to a range of primary care services provided by the NP. Nurse practitioners represent a highly valued and cost-effective health care resource in terms of meeting the great need for primary care among uninsured and underinsured persons in underserved rural, semirural, and urban communities.

It is significant that this high level of statewide consumer support for the advanced practice nurse role is documented in Missouri, the sixth most rural state in this country and one with demonstrated shortages in primary care services in both rural and urban areas (Morgan et al. 1993). Vulnerable, underserved populations are shown to be as receptive to primary care services provided by NPs as are less vulnerable groups.

Those above poverty level were more accepting of the health history or physical assessment role of the NP (and perhaps more apt to seek preventive care than those of lesser financial means). Conversely, those without insurance were more accepting of the role of the NP in deciding whether a doctor needed to be seen. This finding may be related to issues of choice, in that those who are uninsured are less apt to have a primary care provider and to practice preventive care. When faced with the option of emergency room care for an acute, nonemergency medical problem, as many uninsured are, the triage function of the NP in assessing the need to be seen by an MD (and perhaps in conserving scarce health care resources) may be more acceptable.

Gender was predictive of acceptance of NP functions of health history or physical assessment, follow-up after acute illness and management of chronic illness, and of borderline significance with the role of routine prenatal and well-baby care. In each case, males expressed higher approval than females (89% versus 82%; 83% versus 74%; and 81% versus 74%, respectively). There was no significant difference by gender in the area of decision on whether the patient needed to be seen by an MD (56% for males versus 54%). The gender difference bears further examination, with implications for targeting those more amenable to NP services for pilot projects and for educating those less amenable. Historically, members of one predominantly male group at risk, rural farmers, have not engaged in health promotion, disease prevention, or early detection programs. Receptivity of male consumers (including rural middle-aged males) to NP-provided services potentially provides a key to reaching this vulnerable population.

Some variations across groups in support of the role of NPs occurred because of responses of "uncertain" (range of 4% to 8% across roles). The highest percentage of "undecided" or "uncertain" responses was found with the NP role of providing routine prenatal and well baby care. This finding may account for some part of the gender differences noted earlier, as certain older female respondents chose the "uncertain" response with some roles, such as NP provision of routine prenatal and well-baby care. Members of this older generation may have experienced firsthand or witnessed complications associated with limited prenatal care, as well as complications of home or lay-assisted deliveries. They may have been educated that there are lesser risks associated with MD-assisted prenatal care. Therefore, they may be uncertain about the appropriateness of this NP role. This finding has implications for education of the health care consumer about appropriate roles of primary care providers, particularly in the face of too-often limited access to primary care among vulnerable populations such as rural and minority groups. With appropriate information and education, it is highly possible that some of those who were uncertain would become supporters of the advanced practice nursing role.

The consistently lower percentage of support for the triage role of the NP in determining whether a MD needs to be seen calls attention to the need for education and careful marketing strategies as health policy planners and providers look at the realities of managed care. This finding supports other research in this area (see, for example, Armer 1993). Choice is extremely important to the American public, both in terms of choice of MD, with, as reported elsewhere (Armer, in review), only 16% of Missouri respondents supporting and 84% opposing health care reform that involved losing choice of personal MD) and in terms of people wanting to see a doctor when they believed they needed to be seen, with 45% resisting the role of a nurse in triaging doctor visits.

The description of the relationships between and among the studied variables contributes to the development of a fuller understanding of the consumer's response to the health care scene. Outcomes of this study provide meaningful and relevant data for local, state, and federal health providers and policymakers.

IMPLICATIONS FOR THE FUTURE: A MODEL FOR CONSUMER PARTICIPATION IN NURSE PRACTITIONER–PHYSICIAN COLLABORATION

Research to evaluate the perceived expectations and effectiveness of current programs and services in the eyes of the consumers is particularly timely as we strive to understand public health needs in the context of state and national health care issues. Consumer responses to a survey have the potential to assist policymakers and health care planners and providers to act in ways that will better represent the views of the citizens and better meet the community's long-range needs (Blendon and Donelan 1991, Blendon et al. 1993). Sharing these research-based data with local, state, and national health care providers and planners can serve to influence the continuation and development of present and future programs and services in the state of Missouri and in this country.

The need for education of the consumer concerning the potential roles in primary care that are competently carried out by the nurse with advanced education is also identified; public opinion survey methodology performs an informative, educative function in and of itself as it serves to increase awareness of the potential alternatives that exist (Aday et al. 1977). The targeting of underserved communities with overall positive attitudes toward the prospective changes enhances the opportunity for a cost-effective, successful demonstration project that has potential to be replicated throughout the state and the country. In the current climate of governmental cost constraint and spiraling health care costs and concerns, such research-based strategies are essential.

The constituency of consumers—of elders and other community-based vulnerable populations, including minority groups—is a powerful partner for potential collaborative endeavors, a natural ally for nursing and other health providers in planning and initiating a health care delivery system that supports a successful model such as APN–MD collaborative practice. As a singular example, at the 1994 Midwest Nursing Research Society Health Policy preconference in Milwaukee, a community health nurse–political activist reported on her work as convener of the task force on healthcare reform for the frontier state of North Dakota. This nurse activist described the power of silver-haired senior citizens marching into the state capitol to demand reimbursement for NP services under health care reform because nurse practitioners were the group who would meet the health needs of rural North Dakota residents. Legislators responded with a positive vote representing the views of their elderly constituency. Such partnerships with consumers, APNs, and other primary care providers can provide a solid foundation for imminent health care reform.

As nurses, physicians, and other health care providers and planners consider how best to meet the health care needs of communities now and in the future, research-based data and renewed attention to the perspectives of the consumer are essential. The examination of receptivity of health care consumers to proposed alternatives is a crucial step in planning and implementing a program of health care reform that will meet current and future health needs of the citizens of this state and the country. Similarly, the inclusion of consumers as allies and collaborative partners in care is essential to the successful redesign of a health care system that will meet needs in the decades ahead.

Acknowledgment:

Grateful appreciation is extended to Toni J. Sullivan, RN, Ed.D., FAAN, for editorial comments, and to Richard Lister, MSN, RNCS, FNP-C,

Cathy Schafer, RN, BSN, MPA, and Lynn Parshall, RN, BSN, MS(N) for their technical and literary assistance and support. Chapter findings reprinted with permission from National League for Nursing Publishing Company, *Nursing and Health Care: Perspectives on Community.*

References

Aday, L. A., Andersen, R., and Anderson, O. W. (1977). Social surveys and health policy implications for national health insurance. *Public Health Reports, 92,* 508–517.

Aiken, L. H. and Salmon, M. E. (1994). Health care workforce priorities: What nursing should do now. *Inquiry, 31,* 318–329.

American Nurses Association (1980). *Nursing: A Social Policy Statement.* Washington, D.C.: American Nurses Association.

Andersen, R., Kravits, J. M., and Anderson, O. W. (1971). The public's view of the crisis in medical care: An impetus for changing delivery systems? *Economic and Business Bulletin, 24,* 44–52.

Andersen, R., Lion, J., and Andersen, O. W. (1976). *Two Decades of Health Services: Social Survey Trends in Use and Expenditure.* Cambridge: Ballinger Publishing.

Armer, J. M. (1997, March/April). Missouri responds to the advanced practice nurse role. *Nursing and Health Care: Perspectives on Community, 18*(2), 86–90.

Armer, J. M. (1993). A social survey: Public perception of crisis in health care and response to advanced nursing role. *The Nurse Practitioner: The American Journal of Primary Care, 18*(10), 15–20.

Banahan, B.F, III, and Sharpe, T.R. (1982). Evaluation of the use of rural health clinics; knowledge, attitudes, and behaviors of consumers. *Public Health Reports, 97*(3), 261–268.

Betancourt, J.C., Valmocina, M., and Grossman, D. (1996). Physicians' and patients' knowledge and perceptions of the role and functions of nurse practitioners. *Nurse Practitioner: American Journal of Primary Health Care, 21*(8), 13–15.

Blendon, R. J. and Donelan, K. (1991). Interpreting public opinion surveys. *Health Affairs, 10*(2), 166–169.

Blendon, R. J., Hyams, T. S., and Benson, J.M. (1993). Bridging the gap between expert and public views on health care reform. *Journal of the American Medical Association, 269*(19), 2573–2578.

Bocchini, C. A. (1990). Capitol Commentary. *Nursing Economics, 8,* 60–61, 120, 274–275.

Boston, C. M. (1990). Healthcare Reform. *Journal of Nursing Administration,* *20*(7/8), 8–9.

Cahill, J. (1996). Patient participation: A concept analysis. *Journal of Advanced Nursing, 24*(3), 561–567.

Chang, B., Uman, G., Linn, L., Ware, Jr., J., and Kane, R. (1984). The effect of systematically varying components of nursing care on satisfaction in elderly ambulatory women. *Western Journal of Nursing Research, 6*(4), 367–386.

D'Angelo, L., Reifsteck, S., and Green, R. (1984). Nurse practitioners co-providers of health care. *Medical Group Management, May/June,* 38–44.

Evans, J. (1994). The role of the nurse manager in creating an environment for collaborative practice. *Holistic Nurse Practitioner, 8*(3), 22–31.

Evans, L., Yurkow, J., and Siegler, E. (1995). The CARE program: a nurse-managed collaborative outpatient program to improve function of frail older people. *Journal of the American Gerontological Society, 43*(10), 1155–1160.

Flexner, W. A., McLaughlin, C. P., and Littlefield, J. E. (1977). Discovering what the health consumer really wants. *HCM Review,* 43–49.

Garrard, J., Kane, R., Radosevich, D., Skay, C., Arnold, S., Kepferle, L., McDermott, S., and Buchanan, J. (1990). Impact of geriatric nurse practitioners on nursing-home residents' functional status, satisfaction, and discharge outcomes. *Medical Care, 28*(3), 271–283.

Hogan, K. and Hogan, R. (1982). Assessment of the consumer's potential response to the nurse practitioner model. *Journal of Nursing Education, 21*(9), 4–12.

Hueston, W. and Rudy, M. (1993). A comparison of labor and delivery management between nurse midwives and family physicians. *The Journal of Family Practice, 37*(5), 449–454.

Johnson, R. (1993). Nurse practitioner–patient discourse: uncovering the voice of nursing in primary care practice. *Scholarly Inquiry for Nursing Practice: An International Journal, 7*(3), 143–157.

Kviz, F., Misener, T., and Vinson, N. (1983). Rural health care consumers' perceptions of the nurse practitioner role. *Journal of Community Health, 8*(4), 248–262.

Kweskin, S. (1979). Innovations in patient care focusing on the benefits of NPs in primary care. *Patient Care, October 15,* 194–204.

Linn, L. S. (1975). Factors associated with patient evaluation of health care. *Health and Society,* 531–548.

Mackay, R. C., Alexander, D. S., and Kingsbury, L. J. (1973). Parent's attitudes toward the nurse as physician associate in a pediatric practice. *Canadian Journal of Public Health, 64* (2), 121–132.

Mauksch, H. O. and Campbell, J. P. (1987). The nursing presence examined by assessing joint practice. In *Perspectives in Nursing 1987–1989 (National League for Nursing) (41–2199),* 157–175.

Miccolo, M. and Spanier, A. (1993). Critical care management in the 1990s: Making collaborative practice work. *Critical Care Clinics, 9*(3), 443–453.

Mitchell, P. H., Krueger, J. C., and Moody, L. E. (1990). The crisis of the health-care nonsystem. *Nursing Outlook, 38,* 214–217.

Molde, S. and Diers, D. (1985). Nurse practitioner research: selected literature review and research agenda. *Nursing Research, 34*(6), 362–367.

Morain, C. (1992). On her own. *RN, July,* 28–32.

Morgan, K., Morgan, S., Quitno, N. (Eds). *Health Care State Rankings 1993.* Lawrence, KS: Morgan Quitno Corporation.

Norsen, L., Opladen, J., and Quinn, J. (1995). Practice model: Collaborative practice. *Critical Care Nursing Clinics of North America, 7*(1), 43–52.

Nugent, K. (1992). The clinical nurse specialist as case manager in a collaborative practice model: Bridging the gap between quality and cost of care. *Clinical Nurse Specialist, 6*(2), 106–111.

Oakley, D., Murtland, T., Mayes, F., Hayashi, R., Petersen, B., Rorie, C., and Andersen, F. (1995). Processes of care: Comparisons of certified nurse-midwives and obstetricians. *Journal of Nurse-Midwifery, 40*(5), 399–409.

Ohliger, J. (1985). Factors related to women's preferences for obgyn care providers: and explanatory survey. *Health Care for Women International, 6,* 327–340.

Olade, R. (1989). Perception of nurses in expanded role. *International Journal of Nursing Studies, 26*(1), 15–25.

Office of Technology Assessment 1986. *Nurse Practitioners, Physician Assistants, and Certified Nurse Midwifes: A Policy Analysis. HCS 37.* Washington, DC: Congress of the United States Office of Technology Assessment, 12(86).

Olsen, D. M., Kane, R. L., and Kasteler, J. (1976). Medical care as a commodity: An exploration of the shopping behavior of patients. *Journal of Community Health, 2,* 85–91.

Patzel, B. and Smith, B. (1994). Collaboration: directions for advanced practice. *The Kansas Nurse, 69*(9), 3–4.

Preziosi, P. (1989). *Developing a national health plan. Why now? Why nurses?* New York: National League for Nursing.

Ramsey, J. A., McKenzie, J. K., and Fish, D. G. (1982). Physicians and nurse practitioners: Do they provide equivalent care? *American Journal of Public Health, 72*(1), 55–57.

Reed, C. and Selleck, C. (1996). The role of midlevel providers in cancer screening. *Medical Clinics of North America, 80*(1), 135–144.

Reifsteck, S. and D'Angelo, L. (1990). Physician–nurse relationships. *Top Health Care Finance, 16*(3), 12–21.

Saur, C. and Ford, S. (1995). Quality, cost-effective psychiatric treatment: a CNS–MD collaborative practice model. *Archives of Psychiatric Nursing, IX*(6), 332–337.

Sebas, M. (1994). Developing a collaborative practice agreement for the primary care setting. *Nurse Practitioner 19*(3), 49–51.

Shaffer, J. and Wexler, L. (1995). Reducing low-density lipoprotein cholesterol levels in an ambulatory care system. *Archives of Internal Medicine, 155,* 2330–2335.

Shively, J. P. (1975). The role of the nurse practitioner. *American Journal of Obstetrics and Gynecology (June 15),* 502–507.

Sovie, M. D. (1990). Redesigning our future: Whose responsibility is it? *Nursing Economics, 8,* 21–26.

Spitzer, W. O. (1984). The nurse practitioner revisited. *The New England Journal of Medicine, 310*(16), 1049–1051.

Stewart, M. A., and Wanklin, J. (1978). Direct and indirect measures of patient satisfaction with physicians' services. *Journal of Community Health, 3,* 195–204.

Stoller, E. P. (1977). New roles for health care consumers: A study of role transformation. *Journal of Community Health, 3,* 171–177.

Stone, P. W. (1994). Nurse practitioners' research review: Quality of care. *Nurse Practitioner* [Letter to the editor], *17*(June), 21,27.

Thompson, R., Basden, P., and Howell, L. (1982). Evaluation of initial implementation of an organized adult health program employing family nurse practitioners. *Medical Care, XX*(11), 1109–1127.

Velianoff, G., Neely, C., and Hall, S. (1993). Developmental levels of interdisciplinary collaborative practice committees. *Journal of Nursing Administration, 23*(7/8), 26–29.

Wakefield, M. K. (1990). Perspectives on health policy. *Nursing Economics, 8,* 121–123.

Zikmund, W. and Miller, S. (1979). A factor analysis of attitudes of rural health care consumers toward nurse practitioners. *Research in Nursing and Health, 2,* 85–90.

Consumers in Health 18
Care Part I:
Consumers Speak Out[1]

Toni J. Sullivan

INTRODUCTION

The purpose of the focus group research and literature review reported on in Chapters 18 and 19 is to find out about the attitudes, beliefs, and perceptions of the grass roots concerning participation in health and health-related coalitions in communities and concerning participation in health care delivery both as patients and as citizens attempting to influence health care policy. Focus group participant data are reported on in this chapter and literature review data are reported on in the next chapter. The end of Chapter 19 contains a discussion and conclusions section that pertains to the data presented in both chapters. This major topic is divided into two chapters for ease of reading and study.

The need for a focus on citizen participation in health care has already been touched upon in the discussion in Chapter 9 on coalition formation and conduct. In that chapter, the characteristics of the members of coalitions (professional or grass roots or combination), the characteristics of their participation in coalitions (voluntary to mandatory), and the nature of the partnership (equal authority in decision making or less than equal authority) were all identified as important determinants of the nature of coalitions and the success of coalitions in meeting their goals and generally achieving successful outcomes.

---

[1]Chapter 19 constitutes Part II of the focus on consumers in health care.

Although the literature authored exclusively by professionals (see Chapter 9) and the conclusions drawn by this author were uniformly positive concerning full or equal grass roots participation with professionals in coalition formation and conduct, there was no evidence of citizens reporting on their own involvement, nor were there any consistent references to indicate who were the grass roots participants. The question was raised in Chapter 9 as to whether the term *grass roots* referred only to individuals or to local organizations as well. The literature is silent on that question. This author believes that this is a contextual issue: A federal view of a locality might label both individuals and organizations as grass roots, whereas a local view might label individuals as grass roots but define organizations as professional bodies. The literature is equally silent on how to label grass roots participants. Terms used in Chapter 9 (both by the author and the scholars in the cited literature) to describe grass roots participants included *advocate, citizen, citizen activist, the community, community activist, consumer, consumer participant, grass roots citizens, lay people, lay persons,* and *volunteers.*

In wanting to advance the ability of professionals to work more effectively and productively with citizens in coalition formation and conduct, one is then left to ponder many questions about how people who are not health professionals but have a major stake in health care in all its manifestations view their roles and their involvement. The term *community activist* seems to be the term that best captures the active and involved relationships these citizens have with their communities and the overall community welfare. Health promotion, policy advocacy, health care planning, intervention research, patient care delivery, networks to increase access to care, and health care costs and financing are but some of the major reasons why citizens would choose to serve as community activists and be actively involved in health care and health-related coalitions. Focus group research was selected as the most appropriate way to learn what citizens' thoughts were on these matters of such direct concern to them.

METHODOLOGY: FOCUS GROUP

The methodology used is focus group research, and following completion of the focus group study, a literature review of concepts identified by the focus group participants was conducted.

Focus Group Description

The methodology of using a focus group is a qualitative research technique borrowed from marketing and psychology. It is an informal session that brings together participants to share their thoughts on a specific subject. The method is especially useful in determining the attitudes, beliefs, and opinions of target populations. It is a way to learn the language and colloquialisms of a particular population group. It also is a way to learn how strongly (representatives of) a group feels about a particular issue or topic.

The knowledge gained from a focus group provides insights regarding how participants view a particular topic. Such knowledge is useful for program planning, as a preliminary step in research, as a backdrop for quantitative research design, and as an educational vehicle for one group to better understand another group. As a technique, focus group research has the limitations of qualitative research. Focus group findings cannot be generalized to the larger population of which the group is a representative sample. It is also important not to assume "knowledge of the magnitude of the attitude" (Ramirez and Shepperd 1988, p. 83) displayed by the focus group participants (Eriksson 1988, Palm and Windahl 1988, Ramirez and Shepperd 1988).

Sample and Procedure for Sample Selection

Twelve active citizens were invited to participate in a focus group session to share insights about their involvement in their communities in health and health-related matters; 9 accepted, and 8 were able to attend the focus group session as scheduled. The participants were nominated by reputation as involved active citizens. The investigator (the author) began the process of invitation by inviting two people with whom she had interacted professionally in a community coalition. She nominated them and sought additional nominations from them. Thus, most of the participants came from nominations by citizens themselves.

Seven of the eight participants are retired or semiretired and active in community or consumer advocacy organizations primarily concerned with the elderly; one participant was fully employed by an advocacy organization for the disabled and is herself disabled. With the exception of one husband and wife, these participants were known to each other only in the capacity of their community activist roles. Three of the eight were previously known to the researcher, but only in a professional capacity. The group, as is recommended by authorities in focus group research, was quite homogeneous and, other than the one exception noted, was not comprised of friends or family of the researcher or each other. Each participant completed a brief questionnaire in which they listed three of the community organizations in which they are active. Table 18-1 provides an outline of their multiple involvements and verifies their status as active involved citizens.

A research assistant for the investigator contacted each potential participant by telephone, briefly explained the study, and invited their participation 4 weeks before the scheduled focus group session. A confirming letter was sent 3 weeks before the session giving information about time, place, parking, and the like. One week before the session, a list of topics for discussion was sent. The intent was not to prepare formally, but to enable the participants to have the opportunity to reflect on the likely discussion topics before the session. Discussion topics listed were community activism and how to define it or related words, motivation for active involvement in the community, biggest issues in health care today, ways in which they can best contribute to community and health care collaborative efforts, roles as active members of the community in influencing community health and health care, suggestions for health professionals and community influentials in working with active citizens, and advice for would-be community activists.

The study plan and topics list received human subjects exempt status from the University of Missouri Institutional Review Board. Before beginning the session, the participants signed release forms allowing the investigator to use the data in aggregate form and to quote the participants verbatim as long as they were not named.

Data Collection

A 3.5-hour session was held in an attractive and comfortable conference room at the University of Missouri. A buffet luncheon was served first during which participants introduced themselves and told a little of their backgrounds. The moderator (the investigator) explained that with the permission of all participants, the session would be tape recorded. She requested that participants speak only one at a time and indicated that

Table 18-1. Organizations and Roles of Participants

Participant	Organization	Role
1.	Local Chapter Missouri Disability Rights Coalition	Member
	Assoc. of Programs for Rural Independent Living	Member
	Home of Your Own Advisory Board	Member
2.	Missouri Coalition for Quality Care	President and Founder
	Hospice of Jefferson City and Mid-Missouri	Member
	National Coalition for Nursing Home Reform	Member
3.	Visiting Nurses Assoc. of Central Missouri	Board Member and Founder
	Boone County Council on Aging	Member
	Missouri Assoc. of Home Care	Member
4.	State Legislative Committee of American Assoc. of Retired Persons (AARP)	Chair
	Homemaker Health Care Board	Member
	Local Chapter, Missouri Assoc. of Social Workers (MASW) Health Watch	Member
5.	National and State Silver Haired Legislature	Member
	Northeast Missouri Area Agency on Aging	Chair and Board Member
	AARP	Tax Aide and Instructor
6.	Missouri Silver Haired Legislature	Speaker of the House
	National Silver Haired Congress	Representative
	Lincoln County Council on Aging	President (Former)
7.	University of Missouri Retirees Assoc.	Member
	Boone County Chapter, AARP	Member
	Senior Services of Boone County	Member

she would state each person's name before they spoke. These procedures help to capture fully each participant's contributions to the discussion. In addition, participants were assured that there were no "right or wrong answers" and that the investigator was far from an expert on these topics. In this way, participants were made to feel comfortable sharing their opinions and experiences.

A follow-up contact was made with each participant within 10 days of the session to inquire whether the participant had any follow-up thoughts they would like to add. This activity was deemed necessary because only one focus group session was held. Only one participant offered a further observation; all others reported feeling satisfied with the completeness of their sharing. The recorded session was transcribed verbatim; the procedures used to ensure clear tape recordings were effective. All the data were captured, with the exception of an occasional indecipherable word.

Data Analysis

The data were reviewed and rereviewed repeatedly by the researcher. First, the data were separated by topics discussed and then sorted into segments. Segments were then reviewed for themes and trends. The minimum unit of analysis was the sentence. Whole segments (usually paragraphs) were also used when, in the researcher's judgment, this extension was necessary to capture the meaning intended by the speaker. Care was taken not to reach conclusions about the data too early in the analysis process. The research assistant was asked to review the themes and trends identified, along with the supporting data, to add to the validity of the conclusions reached by the researcher.

METHODOLOGY: LITERATURE REVIEW

The literature review, which may be defined and used in myriad ways, is defined and used here in accord with the classic literature review function of organizing and summarizing a representative sample of the literature on a selected subject in order to provide a firm foundation for further research or new understanding of a well-known concept or construct (Polit and Hungler 1991, p. 105). In this case, the literature concerning the defining labels these focus group participants used to label themselves was surveyed in order to compare and contrast the understanding of professionals or scholars with the understanding of the citizen participants in the focus group.

Sample Selection

The literature search was conducted to review key constructs related to citizen participation in coalition building, particularly from the broad perspectives of consumer and advocacy. Key words used for the search were *advocacy–advocate* in the context of patient or community, *community activist* or *activism* or *involvement*, and *consumer participation*.

A two-phase search was conducted using the databases of ABI/Inform, Cumulative Index of Nursing and Allied Health Literature (CINAHL), and HealthStar. Within ABI/Inform, the search was limited to 1993 to June 1997; within CINAHL, the search expanded to 1982 to 1996; and within HealthStar, the search was limited to 1990 to the present. Health-Star and CINAHL databases have health as an overriding context of all noted articles. Within ABI/Inform, however, health was used as a combining word initially to sort out concepts that were within the context of health care. Listings of just key words independently were also used.

Across the three databases queried, 396 potential articles were noted with the key word of *consumer* (or *consumerism*); 254 potential articles were noted with the key word of *community involvement;* and only one potential article was noted with the key word of *community activist.* From this initial search, 22 articles were found across all three databases that were deemed appropriate for the discussion of citizen participation in coalition building or citizen influence of health care delivery policy and practice. Many of these articles were preoccupied with consumer interactions with managed care models of health care delivery.

The second-phase search focused on the constructs of advocate and advocacy, using the body of literature described above, and resulting in over 5000 articles. Reduction of the search was accomplished by key words, particularly relating *community* and *consumer* as modifiers of the word *advocate* or *advocacy.* This query resulted in approximately 70 articles to be reviewed for relevance to the topic. By relating these abstracts to advocacy within health care situations, the number of articles to be used was reduced to 19.

RESEARCH QUESTIONS

The research questions posed were as follows:

1. How do citizens who are laypeople and who are active volunteers perceive themselves and their responsibilities and actions in actively influencing health care in the community or health care as available to the people (citizens)?
2. How are laypeople defined in the health sciences literature; what does the health sciences literature describe the opportunities, responsibilities, and actions of citizens who are laypeople to be in actively participating in and influencing health care in the community or health care as available to citizens?

Research question 1 is addressed by the focus group findings in the next section. Research question 2 is addressed by the literature review findings and is found in the next chapter. Also found there is a discussion that compares and contrasts the focus group and literature review findings. Tentative future predictions are offered concerning the future direction of health care in the United States and the developed world as a result of the playing out of tensions between consumers and organized professional and corporate health care interests.

PRESENTATION OF FINDINGS: FOCUS GROUP

The participants were remarkably articulate, informed, and assertive in sharing their informed opinions and their expertise. As seen in Table 18-1, these participants are all extremely active in myriad volunteer roles in their communities and in lay organizations. Because the researcher wondered whether this group was an exceptionally well-educated group in relation to their age cohorts, they were queried as to their educational backgrounds. Four of the participants had "some college," one had postsecondary training in a vocational program, one had an undergraduate degree, one had a master's degree, and one had a professional doctoral degree. It seemed correct to conclude that this group was relatively well educated and well positioned to provide leadership to their age cohorts.

Table 18-2. Topics and Themes of Focus Group Data

Topical Area	Theme	Units of Analysis
Consumer advocacy	Call me advocate or consumer	16
	Consumer advocacy roles	50
Motivation	Concern for others	11
	Personal satisfaction	07
	Mission\Vision\Goals	06
	Personal life stories	04
Reaching out	Mentoring\Recruiting\Involving others	08
	Concern for next generation	02
	Advice to Professionals	04
Health care	Dissatisfactions	22
	Horror stories	12
	Satisfactions	06
	Sympathy for health care professionals	05

Four broad topical areas are encompassed in the data: consumer advocacy, motivation, health care, and reaching out. Twelve broad themes are present, and the themes show numerous trends that the presentation of data aims to capture. Table 18-2 outlines the topics and themes, and lists the number of units of analysis identified for each theme. It is important to note that each unit of analysis was only coded in one way; codes were often changed as the researcher struggled to decide which theme was paramount in these complex statements. The total number of the units of analysis is 153.

Consumer Advocacy

Call me *advocate* or *consumer*

This group generally did not favor the term *community activist*, and several of its members had a strong negative reaction to the term. "I have a little problem with the term *community activist*." "*Activist* brings up all sorts of negative feelings to me." "An activist to me . . . would picket in front of some place." "*Activist,* I agree, I did not like the term *activist*."

"I really strongly object to the connotation of the word *activist,* because I consider that the next step to *terrorist* or *terrorism.*" "The term *activist* implies to me more of a confrontational approach to things." Two group members tried to be fair to the term: "*Activism* is [defined as] taking a positive direct action to achieve an end. I think I kind of like that . . . so I guess I'm an advocate for activism." "I don't agree that [use of the term] *activist* is necessarily a bad thing."

These participants defined themselves as *advocates,* a self-defining term they all appeared comfortable with: "I would think of us more as advocates [than activists]." "An advocate is someone who is doing something out of pure concern or feelings for whatever the issue is." "Helping others to help themselves would be advocacy." "An advocate is one who pleads the cause of another." "In the disability community our purposes are advocacy, advocacy, advocacy—not necessarily in that order."

Part of the way through the discussion of advocacy and activism, the term *consumer* was raised by one of the group and then became either integral or dominant in the balance of the discussion concerning how to regard one's active roles in the community. The group was not entirely pleased with the term *consumer,* but they seemed to attribute their dissatisfactions with the term more to health care system inadequacies than to the meaning of the term itself. It also was noted by this researcher that these participants did not label themselves as *consumer* advocates. What becomes very apparent, however, is that the focus of their advocacy is on consumer issues and the beneficiaries of their advocacy are citizens, including themselves, whom they label as consumers. "I have a little problem with consumerism [along with activism] because the whole health care system is set up so that it's difficult for anybody to be a true consumer who makes choices. There's limited access." "The Governor's Advisory Council [of which this respondent is a member] has turned the consumer into customer, because we as a customer are buying the service, whether it's through our insurance, Medicaid, or whatever." "The thing that bothers me about *customer* or *consumer* is that both of those [terms] imply available information that people are not provided when they go into the health care marketplace."

The opportunity to make choices was clearly the essential attribute of being a consumer to these citizens. "We as a consumer or customer, when we make the decision that it's our choice, we're a much happier camper than if we're told we have to accept something that someone else thinks we need, and maybe it's not what we need at all. . . ." "We are consumers or customers . . . and we want to ask for what we can get . . . to have free choice as a customer, and if you don't like what one grocery store has . . . you have the ability to go to a different grocery store." Again, the analogy to shopping for groceries: "When I go to the grocery store, I see price tags on the shelves and I can make choices. . . . We don't have that kind of price knowledge in the health care field, so it's a little hard to be a good customer." A respondent bluntly stated, "Don't tell us what you think we need, tell us what we need to know and let the choice remain ours." A related term for *consumer* was suggested: "I like the term *purchaser* more than *consumer* . . . when you say *consume* you eat it up and swallow it . . . where a purchaser [is] actually buying something."

As the group discussed the labels of *activist, advocate,* and *consumer,* several participants began to relate the terms to each other in some very interesting ways: "I see them [activist and advocate] as very different roles. If there isn't anything here . . . but there is a need, then there's time for...activism or activists. Then to keep things going we have advocates. And then activists . . . continue in their roles—stimulating, exciting, developing—so [that] the advocates can continue to support the . . . need." Another respondent defined activism as a tool of the advocates: "[A]dvocacy [is] the first thing as you . . . work with people [community or government influentials], you try to make them understand how what we're trying to get them to do is going to work for them, too. But we have all different ranges. If it takes picketing. . . . If it gets to the point where nothing else . . . works . . . then as an advocate those are your extreme resources."

Another comment integrated the notions of consumer and advocate: "I'm both. I'm consumer and user and purchaser. . . . I'm an advocate because I believe we all have the right to health care the way we need it. . . . I know what I need, and when I go to use the system, I pretty much have expectations at this point of being listened to. When I'm not I don't go back to that person. . . ."

Consumer Advocacy Roles

This theme proved to be the most prevalent, with 50 units of analysis falling into this category. Teaching, lobbying, forming and conducting coalitions, and leadership are the dynamic roles these citizens play. "One of the goals of the organization I'm involved in [which speaker founded and leads] is to teach the consumer how to evaluate health care facilities . . . as far as quality indicators and not just cost, but quality indicators that we want to teach people how to use." "Day in and day out I run into seniors who need more information. . . ." "We are holding forums around the state this year, to try and get information to seniors so that when the time comes that they have to make a decision, they have some information and make better decisions on the type of health care they're purchasing." Teaching others in order to swell the ranks of consumer advocates is understood to be an important role: "We teach people how to work with the legislators, how to write letters, how to make phone calls, how to go down there and talk to them."

"What we're talking about is getting groups together. . . . [A] lot of coalitions have been going on these last few years." "We [seniors federation of advocacy organizations] put a push on the managed care thing[,] and the governor got a thousand letters from senior citizens." "The federation of aging organizations . . . I think there's 20 . . . retired teachers, retired professors, the Jewish community . . . retired federal employees, silver haired legislature. . . . [W]e all band together. . . . [W]e voted that we were going to stay together and we're going to continue to work as a common front for all of these issues that we're talking about." "We get together to share legislative information so we're all on the same track. If we can go in and say to legislators that we are focused [within the federation] on this issue, we are far more effective."

Membership in the coalitions discussed seems to be composed primarily of diverse groups of volunteers. Most of the membership in the seniors organizations are likely to be volunteers. Health care professionals and other professional or managerial workers do not seem to be members of these coalitions as part of their daily professional or managerial responsibilities. All persons who share in the mission or goals of a particular advocacy organization or coalition are, however, welcome to join. "There's a mixture of professionals, there's PhDs, whether they are in education or something else. There's people who're non-professionals, as such. . . ." Another respondent stated, "At least in this organization that I'm involved in, there is a very clear place . . . for the health care professionals who care about quality of care. . . ."

The coalition activities, advocacy roles, and general expertise of the group members added up to their being leaders in their communities and with their reference groups. "And it seems to me we need to work on getting the whole community to know what's going on so that we don't have a lot of duplicate efforts, but rather have collaborative efforts. . . ." "One of the things I see is the need for knowledge about the policy and laws and what is actually happening." Often new members of organizations need to be educated about what is really going on. "[A] retired state representative spoke to [the federation on aging] last month about forming another organization that would deal with not-for-profits. . . . Everyone in the group was not sure we needed another group to belong to. . . ." The informant goes on to say that she, as the leader, discussed this with her [the former legislator] personally and informed her about where to obtain information that she needed to have to understand the activity and organization already occurring. She concludes by saying: "[T]his is someone newly into this network . . . who's having to educate herself as to what all does exist."

One informant spoke of the advocacy leadership that he and his wife share with their fellow citizens in their county:

> What we have done in our county, and [what] Beth [assumed name] and I have done on numerous occasions, is when people come into the senior center, they sort of look for us. So we're their advocate. And they'll bring in a box of these bills. And we have sat down, I don't know how many times, at the kitchen table or dining table and sorted all these out and put the Medicare and what it will [cover] and the supplemental bills [and what they'll cover] and we'll staple them together. And we'll come out with what's left. And nine times out of ten they don't owe anything, but . . . this generation, we have been so trained that you pay your bills. You almost have to fight with some of these little old ladies about don't pay it, wait two months, wait six months. And by that time it will all resolve itself. Regardless if they say they are going to turn it over to a collection agency or get a lawyer. Well, just say your lawyer can talk to my lawyer. That's your standard answer, see. But don't pay anything for six months . . . because it always resolves itself out.

This group is highly expert and savvy in political action as well as advocacy, and through their organizations and federations, they have access to expert analysis of legislation:

> When we have bills we send them to Washington D.C. for professional analysis and they come back, you know, this is a fair bill but it certainly does not provide all we need. . . . You grab what you can this year and work on that and develop it and just hope that you can be influential

enough to take out the parts that are detrimental and work on the good parts. . . . It's rare that legislation is passed the first year it's introduced[,] and you have to work with what you have to work with.

Another participant stated:

You have to stay abreast of the legislation as to what's actually hidden in there . . . as well as to the funding formula. . . . So you have to watch the legislation, you can't take it as a whole. And after you look at it and evaluate it and talk to others, then you have to go up there and talk to the legislators . . . and get them to amend, in other ways water this bill down, keep the good points but water down the hard points.

The members of this focus group shared of their expertise and savvy in communicating with and influencing the legislature. "We make a point when we [go] to the capital . . . not looking for any support in a bill . . . we stick our head in the door, we leave our card . . . and wish a good day. Or check in with the secretaries . . . they run those legislators lives. . . . And if you get to know them on a first name basis you can accomplish a lot. . . ." "One hand written letter is worth I don't know how many computer generated letters, but it's a lot." "And I think what you have to do is ask them to listen. And it's important for you to listen to what they have to say. And if at the end you still can't come to agreement you thank them for their time and hope to get together with them on some other issue." "When you go to your legislators, make sure you've got your facts straight."

They also shared examples of successful outcomes of their political action. "If we go to testify, most of [the legislators] have recognized us in the capital, that we're a member of silver haired[,] and . . . the chairman of that committee . . . when the issue comes up will ask what does silver haired feel about this issue. So they do respect our views." Another shared:

It was a major issue we were dealing with. He [a legislator] always supported most of our issues but this one, he wasn't going to. And it was going to come to a vote. We knew he wasn't going to vote for us. So we just said can you just be gone out of the room when they vote so you won't be put down as a no. And he did it. So we couldn't get him to say yes. But at least we got him [not to] vote against us. That's almost as important.

Several examples were shared of how important it is for influentials—legislators or others—to feel the implications of a given bill or issue:

What we try to do is make it real personal . . . just bring it home to them . . . we . . . use the aging population, and with that comes your family. . . . Your eyesight grows dimmer, your hearing, all those things start happening. All of us are going to have to deal with it one way or the other. So that's why we make it real personal. Like, maybe you don't have to deal with this now, [but] it's coming sooner or later.

During those [managed care] hearings . . . everybody was there—the consumers, the insurance reps were there. . . . They got a call from one of the reps who was supposed to be there. . . . He was experiencing the same problems [we were discussing] in the last two days and I thought this is good. And we were laughing about it, they [the insurance reps] were too [and the sides came closer to agreement].

When we were trying to get legislative support for an upgrade of the nurse practice act, a . . . [nurse] . . . was in the capitol building when the presiding senator of the hearing about the bill, his secretary tripped and fell on the capitol steps and Jane [assumed name] was the first one to his assistance. Somehow, his attitude about nurses changed.

Many comments directly addressed the burden on consumers imposed by the current health care delivery systems. Both consumer advocacy for vulnerable others as well as self-advocacy and self-responsibility were recognized as the ways to deal effectively with these considerable burdens: "But my mother says [spoken by a retiree], I never could keep track of things like this [piles of bills and statements from insurers], if I didn't have you. I think you have to have some knowledge. . . ." "Know what coverage you have, read your policy and see what they cover and what they don't." "Sometimes you think you understand what is going on [but] it is so complicated. People with serious disabilities, they just can't do it." "It begins with each individual, [we] have to do it ourselves." "I think that health care and the charges on health care are my responsibility first." This respondent goes on to say that those who are able must monitor their health care charges and question any they don't understand *at the time services are provided.*

One participant tells of her story at self-monitoring her health care costs:

I have a little pocket notebook and in it I write down every time I go to the doctor and if I have lab, x-ray, you know, whatever I had. Last year I sat down and I made up a little form . . . and I wrote down all of the services I'd obtained and then I checked off as the Medicare things came in. Well I got one from Medicare and I looked at it and I said, "that's not me." I went back to my little notebook and I checked. No I didn't have any of that kind of stuff on that day. In fact, I got one [bill] for a day that I wasn't even in town. . . . So I go trucking into the patient accounts representative and I said, "I'm sorry . . . but I'm being charged for things I didn't get. They looked it up and what had happened was . . . somebody else's bill had been submitted under my claim number. So they got that sorted out. Then I also pulled out three other Medicare things and I said, now this one is from April and this one is from May and I haven't gotten anything from my insurance [other carrier] on them. Have they been billed? They looked, they'd forgotten to bill the secondary on those things. So I think we have a responsibility to track and be sure that the care provider does get paid for the things they provide, but they don't get paid for the things that . . . they didn't provide.

Consumer advocacy for those who are vulnerable, however, is vigorously provided—and with impressive results. "When we find out something we pass it on. Just like division of assets. This last week when I was attending a meeting, one lady came over to me and says, 'I want to thank you for telling me about the division of assets.' She said, 'that saved me my house and my car.'" "I looked at one bill, and I said, 'They are overcharging you. Medicare cannot charge you over 15% of Medicare allowable.' So [I] called the office and the little girl [clerk] said, 'Oh, I didn't know that.' And we did get the money back. . . ." "So as community advocates and activists, it really would behoove us to work very actively, in somehow or other making our fellow citizens knowledgeable of the system . . . I think the problem with a lot of people . . . the services are there, [but] they don't know how to cope with the third party payment system."

A perceived component of advocacy for the self or others is learning how to manipulate the health care system. "[Y]our insurance or Medicare will not pay for them [services] unless you have physicians orders saying so . . . [i]f you can convince your physician that this is what you need, then your insurance will pay for it." "And my question was does the anesthesiologist bill me as the patient, or bill the hospital? [I was scheduled to have an operation and needed an anesthesiologist. I started calling], because my insurance covered as out patient 100% of the hospital bill. . . . The sixth one [physician] billed the hospital, so naturally I accepted him."

"There is a 1-800 [toll-free telephone number] which is available seven days a week, 24 hours a day for patients . . . admitted·to the hospital [for Medicare]. By law that information must be given to every patient in their admission package and you sign it. Now, when you go in and you sign it you have no idea what you are signing. . . . If you just call that number, the hospital, by law . . . cannot discharge you until there has been . . . an investigation and follow up." The group members then shared several other help line numbers that covered commercial insurance complaints, home care complaints, and Medicaid complaints. All explained that they would use these numbers and also provide them to their friends and colleagues.

Motivators

Concern for others

These active citizens expressed passionate concern for others and shared vignettes that told how they were raised to be involved with the welfare of their fellows. "At 16 I was a legal orphan, and other people helped me, and I think it's payback time." "Sometimes your family influences how you behave. . . . I happened to have a mother who did things like be on the board of The American Bible Society. . . . I paid very little attention at the time . . . but it probably had some impact on me and my attitude towards making a contribution in some way or another." "I'm part liberal. I think I was born that way. I don't think I ever considered any other choice . . . when you look around and things aren't right." "There but for the grace of God go I. I think that is our sole motivation. That is our mother. That is our father. That is our handicapped sister. . . ." "We were seeing things that we didn't like. We didn't want them to continue. We wanted to make change and with that kind of motivation we had the strength to leave comfortable environments and start doing other things."

The concern for others was shared universally and expressed again by three respondents: "My motivation was partially through need, but also through interest in my fellow man." "We are our brother's keeper. We need to be concerned because our country is only as good as its weakest link. We need to help those who need help." "People motivate me like crazy. There are wonderful people out there. You don't hear it on the news, but when you're out working in the community, you find it."

The group members spoke about how their volunteer work capitalizes on the skills and knowledge they have gained in their salaried working lives. "[T]he reason I'm working at this level is to use my knowledge and skills. . . . There are people who help in their own ways, whether it's driving or doing things of a different variety. I have a background of an organizational variety, and therefore I can help in a certain way. It's like serving on the board of the hospice is something I can contribute to. . . ." "I retired from home care, all the time I was working I saw the need for more involvement in this, which I didn't have the time for when I was working, so as a result I have continued in this area since I retired." One respondent eloquently links the advocacy role to her knowledge and skills and attempts to speak for others as well as herself:

> I think that other community advocates have motives that are very similar to mine, not 100%, but the majority of them have quite similar motives, mine being helping fellow mankind [by] sharing my knowledge with those that didn't have the benefit or exposure to further enhance their lives.

This same informant shared her conviction that "the Medicaid recipient is particularly handicapped in terms of access to services, and they ought to have the same choices and same rights as a middle income or upper income person. That was my motivation."

Personal satisfaction

Seven of the eight respondents also identified personal satisfaction as a key factor in their being active community advocates. "That's why you do it. It's so rewarding." "I think I would be amiss if I didn't say . . . that I didn't also get a great deal of satisfaction out of my successes . . . each success is so rewarding." "I have always felt . . . that I've gotten far more out of it [everything I've done] than I've been able to give." "If people would just get themselves involved . . . they would find a lot of self-satisfaction." "I've gotten myself in some real messes, and they always work out . . . and you feel good about it." "So the rewards are there." "I think we all do it [volunteer work] to some extent for self-satisfaction, but I don't look for any halos . . . because if I climb one rung up I slip two rungs back, so eventually I think I'll be shoveling coal."

It is evident from comments already shared that these participants are acting out of spiritual, humanistic, and/or political convictions. They experience feelings of pleasurable self-satisfaction when they achieve successes for their efforts. Not surprisingly, these citizens spoke about their goals and their commitment to a cause or a vision.

Mission, vision, or goals

Many of the group members articulated a highly developed sense of purpose in statements of mission, vision, or goals. "I wanted in-home services. I called it one stop shopping. One place you could go and get the help you needed to stay in your own home as long as possible." "If we don't get involved in the process, nothing is going to get accomplished." "[C]oncern needs to be that we get quality care and adequate care, and that the consumer has a voice in it." The participants were shrewd, and they persevered in pursuit of their goals. "Don't ever accept failure or defeat. . . . [T]ake any small crumb you're given. Take one small block and then build on it." "You don't have to get the whole building, just get the first brick. . . . [I]f they won't give you the building, take the brick."

These respondents have a vision of a desired future they are working toward. "I guess I believe that it [managed care]'s a step in the process, a movement away [from the old system] to a single-payer system; that it's a transition. There has to be this upheaval period that we're going through. . . ." "I think it's a transition, too. . . . We will end up eventually, whether we call it national health insurance, or whatever. . . ." "One thing I think, we are living longer, . . . and if we do preventive care it's a lot better keeping someone healthy than . . . trying to bring them back to health . . . you know, the band-aid approach."

Personal life stories

Many of the respondents also shared personal anecdotes or brief life histories that underscored their visions or sense of mission in pursuing their active roles in their communities and chosen reference groups. "I went through [care of] my mother and father in a variety of settings. . . . I was a sophisticated consumer. I knew the systems. . . . And to try and get it, to access it was a major challenge for me, but I was able to . . . for the benefit of my family. But almost no one would have the same kind of understanding…that I happened to have had because of my professional connections." "I had done a lot of volunteer work, this is many years ago, and in a lot of areas with my children and my church, and my husband was killed. . . ." (This woman went on to establish a home health agency.)

Reaching Out

Mentoring, recruiting, or involving others

The respondents were universally active in these networking processes. "I'm always recruiting people to work. . . . [A]fter you get someone involved in something I think they feel the way we do on a lot of these things. You have to expose them. . . ." "The people to recruit are recent retirees before they get involved in 20 things. . . ." "I invite them to go with me. . . . You don't tell them; you let them experience it . . . and ask them to help." "[M]ake an overt effort to get others involved, . . . this really is the most important thing. We can stay in our own isolated do-good roles and get our warm fuzzies from succeeding, but the greatest thing we can do is get others involved in the dissemination of information." "That is the important thing—networking."

The group members clearly believed in the power of numbers. "I think the dominant need for the grass roots level is in the numbers. Most of what we're talking about today is impacting on legislation to try and make changes where we as advocates believe [change] is needed and numbers count—numbers are votes and votes are what really make the difference." "[W]e get to the grass roots. We can run around the capital and contact [legislators], but it's the people back home you need to inform of the need for them to contact their own representative . . . get out the grass roots. . . ."

Concern for the Next Generation

A legacy for future generations was an apparent focus: "[W]e have this huge group of baby boomers coming, that are all of a sudden having to cope with care of older parents and that is a group we need to work with. I get called [by people] all of a sudden having to cope with a situation, 'Where do I go?' 'What do I do?' . . . We need to include them." "I know that with our children, I think they are all scared to death by what has been happening these last couple of years. They don't know what's going to be left, and I think it's our duty . . . I know things are constantly changing, but I have enough confidence in this country and in our government that it is not going to be as bad as some people say. . . . I think we need to get across to our children that there is going to be something out there when you get there."

Advice to Professionals

As would be expected, this group of consumer advocates was not hesitant to offer advice to professionals. Listening seemed to be the major attribute required. "Listen and simplify the system and not make it more complex than it already is." "I'd say listen, listen, listen." "I believe in the kiss system. Keep it simple, stupid." "I guess involvement of themselves . . . they need to be involved with the community themselves, and they'll get a perception of what the community needs."

Health Care Themes

Dissatisfactions with health care

It became very apparent that the members of the group believe they have a fertile field on which to focus their attention as consumer advocates. "I think . . . that we have all acknowledged that health care now has become a payment-driven industry . . . rather than health care . . . so you're getting total fragmentation of care and you're getting this assembly line environment, which I don't think is care." "I think the issue here is we don't have health care. The word care in any dictionary, I'm sure, means care. But service doesn't. Service can be good or bad and we now have a health care industry that provides a payment-driven service." "I've long said we don't have a health care delivery system, because delivery implies that it's brought to you as a service. If you need health care these days, you have to go out and get it. It doesn't get delivered. On top of which, . . . you have to sit in a waiting room as if your time was immaterial. But the health care provider's time is valuable." "Once that legislation was passed [presumably Medicare DRG legislation] the outpatient care is more profitable. And so exactly that time we saw this tremendous emphasis towards outpatient care—100% money-driven."

"Unfortunately [health care] is the managed care concept. I think we have got away from care . . . the system today doesn't provide care. It continues to provide services for a price, and then it, the system, makes the decision, not based on the patients needs, but unfortunately based on the cost of what it's going to provide. That's it in a nutshell. Health care today." "I agree. It's not based on the patients needs or the physician's or the health professional's recommendation. Those are totally disregarded." The Kennedy-Kassebaum legislation to increase portability of insurance was not looked upon favorably. "Well, I don't think that bill covered any cap on the premiums . . . I'd say it is a pretty useless piece of legislation." "I think that the state has to watch how they implement that . . . how the bill is implemented will have good or bad effects."

The respondents believed that managed care could increase illness prevention efforts:

> Theoretically it could. Theoretically, they want to keep people healthy. Theoretically, you would be reimbursing people for ongoing routine kinds of care to pick up on in the early stages, things that would be very expensive. Unfortunately, it doesn't seem to be working properly . . . The whole effort at assisted suicide, at attempting to convince people that the funding for Medicare hospice [needs to be cut] and technology is keeping people alive.

"I think under the guise of preventive care, managed care today is choosing a less costly alternative, is giving lip service to preventive care." These respondents seemed almost fearful of the health care system. In addition to inferring that assisted suicide is actually being seen as a cost-saving measure by managed care companies, at least one participant sees the system as geared strictly to financial gain:

> I am frightened with these HMOs. It is my understanding . . . that the doctors are employed, . . . by the HMO and they're told . . . that they have x number of dollars per year to spend on each patient. If that goes over, then it comes out of what they make. Now I am 72, soon to be 73, I have a heart condition. Now, my doctor, maybe in his wisdom, since he might have a multimillion dollar home and a couple of kids going to medical school, might decide that I didn't need this extra catheterization for my heart, because I am going to die anyway. Now that to me is frightening.

The economics of health care are clearly on the minds of these consumer advocates:

> Of course when we go into the whole economics of . . . health care . . . you'll find that you have CEO's of these companies being paid millions of dollars. The general public doesn't go for it. My mother says, "Ain't no man around that can work hard enough to earn that much."

"There are monopolies evolving, which means there's less choice. Which . . . drives up prices . . . and cuts down on competition." "It's the for-profit mentality and operating at the lowest possible standard."

These consumer advocates had definite expert opinions about what are the core problems in managed care. "Now as to HMOs . . . , we have to get rid of the connotation of case management. We would like to see *care* management for consumers or customers, not just a case and a number. We're not a number, we're a human being, a person . . . [emphasis in original]." "One of the major issues is cost containment, but at the expense of older people. You set arbitrary ages of 70 or 75 years old, not tied to quality of life, you have a scary scenario." "[T]here's been a great adulteration . . . of the concept of public health. The majority of people today don't understand what public health means. . . . Public health . . . has become a primary care giver for welfare recipients or persons without insurance."

"[T]he biggest issue is inaccessibility. . . ." "[T]he biggest issue in health care today, I would say is access. In hospital care, a biggy I think, is the increase in outpatient surgery and the increased tendency to send people home with a lot of sophisticated things to do at home." "I think . . . a big problem is communication . . . the lack of people listening to what you have to say. We all know our bodies best . . . they just won't listen to you."

One of the group members shared his concern about nurse–patient staffing ratios in hospitals:

> I'm scheduled to go into the hospital , and I'm scared to death, downsizing RNs, and there's no tags to tell you [who's who]. Their name can be anything, but I'd like to see whether it says RN, LPN, or CNA. It scares the hell out of me, because I know it only takes a small time for a CNA [certified nursing assistant] to be certified . . . and they can hire three CNAs for the price of one RN, and if there's CNAs taking care of me, the price is the same [as if RNs were caring for me]; they're not downgrading the price of my care, but they're downgrading the quality of care. That's my main concern. If I'm in there and my life is on the line, I want to know the alphabet behind the name of who's taking care of me.

Horror stories

All the respondents told at least one horror story concerning interactions of family or friends or themselves with the health care system: "[I]n our age group, it's a panic situation. . . . Someone breaks a hip. Suddenly someone has a stroke. . . . [I]f there's no place to go to get the information, . . . how can we make an educated choice?" "One case is a sister who shouldn't have been in home care. . . . She became impacted [severely constipated] and died before anybody could do anything. Who makes these kinds of judgments?" "I've had physicians tell me I don't need an answer to my question; they're the doctor; they know. Well, . . . I'm not going back to those people. You hear over and over . . . what some health professionals have done and how they have disregarded people's dignity."

> My husband had a heart attack last fall and had surgery and was in three hospitals . . . he had good supplemental insurance, but the bills that come, there is no way of telling what they are for. And I have kept track of it because Medicare does send to the other insurance. . . . I have a stack that high [raises hand one foot above table] . . . and they're still coming. I don't know what we're going to do to get through all this. . . .

The horror stories about the complexity of managing the finances following an illness episode were numerous. Also, as previously reported, the issues surrounding payment for services permeated many of the themes. The group took on the subject of clinical pathways, finding them less than satisfactory:

> My husband had bypass surgery. . . . He was a person of 78 and they treated him like he was a 50 year old. Now granted, he was a very active person prior to this but he was discharged from that hospital in four days. I asked to meet with [the doctor] when they [cut down on his time in ICU from 48 to 24 hours], but they obviously had a tracking system, like on day one you do this, day two you do that. I became aware of clinical pathways around that same time and I could see what was happening to him, but they put him into a track that fit for a much younger age group, and as a result, when he was discharged he got worse. Asked for home health care, oh you don't need that. And he ended up having to go back in the hospital for another eight days, which was totally unnecessary if the original care had been [appropriate], in my opinion, and it was an incredible experience. The second time I was orchestrating things, and the doctor was humble enough to let me say he needs this and he needs that and he'll stay until he gets better.

Satisfaction with health care

The participants were very open to identifying those aspects of the current health care system that pleased them. "I can't tell you how pleased I am by the people over there [rehabilitation hospital], because the people who've been through this, as users of the system, we know what's going on; they [health professionals] are including us in that process of getting information to improve what they're doing." "I am pleased with the increased technology and things we have available to us today." "I see the movement towards the involvement and participation of the consumer in quality assurance systems [as positive]."

One participant related technology with payment systems in a positive way:

> Advanced technology is incredible and I'm very happy that's there . . . for my fellow Americans . . . and for me should I need it. But I'm also grateful for the third party payment system out there. Because, certainly with the advanced technologies as they exist today, in our advancing years, we are going to need to avail ourselves of those. And even though the third party payment system isn't perfect, it is available to us, and many of us couldn't avail ourselves of these wonderful facilities and services if it wasn't there.

Sympathy for health care professionals

The group took the position five times that health care providers were being controlled by business interests and, therefore, deserved sympathy and understanding. "What we've gotten away from is allowing health professionals to give their full measure of care. . . . [B]ean counters who are far away from the people they serve and think in terms of numbers, not people [are making decisions]." "I think the professionals themselves are going to have to take this industry back." "[M]y doctor says, 'I am a doctor and I want to be able to doctor,' but he says 'I have to hire an attorney to advise me how to doctor to keep malpractice suits down.'" "The physicians are as angry as we are about this. The physicians, the nurses, the other therapists involved are all angry." "I think some of us can't even imagine some of the frustrations that they [physicians] face with the HMO situation."

References

Eriksson, C-G. (1988). Focus groups and other methods for increased effectiveness of community intervention—A review. *Scandinavian Journal of Primary Health Care Supplement I,* 73–80.

Palm, L. and Windahl, S. (1988). Focus groups: Some suggestions. *Scandinavian Journal of Primary Health Care Supplement I,* 90–98.

Polit, D. F. and Hungler, B. P. (1991). *Nursing Research: Principles and Methods.* Philadelphia: J. B. Lippincott.

Ramirez, A. G. and Shepperd, J. (1988). The use of focus groups in health research. *Scandinavian Journal of Primary Health Care Supplement I,* 81–90.

Consumers in Health Care Part II: Expert Viewpoints[1] 19

Toni J. Sullivan

PRESENTATION OF FINDINGS: LITERATURE REVIEW

Introduction

The research questions posed were as follows:

1. How do citizens who are laypeople and who are active volunteers perceive themselves and their responsibilities and actions in actively influencing health care in the community or health care as available to the people (citizens)?
2. How are lay people defined in the health sciences literature; what does the health sciences literature describe the opportunities, responsibilities, and actions of citizens who are laypeople to be in actively participating in and influencing health care in the community or health care as available to citizens?

Research question 1 was addressed by the focus group findings explored in the previous chapter. Research question 2 is addressed in the health sciences literature. The central idea in the literature with respect to describing laypeople who are active in their communities is the idea of the individual as consumer. The individual as community activist or

[1]Chapter 18 constitutes Part I of the focus on consumers in health care.

citizen activist is barely mentioned in the health sciences literature (five articles). The idea in the health sciences literature of the layperson as advocate is more present in the literature (19 articles), but not to the extent of the notion of consumer. Moreover, the concept of advocacy is more often linked to related fields (ethics or law) or to related terms *(devil's advocate or court-appointed advocate)* than it is to community action. As with the focus group participants, consumer (preferably linked to the term *advocate* as *consumer advocate)* is clearly the current term of choice in which to couch the behaviors of active laypersons as they engage in activities to influence societal institutions.

The evolutionary approach to concept analysis, which recognizes that the meanings and usage's of concepts are dynamic and changing over time (and even by different users at the same time), is entirely legitimate in the analysis of the concept of consumer. The fundamental meanings of the term, that is antecedents or underlying values and needs, attributes or characteristics, references or uses, and consequences or outcomes are variable and evolving. Their evolution, as well as the larger society in which they are evolving, is extraordinarily dynamic and even chaotic. Defining the term *consumer* is, therefore, an impossible task. The author instead presents a series of ideas concerning consumer and consumerism (goal-directed behaviors by consumers) that is organized as follows:

- Philosophical beginnings of concept of consumer
- Historical overview of consumer laws in United States from 1790 to 1980
- Generally accepted attributes of concept of consumer
- Political tensions in conceptualizations of consumer concept
- Comparative attributes of the concept of *consumer* and related terms
- Current status of consumer protections in United States
- International perspectives on consumers and consumerism
- Advocacy and consumer advocacy
- Consumers or consumerism and managed care
- Potential consequences of consumer actions on society

Philosophical Beginnings of the Concept of Consumer

Two towering political and philosophical thinkers of the 18th century, Adam Smith and Thomas Jefferson, can be credited with giving meaning to the notion of a consumer as essential to an economic system of free enterprise embedded within a democratic society (Turner 1995, Warne 1993). The consumer voice, as conceptualized by them, although focused largely on marketplaces, spoke the language of democracy. Adam Smith wrote in the *Wealth of Nations,* "Consumption is the sole end and purpose of all production, and the interest of the producer ought to be attended to, only in so far as it may be necessary for promoting that of the consumer" (Lerner 1937, p. 625, quoting Smith as cited by Turner 1995, p. 3). Thomas Jefferson wrote in the *Declaration of Independence,* "All governments derive their just powers from the consent of the governed" (cited in Turner 1995, p. 3). Jefferson also wrote in the *Declaration* of the governed having an entitlement to life, liberty, and the pursuit of happiness.

Both Jefferson and Smith, Turner (1995) points out, challenged political and economic systems in which power of kings or deities flowed from the top down and promoted a system in which power flowed from the bottom up to the people as voters or consumers creating and supporting both governments and markets. Life, liberty, and the pursuit of happiness in this new society required freedom of choice for goods and services as well as freedom to vote. "A certain kind of society, a certain kind of awakened spirit" (Turner 1995, p. 3) was deemed essential to achieving these towering rights within a political and economic system—the idea of which was previously unknown in history. The ideas of the worth of the individual, of acceptance of responsibility for one's actions, of freedom of choice, of valuing the life of the intellect, of vocation or choosing one's life work, of personal growth and development, and of achievement and recognition for achievement were all heady new ideas spawned by the new political and economic systems.

These central ideas forged what in 1937 the great political theorist, Max Lerner, called "the new doctrine of economic liberalism and freedom from governmental interference" (cited in Smith 1937, foreword, as cited in Turner 1995, p. 3). These philosophical underpinnings (according to Turner 1995) explain why consumer theorists of the 20th century such as Morse and Warne assert that the consumer is to economics what voters are to politics—and that the two are melded together. They believe that "[t]he central faith of the consumer movement is that free choice lies at the very core of democracy in an economic system" (Turner 1995, p. 2). Colston Warne (1993, cited in Turner 1995, p. 2) links free choice by persons inextricably to behaviors of free markets in a democratic society. He states:

But free choice depends upon a fair exchange of knowledge—knowledge of price, knowledge of quality, knowledge of quantity, and knowledge of the limitations associated with the product for which we exchange money. If this freedom of choice is to serve as the mainspring of our economic system, it must be informed choice upon which the consumer can rely. No advertiser can justly boast of a consumer vote of confidence in his product when the voter [purchaser] has been denied the knowledge essential to such a rational choice. Uninformed choice is not free choice.

These philosophical and political ideals contain the roots of recognition that the citizen is a consumer, and more important, perhaps, that the consumer is a citizen and acts as a citizen in the pursuit of fair and open markets. Markets that withhold information, promote inequities, or encourage exploitation of weaker or poorer by the stronger and richer are not to be tolerated by consumers as citizens in a democratic society.

Historical Overview of Consumer Laws in United States From 1790 to 1980

Consumer protection laws and protections at the federal level date to the 1790s. During this era when most Americans lived and toiled on farms and the remaining few ran small businesses, Jefferson recommended and Congress passed a set of standards for weights and measures, inaugurating consumer protection. Jefferson thus acted on his belief that economic dependence denies political freedom (Turner 1995).

In 1887, after a boom and bust cycle followed the Civil War, and following robber baron excesses and political corruption, Congress, using clear consumer rhetoric, passed the Interstate Commerce Act (Turner 1995). Between 1887 and 1916, in the era known as the Progressive Era, Congress passed 56 consumer laws. This era is noted for the development of factories and large industries in the United States. The automobile, clothing, and food processing industries are a few of the major ones. The influx to American shores of hundreds of thousands of poor European immigrants who worked in these factories is another major characteristic of the Progressive Era. In 1906, Upton Sinclair published *The Jungle,* his stinging indictment of the meat-packing industry. Shortly thereafter, in response to public outcry, Congress passed a series of pure food laws (Simon 1996, Turner 1995).

Between World War I and World War II, in the 1920s and 1930s, Congress passed 73 new consumer protection laws (Turner 1995). In response to a series of deaths attributed to pharmaceuticals, Congress passed a series of laws requiring pharmaceuticals to be safe. At that time, legislation did not require pharmaceuticals to be *effective;* but they had to be *safe* (Simon 1996).

After World War II, from 1951 to 1980, Congress passed 227 new regulatory laws aimed at protection of consumers (Turner 1995). This was an era in the brief history of the United States of unparalleled consumerism. The 1960s, known by many labels, is sometimes called the decade of the Consumer Movement (MacFarlane 1996). In 1962 President Kennedy announced a Consumer Bill of Rights, proclaiming four basic consumer rights: safe products, full product information, freedom of choice in product availability, and voice in the development of consumer policies. The Kennedy message highlighted modern consumerism. The United States was no longer a nation of farmers—only 6% of citizens toiled or lived on farms. Americans worked primarily for large corporations or for government. They expressed their economic stake in the society through consumer purchases.

The consumer movement picked up speed with the emergence of Ralph Nader, who became famous with his 1965 expose of unsafe automobiles. Between 1965 and 1980, Congress passed myriad laws that set tough (perhaps arguable) safety standards for cars; banned dangerous toys; required that pharmaceuticals be proved *effective;* and gave more information on food content, borrowing costs, and sales practices (Simon 1996). Moreover, the President and Congress established the Consumer Product Safety Commission.

On the basis of prior history and using statistical projection models, Turner (1995) projects 350–450 new consumer laws between 1989 and 2018. This is by no means a sure projection, however, as the 1980s began the current era of deregulation. As is outlined in a later section of this chapter, many consumer gains are being reversed. Moreover, the world is changing so rapidly that it is, perhaps, foolish to base future projections in a world now gone. Increasingly, knowledge, not wealth or even force, defines power in the marketplace. The consumer concerns of the present and the future are and will be focused in access to and control of information along with the more traditional concerns. "For example, policing the Internet, finance, trade, safety, quality, and price information, and protecting privacy, speech, and intangibles are all matters of hot debate even as we observe so-called deregulation" (Turner 1995, p. 8). Before considering the status of consumers and consumerism in the present and for the future, it is necessary to consider further *what is a consumer.*

Widely Accepted Attributes of the Consumer Concept

This author searched for meanings of *consumer* that would likely be acceptable to all scholars, regardless of the particular perspectives each holds of the term. The resulting listing is not lengthy. First and foremost, *consumers are shoppers.* Shopping around in order to make the best purchase requires energy, knowledge necessary to make informed and free choices, and motivation to engage in the hard work involved. *Motivation to act on one's own behalf or on behalf of another* is thus another attribute of consumer. *The ability to act on one's own behalf in terms of energy level and physical stamina* is yet another attribute. Again, shopping around is hard work. *The intellectual ability to seek and process and use knowledge and information regarding products and services* such as quality, quantity, price, and cost benefit is another attribute. Motivation, energy, and intellectual ability are thus three enabling attributes that empower consumers for "going shopping."

Freedom of choice is the second defining attribute of consumer. As shown in the Warne quote in the earlier section on philosophical foundations of consumer, free choice depends on a fair exchange of knowledge. It must be *informed* choice in order to be free choice. *Consumers make purchasing decisions;* they act on freedom to choose and express their individuality through their purchasing decisions or selections. They can be defined, in part, by the free choices they make in the marketplace. Consumers, according to some researchers (Hayes 1991, Thorne and Robinson 1989) are *skeptical of claims made by salespeople and by advertisers.* They prefer to verify the quality or other attributes of a product or service for themselves, and they are competent to do so. *Consumers are frequently familiar with consumer laws and know their rights within the law* (Lang and Gabriel 1995).

Theoretically, the consumer is classless, ageless, sexless, and of no particular racial or ethnic group (Symonds 1994). In reality, this is not so. The person of the consumer exists in a set of economic, social, and intellectual power relationships. All consumers are not equal. *Consumer power includes having financial resources to expend, having the social and political clout to access resources, and having the knowledge of resources available in a society.*

The ability of citizens to act as consumers presupposes a society that enables consumer behaviors. There must be choices available to make in the marketplaces of goods and services. There must be information available about those goods and services. Product information, labeling, safety data, and the like are essential to consumers making free choices. An educated citizenry, both in general education and consumer education, enables wise choices while discriminating among products and services. Another presupposition is that the political system allows freedom of choice; persons are not punished or sanctioned in any way because of their exercise of freedom of choice. Another presupposition is that the economic system is able to offer goods and services for purchase in the marketplace and that the citizens have the economic means to exercise freedom of choice when making purchasing decisions.

Political Tensions in Conceptualizations of Consumer

The evolution of the term *consumer* is fraught with tensions pulling the term in one political direction or another. As seen in the philosophical foundations section, the idea of the consumer is embedded within a democratic society with a free market economy. Freedom of choice in purchasing goods and services would seem to be central to democratic ideals. Warne (1976) believed especially that the consumer voice should focus on the language of democracy. This model would hold true for the future if, as Turner opines, "As knowledge power grows, Jefferson/Smith economic liberalism and freedom from governmental interference expands" (1995, p. 8). How this freedom plays out, however, is the topic of heated debate in the literature. The stakes are high for both consumers and producers and for societies.

The first debate is between the notion of *citizen* and the notion of *consumer.* Some believe that the consumer has replaced the citizen in free-market societies. Others believe that the citizen with consumer attributes is the new ideal. Lang and Gabriel, British scholars, are particularly convinced that the consumer has replaced the citizen: "The term consumer has the authority of modernity. Consumers are free, able to choose, allowed to express their individuality" (1995). They ask, "The term citizen, is it obsolete? We think not, although the term *citizen* does have a rather quaint old-fashioned ring to it; citizenship was what liberal political theorists referred to, . . . what children were or are taught in class" (Lang and Gabriel 1995, p. 11). Table 19-1 compares and contrasts the idea of consumer and the idea of citizen in accordance with the characteristics presented by some theorists.

Similar to the consumer versus citizen dichotomy is the left versus right political dichotomy. Both left and right politically leaning thinkers seem to be battling for "the heart and soul of the consumer" (Lang and Gabriel 1995). Understanding these political directions as they manifest themselves in consumers and consumerism and consumer protections can assist greatly with understanding various arguments by members of societal institutions such as government or health care organizations as they compete to have their perspectives dominate public policy and the health care marketplace. This researcher concludes that the international literature, as compared with the literature from the United States, is particularly overt in its criticisms of the left by the right or of the right by the left. The American (United States) literature, on the other hand, deals with the subject more subtly, and more conservative rhetoric (right) is dominating the American literature, particularly with regard to health care and managed care.

Lang and Gabriel (1995) assert that the left, having little faith in "right-wing economics" has sought to enlarge the consumer into a responsible, socially aware person who may occasionally sacrifice personal pleasure for communal well-being. This person is then the consumer as citizen. Lang and Gabriel opine that this role had been pioneered in developing countries by the Consumers International and in the United States by Ralph Nader and the organization he founded, Public Citizen. The only route to rebuilding citizenship is through involvement with others. (It is logical to agree with Jefferson and Smith that the philosophical and historical foundations of the concept of consumer are, in fact, of the consumer as citizen. This view, however, is by no means universally accepted in the literature. The concept of consumer, although clearly an economic concept, seems to be so embedded in political thinking that the concept becomes ipso facto a political concept, as well, and subject to the vagaries that exist within schools of political thought.)

The right, speaking from the left, developed the idea of the purchase as analogous to the vote. Consumers vote with their pocketbooks (Lang and Gabriel 1995). The more wealth a consumer has the more "votes" he gets. The market becomes a surrogate for political discourse and may render political discourse redundant. Market surveys become the nearest

Table 19-1. Citizen Contrasted With Consumer

Variable	Citizen	Consumer
Foundation of idea	Athenian democracy, reinvented or expanded by French and American Revolutions; a political concept.	Ideal of economic man; an economic concept articulated by Adam Smith.
The good life— or happiness	Attained through political action in and with the community.	Attained through economic action in the market-place and the purchase of goods and services.
Responsibilities	Has social responsibilities in and for the community; may have to sacrifice personal wants for the common good.	Unencumbered by social responsibilities and duties; no sacrifices for others required.
Rights	Inalienable rights to one's own views and to criticize the government.	With money may acquire privileges; may, perhaps, buy citizenship.
Membership in society	Equal member of society; unable to achieve full individuality and happiness except as part of whole.	Need not defer to, or belong to, any collective of society.
Freedom of choice	Citizens are prepared to listen to views of others, and to defer to the will of the majority.	Consumers act on their own behalf without regard to the will or preferences of others.
Moral imperative	Citizens must confront the implications of their choices; their meaning, their values, their impact on others.	Consumers operate in impersonal markets where they make choices unencumbered by guilt or by social obligations.
Discrimination	Persons lacking citizenship, or perhaps considered as less worthy citizens may experience discrimination or exclusion.	Consumers experience no discrimination or exclusion as long as they can pay the price required for the goods or services—including the price of admission.
Social bond	Citizens have a bond with society based on a sense of responsibility for the society and a sense of loyalty to the society.	The focus on money as the driving force dissolves all social bonds.

Sources: Appleby 1995, Lang 1995, Turner 1995, Warne 1993.

thing to political will. Public places become marketplaces—not social places. Behemoth shopping malls and Disneyland-like commercial amusement parks replace public parks and community recreation facilities. Rieff (1993, pp. 66–72) asserts: "The U.S. citizen is a supermarket cultural browser. For better or worse, ours is a culture of consumerism as spectacle, of things and not ideas" (cited in Lang and Gabriel 1995, p. 15).

These conservative views of consumers and consumerism in their relationship with the marketplace have led to a movement for deregulation (which will be overviewed in a later section of this chapter). More liberal or left-leaning thinkers lament this movement. Some contend there is a new lack of sympathy for consumers and their problems obtaining information sufficient to make good purchasing decisions, or having quality—or even safe products available in the marketplace. Bernice Friedlander, Acting Director of the U.S. Office of Consumer Affairs in the Clinton administration describes the attitude of the 104th Congress as "Let the buyer beware" (Simon 1996, p. 2). This left-leaning position is countered by those who contend that it is consumers who benefit as costs and taxes are reduced. Consumers can vote with their feet if they do not like a particular service or product. With respect to health care, it has been a premise of the left that health care is a right of all Americans. This has also been a well-established premise underlying health care in many European democracies. Many now assert, in both the United States and other nations, however, that "unlimited or uncontrolled use of health care is no longer a . . . right" (Copeland 1993, p. 4).

The left contends that the new business orientation to health care makes the poor look like failed citizens who mishandled their exercise of choice and are now forced to accept the states' choices, or withdrawal of choices, regardless of their preferences (Lang 1995). The left contends that the buzz word, *empowerment,* is just that—a buzz word. It promises rights for users or consumers of services, but does not shift any power to consumers. In fact, new health care arrangements are designed to limit consumer choices and options systematically (Lang 1995, Rodwin 1996, Simon 1996). It is not surprising, therefore, that consumers are increasingly seeing themselves as "victims in a difficult search for affordable, accessible, quality health care" (Copeland 1993, p. 1). "Nonsense," say conservatives. The consumer movement escaped health care education and "incentives to be good health care consumers" (Copeland 1993, p.1).

Comparative Attributes and Related Terms

It is a logical extension of the politicization of the concept of consumer that the notion of "good consumers" and "bad consumers" would follow. With respect to health care, a good consumer is one who strives for mastery over his or her own health needs (Pittman 1992); they are patients with the ability and desire to seek out health care of good quality and reasonable cost, and furthermore have the ability and desire to shop around to obtain the best deal (Donaldson et al. 1991). Good consumers have a responsibility to self-manage their care and to prevent contemporary lifestyle health problems (Pittman 1992).

A bad consumer is one who is poorly informed or who passively reacts to the health care system (Pittman 1992). The elderly are an interesting case in point. They can act as good consumers, but they often do not want to or do not have the energy to do so. They want to be trusting of their providers, loyal; they do not want to be perceived as confrontational when interacting with their providers or with the system (Donaldson et al. 1991). A bad consumer is one who thoughtlessly or selfishly or carelessly uses too much of the limited health care resource. Copeland captures this mind-set well (1993) in speaking of employees as the recipients of a health care benefit from employers. She asserts sharply:

> Employees must learn that health care is not a bottomless pit, a cookie jar with unlimited cookies. Immoderate consumption of health care will be tolerated no longer. Employees must learn to shop and compare just as they do when buying a new car (p. 2).

Several related terms help to explain a particular aspect of consumer or consumerism. No surrogate terms stand in for the term *consumer*. *Macro-consumer* is the United States term used to describe or label the large purchaser of health care services. Usually employers, they have become negotiators for the best price with managed care companies or directly with health care providers. They have also become arbiters of health care information and data concerning quality and cost-effectiveness of care provided by managed care companies. As major purchasers of services for their employees, they have been catered to by managed care companies, perhaps to the neglect of the employees and primary recipients of the health care services purchased. Macro-consumers are also middlepersons in health care purchases, standing between the managed care company and the consumer (employee) or standing between the providers and the consumers.

The *micro-consumer* is the individual employee and his or her family. Many would argue that the micro-consumers, not the employers, as the users and recipients of services, as well as the payers through their employee contributions and their labors, are the real consumers of health care. The opportunities for micro-consumers to come to the head of the table in negotiating health care services as savvy consumers have increased. Consumers are seeking and obtaining better information. Better information channels, such as the Internet, are readily available to a mass market. Micro-consumers, along with macro-consumers, are beginning to join forces to negotiate better terms on behalf of micro-consumers (Appleby 1995, Burke 1996).

The British use a dichotomy to differentiate between those whose services are paid by taxation and those whose services are paid by individuals out-of-pocket or with a third-party payer with the premium paid by the individual. This use of related terms provides a different perspective. That is, those who receive public services are also viewed as consumers with the rights and status accorded to consumers. In addition, it is recognized that all services to all people with a legitimate need for those services cannot be treated in accordance with market-based approaches or criteria.

Dunleavy (1980) defines two sectors of consumption: *collectivized social consumption and individual private consumption.* In collective, services are allocated out of taxes and decided in accordance with non-market criteria. In individualized, services are purchased using market criteria (cited in Symonds 1994, p. 6). Collective consumers are more likely to be vulnerable populations; that is, those with the least social power or financial power. They are likely to be the frail elderly, the poor, the disabled, children of the poor, and those who may be disenfranchised in a society (Symonds 1994). Recognizing this collective group as consumers can help them and those who advocate for them to be more successful in achieving a bigger share of scarce resources.

Citizen participation is the term put forward by Macfarlane (1996), a Canadian author, as the term growing out of the consumer movement of the 1960s to recognize organized and active citizen participation in public policy development. The 1960s saw the unraveling of the medical model in Canada, along with the rise of consumerism. This era, according to Macfarlane, began the dispersion of power vested in health care providers and saw the rise of influence by many stakeholder groups and large numbers of stake-holders, all influencing and shaping the nature and directions of health care in Canada.

The *citizen as expert* is another related term for consumer advanced by Macfarlane. By 1996 Macfarlane states:

> Changing perceptions about health care, along with the rise of consumerism, and the demand for greater accountability in the use of public health resources, are propelling governments and consumers toward ever broader citizen as expert participation in difficult health care choices (p. 32).

The citizen expert is usually well organized and has an agenda and strong opinions which he or she articulates well. The involvement of the citizen as expert, it is important to note, alters the existing power relationships.

Pittman (1992) speaks of *consumer activists* as effective consumers assertively pursuing their own agendas. Consumer activists 1) acknowledge their own expectations during health care encounters, 2) discriminate in the selection and usage of professional services, and 3) self-manage their own health care. Alternatively, Pittman (1992) also uses the term *pro-consumer* as meaning a savvy or smart or strategic or effective consumer.

Finally, the last related term to share from this body of literature is *consumer satisfaction*. With respect to health care, it means that the patient receiving the care has no complaints about the care. This judgment can be applied to any number of patient care variables—both process and outcome. It is for the patient to decide what the variables are. Health care professionals tend to define the elements of patient satisfaction as mainly service components such as waiting time, courtesy, and food quality. The movement by both macro-consumers and micro-consumers, however, is toward a far more complete and sophisticated inventory of both process and outcome measures that concern the quality of care along with the styles of care delivery. It is now widely recognized, if not happily embraced by providers and insurers, that care cannot be high quality unless the consumer recognizes it as satisfactory (Williams 1994). The idea of consumer satisfaction is widespread in the literature, as is the recognition of its growing importance to current and future collaborative relationships between consumers, providers, and payers as health care evolves in the future.

Current Status of Consumer Protections in the United States

The United States is currently experiencing a movement toward deregulation in myriad areas of consumer protections. Perhaps the most widely known area is in air travel, where deregulation has made dramatic changes in the airline industry. The consumer has arguably benefited from lower air fares and has been disadvantaged by a noticeable decline in dependability of schedules and baggage handling, for example. Perhaps the first event signaling the era of deregulation was the defeat by Congress in 1978 of the creation of a cabinet-level consumer protection agency.

In 1981, President Reagan began slashing funds for consumer protection, contending these cuts would ultimately benefit consumers, as product costs would be reduced and taxes would be lowered. Consumers would, of course, be free to choose their purchases and could refuse to purchase products or services that were not satisfactory to them. Between 1980 and 1985, the two major federal consumer protection agencies, the Consumer Product Safety Commission and the Federal Trade Commission lost 40% and 50% of their funding, respectively. In 1989, the Federal Trade Commission suffered a sizable budget cut. In 1994, the Consumer Product Safety Commission budget was cut another 6%; the Environmental Protection Agency budget was cut 25% for enforcement of laws, and 33% specifically for enforcement of worker health and safety laws (Simon 1996). These federal agencies are reportedly still led and staffed by persons who are very committed to aggressive consumer protection. Their meager budgets simply hamper their efforts. They lack investigative personnel and modern testing equipment. "Consumer protection is a shadow of its former self" laments Richard Hesse, consumer lawyer (cited in Simon 1996, p. 3).

Simon (1996) reports, too, that consumer laws are also being undermined by state legislatures. In combination with federal law, the result is that protections Americans have taken for granted are disappearing. Four major areas of concern emerge. Americans are or will be facing major consumer protection issues in these areas.

1. Eroding bank laws,
2. Return of nursing home horrors,
3. Dangerously lax food standards, and
4. Virtually no regulation of managed care (p. 6).

It is important to note that two of the four areas of concern are in health care, and the remaining two have major direct or indirect implications for either the cost or the quality or both of health care delivery. The idea of references in concept analysis addresses the uses to which a concept is put. In the case of the concept of consumer, these extremely broad areas of social concern—banking and finance, health care, food and food processing—cover the entire society to which they are addressed. Consumer protection would seem to be one valid purpose of consumer behaviors. Consumer choices by individuals on behalf of themselves and their families, and any other reference group for whom they are acting as a consumer advocate would be made in relation to these important reference areas.

The face one puts on the current status of consumer protection in the United States depends on one's political position to the right or the left. In the present environment, Ralph Nader states:

> Stand up for your rights and if you care about these issues, speak out for consumer protections . . . about the best the consumer can do in the current environment is redouble their efforts to shop more wisely (cited in Simon 1996, pp. 11–12).

International Perspective on Consumer and Consumerism

At about the same time as the deregulation movement began in the United States, many of the developed nations of Europe and North America began to deal with a process of increasing privatization of services, including health care. Services that had been provided almost exclusively by central governments and financed by taxation came under scrutiny. Mainly, they were defined as increasingly costly and unaffordable by governments at the levels and in the ways they were currently being offered.

> Throughout Europe and many other parts of the world governments are rethinking the balance between state and family for the provision of social and health care. Increased emphasis on family and community responsibility is having profound implications for the traditional separation between employment and home/family life, and for the kinds of support employers will have to ensure exists if staff are to be both successful

employees and parents and carers . . . . There are increasing demands on fewer state resources and if we persist in old patterns we will fail (Statham 1994, p. 17).

Concern for consumer protections, as well as debate concerning how to define the consumer, is rampant in the international literature. Some of the debate has already been presented in the discussion of the right versus left dichotomy. In short, the left sees privatization as making the receipt of services as contingent on ability to pay, thus diluting the rights of citizenship, whereas the right sees privatization as a way for consumers to get better value for their money (Lang 1995).

Much of the literature defining consumers focuses on empowering consumers to be able to make choices, especially good choices. The modification of power structures between government, private industry, and people—workers, community dwellers— plays a major part in how to define consumers. Many lament that the rhetoric of politicians and policy-makers talks of empowerment but does not shift any power to consumers (Donaldson et al. 1991, Kim et al. 1993, Kindra et al. 1995, Lang and Gabriel 1995, Macfarlane 1996, Statham 1994, Symonds 1994, Winn and Quick 1990).

Winn and Quick ask, "Are users of services seen as passive consultees or as active partners in the process of change [privatization]? The answer has important implications for information sharing and processes [of care provision]" (1990, p. 90). Kim et al. (1993) report on a five-nation study in which they learned that "a consumerist attitude" had to be developed in health care providers before patients or recipients of services could become decision-makers concerning their health care. The greater the consumerist attitude by staff, the more likely patients would be to act as consumers.

Symonds (1994, p. 7) summarizes the issues in the United Kingdom by stating, "The three main issues regarding patients as consumers are: 1) The identity of the consumer, 2) The change in power structure of the traditional patient/professional relationship, and 3) The place of consumer power in the National Health Services." She argues that the consumer, in the sphere of the National Health Services, is an individual and is relatively powerless. The real consumer in the National Health Service, she asserts, is the purchaser. The purchaser is the one with the power. Although coming from opposite directions, it seems that the United States and the rest of the developed western nations are coming together on their approaches to health care and to consumers. All are increasing the role of the private-for-profit sector, and all are requiring consumers to assume larger responsibility for minimizing their use of health care resources and for paying a larger share of the costs when they do consume them.

One group of Canadian economists, Kindra et al. (1995), explain how to *demarket* services that have been marketed too well in the past. The intent is to reduce services and service utilization. When an entity, for example, Canada's Health Service, wants consumers to use less of their product they have four demarketing options:

1. Increase the price to consumers through co-payments or user fees.
2. Reduce the level of services through managing the care.
3. Promote reduced utilization.
4. Lessen the convenience of existing or potential services.

Consumers are going to have to become far more active, organized, and politically savvy in order to gain power and voice in shaping the current and future health services in the developed western nations, including the United States. Steve Wetzell, Executive Director of The Business Coalition in Minnesota (a group of large corporations representing 250,000 employees who are about to begin purchasing their health care directly) states, "Consumers are going to have to take control. They're going to have to be much more sophisticated . . . the consumer should drive the market" (pp. 2–3). Whether the consumer is perceived as and acts as a passive recipient of services, or whether the consumer is perceived as and acts as an active participant, is very important to the future nature of health care in the developed world (Winn and Quick 1990).

Advocacy and Consumer Advocacy

Advocates have a point of view; they approach a topic as a cause, and they interact with others by pursuing their agendas (Barney and Black 1994). Advocacy requires skills in the art of persuasion. Advocates are not always objective; they may use facts and data selectively to further their agendas. Consequently, the ethics of advocates can be called into question. Effective advocates, those who achieve much of their agendas while also achieving the respect of those who may disagree with them, are to be applauded and emulated. Such esteemed advocates are usually exemplary representatives of the causes they espouse, evidence no self-serving agendas, and show a respect for truth—even though selective.

Effective advocates are found among the humble and the celebrated. (Rose 1995; Rusin 1996). The focus group representatives reported on in Chapter 18 represent the humble. The famous may become famous because of their advocacy, such as Ralph Nader, or those famous in other walks of life may choose to lend their celebrity to causes. The late Joseph Cardinal Bernardin, for example, was a passionate advocate for not-for-profit health care (Japsen 1996). The late Bob Keeshan, also known as Captain Kangaroo, was the dedicated spokesperson of the Coalition for America's Children, an alliance of 250 national, state, and community-based organizations working to elevate the status of children's issues on the United States public policy agenda. He was seen as a strong advocate of health promotion for children and of hospitals providing such services (Sabinto 1993).

A formal advocate, within the organizations with which laypeople interact to receive services, may be mandated by law, regulatory law, or certification standards. Patient representatives, for example, are institutionally employed advocates by hospitals to comply with 1990 Joint Commission on Accreditation of Health Care Organizations requirements that every organization have established and public grievance procedures. Health professionals, such as nurses and MDs, are another large category of workers who have unbroken ties to organized health care. They are employed by or compensated by payer organizations, yet consider patient advocacy to be a core value of their professions.

Under managed care or other cost-containment models of health care compensation, patient advocacy by professionals is increasingly compromised. Although ethically, few would argue the premise that it is wrong to let the amount of money someone has or whether someone has health insurance coverage dictate how much health care they receive, this is exactly what health care providers are contending with. The day-to-day cases they are concerned with are not political abstractions by the right or the left; they are, to the contrary, real people with real needs who are being denied access to professionally determined needed health care services (Slomski 1994).

Because advocates are, by definition, linked to a cause, it is the norm to qualify the term *advocate* with a defining adjective, such as *children's advocate, environmental advocate, advocate for the disabled,* or *consumer advocate.* With respect to health care, the literature, when speaking of the involvement of laypersons in health care, commonly uses the term *consumer advocacy,* just as do the focus group participants. The American Organization of Nurse Executives thus speaks of their vision of quality health care as a new order with empowered consumers, interdependent systems, and healthy societies (Beyers 1996).

Consumers and Managed Care

This section of the chapter presents a story of tensions and pressures between the principles of cost containment, especially within managed care, and the consumers of health care. The playing out of these tensions with resulting easing of tensions will likely define the future of health care in the United States and much of the developed world. The major actors at present are the managed care companies and the purchasers of services, usually large employers including government. In the not-too-distant future, the actors will likely expand to include providers of care, consumers of care, and government as a representative of vulnerable populations (and as a greater funder of services). The managed care companies and the large purchasers will likely exercise less power and control over pricing and service than they currently enjoy. These trends can be cautiously predicted on the basis of what's already beginning to occur.

Managed care is transforming the health care marketplace in ways that few would have predicted even 5 years ago when the Clinton administration's Health Security Act was being hotly debated by Congress. The changes that are occurring are more far reaching than any proposed in that plan. Rodwin (1996) uses a term coined by the economist, Joseph Shumpeter, (1976, cited in Rodwin 1996) to describe the changes occurring. The term to describe the changes in health care is *creative destruction.* At its core is the creation of the managed care system and the dissolution of the traditional fee-for-service illness-focused system. In a remarkably short period of time, managed care approaches to health care have come to dominate the marketplace. They have provided disciplined and efficient approaches to the provision of services and the control of costs. Burke (1996), in an exercise to list all the reasons why managed care is a sane and efficient way to offer health care, identifies high technology that can be used in outpatient settings, telemedicine, macro-consumerism, micro-consumerism, managing demand, managing disease, and direct contracting (purchasing services directly from providers).

Despite the positive performance of managed care in being cost-efficient and in increasing attention to health promotion and prevention of disease, managed care poses three sets of problems for consumers:

1. Managed care systems are organized to create incentives for providers to skimp on services.
2. Managed care plans are vulnerable to organizational pathologies, as are all formal organizations.
3. Managed care plans restrict consumer choice by primary care gatekeepers or by utilization review (Rodwin 1996, p.2).

Moreover, these problems assume consumer inclusion in managed care. Rodwin (1996, p. 2) notes, however, that the uninsured and underinsured in the United States by some counts now total 75 million people. He points out that the private health care system cannot behave more equitably and efficiently at the same time. The poor and vulnerable will increasingly be excluded from health care benefits unless other forces and approaches intervene.

The managed care industry has grown up virtually overnight. Moreover, the climate in which this explosive growth occurred has favored the growth of business and the absence of regulation. Managed care is largely an unregulated industry at present (Rodwin 1996, Simon 1996). Four types of regulatory changes are widely proposed in the literature:

1. Increased information and choices for consumers,
2. Standards for services and marketing,
3. Administrative oversight (holding plans accountable), and
4. Procedural due process for consumer complaints.

Such changes would enable consumers to be more discriminating in their choices of providers and services and would allow consumers to acknowledge their expectations for services and generally take a proactive approach to their health care (Pittman 1992, Rodwin 1996).

These improvements, although positive, are believed to be insufficient to address consumer needs and concerns regarding managed care. Many reasons are posited for the insufficiency. The rapid pace of change in health care is itself sufficient to explain the great confusion by consumers about managed care (Graham 1996). Second, consumers are aware that health management organization (HMO) gag rules have or had prohibited MDs from talking about financial arrangements. Such approaches are the antithesis of openness and information sharing (Graham 1996). Coupled, these two factors alone account for both anger and distrust with managed care providers.

Another reason why the modest improvements usually posed will not be sufficient is that "market changes and attacks on government that limit funding, authority, and public support challenge the system of [regulatory] oversight" (Rodwin, p. 3). Additionally, there is no active role for consumers in running managed care plans. Nor, asserts Rodwin, is there a sufficiently powerful consumer movement. Several scholars lament the lack of a powerful consumer movement and/or the consumer lack of empowered roles within the design and conduct of health care.

Yet another reason why the commonly proposed changes are insufficient is that the process of providing and sharing information to consumers is primitive, at best. Experts really do not know what information to provide to consumers. Report cards have been used to rate various services or service settings but have only achieved mixed reviews by consumers. Currently, purchasers of care (macro-consumers) are partnering with their employees (micro-consumers) to improve quality and control costs (Graham 1996). The consumer ultimately will have to be queried about needed information and data. This will occur in individual patient care encounters, and it will occur through organized consumer groups.

As tensions mount between consumers and managed care companies, the health care industry has started to listen more to consumers. Government is also beginning to listen. Both of these major stakeholders are to date reluctant listeners, but they are listening. There is a heightened emphasis by the health care industry on patient-centered care and on providing easy access to medical information. Patient-centered care is defined by the Picker Institute as "making consumers an ongoing part of Quality Improvement efforts by using their feedback and participation to build better health care systems" (Graham, p. 7). Managed care providers and purchasers are engaged in major "consumer education and information-sharing efforts to get consumers to be more thrifty users of managed care services" (Graham, p. 7).

The various approaches and solutions put forward by experts to reduce tensions while strengthening managed care are influenced by their perspectives from the right or the left of the political spectrum or by whether they are advocates for the managed care companies or advocates for consumers. The solutions and directions they propose serve to advance their point of view. *Demand management* is an approach to allocation of health care resources that relies on four behaviors by consumers, usually encouraged by employers of employees. Employees must:

1. learn to manage their own and their family's health more effectively.
2. learn to curtail health care overconsumption.
3. understand about and actively address any potentially serious health care risks.
4. be aware of costs and make cost a key factor in all health care decision making (Copeland 1993, p.1).

Demand management addresses "consumers' insatiable desire for medical care" (Graham 1996, p.7). The idea is to let the consumer know that "their immoderate consumption of health care can no longer be tolerated" (Copeland, p.1). Employees are therefore engaged in a rigorous educational program to help them to be "good health care consumers" (Copeland, p.1). To date, most educational programs rely on basic technologies such as the *HealthWise Handbook,* which has eight million copies in print and is widely distributed by employers and by managed care companies (Graham 1996, p. 8). Graham reports that demand management appears to increase patient satisfaction while decreasing utilization of health care services. It is asserted that demand management can help to avert rationing of health care by emphasizing consumers' responsibilities, as opposed to the consumer's rights and entitlements. These responsibilities include having a healthy lifestyle, using health care services wisely, and adjusting unrealistic expectations regarding medical science (Borland et al. 1994, Burke 1996).

Disease management, another approach to providing needed care while maximizing scarce resources, is case management of chronic illness, usually by heavy utilizers of care. Its goal is "the judicious use of resources on chronically ill people at certain stages of disease in order to prevent catastrophic episodes and improve overall quality of life" (Burke 1996, p. 7). Overall responsibility for monitoring complex patients—and their use of services—is assigned to case managers by the managed care companies. Disease management is perceived by managed care organizations as the critical bridge between health promotion and the effective coordination of care. Kevin Butler, Director of the GM Health Care Initiatives Program, states, "We are certain if we do nothing on this dimension [disease management], we're going to see a substantial increase in the cost of care" (cited in Burke 1996, p. 8).

Consumer education in direct contracting models presents as a more collaborative effort between employers and employees. Two such models are reported in the literature. The Business Health Care Action Group is a coalition of self-insured major corporations in the Minneapolis region with about 250,000 employees. Starting in 1997, they are giving their members' employees cash vouchers for buying their health care coverage. They reason that they do not tell their employees where to shop for other goods and services, so why should they do so with health care. They are therefore removing the employer from the middleperson position between consumers and insurers or providers. The employees may choose from among all of the plans available on an individual basis. Even within the same families, persons may choose multiple plans. The coalition intends to continue to provide consumers (their employees) with all of the standard information available on the competing plans. In this model, the consumers (micro-consumers) will drive the market. The various competing plans will be accountable to the consumers. Plans will compete with data on such variables as price, quality, access, and consumer satisfaction (Appleby 1995).

Another model, The Employers Health Care Alliance Cooperative (The Alliance), founded in Madison, Wisconsin, in 1990, is structured to assist employers to access quality, cost-effective health care for employees. The Alliance has grown from seven founding members to over 70 employers representing over 60,000 insured lives. By aggregating purchasing power, The Alliance increases its clout regarding both quality and costs of care. The Alliance also supports a consumer education and consumer advocacy department. Alliance staff nurses orient new employees to the mission of The Alliance and the services it offers such as The Alliance Healthy Answers Hotline. They also develop and offer a customized consumer education program at the work sites. Another program, Baby Love, provides an array of educational programs for expectant parents. Low-cost health-risk appraisal programs are also offered followed by the custom design of health promotion programs, if requested. This model, it is reported, has saved money and has kept workers healthier without having to engage in some of the practices that are, perhaps, more objectionable to consumers (Borland et al. 1994).

Winn and Quick (1990), in writing about the increasing privatization of the National Health Service in the United Kingdom, simply notes that it is pointless to talk about what consumers want in health care without including them in planning health care and without simply asking them what they would like. Surveys and focus group sessions are recommended strategies. In a more formal approach, Winn suggests that membership on planning committees or advisory committees be widely used. If consumers are to be truly consumers, then they must be viewed and treated as active participants in health care decision making and not merely as passive recipients (Symonds 1994, Winn 1990).

Many believe that in the developed world, as well including the United States, increased regulation will be essential because not all consumers are good consumers and because insurers do not have the consumers welfare as their top priority. In the United States, Rodwin (1996) asserts, consumers will have to organize to represent their own interests before Congress and in statehouses before there can be any significant increase in oversight. "Effective consumer protection requires organized consumer groups that are strong enough to respond to their interests and to maintain quality, to monitor performance, to marshal political resources, and to form strategic alliances" (p. 3).

Rodwin outlines a three-point scenario for the future that is well supported by many of these scholars. He is saying that although organized consumer advocacy could be very effective, consumers have a very difficult road to travel to achieve satisfaction in the health care marketplace. He is also saying that consumer action, while essential, is insufficient by itself.

1.   Powerful consumer organizations and alliances do not exist yet because formidable obstacles make it difficult to organize disparate individuals with diverse interests. Creating and sustaining such organizations will be difficult and might not occur.

2.   Organized consumer groups, although useful, will be insufficient. Government agencies will still have an important role to play in setting standards, monitoring compliance, and penalizing illegal conduct.

3.   When scandals begin to mount, the public is likely to call for the government to recreate the regulatory system that Congress and state legislatures are attempting to dismantle. A new and better oversight system will be created if vigorous, non-governmental consumer organizations promote it and then monitor it (1996, p. 12).

DISCUSSION AND CONCLUSIONS

The focus group findings (see the previous chapter) and the literature search findings just discussed are in substantial agreement that laypersons are defining themselves and their involvement in health care both as recipients of care and as citizens working to influence care as consumers and as consumer advocates. Both the focus group participants and the professional literature are consumed by the transformation of health care from the traditional fee-for-service illness-focused model (or in the other developed nations from a government service) to a market driven model, usually some form of managed care. Both recognize the magnitude of the transformation and are energized to analyze the changes and influence their shape for the future.

The concept of consumer turns out to be one of extraordinary complexity and richness, woven into the texture of democratic society and the conduct of human affairs. The topic of the relationships between consumers and market driven health care, as evidenced by both the focus group findings and the literature search, is one of both detail and dynamic complexity. This is not surprising as all of the topics surrounding person-to-person or person-to-organization working together to achieve complex, often disparate, health care and health care finance goals have proven to be richly human high-stakes subjects. Systems thinking and systems approaches are mandated for successful integration of seemingly disparate, but mutually interdependent interests.

This focus group and literature review study has two limitations that are particularly noteworthy. The first is that the focus group research reports on only one focus group. The findings will be strengthened by the addition of research findings from more focus groups responding to a similar set of topic areas. A second limitation concerns the literature review. While as current as the published literature allows, it fails to capture day-to-day events. The managed care environment is so dynamic that one would have to track the mass media news reports and the federal and state legislative reports daily to capture the many actions being taken and changes occurring that are influencing managed care approaches and consumer behaviors. Many of the shortcomings listed or actions recommended are, in fact, beginning to occur in many of the states.

The focus group findings lead to an optimistic assessment of the consumer level of sophistication and their level of commitment in the current arena. The consumers in this focus group are most impressive. They belie the literature, which is more pessimistic about the extent and strength of consumer empowerment and participation. If this focus group is representative of other consumers, there is reason for optimism. Rodwin (1996) has argued that organized consumer groups, although useful, will be insufficient to improve managed care systems, that the government will have to play an important role. This is perhaps true, but it must be pointed out that it is likely to be the organized consumer groups that rally the government to action.

The consumer as citizen is the consumer advocacy model put forward by the focus group participants. They were concerned for the welfare of their peers and of others, including other population groups. These consumer advocates were all members and leaders of myriad consumer advocacy organizations, many of which they had helped found. It was especially notable that they carried forward into their volunteer activities the professional knowledge and skills they had honed in their salaried positions. This finding is promising, as unprecedented numbers of well-educated, healthy older Americans will increasingly be available to lend their talents and energies to consumer advocacy roles.

Additional research concerning consumer perspectives on health care, assessment of their needs and expectations for health care, and their understanding of health care issues is badly needed. What consumers say they want in health care as opposed to how they actually behave is another fruitful area for research. Consumers often report that they value health promotion and disease prevention, but they choose plans with the fewest illness care problems. Their decisions, therefore, are risk averse in practice (Williams 1994). Patients, Williams reports, will also often be far less critical when responding to surveys than they are when responding to an interview or within a focus group (1994).

Clearly, it would be advantageous to conduct far more research that asks consumers directly what they are thinking (Graham 1996, Williams 1994). Survey research is an important way to gather data from large consumer samples, such as the enormous 5-year project of the Agency for Health Policy Research, Harvard Medical School, the Rand Corporation, and the Research Triangle Institute to develop and test a standardized consumer assessment survey that could be used nationwide in inpatient, outpatient, long-term care, and home health settings along with other standardized measures for assessing quality and plan performance (Graham 1996, p. 6).

It is, perhaps, shortsighted to seek to learn from consumers merely how health care providers and insurers can satisfy consumer wants for specific services. Research and study to learn consumers' visions, missions, and goals could prove to be both fruitful and prudent. Again, focus group research offers itself as one excellent method for learning what is on the minds and the agendas of individual consumers and consumer advocacy organizations, respectively. Study of and participation in consumer advocacy organizations is another important way to gain insight into consumer behaviors and agendas.

Consumers and managed care seem to be on a collision course. It appears to be inexorable that consumers will make major gains in responsiveness of managed care providers, specifically, gains in the choice and quality of services provided. How long it will take and what exactly will be the specifics of the changes is up for speculation. The future face of health care in the United States and perhaps throughout the developed world will be very different than it is today. The future paradigm will, perhaps, be defined within 5 to 10 years. Of particular concern to advocates for the vulnerable populations is the question of how will the clash of market forces and consumer advocacy impact the availability and accessibility of health care for those vulnerable populations outside the system? What will the citizens of the United States and its representative governments do about health care for the 75 million citizens who are uninsured or underinsured and who therefore lack access to affordable health care? How will the health care financing system be changed to both provide access and assure affordability for a large majority of citizens?

Many of the preceding discussion points and recommendations presume that consumers have a legitimate role in shaping systems and services, including health care delivery systems, and in shaping social policy. Certainly, the idea of a symbiotic relationship between consumers and producers (or insurers and providers) dates to the founding of the nation when Adam Smith and Thomas Jefferson conceived of the great experiment of a free-market economy in a democratic society. Throughout much of modern history, the symbiotic relationship of management and labor has been the focus of attention by scholars, policy-makers, and advocates for one side or the other (Turner 1995, p.17). The developed world is into a new era, however. As the global economy moves into cyberspace and the 21st century, the world will become much more apparent from the consumer point of view. Certainly, myriad examples already abound. For example, we are surrounded by products we have purchased from other nations, despite exhortations by many to buy U.S. goods only.

In the global society, the role of consumption and the behaviors of consumers take on new meanings. Consumers are increasingly likely to use markets to shape the social agenda. If consumers fail to do so, they will assure that the balance of power tilts in favor of producers. (In the case of managed care, the balance of power will side with the insurers and, perhaps, the providers.) When thinking people consider the topic in the context of the new societal paradigm and consider, too, the rich sociopolitical and socioeconomic history and conceptual meanings of consumer and consumer advocacy, it is hard to envision such an unbalanced power relationship of consumers and insurers in favor of insurers in the long term.

Consumers and health care providers often, albeit not always, have a common cause. It is predictable that providers and consumers, both desirous of an open and caring health care delivery system that is not driven exclusively by market forces, may join forces in alliance to advocate for health care reforms that will please both groups of stakeholders. At the risk of sounding biased, this investigator hopes so.

References

Appleby, C. (1995, June 5). The middle no more. *Hospitals and Health Networks, 69*(11), 96, 98.

Barney, R. D. and Black, J. (1994). Ethics and professional persuasive communications. *Public Relations Review, 20*(3), 233–248.

Beyers, M. (1996). Creation of new order. *Nursing Management, 27*(4), 48.

Borland, M., Smith, C., and Nanakivil, N. (1994). A community quality initiative for health care reform. *Managed Care Quarterly, 2*(1), 6–16.

Burke, G. (1996). And now the good news. . . *Health Systems Review, 29*(4), 21–24.

Charters, M. A. (1993). The patient representative role and sources of power. *Hospital and Health Services Administration, 38*(3), 429–442.

Copeland, J. (1993). Health care needs a proconsumer movement. *Business and Health, 11*(7), 80, 79.

Donaldson, C., Lloyd, P., and Lupton, D. (1991). Primary health care consumerism amongst elderly Australians. *Age and aging, 20,* 280–286.

Graham, J. (1996). The rise of the health care consumer. *Business and Health* (Suppl. State of health care in America), 49–53.

Harvey, C. A. (1989, August). Older patients and medical consumerism. *Consultant, 89–91.*

Hayes C. (1991). The white paper and the consumer. *Senior Nurse, 11*(1), 11–13.

Japsen, B. (1996, November 18). Cardinal Joseph Bernardin, advocate of not-for-profit health care dies at 68. *Modern Healthcare, 26*(47), 3, 6.

Kelly, J. M. (1994). Mandate reimbursement measures in the states. *American Review of Public Administration, 24*(4), 351–373.

Kim, H. S., Holter, I. M., Lorensen, M., Inayoshi, M., Shimaguchi, S., Shimakzaki-Ryder, (1993). Patient–nurse collaboration: a comparison of patients' and nurses' attitudes in Finland, Japan, Norway, and the U.S.A. *International Journal of Nursing Studies, 30*(5), 387–401.

Kindra, G. S., and Taylor, D. W. (1995). Demarketing inappropriate health care consumption. *Journal of Health Care Marketing, 15*(2), 10–14.

Lang, T. and Gabriel, V. (1995). The consumer as citizen. *Consumer Policy Review, 5*(3), 96–102.

Lerner, M. (1937). Introduction. In Smith, A., *The Wealth of Nations,* The Modern Library Edition. New York: Random House, Inc.

Macfarlane, D. (1996). Citizen participation in the reform of health care policy: A case example. *Healthcare Management Forum, 9*(2), 31–35.

Pittman, K. P. (1992). Awakening child consumerism in health care. *Pediatric Nursing, 18*(2), 132–136.

Rodwin, M. A. (1996). Consumer protection and managed care: The need for organized consumers. *Health Affairs, 15*(3), 110–123.

Rose, N. (1995, November 15). The advocate's art. *International Commercial Litigation.*

Rusin, K. (1996). Serving the children. *Life Association News, 91*(10), 160–161.

Sabinto, F. (1993). The "Captain" charts a steady course: Advocacy for children's issues. *Trustee, 46*(6), 10–11.

Siedman, E. (1996). Renascent retirement: The fourth career. *Public Manager, 25*(2), 41–42.

Simon, R. (1996). You're losing your consumer rights. *Money, 25*(3), 100–111.

Sinclair, U. (1906). *The Jungle.* New York: Amereon.

Slomski, A. J. (1994). Think today's ethical issues are tough? Just wait. *Medical Economics, 71*(8), 38–59.

Statham, D. (1994). Working together in community care. *Health Visitor, 67*(1), 16–18.

Symonds, A. (1994). Patients as consumers: A case of packaging only? *Management Research News, 17*(7,8,9) 83–85.

Thorne, S. E. and Robinson, C. A. (1989). Guarded alliance: Health care relationships in chronic illness. *Image Journal of Nursing Scholarship, 21*(3), 153–157.

Turner, J. S. (1995). The consumer interest in the 1990s and beyond. *Journal of Consumer Affairs, 29*(2), 310–327.

Valachich, J. S., and Schwenk, C. (1995). Structuring conflict in individual, face-to-face, and computer-mediated group decision making: Carping versus objective devil's advocacy. *Decision Sciences, 26*(3), 369–393.

Warne, C. (1993). *The consumer movement.* Manhattan, KS: Family Economics Trust Press.

Williams, B. (1994). Patient satisfaction: A valid concept? *Social Science Medicine, 38*(4), 509–516.

Winn, L. and Quick, A. (1990, April). User friendly services. *Health Services Management,* 90–91.

Collaboration:
An Imperative Journey

Collaboration: More 20 Than a Practice

Daryl Hobbs

INTRODUCTION

This book has been about more than improving working relationships among professional health care providers, however meritorious and beneficial that purpose might be. It goes beyond management practices and technique; it is also a book about values and improving the connectedness of values and practices in the world of work and beyond. Implicitly, it is a book about an American society caught in the throes of a transition from a corporate culture and the mass industrial society it spawned to a new era that is sufficiently different that we have not quite settled on a name for it yet, other than ill-fitting terms like *postmodern* and *postindustrial*. It is this transition that helps explain why collaboration (and all the meanings one can read into that term such as community, cooperation, and connectedness) has only recently emerged as a research and intellectual focus. Collaboration is one of many concepts whose greater currency seems to reflect a larger societal search for meaning beyond individual achievement and technical efficiency.

The concerns and issues cut across all sectors of contemporary society. For all the research reviewed in this volume focusing on collaboration in health care, an equal or greater amount could be found focusing on collaboration and other similar changes in the organizational culture of corporations, education, government, and social services, as well as the family and community. It is not that collaboration is a new idea (in some respects, it seems to be an effort to revive what is presumed to have

593

been common practice in an earlier and simpler day), but rather that organizational complexity and impersonality have contributed to many workers, both professional and nonprofessional alike, feeling a greater need for integration and connectedness at work, at home, and in other domains of everyday life. Those problems of meaning and connectedness have surfaced even as new technologies continue to amaze and as private and personal wealth accumulates for many. But quantitative achievements seem to be insufficient. More money than ever is being spent for health, education, and other public services, yet neither providers nor consumers seem content with the outcomes, reflected in part by a general decline in public trust and confidence in most institutions.

A BROADER FOCUS

This chapter does not focus much further on collaboration among professionals in the institutional settings in which most health care is delivered; the preceding chapters have covered that thoroughly and well. Rather, it concentrates more on collaboration and cooperation as emerging themes and processes in and of the larger society. There are two reasons. First, health care, although a unique sector, is affected by, and is indeed based on, many of the norms, values, assumptions, and beliefs that are endemic to American society at any point in history. Although health care has become increasingly uncoupled from other institutions, it is still an American system, and if changes occur in American society, those changes will affect health care and how, where, and to whom it is supplied. That is clearly happening now, to the accompaniment of substantial uncertainty about the health care system of the future.

The other reason is that there is growing public, professional, and even policy interest in health, as well as health care. There are many reasons for that interest, including a widening belief that a healthier population may be the most effective way of paying for the present and future health care system. Changing the definition of the problem from providing health care to improving health would involve a different set of players and would reflect a need for greatly expanded collaboration across a broader front. Indeed a societal focus on health could become an important mechanism for achieving greater integration and connectedness among institutions. Although health care is generally the exclusive domain of the health care institution, individual and collective health is a product of, and is affected by, all aspects of society especially including education, religion, families, work, and communities. If improving health were to become an objective shared by all of those institutions, collaboration would undoubtedly be effective in improving health; but collaboration in pursuit of a common goal would also contribute to restoring greater connectedness among institutions that have become increasingly uncoupled as this century has worn on.

THE VALUES OF COLLABORATION

Ideally, collaboration in the contemporary context is more than a formal, or even informal, division of labor for performing some task. Beyond being a specific practice, a norm of collaboration can become a value of an organizational culture, valued not only for efficient accomplishment of a task but also for the interpersonally rewarding relationships that can accompany collaborative performance. Such a norm of collaboration is suggestive of a concomitant sense of community that transcends individual achievement. Later in this chapter, a connection between collaboration as a practice and social capital as a resource is explored.

A recent analysis of American society (Bellah et al. 1985) explored, through community study and intensive interviews, the current state of the American mind. That book, *Habits of the Heart,* borrows its title from the expression employed by Tocqueville to describe the mix of traits fundamental to 19th century American national character. Bellah et al. explore the currently relied on traditions to try to make sense of our lives and to delineate, as a current moral dilemma, the conflict between our continued dedication to individualism and our expressed need for community and commitment to one another. The authors contend that an accumulation of social changes has created a need for a new social ecology—a new set of interrelationships between people and between people and their environments, both social and physical. Such a social ecology would reflect a set of shared values and their connection to practices of work and everyday life. The challenge is not so much one of devising new values, but rather to link existing values with our practices more effectively. Greater meaning is produced in our lives when what we believe and what we do are in greater harmony.

We can infer values from what people say and do, but we can also gain insight into people's values from what they say is missing in their lives.

We do not miss something we do not care much about. Therefore, when people talk about emptiness, shallowness, or a lack of meaning in their lives, they seem to be reflecting a lack of connectedness between the values they profess and the practices they find themselves employing. Much of the research reported in this volume has focused not only on the functional effectiveness of collaboration for accomplishing tasks, but also on the feeling of gratification and worth it induces among the collaborators. Meaning and gratification are to be found as much in the process as in the accomplishment.

To establish further a frame of reference for the remainder of this chapter, collaboration continues to be viewed not as a value, but as a practice; a form of relationships and doing things that can be applied to a wide range of circumstances and purposes. If the expectation of collaboration becomes a part of a group, organizational, or even institutional culture, that is an important step toward attaching greater meaning to participants' efforts. More specifically, it is suggested that when collaboration has become normative for any group or organization, it is simultaneously an expression of several values fundamental to a new social ecology. Although the following list of values is not by any means exhaustive, each is a value that is embodied in effective collaborative activities (Hobbs 1990). These four values intentionally contrast with individualism. It is the sharing of values that makes them powerful.

1. *Community*—A value that is expressed by kinds and styles of human relationships and transactions that emphasize integration more than separation; relationships that contrast with excessive individualism, but not at the expense of individuality. Later, community, not only as a value but also as a social mechanism for improving health, is discussed.
2. *Fairness*—Fairness implies an emphasis on interpersonal respect in an atmosphere devoid of prejudice. Fairness does not equate with equality, but it is egalitarian. Many examples in this book focus on the physician–nurse game and on other health care relationships that reflect hierarchy or power imbalances. What subordinates seem to find dissatisfying about such relationships is not an absence of equality, but rather a perception of being treated unfairly or not having one's expertise respected. In those circumstances in which high-technology health care is delivered, it is not practical or effective to think of all participants as bringing equal

levels of skill or knowledge to the task. But successful outcomes are achieved by the effective integration of those skills. Participants are most likely to believe that they have been treated fairly if their contribution is valued and the outcome is a shared accomplishment. Community does not and cannot coexist with unfairness.

3. *Work*—Not merely as a means of making a living or even achieving status, but as an activity that is both productive and contributory to feelings of personal worth; work that is intrinsically and extrinsically useful. It is through their work that the contributions of collaborators are recognized and valued. All commercial organizations financially reward workers for their efforts; but not all organizations place workers in positions where their work contributes to feelings of self-worth. As stated by Bellah et al.: "The satisfaction of work well done, indeed the 'pursuit of excellence' is a permanent and positive human motive. . . . [I]n a revived social ecology, work would be a primary form of civic virtue" (1986, p. 288). Embedded in a new social ecology, work as a value is one of the important means for mending the splits between public and private, work and families that have grown over the century.

4. *Choice*—As a paraphrase for freedom. It is difficult to conceive of freedom in the absence of choice. A recent summary of job satisfaction literature reported that workers are satisfied with their jobs to the extent that they feel they have some autonomy and/or opportunity to make decisions. Beyond the world of work, recent authors (for example, Theobald 1997, Kemmis 1990) have suggested that to restore a sense of civic responsibility in our society, it is important to think of freedom not only as freedom *from* (fear, coercion, responsibility), but more as freedom *to* exercise the rights and responsibilities of citizenship in a free society. There has been a recent tendency to think of freedom as the freedom to do what we want rather than freedom to do what we should. Freedom and choice are fundamental to effective collaboration and shared responsibility.

Within the context of this discussion of collaboration as a practice, the term is also used in the sense of reflecting values essential to a new social ecology that overcomes some of the adverse consequences of excessive individualism and hierarchy.

This concluding chapter focuses on how and why society is increasingly concerned not just with the costs and benefits of health care but also with social, emotional, and physical health. There is a growing realization that essential components of quality of life, such as health and education, are to be gained not solely from large organizations with impressive technical capabilities but also from the quality of relationships beyond the venues of formal health care and education.

Before proceeding, a brief assessment is offered of why, despite unprecedented economic growth and technological accomplishments, we arrive at the end of the 20th century in a state of social and institutional uncertainty, if not disarray.

THE FOUNDATION FOR OUR PRACTICES

Social change occurs when the basic rules, assumptions, and premises that we live by change. Although not usually formalized, those rules, which evolve from experience, practice, success, and values in a cultural and historical context, are nonetheless powerful, and are the foundation of social existence. When the rules become the basis for the organization and practices of society's major institutions, the rules become "self-evident"; it is the way things are done; it is the "American Way." They are thus taken for granted, and as one philosopher has noted, nothing so persistently evades our attention as that which we take for granted. We do not debate the "self-evident" rules. We generally just follow them. We reify the rules and principles in ongoing practices. As long as things are working reasonably well there is little pressure for change.

Ongoing small-scale changes and refinements are a part of the cultural pattern for any society. There are periods, however, when for any number of reasons (North 1990, Kuhn 1962), an accumulation of changes or discoveries brings into question the validity of existing rules and the assumptions and beliefs on which they are based. Conditions contribute to the formation of new rules and assumptions, and for a period of time there is uncertainty and disarray as both the new and old rules coexist. The United States is currently working its way through such a period. When the new rules have become hegemonic, a paradigm shift has occurred. Although the current pervasive use of the term *paradigm shift* in both academic and popular publications has reduced it to a virtual cliché, nevertheless when the change of rules is profound and affects all aspects of society, the societal paradigm has changed.

During the 20th century, the United States has gone through one paradigm shift and is in the midst of a second. We began the century as a largely agrarian society with relationships generally confined to communities and neighborhoods owing to the limits of transportation and communication technology. During this early era, community residents knew a great deal about where they lived and not much about the world beyond. In the small towns and urban neighborhoods, it was obvious that the work of each person contributed to the good of all; that work was a form of mutual obligation, not just a source of material or psychic rewards. In that fashion, work contributed not only to production and therefore survival, but it concurrently sustained a sense of community. The community and its rules affected the way work was done and work was a defining attribute of community. One's work was a principal means of establishing one's place in the community. One's sense of self and worth could not be separated from one's work. Those conditions applied also to the work of the professional providers of health care and education. The physicians and teachers not only provided their professional services to a local clientele but were, at the same time, their friends and neighbors. Relationships overlapped, and the ongoing face-to-face relationships ensured that the different aspects of community life were connected. Communities were necessarily holistic, and cooperation was normative. Communities and neighborhoods were, quite literally, little societies.

But changes were occurring quickly, and not long after the 20th century began, the era dominated by communities and neighborhoods was giving way to an industrial era that would become the foundation for a mass society. It was not far into the 20th century before work was to become separated from community and household, and accordingly, the social meaning and value of work would change.

The 20th century transformation from an agrarian to an industrial world is called by some social scientists the Fordist Era in recognition of Henry Ford's contributions to industrial organization and production. It was Ford who elaborated the idea of the assembly line on the basis of the organizational principles of specialization, centralization, and standardization. The objective was to increase the efficiency of mass production of standardized products. Production became more efficient as each worker performed a specialized task while the product under construction moved along the assembly line. The outcome would be a standardized vehicle exactly like the one that preceded it and the one that would follow. In order for specialized labor inputs to result in a completed machine, it was necessary for a large number of workers to be present at the same location; hence centralization. The premise of these principles was economic; it was about efficiency, especially labor efficiency. Ford's economic aspiration was that through the efficiency of mass production, it would be possible to increase wages and lower the cost of the automobile so that workers who helped build cars could afford to own one.

These principles were of course not new; they had been described and analyzed by many philosophers and social scientists in the 19th century in the context of an industrializing Europe, but their full implementation in the United States ushered in a period of academic attention to scientific management. Industrial organization became an object of research and engineering. Organization researchers focused their analyses on designing organizations to increase the efficiency of production, especially increasing the span of control of managers so that unit cost of production would diminish. These developments, beginning in the 1920s, would lead to the United States becoming the world leader in scientific management, which was the foundation for the prototypical industrial economy.

With the coming of large-scale industrial society, it became more difficult to see work as a contribution to the whole and easier to view it as a segmental, self-interested activity. Where one lived and where one worked became separated, not only by place but by social significance as well. The wholeness of the earlier, simple community was being lost, replaced by a world of pervasive specialization and corresponding fragmentation. This new industrial world involved more than moving production from household to factory; new institutions were being created along with the rules governing their performance. The underlying premises were largely economic, with efficiency as the criteria for effectiveness and labor as a market commodity. The accompanying forms of organization for producing machines and goods and, eventually, for education and health care were expressed in organization charts showing a pecking order of roles, not persons. The chart was a pyramid. The decision making that accompanied the new industrial model was removed from workers and placed in the hands of managers. It was an authority system that was designed to minimize judgment at lower levels of production. The focus of engineering was to make production workers into more effective cogs of the organizational machine. It was the structure of the organization that was responsible for productivity more than the individual role players within it. The layers of authority, pyramid forms of organization, and bureaucracy had become the genetic glue of the industrial economy, of society.

Concurrently, the hierarchically structured industrial organizations were becoming larger. Growing research attention was being paid to the contribution of economies of scale to economic efficiency. Generally, the unit cost of production would go down as the volume of production increased. Following that principle, big corporations were becoming bigger and labor was becoming more organized. Bigger as better was becoming a dominant cultural conviction: a conviction that would extend beyond the industrial sector to health, education, and other institutions as well. Another piece of the industrial society was falling into place.

Although industrial work was becoming depersonalized, compensation for it was increasing. A result was a rapidly growing middle class. The increasing rates of wages were enabling greater numbers of blue collar workers to ascend to the middle class and relocate from the city neighborhoods to the new suburbs. Changes in social organization and lifestyle were pervasive. Following World War II, the declining relative prices of consumer goods, along with increasing real wages, were contributing further to consumption and materialism as a feature of middle-class lifestyle. Robert Reich (1992) refers to the 1950s and 1960s as reflecting a social contract between big corporations, big labor, the government, and the middle class. The industrial era had reached its zenith. The recent demise of that social contract is one of the signals of the emergence of a new set of economic and organization rules and the advent of another paradigm shift.

THE EXTENSION OF INDUSTRIAL PRINCIPLES

Had the principles of efficient mass production of standardized goods remained confined to the factories, they would not be relevant to our analysis in this chapter. But as a result of impressive growth in industrial productivity and corresponding growth of the middle class, the United States was increasingly becoming a mass society, extending the principles of mass production beyond the factories to other sectors as well. By the 1960s, both health and education had changed dramatically from their earlier community base, and the more hospitals and schools changed, the more they organizationally resembled the world of corporate mass production. Medicine was becoming more specialized, and as it did, the more it became imperative to concentrate the services in larger organizations. In the name of improvement, public education also became the domain of specialists and schools also were reorganized in order to be able to offer the full range of specialized educational services cost effectively. Following the principles of efficiency, the more specialization the greater the centralization and the greater the size of the organizations. Schools and hospitals increasingly became large organizations, and the principles of management of large organizations became applicable to each. Health and educational services were thus being restructured and reorganized using economic efficiency considerations. Large hierarchically structured organizations increasingly became the locus for providing health and education services. The industrial model and the rules on which it was based left few sectors of the society untouched.

As the health care and education organizations became larger, they all began to look alike. What had been a society of great local institutional variation had become a society of great institutional homogeneity. It became fashionable in the 1960s for social scientists to produce analyses of what had become the *mass society*. The analyses were presented as a kind of zero sum game: the more the society followed the rules of mass (mass media, mass production, mass education, mass merchandising), the less it was a society of socially and economically viable communities and neighborhoods. Whereas at the turn of the century, people's fortunes were greatly affected by their locality, that became less so as citizens of the mass society had become highly mobile. People moved in response to what they perceived to be the best market for their skills and labor. Social attachments and obligations were typically left behind. This mobility further reinforced the uniformity of institutional practices across the country. All of those features of our common existence as citizens of the nation were being proclaimed and reinforced by the mass media. The mass media played a major role in culmination of the mass society by providing citizens with the opportunity to become better informed about distant locations and events, often at the expense of what was happening in the communities and neighborhoods. Localities became less and less relevant, and what had been a rural–urban nation was increasingly becoming a suburban nation. A concurrent move, however, especially of displaced rural

African Americans to the cities was prominent in the creation of poverty-stricken inner cities. Rather than being citizens of places, people had largely become social, economic, and political citizens of the nation, redefining their personal identities and social attachments in the process.

A concomitant change was the increasing specialization of institutions and a corresponding separation of their purposes. Accordingly, public policies and issues became redefined in terms of the institutions rather than as problems of the society. The welfare of institutions often seemed to take precedence over attention to the social needs that were their purported reasons for being. Instead of being synergistic, the institutions had become *antergistic,* a term used in Chapter 3 to indicate a whole comprising less than the sum of its parts.

Douglas North (1990), a recent winner of the Nobel Peace Prize in economics, has observed that it is the interrelationship between institutions in a society that is the basis for economic growth and cultural dynamism. North observes that throughout history there have been epochs when societies were creative. Those periods he refers to as *learning societies*, periods when the institutions of a society were integrated and collaborative. By contrast, societies whose institutions have become separated, with each focused on maintaining its own role and on survival, he refers to as being *stuck.* American society has recently been experiencing the consequences of being stuck as public attention has become focused on each institution separately, rather than their interrelationships with each other and with the whole society.

Among the many consequences of institutional fragmentation has been a growing tendency toward sector-specific public policies: public policies that seek to solve societal problems through individual institutions. Public programs and legislation (both state and federal) pertaining to health care provide a clear example. Health care legislation and funding have greatly affected the institution of health care and the kind of services that are provided, who provides them, and under what conditions. But those policy initiatives have been advanced and implemented with little attention to effects on other institutions and sectors of society. As emphasized later in this chapter in the discussion of community, reestablishing connections among institutions at a community level is becoming an increasingly important objective of community development efforts. The benefits of collaboration pertain to institutions and organizations as well as among individuals.

INDIVIDUALISM

Although smaller communities and neighborhoods were dominant features of early 20th century social organization, that should not be misconstrued as reflective of a society based on communitarian principles. Those communities were more a product of practical necessity, imposed by limits of transportation, than a reflection of a societal commitment to community as the foundation of social life. From the outset, American society has been committed to a social philosophy that views the public good as a product of the aggregate of individual achievements. The American focus has been an individualistic but egalitarian society, emphasizing each person's rights and liberties held in balance by contractual obligation and reciprocal exchange.

The emergence of the mass society built on industrial principles did not occur over the protests of a population decrying the concurrent demise of community. Rather, the industrial society provided the means and reinforced the pursuit of individual achievement. Theobald (1997) summarizes the consequences as follows: "[T]here has been an undue focus on the self in our society and the predictable result has been disintegrating neighborhoods and a vanishing sense of community. . . . [W]e have become a society marked by few allegiances and almost no propensity to shoulder mutual obligations" (p. 12).

Americans were not generally forced from their communities and neighborhoods, except in the sense that economic growth and opportunities were unevenly distributed geographically—the growth was in the cities. Millions of Americans perceived greater opportunities for individual gain by leaving rural communities behind and joining the march toward the centers of economic growth. Small communities not only declined as a lifestyle but were declining in economic sustainability as well. These migrations and relocations, which were built substantially on the pursuit of individual success, were important contributors to reinforcing the impetus of a growing industrial and mass society. The historical commitment to individualism and individual achievement and success had produced willing participants in the advancing industrialization and its opportunities for improving income and enhancing status. Individualism was compatible with the industrial organizational structures and the incentives they offered. As Theobald (1997) suggests, "[I]ndividuals increasingly began to think of themselves as actors in the world unencumbered by communal obligations or traditions" (p. 45). Freedom increasingly became freedom to do what we want. Many authors, each using somewhat different language, have observed that what became a contractual basis for interpersonal relationships in much of professional and managerial work could not carry the weight of sustained and enduring commitments.

The institutions of the mass society have been a highly effective mechanism for reinforcing individualism and incentives for individual achievement. Most institutions are structured to serve the needs of individual clients and have implemented reward structures that sustain individualism; there have been few mechanisms for rewarding collaboration. There is no better example than public education, in which all assessments of performance, except perhaps for extracurricular activities, are individually based. Likewise, in universities, it is the performance of individual students and individual faculty members that is evaluated and rewarded. That practice continues, even though there is growing recognition that much of the best research is being done by teams of researchers, often from different disciplines. Despite the acknowledged benefits of collaboration and synergism, when faculties are evaluated for tenure or promotion, it is the accomplishments of individuals that are required to be submitted for evaluation. From the preceding chapters, it is clear that those norms, at least until very recently, have prevailed in the training of health care professionals as well.

Bellah et al. (1985) observe how the persistent emphasis on individualism has contributed to what they describe as a therapeutic society—a society that has turned to professional specialists for the resolution of most of life's problems. The therapeutic self that emerges from that society is "[d]efined by its own wants and satisfactions, coordinated by cost–benefit calculation" (p. 127). A variation of the therapeutic society is that we have become a society inclined to seek expert assistance no matter what the problem might be. It is not that outside expertise may not be pertinent or helpful, but that the inclination to turn unreflectively to expertise for assistance in problem solving sustains our tendencies to overlook the problem-solving benefits of collaboration.

Perhaps we have devoted excessive attention to tracing the origins of our industrial and individually oriented society, but we have been seeking to understand why, despite all the attractive benefits of collaboration enumerated in this volume, that practice is still in the process of gaining acceptance. Our institutionalized commitment to individualism remains an impediment to more routine collaboration despite evidence that many Americans are seeking more than status and salary from their work and their relationships. Although the pyramid form of organization is losing favor in corporate America (Reich 1992), it still remains the dominant organizational form in our most prominent public service institutions, including health and education. Although many managers and participants intellectually understand the social and production benefits from collaboration that practice has not yet become a "habit of the heart." Thus, many of our routine practices are not yet delivering on the potential of collaborative work and community to link practices with values.

PARADIGM CHANGE: NEW RULES OF ORGANIZATION, NATION, AND COMMUNITY

Evidence of the transformation of the prototypical industrial society has been accumulating for several decades. Notable to most older Americans is the demise of what Reich (1992) refers to as a social contract that was securely in place through the 1960s. Over the past 30 years, the industrial foundation for that social contract, namely, factories efficiently mass producing large quantities of standardized goods, has largely left the United States in favor of cheaper wage rates and lower costs of production elsewhere. Their destination has most often been to countries formerly called Third World, but because of extensive relocation of factories, many are now referred to as newly industrializing nations. Those countries that offer political stability, tax breaks, and a cheap and dependable labor supply have become the producers of much of the world's supply of consumer goods (Barnet and Cavanagh 1994). The goods are produced cheaply but not without problems, as exemplified by recent concerns about widespread use of child labor. With globalization of the economy, the United States no longer enjoys a comparative advantage in the production of mass-produced standardized consumer products: the role of the U.S. economy has changed.

As a consequence, most consumer products, formerly bearing the label "Made in the USA," now arrive here from numerous offshore locations. Many of those imports actually originate with corporations traditionally thought of as American, but whose operations are now global. The corporate (global) headquarters may still be here, but their production facilities are geographically dispersed. The role of the global corporation is to coordinate a global production, distribution, and marketing system. Production and markets have become uncoupled from nations. In the new economy, very few goods are being produced exclusively for national markets because both the markets and production facilities have become global. National corporations have become global corporations with little allegiance to any national flag. These changes have affected our national identity as well; Reich (1992) devotes a chapter in his book to addressing the question that has evolved, "Who Is Us?"

These global corporations are operating by very different rules and with very different objectives and obligations than the national economies of our recent experience. The changes are sufficiently profound and comprehensive that McMichael (1996) and numerous other authors describe the emergence of a global economy as a paradigm shift. The global economy operates in an environment of nearly unlimited mobility of capital made possible by extensive dependence on telecommunications technologies. Whereas in the industrial era, labor and capital were generally joined, today they have become extensively uncoupled as well. Although capital is highly mobile, labor is not, placing the labor force at any location at risk of losing its basis for existence. These global relocations have contributed to the demise of the 1960s' social contract and have been accompanied by significant changes in the distribution of income and the social class structure.

The chronology of these changes has been widely documented and described but can be symbolized by three books authored by Alvin Toffler appearing at the beginning of each of the past three decades. In 1970, Toffler's book *Future Shock* described the beginnings of a postindustrial society; that was followed in 1980 by the *Third Wave,* which described a paradigm shift as profound in its implications as the industrial revolution's; and in 1990, came *Power Shift,* which described how speed and flexibility have become the operating principles of the global economy.

In the context of global markets and global production, the rules by which large corporations are now operating have changed greatly. By the late 1970s and early 1980s, a number of major American corporations who were producers of widely known brand names were having difficulty remaining domestically and internationally competitive. Much national worry was generated about losing market share to Japanese and European producers. Although the competitive environment had changed, many United States-based corporations were still organized as pyramids and operating by the principles of standardized mass production (Reich 1992). Typical was the American automobile industry, which was piling up large losses in the early 1980s: over the past 15 years, the industry has made a remarkable comeback. But the automobile industry of today is dramatically different organizationally from the industry of a decade ago. The new auto industry is much more organizationally flat, decentralized, and geographically dispersed.

In the new global economy, effective industrial organizations are now defined by their ability to innovate, adapt, and change. Effective organizations are increasingly flexible and rely extensively on small groups of collaborators possessing different but complementary skills. For American industries, the transition has been from corporate structures producing a *high volume of goods* to firms increasingly focused on producing *high-value goods*. High-value organizations operate by very different principles. Reich (1992) refers to the new organizational forms as "webs of enterprise"; the organization chart resembles a spider web more than a pyramid. The web is a series of horizontal linkages across numerous small nodes of productive activity. Rather than a vertical chain of command, the smaller nodes tend to be relatively autonomous and function with a high level of collaboration both within and between the nodes of production. Some of the webs have become so geographically extensive that they form global commodity chains (McMichael 1996). *Collaboration is no longer only a tactic for improving employee morale: it has become a defining principle of organization in the global economy.*

High-value organizations (health care is a high-value form of service and enterprise) depend on, and expect, workers at all levels to be capable of making decisions. It is the ongoing uniqueness of enterprise that is a distinguishing characteristic and the basis for organizing work, rather than efficiency among relatively low-skilled production workers. Reich refers to that whole class of "knowledge workers" as *symbolic analysts*—their work is primarily mental and requires judgment. They are the workers who, in the current economy, are making higher wages and are generally employed by organizations who are competitive. It is knowledge and judgment that has become the key to competitiveness, not the former industrial mode of labor efficiency. The high-volume enterprises that depend on labor performing repetitive tasks are the ones that have transferred offshore.

Not coincidentally, it was the economic production sector that was at the forefront of developing and elaborating the roles and principles of the industrial paradigm, and now again it is the economic sector that has been pioneering organizational adaptations to a global economy. Following the lead of the commercial sector, the industrial organization model was, over a period of time, adopted as the model for health, education, and other social services. The same sequence is occurring again. The recent innovations in organization, production, and management have come from the commercial sector, whereas government, education, social services and, to an extent, health care remain substantially committed to the organizational structure and practices of the industrial paradigm. Collaboration has become routine, normative, and productive in high-value enterprises, but little of the work in education, whether in public schools or colleges and universities, either teaches or requires collaboration. The typical public school still significantly resembles a factory both in appearance and methods of operation. It is noteworthy, however, that changes seem to be further along in health care. Several chapters in this book have described collaboration in health care. Nursing education has, for example, become more frequently linked with practice.

SOCIAL IMPLICATIONS OF ECONOMIC CHANGE

Movement toward a new global paradigm has been accompanied by pervasive social change. There has been widespread societal concern about change in family organization, economic opportunities, and civic responsibility in a context of such public concerns as rising rates of substance abuse and violence among youth, teenage pregnancies and rising crime rates. These and many other social concerns have surfaced concurrent with unprecedented levels of personal wealth for a growing number of people. While many citizens have sought explanations for these changes by declaring them to be a consequence of "loss of traditional values," there have been a number of objective changes that have affected families, communities, and the social class structure.

Space does not permit an enumeration of more than an abbreviated list, but the following make it clear that no aspect of contemporary society has been left untouched by the economic restructuring that has accompanied globalization. Many of these are producing important implications for health care and how health care relates to other social issues and concerns.

- Whereas bigger is better was a widely held conviction a generation ago, many of the recent changes negate that conviction. Since the late 1970s, research studies have reported that most of the new employment in the United States has been generated by small employers rather than large corporations. Part of that is attributable to changes in the structure of large corporations, which have turned extensively to outsourcing for many of their functions. But concurrently, entrepreneurship has been widespread and new business startups have been much higher than in previous decades. A consequence has been a diminished rate of employer-supported health insurance. Large employers are more than twice as likely as small employers to offer health insurance as an employee benefit.

- The typical family in the era of Reich's social contract was supported by the work of one family member. Today more than three fourths of all women having children at home are employed outside the home. Child care has become an essential and prominent national industry, and the health of children is becoming a growing issue as it affects their educational performance.

- In the era of the social contract, about 40% of workers were labor union members. Today, labor union membership claims about 10% of the workforce. Real wage rates have declined as competition for industrial plants has become international. A consequence has been declining real income for the bottom half of wage earners.

- The middle class has been shrinking. To paraphrase one recent analysis, the social class structure now comprises an overclass, an underclass, and a nervous class (Ehrenreich 1990). Even with two or more workers per household, about 60% of U.S. households experienced a decline in inflation-adjusted family income from 1970 to 1990.

- There is no doubt that the economic changes have produced winners and losers with a corresponding impact on the national psyche and the need for, and the ability to access, health care services.

THE SOCIAL IMPACT OF TELECOMMUNICATIONS TECHNOLOGY

The role of telecommunications technology in facilitating qualitative changes has been so significant that some analysts (for example, Allen and Dillman 1994) describe the new paradigm as a global-information era. Telecommunications technology is enabling greater decentralization of production and services and simultaneously making possible continued centralization of decision making and control. Telecommunications technology is currently also contributing to significant relocation of population in the United States and is just beginning to become a more widely utilized means of providing health and education services. These are important changes because technologies of most of the 20th century led to greater concentration of population, services, and production.

Both change in what the U.S. economy is producing and how the new products are being transported are having important implications for where new economic investments are occurring. Firms that produce information products (some estimates report that more than half of the U.S. workforce is employed in information-related jobs) and therefore can utilize telecommunications technology to transport their products are free to change the criteria they employ in deciding where to locate their business. Connecting links of the webs of enterprise are predominantly electronic: the nodes of production can be both organizationally and geographically dispersed and remain in effective collaboration.

Evidence of the results of changed criteria for location of productive activities has been accumulating for the past few years. Since 1990, there has been an important relocation of U.S. population. States that experienced significant in-migration and, therefore, great population growth during the 1980s, such as California, New York, Connecticut, Massachusetts, and New Jersey, have experienced significant out-migration since 1990. In direct consequence, states that had experienced little or no population growth during the 1980s, such as those in the Mountain States and in the Midwest, have experienced significant in-migration during the past six years. Every state in the mountain region has experienced at least a 15% increase in population since 1990 and states in the Great Plains have led the nation in income growth since 1990 as well. People from the East and West Coasts are moving inland. These are trends directly contrary to those experienced during the industrial era. Population change since 1990 suggests that the lower cost of living and the higher quality of life and rural residence, facilitated by telecommunications technology, are contributing factors to changing location of economic activity and, therefore, population. Increasingly, people are freed to make residential location decisions independent of where they might do business. In an era of widespread use of Internet technology, it is possible for a person's body to be located anywhere and for their mind to go forth and make a living. That possibility is being enacted by a growing number.

Important for future demand for health care is that there continues to be a movement of retired people from larger metropolitan areas to rural locations, especially in areas offering environmental amenities. Communications technologies are also beginning to change the way health care services are offered. Throughout the industrial era, it was a foregone conclusion that it was necessary for health care consumers to travel to increasingly specialized, and therefore centralized, services. An observer during that era suggested that one of the greatest public investments in rural health care was roads, enabling rural residents to drive further to avail themselves of the more centralized services. But the evolving utilization of telemedicine may contribute to important restructuring of where and how health care services are accessed and how often communication will substitute for travel as a means of obtaining the services of professional health care providers. In terms of the focus of this book, an implication is the extent to which future collaboration of health care professionals will take place electronically.

Different from describing the industrial paradigm of the past, the preceding discussion has been devoted to describing changes in conditions that are leading to the emergence of new forms of organization, new forms of delivering services, and new ways of relating to each other, both at work and at home. A new paradigm is emerging, but we are not there yet. Consequently, we see all around us the paradoxes of the co-existing old and new rules stimulating discussion, debate, and uncertainty, even as the society is in the process of remaking itself. Optimism and pessimism about the future coexist not just between different people and their viewpoints but also within the mind of each person.

TOWARD A NEW SOCIAL ECOLOGY OF COLLABORATION

Our purpose in the preceding pages has been to emphasize that a transition to collaboration becoming normative is not simple; it involves more than a change in behavior and practice simply because it works better. Collaboration is based on an integration of values and practices embedded in a society. The rules of the industrial society, which were adopted and practiced because they worked and produced significant economic and status benefits for many, strongly emphasized individual success and institutionalized rewards for it; thus, in practice, collaboration was discouraged. Hierarchy and the "organization man" were the prototypes.

If the focus of the industrial society was reductionism, an emphasis on identification and improvement of the parts, the emphasis of the emerging paradigm is on integration. That emphasis includes not only integration between parts of organizations but also restoring connections between the different institutions of society. But even with growing attention to integration, there has been a concurrent emphasis on social, economic, and professional pluralism. The mass society is giving way to greater uniqueness, locality, culture, and community, with a corresponding emphasis on societal diversity. In such an environment, flexibility and adaptation are prized more than uniformity and standardization. The emphasis on integration is being advanced as a way of achieving sustainable distinctiveness. For a community to generate a sustainable identity, there must be recognition of a common interest and for integration of the disparate parts in order to advance the common welfare (Theobald 1997).

In our treatment of collaboration, we have typically linked it with community, either as a value or a set of relationships reflecting common identity and reciprocal obligations, or both. A part of society's growing attention to collaboration and community arises from the search for meaning and connection that have been reported casualties of the excessive 20th century emphasis on individualism (Bellah et al. 1985, Theobald 1997, Kemmis 1990). But part of that renewed attention to community is also attributable to the effect of globalization on the role of nation-states and national governments. The 20th century has been described by some authors as an era in which national governments played a dominant role in instigating and reinforcing modernization and industrial organization: an era described by McMichael (1996) as the development paradigm. National governments were the instigator in devising strategies and making investments to stimulate national social and economic development. Correspondingly, Chirot (1986) notes that nationalism has been the dominant ideology in the world during the 20th century. McMichael (1996) asserts that the global paradigm is displacing the development paradigm and that as the global economy has gained hegemony, the relative prominence of nation-states has diminished. It is in this context that cultures and localities are beginning to take a more dominant part as a determinant of the relative well-being of their citizens. In observing this shift, Barnet and Cavanagh (1994) draw the following implication regarding the effect of globalization on community:

As traditional communities disappear and ancient cultures are over-whelmed, billions of human beings are losing the sense of place and sense of self that give life meaning. The fundamental political conflicts in the opening decades of the new century, we believe, will not be between nations or even between trading blocs but between the forces of global-ization and the territorially based forces of local survival seeking to pre-serve and to redefine community (p. 22).

Although in the United States, the national government remains a central player in most societal arenas, there are nevertheless indications of a shift in perspective regarding where and how public policies should be formulated, implemented, and enacted. The recent emphasis on devolution and on enactment of initiatives such as welfare reform emerge from a premise of presumed benefits of decentralization. States and localities are envisioned as playing a more prominent role in affecting the future well-being of their citizens. If the mass society was destructive of communities, the emerging paradigm, on the other hand, appears to be encouraging the restoration of community and the kind of civic respon-sibility that would make that possible.

These changes in the society, no less than those of a half century past, are greatly affecting public perceptions, policies, and practices regarding health and health care. Among the most prominent public questions to have surfaced in this context is how society's health care resources are going to be allocated and rationed. This currently takes the form of debate about paying for the health care system. But that debate has really become a proxy for a whole range of issues concerning health and the public interest, including not only who will pay for the services, but also who will provide them and in which venues and, indeed, what services will be provided and to whom will they be provided. It is a time of experimentation, and new providers participating in new forms of col-laboration have contributed to extending the reach of the health care sys-tem. Concurrently, investments in health are beginning to be understood as a cost-effective and socially beneficial alternative to the problem of growing health care costs.

It is in this social, economic, organizational, and political environment that collaboration has become an integral part of present and future health planning. Neither promoting health nor providing health care is any longer the exclusive domain of the "therapists." It seems very clear that health, along with education and other essential societal purposes, will become more collaborative and will contribute toward reestablishing productive connections among society's institutions. But collaboration will not be confined to any particular setting. It promises to become a practice that will become a routine part of promoting health and providing comprehensive health care in whatever environment those services are delivered.

It is envisioned that collaboration will continue to play a greater role among professional providers in hospitals and clinics delivering both routine and complex services. As the chapters in this book have emphasized, those services have already become multidisciplinary, including professionals having training in social services and other supporting disciplines. In the cause of improved patient care, multidisciplinary and professional collaboration will continue to become more normative. With greater use of communication technologies, it is probable also that more of that collaboration will occur among health care professionals working in physically separated locations. Achieving true collaboration, however, will take time because it must build on mutual trust acquired through experience among particular individual participants. As experience accumulates, collaboration will move beyond a technical division of labor and embody more of the values of collaboration. As these changes occur, it is probable also that the organization of health care will continue its move toward greater resemblance to the "webs of enterprise" organizational model. The emergence of managed care is beginning to change not only the organizational model of health care but the very purposes to which the organizations are directing their efforts.

Beyond professional health care, a feature of a new collaborative social ecology would also include an emphasis on values, norms, and behaviors intended to preserve health. The task of improving and preserving health extends beyond the domain of the health care institution: values and behaviors leading to healthier and more productive lives should be a product of effective families, educational centers, work places, and community social and religious organizations. Such a social ecology would likely include a perspective that would shift the frame of reference from not only healthy individuals but also to assessment of the relative health of communities, neighborhoods, or organizations. Such a perspective would evaluate the health of a population, along with such other characteristics as education, as components of a sustainable social environment. Achieving a healthy community would require extensive collaboration among families, institutions, and professionals.

It would not be unexpected for a community focus on health to produce a different perspective on the attributes of good health than might be produced by health care specialists. Indeed, that is one of the potential benefits of community collaboration toward achieving a shared goal such as a healthy community. Recently, a comprehensive community project was undertaken in a small midwestern city to assess the health of the community and to identify strategic objectives for improving the population's health status. This activity was instigated and organized by the local Chamber of Commerce and other collaborating community organizations. Citizens participating in public meetings were provided statistical information about the community's population. From their analysis and discussion, they identified the following issues as the priority health problems: 1) access to professional health care, 2) high-school drop-out rate, 3) dental health, 4) family nurturance and preservation, 5) senior health care, 6) child abuse and neglect, 7) workforce readiness, 8) low levels of childhood immunization, 9) tobacco use and prevention, 10) poor pregnancy outcomes, 11) substance abuse and prevention, 12) teen pregnancy, and 13) mental health issues. Of pertinence is that several of the problems were not specifically health problems but social problems, which, if not addressed, could lead to poor physical and/or emotional health. Further, few, if any, of the problems could be effectively addressed without substantial collaboration among a number of community agencies, organizations, or professional providers. Important also is that such a process, involving a broad spectrum of the community in identifying problems and developing strategies to ameliorate them, is fundamental to building community capacity. If such relationships are sustained and similar processes employed in addressing other community concerns, that community collaboration, apart from the separate agencies, becomes a resource of social value.

NETWORKS AND RELATIONSHIPS AS A RESOURCE

We have used the concept of community repeatedly without offering a specific definition. Community can mean many different things depending on the perspective of its participants. It may be a place, or it may be a network of persons having common interests and common purposes. Although there are many towns and neighborhoods in the nation that have a name and are often referred to as a community, they lack the extensive social relationships essential to a sociological concept of community. Many have become aggregations of households sharing little or no sense of community and common purpose. It is the quality of relationships, more than sharing a piece of geography, that defines community. Communities do things on their own behalf; places do not.

Although many places are lacking a sense of community, recent social science research has found that there are important exceptions, that is, numerous places where the networks of relationships and shared sense of purpose and responsibility have enabled the residents to accomplish meaningful shared purposes. In those places, the community is not just a place to reside, but is a powerful social resource. It is community as a resource that has contributed to a growing literature on social capital. Social capital, however, is not confined to communities: social capital is a product of sustained collaboration and may apply to any group or pattern of relationships including those involving health care professionals and their work.

A speaker (Barlow 1997) recently observed that in this emerging age of the Internet and communities of networks as well as of places, relationships are coming to have greater value than is ownership. Within the past 10 to 12 years, there has been a growing literature in the social sciences on the value of networks and relationships, with an increasing number of analysts referring to such networks as a form of *social capital*. As collaboration has been described throughout this book, it embodies many of the features of social capital as defined by contemporary theorists. Bourdieu (1986), for example, describes social capital as networks that establish social relationships that are directly productive in the short or long run. Somewhat more precisely, Putnam (1993) defines social capital as:

> the features of social organization such as networks, norms and trust, that facilitate coordination and cooperation for mutual benefit. Social capital enhances the benefits of investment in physical and human capital (p. 4).

The reason for employing the term *social capital* is that the quality of the interpersonal relationships and networks among organizations is a resource that has a positive effect on a wide range of outcomes. Recent research has found that the social capital of families and communities has a great effect on the school performance of students, regardless of resources and other characteristics of schools they may attend (Coleman 1988). Other research has reported great differences in the quality of relationships in communities that have a direct effect on the quality of life of small towns and their ability to achieve economic development (Flora and Flora 1993). Other studies have shown that social capital networks are very effective to people of limited resources in obtaining employment (Green et. al. 1995). One of the classic studies found that local governments in Italy varied greatly in their effectiveness, with the more effective governments being in those communities having the greatest stocks of social capital (Putnam 1993).

Like physical capital, investments can be made in increasing social capital; it can be accumulated (Seipel and Hobbs 1996). But different from either financial capital or human capital (education, skills, health of individual workers), *social capital inheres in relationships* and is not defined by qualities of individuals. Groups and organizations possess social capital; individuals do not. Further, the more social capital is used, the more it accumulates. Inversely, social capital depreciates from disuse. As described by Putnam (1993):

> Stocks of social capital such as trust, norms and networks tend to be self-reinforcing and cumulative. . . . [I]t is according to some a moral resource, that is, a resource whose supply increases rather than decreases through use and which (unlike physical capital) becomes depleted if not used (p. 6).

Thus, social capital represents something of a departure from the excessive individualism that has characterized American society. Although social capital has been carefully defined by a number of theorists, the essence of social capital is embodied in terms like *community, cooperation,* and *collaboration*. In that sense, social capital is a concept consistent with the social changes of the emerging paradigm. The idea of relationships as a collective resource seems consistent with a new social ecology.

CONCLUSION

Important about the concept of social capital is that it provides an alternative way of thinking about collaboration, whether in a work setting such as a hospital or as a resource of an organization or community. Although the term *social capital* has emerged only recently, the idea draws on a number of familiar social science concepts, including social ties, affinity, community capacity, community development, and networks, and links them with the idea of investment. Social capital is accumulated as people interact frequently over a period of time in a way that builds reciprocated trust. This web of relationships becomes a durable resource that can be drawn on for problem solving and accomplishment of group tasks. It offers a source of meaningful connection between work and meaning and values. In many respects, the resource of social capital produces a dual benefit: It facilitates production of important outcomes and simultaneously provides gratification to the participants. As observed by Theobald: "Most people generally recognize that meaning or fulfillment in a human life is inevitably tied to the quality of the relationships a person creates with others" (1997, p. 43).

If we equate social capital with effective and repeated collaboration, then we can think of collaboration, not just as an occurrence, but as an investment in capacity that will continue to yield dividends over a period of time. Collaboration as a resource will diminish in value only from disuse.

As society and health care professionals alike begin to focus on preservation of health and prevention of disease, the idea of assisting towns, organizations, or neighborhoods to become communities through investments in building social capital will become a part of an effective strategy. A community that includes a sense of belonging is in itself an important contributor to health. A strong community generally translates into emotional and mental health among residents as well. In any comprehensive strategy for improving the plight of America's communities, rebuilding social capital is as important as investing in human and physical capital (Putnam 1993).

Although investing in social capital may not yet be thought of as an important component of our future health care strategy, that perspective may gain momentum as we improve our understanding of the multiple sources that contribute to individual and collective good health and how to bring those sources into effective collaboration.

References

Allen, J. and Dillman, D. A. (1994). *Against All Odds: Rural Community in the Information Age*. Boulder, CO: Westview Press.

Barlow, J. P. (1997). *Fast Forward to the Future of Communications*. Keynote address. 34th Annual Winter Convention of OPASTCO. Kauai, Hawaii. January 1997.

Barnet, R. J. and Cavanagh, J. (1994). *Global Dreams: Imperial Corporations and the New World Order*. New York: Simon and Schuster.

Bellah, R. N., Madsen, R., Sullivan, W., Swidler, A., and Tipton, S. (1985). *Habits of the Heart: Individualism and Commitment in American Life.* New York: Harper and Row.

Bourdieu, P. (1986). The forms of capital. Chapter 9 in J. G. Richardson (Ed.). *Handbook of Theory and Research for the Sociology of Education.* New York: Greenwood Press, pp. 241–258.

Chirot, D. (1986). *Social Change in the Modern Era.* San Diego, CA: Harcourt Brace Jovanovich, Inc.

Coleman, J. S. (1988). Social capital in the creation of human capital. *American Journal of Sociology,* 94 (Suppl.) S95–S120.

Ehrenreich, B. (1990). *Fear of falling: The inner life of the middle class.* New York: Harper Perennial.

Flora, C. B. and Flora, J. L. (September 1993). Entrepreneurial social infrastructure: A necessary ingredient. *Annals, ASPSS, 529,* 48–58.

Green, G. P., Tigges, L. M., and Brown, I. (1995). *Social Resources, Job Search and Poverty in Atlanta. Research in Community Sociology,* Vol. 5. JAI Press, Inc., pp. 161–182.

Hobbs, D. (1990). Values worth preserving and building on. Chapter 1 in *Values of a Community Economic Developer.* Madison, WI: University of Wisconsin Cooperative Extension Service, pp. 1–18.

Kemmis, D. (1990). *Community and the Politics of Place.* Norman, OK: University of Oklahoma Press.

Kuhn, T. (1962). *The Structure of Scientific Revolutions.* Chicago: University of Chicago Press.

McMichael, P. (1996). *Development and Social Change.* Thousand Oaks, CA: Pine Forge Press.

North, D. C. (1990). *Institutions, Institutional Change and Economic Performance.* New York: Cambridge University Press.

Putnam, R. (October 1993). The prosperous community: Social capital and economic growth. *Current,* pp. 4–9.

Reich, R. B. (1992). *The Work of Nations.* New York: Vintage Books.

Seipel, M. and Hobbs, D. (1996). Social capital in the production of human capital: Implications for rural economic development. Paper presented at annual meeting of the American Agricultural Economics Association, San Antonio, TX.

Theobald, P. (1997). *Teaching the Commons: Place, Pride and Renewal of Community.* Boulder, CO: Westview Press.

de Tocqueville, A. (1969). *Democracy in America.* J. P. Mayer (Ed.). New York: Doubleday, Anchor Books.

Toffler, A. (1970). *Future Shock.* New York: Random House.

Toffler, A. (1980). *The Third Wave.* New York: Morrow.

Toffler, A. (1990). *Power Shift: Knowledge, Wealth and Violence at the Edge of the 21st Century.* New York: Bantam.

Collaboration, A Health Care Imperative: Reflection on Values

21

Toni J. Sullivan

INTRODUCTION

This book is about planned change and about creating a desired future. Embedded in the many scholarly treatises and discussions are implicit or explicit technical, cognitive, or value-laden arguments for collaboration. Collaboration as a practice has been proved to be a good act; when two or more people or two or more organizations join together to achieve common goals, good things happen (likely successful outcomes). We have even had the temerity to argue that collaboration is an imperative for the future; that the postmodern (global information) age requires the practice and philosophy of collaboration to conduct human affairs effectively.

Collaboration as a way of addressing important social problems and as a philosophy of working or problem solving has been put forth as a, indeed even *the* good way to conduct work in the future. Implicit in all of this push for the good of collaboration is the profound idea that persons need to change, or at least reaffirm, their values (as well as their attitudes and behaviors), to change the way they work and function with others in human organizations and social systems. These weighty notions mandate unbundling and making explicit and orderly the values entangled with the technical and cognitive arguments scattered throughout this book.

What also gives rise to serious consideration is the influence on people and human systems of collaboration itself. Collaboration changes people; collaboration changes systems. It is, therefore, a powerful human and social tool. Reflection on planned change and creating the future is sobering because we come to realize that we may indeed succeed in our efforts to change people, systems, and events. We had best tend to our values.

Values can be defined in many ways. Four meanings of the term have relevance for this discussion: 1) *Values* refer to the social principles, goals, or standards held or accepted by an individual, class, or society; 2) *values* (or *to value*) is to think highly of, to esteem, as in to value one's friendship; 3) *value* is that quality of a thing that makes it thought of as being more or less desirable, useful, or worthy; 4) *value* is that which is desirable or worthy of esteem for its own sake (*Webster's New World Dictionary* 1996, p. 1474).

Reflections on values take four directions. First, a reflection on the ethics of collaboration and a beginning normative ethical model of collaboration. Second, a reflection on the depth and nature of the commitment that occurs in true collaborative partnerships. Third, a reflection on the depth and quality of communication required to achieve true collaboration. Finally, the author offers a reflection on the integration of collaboration into all facets of human concerns and social functioning and asserts again that collaboration is a health care imperative.

REFLECTIONS ON ETHICS

Definitions of Ethics

Ethics may be defined as a system of moral standards or values concerning the good or the good life, and of right acts to achieve the good or the greatest good. *Ethics* is knowledge of the good and of right acts. *Moral* or *ethical behavior* is adhering in practice to a system of moral standards or values. *Moral* or *ethical behavior* is the performance of right or good acts. It may be said that *ethics is knowing* what is right, and *morals is doing* what is right (Sahakian and Sahakian 1966).

Normative ethics is the field or branch of ethics that concerns identifying, specifying, and refining right or wrong characteristics of actions or policies (Purtilo and Cassel 1981). *Moral principles* or *moral obligations* are defined here as the deep-seated human pull or impulse to act in right ways toward others. These obligations are often thought of as *moral duties.* Even though the innate inclination is present, these principles must be learned and the maturity to meet them must be developed and nurtured (Purtilo and Cassel 1981). Six *moral principles* are commonly articulated for health professionals. They are a common foundation for codes of ethics for health care professionals (Pappas 1994, Purtilo and Cassel 1981). These principles may be simply stated as follows:

- *Autonomy*—Patients' freedom to make choices and decisions regarding their care.
- *Beneficence*—Do good.
- *Fidelity*—Keep promises; honor commitments and social contracts.
- *Justice*—Be fair to one and all.
- *Nonmaleficence*—Above all, do no harm.
- *Veracity*—Tell the truth.

Discussion and Ethical Analysis of Values Statements

Premise 1 of the systems model of collaboration states: "Health care professionals desire to provide high-quality care to people in need of their services; they desire to do their best" (Chapter 4). This statement captures the most fundamental health care ethic of health professionals. They enter the field with lofty goals to do good. Most continue to value this ethic highly throughout their careers, although competing interests may intercede to prevent providers from fulfilling their commitment to doing their best for those in need of care. This ethic presents as a social contract with society. People expect, and have a right to expect, health professionals to do their best for those in need at all times, regardless of intervening variables, such as an inability to pay for care. A violation of this ethic, therefore, violates the principles of fidelity and beneficence.

This book contains myriad indicators of what constitutes doing good in health care at present and in the coming millennium. Presumably, the principle of beneficence requires that health care providers be knowledgeable about the current state of the art in health care. If this is so, then health care providers need to be prepared in the aggregate to "the emergence of health, rather than illness, as a national and an international concern along with the growing realization that health is a personal, family, and community concern" (Chapter 3). Similarly, health care providers need to be prepared to respond to the orderly, expressed needs of a community for their health needs. The example, found in Chapter 20, of 13 community top priority health problems *can only be responded to with a collaborative approach.* No one professional discipline has the expertise to care for all of a given community's needs.

Blair (Chapter 13) uses a community values model as a standard for determining the kinds of problem-solving and care-giving responses that coalitions ought to make to communities. She urges that providers and other experts be culturally sensitive to the citizens in need of assistance. Within that context, the experts and *fully participating citizens* need to work together to address quality of care, access to care, and cost benefit of care. These principles mean that the care provided is of the highest possible quality within the framework of what the citizens are able to afford or benefit from (quality). Access to care is provided to as many citizens as is possible, regardless of inconvenience to the programmers or providers. Cost benefit means that the funding is conscientiously used to gain the greatest benefit possible to the largest number of people. The broad ethical principles responded to are fidelity, beneficence, and justice. Bailey and Armer (Chapter 8) report that their interviewed collaborative pairs recognized quality care as a principle driving their collaborative practice decisions. "All of the dyads expressed similar philosophies in their approach to patient care and emphasized quality as their primary goal in providing care."

A similar model to the community values model is reported in a recent article (Cross 1997). In that article, Cross asks us to "[i]magine a practice that defined its mission and core values in the context of patient satisfaction, patient empowerment, cost effectiveness, access, and quality" (p. 16). He continues: "Suppose . . . the health care infrastructure was intrinsically designed to manifest these values in the service of patients" (p. 16). Cross then stresses that each of these values has been documented amply as having major benefits to patients. The model of practice that can be readily imagined is a collaborative multidisciplinary model of practice with full patient or citizen participation. The documented outcomes in Chapter 1 amply demonstrate that patients as well as providers experience feelings of empowerment and of satisfaction in collaborative practice. In addition, several other chapters address either provider or patient satisfaction. These are clearly highly held values, and responsiveness to them fulfills the ethical principles of autonomy, beneficence, justice, and veracity.

Collaborative approaches to health care delivery, education, research, and organizational management have been documented throughout this book as being very effective. In Chapter 4, it is asserted that "there is no known health care situation that would not benefit from a collaborative approach." One of the major findings of the concept analysis of collaboration is that "there is not one negative consequence of collaboration reported between or to anyone" in the literature (Chapter 1). The principles of beneficence, fidelity, and, perhaps, justice would seem to require that health care providers at least seriously consider organizing their practices and programs using collaboration. Those who choose not to practice collaboratively would seem to need an ethically and morally defensible reason for their decision.

Collaboration creates new ways of being, doing, and knowing. This powerful evidence of change that collaboration stimulates is cited in at least three of the chapters, two of which are cited here. Porter et al. note in Chapter 10 that "coalitions based upon a paradigm of cooperation and collaboration, rather than competition and turfism . . . [create an] ethos [that] create[s] the necessary means for organizations to rise above their self-interests and see beyond themselves within a larger continuum of health care necessary for each community." Likewise, Meleis and Johnson note in Chapter 12 that "Knowledge developed through collaborative efforts tends to reflect diversity of thoughts and of goals. As such, it is more congruent with the increasing population diversity that we experience in every corner of the world. Such knowledge is empowering to members of a discipline." Meleis and Johnson also state their belief that such knowledge gained through collaboration acts as a catalyst for increasing acceptance of one another and our diverse values. Again, the fulfillment of the social contract between health care providers and society means that society has a right to expect that providers make every reasonable effort to advance and improve health care delivery, education, and research. Failure to do so violates the ethical principles of beneficence, fidelity, and justice.

In Chapters 3 and 20 especially, we learn that people are yearning for connections. The model of individualism is no longer working; societal institutions organized around individual functioning and achievement are floundering. People worldwide are fearful for the future; they are fearful that their children and their children's children will not be better off than they are. Hobbs, in Chapter 20, points out that we can infer values from what people say and do, and also from what they say is missing from their lives. People are missing a sense of connectedness between the values they profess and the practices they employ. A person may desire to do meaningful work, for example, but find their job to be unimportant. Collaboration, Hobbs points out, leads not only to functional effectiveness, "but also [to] the feeling of gratification and worth it induces among the collaborators. Meaning and gratification are found to be as much in the process as in the accomplishment."

Hobbs (Chapter 20) discusses a new social ecology as part of the global-information age. This new social ecology reflects a set of *shared values* and their connection to practices of work and of everyday living. The suggestion is that "the challenge is not so much one of devising new values, but rather to link existing values with our practices more effectively. Greater meaning is produced in our lives when what we believe and what we do are in greater harmony." Collaboration, again, changes people and systems. Hobbs argues that collaboration ultimately changes our values. "[W]hen collaboration has become normative for any group or organization, it is simultaneously an expression of several values fundamental to a new social ecology. . . . It is the sharing of these values that makes them powerful." (See Table 21-1 for a listing of shared values proposed by Hobbs.)

Meleis and Gray (Chapter 12) identify four principles for working within and nurturing collaborative relationships. They use the acronym MICR to refer to *m*utuality, *i*nvolvement, *c*larity, and *r*eciprocity. These four principles are value laden as *shared* values. Hobbs's set of values of community, fairness, work, and choice, likewise, only exist in the sharing (Chapter 20). Both sets of shared values are most ethical. They respond to the ethical principles of autonomy, beneficence, and justice to a very high level.

Based on the selected excerpts from the preceding chapters, the ethical implications of collaborative models of practice, education, and research become very apparent. Collaboration is highly responsive to the ethical principles that health care providers aspire to live by. It is possible to imagine, and even to witness in practice, models of health care delivery that are designed to manifest core values of patient welfare first, patient satisfaction and empowerment, and provider satisfaction within a context of access, affordability, and quality care. These models of practice are usually collaborative models. This discussion can be viewed as foundational to the creation of a normative model of ethics for collaborative practice.

Table 21-1. Shared Values that Facilitate Communication

Meleis and Gray, Chapter 12

Mutuality: Commitment to shared and agreed upon goals and assumptions; ensuring that all collaborative members have knowledge of both goals and objectives, and that at least some of the goals are shared ones that drive the need for collaboration.

Involvement: Commitment to including all collaborative members in all aspects of planning, establishing, conducting, and finalizing the collaborative project. "Involvement enhances equity in expenditures and rewards."

Clarity: A doctrine of precision in specifying all components of the collaborative plan that may require contracting or recontracting of expectations and goals. Collaborators should not shy away from discussion about ownership, authorship, long- and short-term benefits, and the like.

Reciprocity: Commitment to give-and-take in the relationship and to assuring that collaboration reflects a win-win situation for all collaborating members. Reciprocity is not an exactly equal division of activities or assets nor is it measured in the short term.

Hobbs, Chapter 20

Community: "A value . . . expressed by the kinds and styles of human relationships and transactions that emphasize integration more than separation; relationships that contrast with excessive individualism, but not at the expense of individuality."

Fairness: " . . . An emphasis on interpersonal respect in an atmosphere devoid of prejudice. Fairness does not equate with equality but it is egalitarian."

Work: "Not merely as a means of making a living or even achieving status, but as an activity that is both productive and contributory to feelings of personal worth; work that is intrinsically and extrinsically useful. It is through their work that the contributions of collaborators are recognized and valued."

Choice: " . . . A paraphrase for freedom. It is difficult to conceive of freedom in the absence of choice." "To restore a sense of civic responsibility in our [American] society, it is important to think of freedom not only as freedom *from* (fear, coercion, responsibility), but more as freedom *to* exercise the rights and responsibilities of citizenship in a free society."

REFLECTIONS ON COMMITMENT

Proponents of collaboration highly value the collaborative partnership that is the core of the collaborative arrangement. We learned in Chapter 1 that they express themselves passionately, speaking of *real* partners, *true* partnership, *full* partnership, and joint problem solving as a *way of life*. These are expressions of commitment; they are indicative of feelings of personal satisfaction and empowerment within the relationship. Respecting each other, excellent communications, working together, and trusting each other are some of the top partnership attributes named in the literature (see Chapter 1). These attributes are discussed both as desired processes and as highly satisfying and valued outcomes of the collaborative partnership.

The *process* of developing a collaborative partnership, whether between two or more persons or between two or more organizations or between two or more nations is extremely complex, and it takes time and energy. It takes a *commitment*. Potential partners who value the idea of partnership and who value the likely benefits of partnership must commit themselves to the systematic development of the partnership. The five major elements declared in Chapter 4 as essential to the development of a collaborative partnership are leadership by the larger system, preparation of the potential partners for collaboration, investment of material and human resources, *commitment* of the potential partners to making the partnership work, and investing time and energy into taking first steps in the partnership.

That these are major elements required for establishing a collaborative partnership is asserted over and over again in many creative ways throughout the chapters. Several of the propositions put forward in the systems model of collaboration in Chapter 4 address these major elements. One proposition simply states that "[w]ould-be-collaborators who fail to incorporate all five attributes of the process of collaboration in developing and sustaining a collaborative partnership will probably not succeed in developing or sustaining a collaborative partnership and practice" (Chapter 4).

Conversely, another proposition states: "If all of the attributes of the collaborative process and partnership are present and supported on an ongoing basis, then collaborative system(s) will likely function successfully on an ongoing basis" (Chapter 4).

Kuehn, in Chapter 14, writing about the development of the team of multidisciplinary faculty who design and teach in their collaborative learning activities, states:

> Because the faculty and staff continued to work with each other on state and university task forces, advisory panels, and grant proposal efforts, they began to know each other in a personal way different from the professional formality of previous encounters. They developed a sense of comfort, confidence, and trust to the point where they could truly dialogue without feeling threatened or appearing defensive; this did not, however, happen overnight. It was a result of 4 years of working at learning to dialogue, to trust, and to establish a comfort level that would allow each to speak openly and honestly . . .

The investment in partnership development yields positive results. In a systematic fashion, the first positive outcome is a strong commitment to the partnership. It is stated in a proposition in Chapter 4 that "[c]ollaborators who accord their collaborating partners a high level of trust and a high level of professional respect are highly likely to have a strong commitment to the professional welfare of their collaborating partners." A study respondent quoted in Chapter 10 states: "Forming partnerships is like gaining a new friend. You have to work together, solve problems together, associate with each other, strive to give each other something you both want. Then you do become friends, and once you are friends, you never want to give them up!"

Collaborative partnerships achieve good and positive outcomes in both the technical and ethical meanings of the terms *good* and *positive*, as has been discussed in the preceding section of this chapter. "[A]n activated collaborative partnership, in the presence of a need or problem seemingly requiring collaboration, is highly likely to achieve successful outcomes" (Chapter 4).

Collaborative partnerships change the collaborators by changing their behaviors along with changing their values. It is noted in Chapter 3 that "fundamental transformation of provider behaviors [collaborative, interdisciplinary teams of peer providers functioning within integrated delivery systems] represents a long-term solution to achieving high-quality, cost-effective care."

REFLECTIONS ON COMMUNICATION

The crucial importance or value of communication and the attributes of excellent communications to collaboration and the strong commitment inherent in true collaboration probably have been named and discussed in this volume 100 times or more. In collaboration, as with so much of value in human and social affairs, communication is foundational to success. In the complex processes of formation and conduct of collaborative partnerships between individuals, organizations, or nations, excellent communications are the fuel that makes the engines go.

Would be collaborators must make a strong and enduring *commitment* to *communication*. Moreover, the style of communication required is one of openness, honesty, and mutual respect between two or more persons who are valued for their expertise and competence. Would be partners are recognized as having an obligation to the would be partnership to be technically competent and ready to make a contribution to the partnership. "Collaborators who describe their partners as competent or highly competent are likely to accord them a high level of trust and a high level of professional respect" (Chapter 4). Campbell, in summarizing his extensive research findings, notes: "The importance of . . . mutual respect . . . [and] the acceptance of different priorities and styles emerged as a key ingredient of a successful collaborative practice team. It was under these conditions that learning from each other was a free exchange among colleagues" (Chapter 6).

Campbell (Chapter 6) also notes that something occurs in practice between collaborators. They absorb each other's styles and do more of what each other does best. This is noted as a paradox because each collaborator is also empowered to do more of what each individual does best. Flesner and Clawson (Chapter 7) also learned in their research that it becomes harder to ferret out differences in practice behaviors as partnerships aged. Meleis and Gray (Chapter 12) discuss how continuing, open dialogue among collaborators in international settings both changes the values and perspectives of the collaborators, and acts as a catalyst to the collaborators knowing and accepting the values of their wonderfully diverse international colleagues.

The importance of freedom of choice in entering into the formation of a collaborative partnership is sharply focused in the formation of coalitions between organizations and between nations. A model of voluntariness or freedom of choice is put forward in Chapter 9: "[A] crucial factor in successful coalition formation and conduct seems to be the degree of freedom or voluntariness members have in choosing to participate in the coalition and actively pursue its goals." Closely related to the freedom to choose to participate—and have your contributions respectively listened to and seriously considered—is the degree of involvement one has in the decision to join the coalition. The influence one has at the beginning of coalition formation, when the initial mission and purposes and membership and structure decision making occurs, is a critical predictor of the future involvement members will have in the coalition and its likelihood of success or failure.

In Chapters 10, 12, and 13, the importance of culturally sensitive attitudes and communications was sharply spotlighted. Cultural sensitivities concerning perceived inequalities in resources and expertise were discussed as were misunderstandings that occur when persons or groups hold differing perceptions and meanings for topics of mutual concern. In Chapter 10, the authors indicate that all the smaller organizations reporting, with one exception, spoke of the stress involved in working with larger hospitals in their communities. They spoke of the intimidation of high expectations and of being the tiny partner organization working with a bigger partner organization. All of these respondents, including one who actually sought the relationship with the larger partner, stressed the "challenge of navigating new systems and coming together from different cultures, perspectives, assumptions, and understandings."

Meleis and Gray, in Chapter 12, speak of nurses from different nations initiating collaboration to address internationally "shared clinical issues and . . . developing knowledge that reflects diversity in culture, ethnicity, religion, and language." Their four principles of effective collaboration, presented in Chapter 12 and summarized in Table 21-1 can also be conceptualized as shared values or guidelines for effective communication in forming, implementing, and sustaining a culturally sensitive partnership. Mutuality, involvement, clarity, and reciprocity capture the mutual respect, openness, and honesty that must occur for culturally sensitive communications to flourish.

In Chapter 13, Blair uses Sullivan's coalition formation model (see Chapter 9) and her own community values model to demonstrate that when international partners work together in planning and program development from the beginning of the process, including goal setting and standards selection or formation, and when all would be partners are included in determining the interventions and the allocations of resources, then culturally sensitive models emerge and likely successful outcomes occur. Conversely, when solutions, even those that are resource rich, are put forward in a culturally insensitive way, such as by not including local leaders in planning, then coalitions fail to meet their goals, however worthy they may be. Communication that is inclusive of all interested and legitimate stakeholders and that fosters mutual respect, trust, and feelings of empowerment is a highly valued feature of collaboration and collaborative relationships.

REFLECTIONS ON INTEGRATION

Integration concerns linkages, connections, diffusion or permeation, and perhaps cause and effect of ideas, or purposes and outcomes, or structures and processes. The term *integration,* as used here, is an abstraction to include all of the possibilities named and perhaps others unnamed. As such, it is a big concept for reflection. Collaboration as an idea, as a practice, and as a value for human and social functioning is an integrator. It brings together people, disciplines, organizations, and nations. It brings together processes and outcomes. It brings together old problems and new teams of problem solvers and new approaches to their resolution. It brings together fragmented approaches to societal functioning and problem definition and creates new holistic ways of defining and addressing human needs. The list of statements of integration is long and could be much longer. The linkages and the connections are imperative for health care and other social endeavors in the new millennium.

In the systems model of collaboration, one of the stated premises is, "In the dynamically complex health care world of the present and foreseen future, collaborative systems of health care practice, education, research, and organizational management are the preferred paradigmatic approach to resolving problems, meeting needs, and accomplishing the work to be done; there is no known health care situation that would not benefit from a collaborative approach" (Chapter 4). Collaborative processes in all facets of health care and health professionals functioning are thus linked with positive outcomes. In Chapter 3, it is noted that the new paradigm of health care that will focus on high-quality, cost-efficient care will have as a defining feature "collaborative, interdisciplinary teams of peer providers functioning within supportive and enabling integrated delivery systems." High-quality, cost-efficient care is linked in this concept to collaborative models of care delivery.

Hobbs, in Chapter 20, discusses the potential benefits of community collaboration in achieving a shared goal of a healthy community. In this sophisticated concept, the connections are myriad. The citizens and multidisciplinary health care providers working together in the community define the health care problems in a new way. They then proceed to address the community's health with a new paradigm of shared functioning. In this approach, the community would not be able to function as it is without the collaborative approach. The values and goals for a healthy community that the citizens hold would go unmet. Hobbs notes that "[i]nvolving a broad spectrum of the community in identifying problems and developing strategies to ameliorate them[] is fundamental to building community capacity." Moreover, Hobbs goes on to discuss how the very process of collaboration builds and strengthens the community. "If such relationships are sustained and similar processes employed in addressing other community concerns, that community collaboration, apart from the separate agencies, becomes a resource of social value."

In Chapter 15, Koetter (1990) is cited as asserting that a central feature of modern organizations is interdependence, a situation in which no one has complete autonomy of functioning, and most employees are tied to many others by the work, technology, management systems, and hierarchy. It is noted in Chapter 15 that in patient care delivery, health care providers are increasingly tied together by the complexity of care needs and the integration of care delivery and payment systems. These tightly integrated organizations "cannot change or evolve unless the wonderfully disparate members become unified in their diversity or align to achieve common goals in their quest of their vision."

In the global society, it was posited in Chapter 19, the role of consumption and the behaviors of consumers take on new meanings. The idea was developed that consumers and producers engage in power relationships within the society concerning quality and affordability of, and access to, goods and services. It was suggested that in the near future, consumers would increasingly use markets to shape the social agenda. It was also suggested that in the case of managed health care financing, consumers would have to be more assertive in the political and market arenas that shape health care policy, or the balance of power would likely shift in favor of insurers and providers. It was also recognized that "[c]onsumers and health care providers often, albeit not always, have common cause. It is predictable that providers and consumers, both desirous of an open and caring health care delivery system that is not driven exclusively by market forces, may join forces in alliance to advocate for health care reforms that will please both groups of stakeholders."

Collaboration: A Health Care Imperative

Many chapters of this volume, especially Chapters 3 and 20, which address the topic directly, develop the grand notion that the world is changing; that profound economic, social, and technological changes are transforming the world community of industrial nation states into a global community in a new global information era. We ventured, especially in Chapters 3, 18, 19, and 20, to look beyond health care to the larger world of commerce and human and social functioning. We learned that all facets of life are changing and that collaborative approaches are integral to the new global information era; that collaboration represents a new—and an imperative—paradigm for human functioning in virtually all social spheres.

Hobbs (Chapter 20) builds the theme of collaboration as multifaceted and as core to the global information era. He indicates that collaboration is more than a practice; it is as well a set of values; a state of commitment; *a state of being as well as doing.* The commitment to collaboration that emerges in practice is a commitment to collaboration within the collaborators as well as a commitment to the collaborative relationship. This idea of collaboration as an essential attribute of the collaborators themselves can be likened to Senge's (1994) notion of the learning disciplines as composed of practices, principles, and essences. In Senge's concept, once the learning discipline is mastered in practice and in principle, it becomes so ingrained within its practitioners that it becomes a part of their very being.

The ethical actions and behaviors embedded within collaboration, the deeply held commitment that collaborators hold for collaboration and for each other, the unwavering value that collaborators and supportive leadership hold for exquisite communications to build and sustain collaboration, and the integration of collaborative practices that occurs within ourselves and our society when all these value-laden elements come together are extraordinarily desirable from intellectual, social, eco-

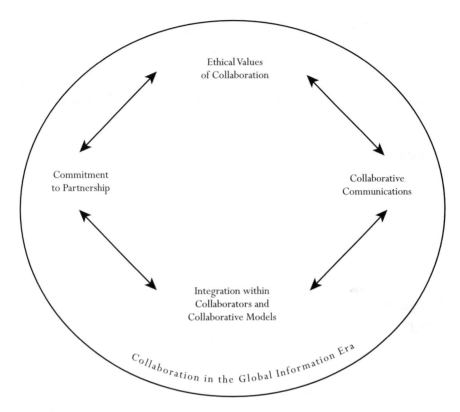

Figure 21-1. *Collaboration: a health care imperative.*

nomic, political, and ethical perspectives. These values and their connectedness form a values-focused model of collaboration. Figure 21-1 depicts this values-focused model of collaboration and links these core values within the global information era.

References

Cross, L. A. (1997). Value-based leadership. *MGM Journal,* May/June, 15–20.

Dyck, A. J. (1973). *On Human Care: An Introduction To Ethics.* Nashville, TN: Abingdon.

Koetter, J. P. (May–June 1990). What leaders really do. *Harvard Business Review,* 103–111.

Neufeldt, V. (1996). *Webster's New World College Dictionary,* 3rd edition. New York: Macmillan, Inc.

Pappas, A. (1994). Ethical issues. In J. A. Zerwekh and J. C. Claborn (Eds.). *Nursing Today: Transition and Trends.* Philadelphia: W. B. Saunders Company.

Purtilo, R. B. and Cassel, C. K. (1981). *Ethical Dimensions in the Health Professions.* Philadelphia: W. B. Saunders Company.

Sahakian, W. S. and Sahakian, M. L. (1966). *Schools of Philosophical Thought.* New York: Barnes and Noble Books. Inc.

Senge, P. (1994). *The Fifth Discipline.* 1st Currency Paperback Edition. New York: Currency Doubleday.

Index

637

ISBN 0-07-063350-9

90000

9 780070 633506